Long-Term Potentiation

A Debate of Current Issues

Long-Term Potentiation

A Debate of Current Issues

edited by
Michel Baudry and Joel L. Davis

A Bradford Book
The MIT Press
Cambridge, Massachusetts
London, England

The following articles have been reprinted with permission of the respective publishers:

Bliss, Clements, Errington, Lynch, and Williams, "Presynaptic changes associated with long-term potentiation in dentate gyrus," © *Seminars in Neuroscience,* December 1990, WB Saunders, Hoxton Square, United Kingdom.

Morris, Davis, and Butcher, "Hippocampal synaptic plasticity and NMDA receptors: a role in information storage?" © *Philosophical Transactions of the Royal Society of London B* (1990) 329, 187–204.

Editorial and production services were provided by Editorial Services of New England, Inc.

This book was set in Palatino by Circle Graphics and was printed and bound in the United States of America.

Library of Congress Cataloging-in-Publication Data

Long-term potentiation : a debate of current issues / edited by Michel Baudry and Joel Davis.
p. cm.
"A Bradford book."
Based on the conference held in 1990.
Includes bibliographical references and index.
ISBN 0-262-02330-X
1. Memory—Congresses. 2. Neuroplasticity—Congresses.
I. Baudry, M. II. Davis, Joel. 1948–
[DNLM: 1. Memory—physiology—congresses. 2. Neural Transmission—physiology—congresses. 3. Neurophysiology—congresses. WL 102 L849 1990]
CP406.L66 1991
153.1'2—dc20
DNLM/DLC 91-11092
for Library of Congress CIP

Contents

Contributors

Simon T. Alford
Department of Pharmacology
School of Medical Sciences
University of Bristol
Bristol, United Kingdom

José Ambros-Ingerson
Center for the Neurobiology of Learning and Memory
University of California
Irvine, California

Laurent Aniksztejn
INSERM U-29
Hopital de Port-Royal
Paris, France

Carol A. Barnes
Arizona Research Laboratories
Division of Neural Systems
Memory and Aging and
Department of Psychology
University of Arizona
Tucson, Arizona

Zafar I. Bashir
Department of Pharmacology
School of Medical Sciences
University of Bristol
Bristol, United Kingdom

Michel Baudry
Neurosciences Program
University of Southern California
Los Angeles, California

John M. Bekkers
Division of Neuroscience
John Curtin School of Medical Research
Australian National University
Canberra, Australia

Yehzekel Ben-Ari
INSERM U-29
Hopital de Port-Royal
Paris, France

Theodore W. Berger
Department of Behavioral Neuroscience
University of Pittsburgh
Pittsburgh, Pennsylvania

Joanna F. Blake
Department of Pharmacology
School of Medical Sciences
University of Bristol
Bristol, United Kingdom

Tim V. P. Bliss
Department of Neurophysiology and Neuropharmacology
National Institute for Medical Research
London, United Kingdom

Thomas H. Brown
Department of Psychology
Yale University
New Haven, Connecticut

Steven P. Butcher
Department of Pharmacology
University of Edinburgh
Edinburgh, Scotland

Brenda J. Claiborne
Division of Life Sciences
University of Texas
San Antonio, Texas

Melanie P. Clements
Division of Neurophysiology and Neuropharmacology
National Institute for Medical Research
London, United Kingdom

Alberto Cobas
Center for the Neurobiology of Learning and Memory
University of California
Irvine, California

Graham L. Collingridge
Department of Pharmacology
School of Medical Sciences
University of Bristol
Bristol, United Kingdom

Françis Crepel
Laboratoire de Neurobiologie et Neuropharmacologie du Développement
Université Paris-Sud
Orsay, France

Stephen N. Davies
Department of Pharmacology
School of Medical Sciences
University of Bristol
Bristol, United Kingdom

Joel L. Davis
Cognitive and Neural Sciences Division
Office of the Chief of Naval Research
Arlington, Virginia

Sabrina Davis
Department of Pharmacology
University of Edinburgh
Edinburgh, Scotland

Pierre de Graan
Division of Molecular Neurobiology
Rudolf Magnus Institute and Institute of Molecular Biology and Medical Biotechnology
University of Utrecht
Utrecht, The Netherlands

Valérie Doyère
Département de Psychophysiologie
Laboratoire de Physiologie Nerveuse
Centre National de la Recherche Scientifique
Gif-sur-Yvette, France

Cynthia A. Erickson
Arizona Research Laboratories
Division of Neural Systems Memory and Aging and
Department of Psychology
University of Arizona
Tucson, Arizona

Michael L. Errington
Division of Neurophysiology and Neuropharmacology
National Institute for Medical Research
London, United Kingdom

Yves Frégnac
Laboratoire de Neurobiologie et Neuropharmacologie du Développement
Université Paris-Sud
Orsay, France

Bruno G. Frenguelli
Department of Pharmacology
School of Medical Sciences
University of Bristol
Bristol, United Kingdom

Willem Hendrik Gispen
Division of Molecular Neurobiology
Rudolf Magnus Institute
Institute of Molecular Biology and Medical Biotechnology
University of Utrecht
Utrecht, The Netherlands

Wim E. J. M. Ghijsen
Department of Experimental Zoology
University of Amsterdam
Amsterdam, The Netherlands

Richard Granger
Center for the Neurobiology of Learning and Memory
University of California
Irvine, California

William T. Greenough
Program in Neuroscience
Beckman Institute
University of Illinois
Urbana, Illinois

Nicholas Hawrylak
Program in Neuroscience
Beckman Institute
University of Illinois
Urbana, Illinois

Serge Laroche
Département de Psychophysiologie
Laboratoire de Physiologie Nerveuse
Centre National de la Recherche Scientifique
Gif-sur-Yvette, France

John Larson
Center for the Neurobiology of Learning and Memory
University of California
Irvine, California

Fernando H. Lopes Da Silva
Institute of Animal Physiology
University of Amsterdam
Amsterdam, The Netherlands

Gary Lynch
Center for the Neurobiology of Learning and Memory
University of California
Irvine, California

Marina A. Lynch
Division of Neurophysiology and Neuropharmacology
National Institute for Medical Research
London, United Kingdom

Zachary F. Mainen
Department of Psychology
Yale University
New Haven, Connecticut

Roberto Malinow
University of Iowa
Department of Physiology and Biophysics
Iowa City, Iowa

Hansjuergen Matthies
Institute of Neurobiology and Brain Research
Magdeburg, Germany

Bruce L. McNaughton
Department of Psychology
University of Arizona
Tucson, Arizona

Cesare Mondadori
Pharmaceutical Research Department
CIBA-GEIGY Limited
Basel, Switzerland

Richard G. M. Morris
Department of Pharmacology
University of Edinburgh Medical School
Edinburgh, Scotland

Roger A. Nicoll
Departments of Pharmacology and Physiology
University of California
San Francisco, California

David J. Perkel
Department of Physiology
University of California
San Francisco, California

Catherine Rédini Del Négro
Département de Psychophysiologie
Laboratoire de Physiologie Nerveuse
Centre National de la Recherche Scientifique
Gif-sur-Yvette, France

Alphonso Represa
INSERM U-29
Hopital de Port-Royal
Paris, France

Klause G. Reymann
Department of Pharmacology
School of Medical Sciences
University of Bristol
Bristol, United Kingdom

Marie-Paule Roisin
INSERM U-29
Hopital de Port-Royal
Paris, France

François Roman
Laboratoire de Neurobiologie des Comportements
Université de Provence-CNRS
Marseille, France

Aryeh Routtenberg
Northwestern University
Cresap Neurosciences Laboratory
Evanston, Illinois

Bernard Soumireu-Mourat
Laboratoire de Neurobiologie des Comportements
Université de Provence-CNRS
Marseille, France

Charles F. Stevens
The Salk Institute
Howard Hughes Medical Institute
La Jolla, California

John G. Taylor
Department of Mathematics
King's College
London, United Kingdom

Richard W. Tsien
Molecular Cellular Physiology
Stanford University
Stanford, California

Christopher S. Wallace
Program in Neuroscience
Beckman Institute
University of Illinois
Urbana, Illinois

Lawrence Weiskrantz
Department of Experimental Psychology
Oxford University
Oxford, Great Britain

John H. Williams
Division of Neurophysiology and Neuropharmacology
National Institute for Medical Research
London, United Kingdom

Mark F. Yeckel
Department of Behavioral Neuroscience
University of Pittsburgh
Pittsburgh, Pennsylvania

Anthony M. Zador
Department of Psychology
Yale University
New Haven, Connecticut

Foreword

LTP—An Exciting and Continuing Saga

Per Andersen
Institute of Basic Medical Sciences
Department of Neurophysiology
University of Oslo, Norway

Long-term potentiation (LTP) has been studied for about 25 years, and we may say it has come of age! It seems highly appropriate to compile a book in which some of the key issues are scrutinized by some of the most active players in this field. An interesting approach was to pit different attitudes and interpretations against each other. The fact that there are a number of opinions is a sign of health in a vigorously active field.

Seen in a historical perspective, it is interesting to witness the truly impressive and accelerating development of the field. Since its discovery by Terje Lømo in 1966, the LTP research was in a descriptive phase for about a decade and a half. Following the seminal discovery by Graham Collingridge, Stephen Kehl, and Hugh MacLennan in 1983 that 2-amino-5-phosphonovalerate (APV) blocked the induction of LTP, the pace of the research quickened appreciably. Particularly during the last few years we have seen a fantastic development, creating an optimism which is nearly tangible.

At the start of this saga, the situation was quite different. First, the number of research groups was quite small, and we all knew each other. In the mid-fifties John Green and Ross Adey in Los Angeles had rediscovered the impressive theta waves in the hippocampus. This activity was first described before the second world war by Richard Jung and Alois Kornmüller in Berlin in an attempt by the latter to make a map of regional electroencephalographic patterns, similar to the cytoarchitectonic maps of Korbinian Brodmann, Constantin von Monakow, Maximillian Rose, and Cécile and Oscar Vogt. Back in the fifties, Thomas Powell and Max Cowan in Oxford started their marvellous companionship with the charting of pathways of the hippocampal and associated structures with the revolutionizing terminal degeneration techniques of Walle Nauta. With the same approach Theodor Blackstad in Oslo showed how precisely the afferent systems were organized, and stimulated the physiologists to take advantage of this arrangement.

At this time, there was only a score of groups that were interested in exploiting the regular structure of hippocampus to study central synaptic transmission and epileptic phenomena, for which hippocampus was known to be prone. The most active groups in hippocampal neurophysiology were John Green and Ross Adey in Los Angeles, Herbert Jasper and Pierre Gloor in Montreal, Eric Kandel and Alden Spencer in Karl Frank's laboratory at the National Institutes of Health, Bethesda, Brian Cragg and Les Hamlyn in London, and Terje Lømo and myself in Oslo. In all groups, the researchers noticed that the hippocampal system was highly sensitive to the rate of stimulation. Too strong or long-lasting repetitive stimulation gave epileptiform after-discharges, while milder stimulation gave well-developed recruitment of signals.

This phenomenon of signal enhancement during frequent stimulation stood us in good use many a time when the preparation appeared to be slowly running down. Often, we could give new life to the signals, just by turning the stimulus rate knob to a higher frequency for a few seconds.

When Terje Lømo joined me in Oslo, he was immediately fascinated by this frequency potentiation, as we called the phenomenon. Before long, he was able to show that the tetanization gave not only a transient improvement, but that the enhancement could remain for a surprisingly long time. In his first report on the phenomenon in 1966, he noted that the recruitment of the population spikes in the second of two tetani (15 Hz, 5 seconds duration) occurred considerably faster than during the first tetanus, and that the population spikes became larger and occurred at shorter latencies compared to the first trial. The stimulation frequency had to be between 6 and 50 Hz, and the enhancement could last for hours. When Tim Bliss came to Oslo, he and Terje Lømo started the systematic analysis which led to the well known paper in the *Journal of Physiology* in 1973. They not only described the phenomenon, but pointed to the cumulative nature of the process, and to the fact that antidromic activation was ineffective, and gave suggestive evidence for input specificity.

Not unexpectedly, the report created considerable interest, both because of the duration of the synaptic enhancement, but also because the process could be elicited by stimulus rates and durations which were similar to those shown by single unit recordings from awake, behaving animals by people like John O'Keefe in London, Jim Ranck in Brooklyn, and Olga Vinogradova in Moscow. Particularly important were, according to my view, the imaginative ideas put forward by Gary Lynch, working in Irvine. Not only did he formulate several interesting and testable theories, but he was instrumental in bringing a biochemical approach to this research area. It is fitting that his main collaborator in this endeavor, Michel Baudry, is one of the editors of this book. The receptor unmasking theory put forward by Baudry and Lynch in 1980 and refined in 1984 has been an essential tool for the LTP research, although the initial results were slightly disappointing. However, we now see that this approach has yielded excellent results, and also colored the way most researchers now look upon the LTP problems.

After the discovery that APV could block LTP induction, the amount of data has escalated and so has the number of people attracted to this field. An important breakthrough was the finding by Wigström and Gustafsson in Gothenburg that blockade of $GABA_A$-mediated inhibition greatly increased the degree of LTP, leading to the discovery that the induction was associated with dendritic depolarization. The natural experiment leading on from this finding was to test whether coupling of synaptic input with artificial depolarization of the postsynaptic cell also would give LTP. The first of these trials was also published by Wigström and Gustafsson, and five laboratories reported similar results within a span of a few months.

The coupling experiments showed that LTP had characteristics required for associative learning, as clarified by Donald Hebb in 1949. No doubt, the important observation of the coupling effect has been instrumental in bringing many new and productive people into LTP research in the last few years.

Naturally, within the large field into which LTP research has developed, there must be room for different opinions. The organizers of the symposium that formed the basis for this book asked the participants to bring such areas of conflict to the fore, not for the purpose of fighting, but to expose the problems in order to search for experimental tests which may settle some of the controversies.

Although there seems to be consensus on the main elements of LTP induction, there is still a hot debate on the machinery behind the expression of LTP and its maintenance.

In addition, we are far from agreeing on the question of whether LTP can be abolished or reduced once it has developed. The discussion as to whether LTP changes are pre- or postsynaptic has been particularly intense, and seems to rage more forcefully than ever. Personally, I feel that there are changes on both sides, and that these changes are interrelated, but expressed with different time courses. However, I am sure that the pre-versus-post debate will keep us busy for quite some time.

Another fierce debate has been over quantal analysis of synaptic responses in LTP. Indeed, some people doubt whether quantal analysis is feasible at all in these synapses. Here, the new technique of whole-cell patch recording offers great hopes for a clarification because it removes a major obstacle, the low signal-to-noise ratio in conventional recording. However, another difficulty is not solved, the large quantal variability of CNQX-sensitive synaptic currents. Only if this variability is unchanged by the LTP process may we overcome this obstacle. The next few years will probably bring clarification on this point as well.

Another controversy in our field has been the relative contribution of various protein kinases in the expression of LTP. Again, the story may be more complicated than we thought a few years back. It may be that several kinases are involved, perhaps in an interdependent fashion both pre- and postsynaptically. Furthermore, the importance of proteases has only been studied on a small scale so far. Judging from other systems, these enzymes may have a significant contribution to the LTP story, as indeed suggested by the work by Baudry and Lynch. The development of the story on retrograde signals will also be exciting. In this context, arachidonic acid is an interesting molecule. However, due to its many roles in the cell housekeeping it may be a bit early to judge its real role in LTP.

Above all, we have to ask ourselves whether LTP represents a single process or a set of intercalated or concatenated phenomena. This also relates to the question of how many variants of LTP there are. Is the NMDA-mediated version fundamentally different from the APV-insensitive form? Are the changes induced by high calcium concentrations for a few minutes the same as standard tetanus-induced LTP? Do the changes expressed as AMPA-mediated responses belong to the same type as those seen as enhanced NMDA-related signals? The top question is probably the relation between LTP and various forms of learning and memory as seen by our behavioral colleagues. These are some of the pressing questions for future experimental attack.

One of the most important aspects of LTP is its possible structural correlate. Many would agree with me that it is perhaps the most important feature. At the moment, the bewildering variability of the structural elements in control tissue represents a sizeable hindrance. In my own view, significant progress in this field requires new techniques and, above all, better control material. However, the sheer number of the many observations at hand fuels the hope of many groups that there may be real changes around the corner. The reward is certainly worth quite some struggle. Again, several new developments in quantitative microscopy, staining procedures, and electronic visualization sustain my hope that real progress in this field may be close at hand.

Looking back on the formidable progress made over the last decade, one has to be thoroughly impressed. Judging from the pace of the new discoveries, and the encouraging similarities with several invertebrate preparations, we are probably in for significant advances at an accelerated tempo. Now that we see the start of a molecular approach to LTP studies, we probably all anticipate spectacular progress.

REFERENCES

Baudry, M. & Lynch, G. (1980). Hypothesis regarding the cellular mechanisms responsible for long-term synaptic potentiation in the hippocampus. *Experimental Neurology* 68, 202–204.

Blackstad, T.W. (1956). Commissural connections of the hippocampal region in the rat, with special reference to their mode of termination. *Journal of Comparative Neurology* 105, 417–536.

Bliss, T.V.P., & Lømo, T. (1973). Long-lasting potentiation of synaptic transmission in the dentate area of the anaesthetized rabbit following stimulation of the perforant path. *Journal of Physiology (London)* 232, 331–356.

Brodmann, K. (1909). *Vergleichende Lokalisation der Grosshirnrinde.* J.A. Barth.

Collingridge, G.L., & Bliss, T.V.P. (1987). NMDA receptors–their role in long-term potentiation. *Trends in Neuroscience* 10, 288–293.

Collingridge, G.L., Kehl, S.J., & McLennan, H. (1983). Excitatory amino acids in synaptic transmission in the Schaffer collateral-commissural pathway of the rat hippocampus. *Journal of Physiology (London)* 334, 33–46.

Cragg, B.G. & Hamlyn, L.H. (1955). Action potentials of the pyramidal neurones in the hippocampus of the rabbit. *Journal of Physiology (London)* 129, 608–627.

Gloor, P., Vera, C.L. and Sperti, L. (1964). Electrophysiological studies of hippocampal neurons. III. Responses of hippocampal neurons to repetitive perforant path volleys. *Electroenceph. Clin. Neurophysiol.* 17, 353–370.

Green, J.D. & Adey, W.R. (1956). Electrophysiological studies of hippocampal connections and excitability. *EEG Clin. Neurophysiol.* 8, 245–262.

Hebb, D.O. (1949). *The Organization of Behavior; A Neurophysiological Theory*, New York, Wiley.

Kandel, E.R., Spencer, W.A. & Brinley, F.J. (1961). Electrophysiology of hippocampal neurons. I. Sequential invasion and synaptic organization. *Journal of Neurophysiology* 24: 225–242.

Lynch, G. and Baudry, M. (1984). The biochemistry of memory: a new and specific hypothesis. *Science 224:* 1057–1063.

Lømo, T. (1966). Frequency potentiation of excitatory synaptic activity in the dentate area of the hippocampal formation. *Acta Physiologica Scandinavia* 68 (Suppl., 277) 128.

O'Keefe, J. (1976). Place units in the hippocampus in the freely moving rat. *Experimental Neurology* 51, 78–109.

Nauta, W.J.H. (1950). Über die sogenannte terminale Degeneration im Zentralnervensystem und ihre Darstellung durch Silberimpragnation. *Schweiz. Arch. Neurol. Psychiat., 66,* 353–376.

Powell, T.P.S. & Cowan, W.M. (1955). An experimental study of the efferent connexions of the hippocampus. *Brain.* 78, 115-132.

Ranck, J.B. Jr. (1973). Studies on single neurons in dorsal hippocampal formation and septum in unrestrained rats. *Experimental Neurology* 41, 461–555.

Rose, M. (1926). Über das histogenetische Prinzip der Einteilung der Grosshirnrinde. *J. Psychol. Neurol. (Loz.).* 32, 97–160.

Vinogradova, O. (1970). Registration of information and the limbic system, in *Short-term Changes in Neural Activity and Behaviour* (eds. G. Horn and R.A. Hinde), pp 95–140. Cambridge University Press.

Wigström, H. and Gustafsson, B. (1983). Facilitated induction of long-lasting potentiation during blockade of inhibition. *Nature* 30, 603–604.

Wigström, H., Gustafsson, B., Huang, Y,-Y. & Abraham, W.C. (1986). Hippocampal long-term potentiation is induced by pairing single afferent volleys with intracellularly injected depolarizing current pulses. *Acta Physiologica Scandinavia* 126, 317–319.

Preface

It will come as no surprise to readers of this volume that the 1990s have been proclaimed (by no less an authority than President Bush) as the "Decade of the Brain." In science, a few areas particularly capture the imagination because of a combination of excitement, substantial technical progress, and implicit importance in affecting the nature and quality of life. The past few decades have witnessed an explosion of information gathering in the neurosciences. Some of the most interesting research strategies have been driven by a search for how neuronal tissue is able to store and retrieve information.

In 1949, D.O. Hebb suggested a synaptic modification for learning that occurs as a consequence of coincidence between presynaptic and postsynaptic activity. Hebb's concept has gained wide acceptance and is often used (albeit frequently modified) as the basis for extensive research and modeling efforts. Since its discovery in 1974, long-term potentiation (LTP) has proved to be a kind of "test-bed" for Hebbian ideas, and various LTP paradigms have generated an explosion of research within the neuroscience community. Simply stated, LTP is a form of neural plasticity (change in synaptic efficacy as a function of some patterns of electrical activity) that seems to depend on both presynaptic and postsynaptic activity. Although the heightened synaptic efficacy produced by afferent tetanic stimulation has now been described in many parts of the brain, it has been best studied, for technical and theoretical reasons, in the part of the limbic system known as the hippocampus.

For many reasons, including the known role of hippocampus in memory processes, the ability of LTP to last for months, and pharmacological evidence, LTP has become the best model for a cellular explanation of biological information storage (memory). The best approaches to understanding the phenomenon have been multidisciplinary, involving neurochemical, neurophysiological, and neuroanatomical approaches. LTP has also provided fertile ground for scientists and engineers interested in describing and abstracting computational ideas for biological information-processing systems.

One measure of a dynamic, evolving science is controversy, and the LTP field continues to have its share. Although some have described LTP as "a phenomenon in search of a function," others have proclaimed it to be the key that provides answers to the major questions in human cognition. The arguments run from the molecular to the behavioral level and reveal the broad spectrum of interest and techniques that are being used.

In 1990, we decided that the time was right to attempt to clarify several issues that had generated intense controversies. To facilitate the exchange of ideas, we thought it would be best to bring together some of the most notable workers in the LTP field. With the great number of meetings and symposia vying for the available time and energy of our invited participants, we felt very gratified at the response (both in Europe and the United States) to our suggestion for an LTP-oriented gathering. Furthermore, we decided that we would try to avoid one typical consequence of a meeting where experts cover different aspects of a subject without any interaction among the participants.

We solved this problem in three ways: all contributors were asked to center their discussion around one (or more) controversial issue in the LTP field. Each author was asked to not simply present his own theoretical position and data but also to constructively criticize "the opposition." Second, because we did not want this book to represent the meeting in archival form, we asked the contributors to circulate a rough draft or position paper before the meeting. The final written contributions were requested after the conference to allow the contributors to respond to challenges and adjust their hypotheses, theories, and ideas in response to meeting activities. Third, through the influence of Drs. Vincent Bloch and Serge Laroche we obtained the ideal setting for this meeting, the chateau on the C.N.R.S. grounds at Gif-sur-Yvette. Neither of us were naive enough to believe that this gathering of minds would provide unambiguous answers (or ambiguous answers, for that matter) to the proposed controversial issues. We do believe that, because of the manner in which the information is presented, and because of the intellectual quality of the contributors, this book will be of great use to those who want a contemporary view of the current status of LTP and of some of the most controversial issues.

Finally, we would like to thank the funding agencies who made this conference possible. They include the Office of the Chief of Naval Research, the U.S. Air Force European Office in Aerospace Research and Development, the CNRS Program in Cognisciences, the firm of Rhone-Poulenc Santé, the Université de Paris-Sud, and UER Scientifique d' Orsay. We are indebted to our host, Dr. Laroche, and his assistants, Mlle Doyère and Mlle Rédini De Négro at the Département de Psychophysiologie, Gif-sur-Yvette, and to the chairpersons and rapporteurs who firmly guided our efforts and provided able overviews and summaries at the end of each panel discussion.

Michel Baudry
Joel Davis

Introduction

Since its discovery in 1972, long-term potentiation (LTP) of synaptic transmission has been popular as a potential memory mechanism. While progress in our understanding of the mechanisms and potential roles of LTP has been relatively slow until a few years ago, recent years have seen an explosion of research in the LTP field. This is probably due to the conjunction of technical and conceptual advances as well as the large increase in the number of scientists working on LTP. It looks as if researchers are feeling that the field is ripe for major discoveries and that definitive answers are at hand. Furthermore, scientists from most neuroscience disciplines have been attracted by the "LTP-mania" as the LTP phenomenon can be studied from the molecular level up to the behavioral level. Trying to cover all the different aspects of LTP in a single volume would have been a very difficult task. On the other hand, several intense controversies have developed in the recent years, and this volume was generated as an attempt to present both sides of the dispute, or in some cases of different perspectives, concerning the themes we thought were most clearly controversial.

1. The presynaptic versus the postsynaptic changes in LTP. At present, two very different types of hypotheses concerning the long-lasting changes underlying LTP exist: one involving a change in transmitter release, and the other favoring an increase in postsynaptic responses. The presynaptic theories are strongly influenced by the findings in invertebrates and thus are additionally justified from evolutionary arguments. This aspect also directs the experimentation along the lines of invertebrate research. This dichotomy has also a profound influence on network modelers and theoreticians who are interested in identifying the rules of synaptic modification. Unfortunately, results found in some laboratories cannot be replicated in other laboratories, some data are overinterpreted, and the hypotheses are often not clearly stated to allow for an unequivocal understanding of the current status. Moreover, the recent application of whole-cell patch recording to hippocampal neurons has provided additional ground for discussion. This new approach has allowed a quantal analysis of transmitter release, and the results contrast drastically with results observed by traditional recording techniques. The first section of

the book covers these issues with several chapters addressing the questions raised by the results of the quantal analysis.

2. The role of different calcium-dependent enzymes in LTP. One aspect of LTP that is confusing at the present time is that of the roles that different calcium-dependent enzymes (particularly kinases) play in the induction or expression of LTP. This particular aspect of LTP is confusing primarily because the experimental approach has been pharmacological, and the particular tools available are never as specific as their users claim. Moreover, there are methodological issues that are often ignored or pushed aside by the investigators. Several of these issues are discussed in the second section of the book.

3. The biophysical and structural changes in LTP. Among the popular theories that try to explain the extremely long duration of LTP are those implicating a structural change in synaptic structures resulting in biophysical alterations of the properties of the synaptic complex that produce an increase in synaptic response. These theories are supported by various data that vary from one laboratory to another. Again the variations in the experimental parameters are often not critically discussed and the general picture emerging from all these studies is far from clear. Bill Greenough has tried to impose some order on this confusing literature and present a cogent update of the subject.

4. The relationship between LTP and learning and memory. Although it is generally assumed that there is a link between LTP and learning and memory, the exact nature of that link is still highly debated. For some, LTP represents only an epiphenomenon resulting from nonphysiological stimulation whereas others are strongly claiming that LTP is the storage mechanism for various types of information. Several chapters in the fourth section of the book review the evidence for or against a causal link between LTP and information storage.

5. LTP rules in neural networks. Computer simulation of neural networks is becoming a very important tool to explore the computational operations of different brain circuitries. A number of laboratories have established multidisciplinary programs to bring together neurobiologists and computer scientists to study the roles of synaptic plasticity in the operation of neural networks. The rules of synaptic plasticity used by different laboratories differ widely as do the resulting performances of the networks. Some of the results and problems provided by this approach are presented in the last section of the book.

We are well aware that this volume will not bring an end to current ongoing controversies and, in fact, may provide some new ones; nevertheless, we strongly believe that it will clarify important issues and give enough critical information to the interested reader to arrive at an independent evaluation.

I Presynaptic Versus Postsynaptic Changes in Long-Term Potentiation

1 Presynaptic Changes Associated with Long-Term Potentiation in the Dentate Gyrus

Tim V. P. Bliss, Melanie P. Clements, Michael L. Errington, Marina A. Lynch, and John H. Williams

The locus of change in hippocampal long-term potentiation (LTP) has been the subject of animated and unresolved debate for several years. The changes induced could in principle be presynaptic (leading to increased transmitter release), postsynaptic (generating enhanced synaptic current in response to a fixed level of transmitter release), or both (Bliss and Lømo, 1973; Bliss and Lynch, 1988). During the 1980s it became clear that the trigger for the induction of LTP in most hippocampal pathways is a postsynaptic event. The powerful depolarization produced by tetanic stimulation activates voltage-dependent channels associated with the *N*-methyl-D-aspartate (NMDA) subtype of glutamate receptor (Collingridge et al., 1983; Nowak et al., 1984). The entry of calcium into the postsynaptic cell through this channel is believed to be the trigger for the induction of LTP (Gustafsson and Wigström, 1990).

In contrast to the general agreement on events mediating the induction of LTP, there is, to put it mildly, no consensus on how or where these events and the signals they generate are transduced into a sustained increase in synaptic efficacy. This chapter concentrates on presynaptic changes in LTP, and in particular on experiments demonstrating a link between LTP and transmitter release in the perforant path, the main afferent projection to the dentate gyrus. The positive correlation we have found raises the question of how the postsynaptic side of the synapse communicates with the presynaptic side. This in turn has led us to postulate the existence of a messenger that is released from a postsynaptic site at the time of induction, and passes retrogradely across the synapse to stimulate transmitter release from the presynaptic terminal. We present evidence that one such signal may be arachidonic acid.

This chapter appeared in *Seminars in Neuroscience* 2:345–354, 1990, copyright © 1990 by W. B. Saunders Company, and is reprinted by permission.

LTP IS ACCOMPANIED BY AN INCREASE IN THE CONCENTRATION OF EXTRACELLULAR GLUTAMATE

Perfusion Studies

Insertion of a push-pull cannula into the dentate gyrus of the anesthetized rat allows the synaptic region traversed by perforant path fibers to be perfused with artificial cerebrospinal fluid (figure 1.1). In this way, transmitter candidates and other substances of interest can be collected and analyzed. Electrodes are attached to the cannula to record population responses evoked by stimulation of the perforant path. Using this technique, we first investigated the release of [^{3}H]glutamate, newly synthesized from [^{3}H]glutamine. Consistent with other biochemical evidence that glutamate is the transmitter in this pathway (Cotman and Nadler, 1981; Storm-Mathisen, 1981), we found a stimulus-dependent increase in release of [^{3}H]glutamate. Moreover, a tetanus to the perforant path sufficient to induce LTP was followed by a sustained increase in the concentration of glutamate in the perfusate (Dolphin et al., 1982). Subsequent experiments to explore the relationship between LTP and the release of endogenous glutamate in the dentate gyrus have confirmed this initial observation (Bliss et al., 1986; Errington et al., 1987; Lynch et al., 1989b). We have seen a similar correlation in area CA1 (Bliss et al., 1990b) but there is disagreement about the extent and duration of the effect in this

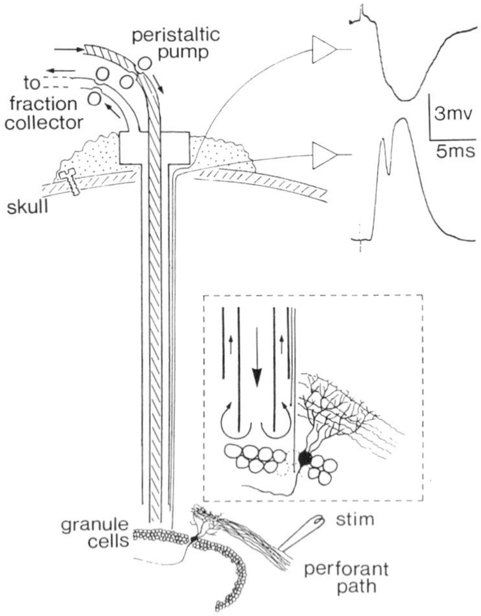

Figure 1.1 Diagram of push-pull cannula with attached recording electrodes used for in vivo studies of transmitter release in LTP. Field potentials recorded in the synaptic layer (upper trace) and cell body layer (lower trace) of the dentate gyrus were evoked by stimuli delivered to the perforant path. The initial slope of the response (the population excitatory postsynaptic potential [EPSP]) is measured as an index of synaptic efficacy. (Reprinted by permission from Errington et al., 1983, *Journal of Neuroscience Methods* 7:353–357.)

region (Bliss et al., 1990a; Aniksztejn et al., 1989). We therefore confine our discussion here to the dentate area. Procedures that block the induction of LTP also block the increase in glutamate release. Examples from three series of experiments, using different procedures to block the induction of LTP, are shown in figure 1.2. In each case, the sustained increase in glutamate release that accompanies LTP fails to occur in animals in which the induction of LTP is blocked.

We have recently extended our measurements of glutamate release to the dentate "minislice" preparation (conventional transverse hippocampal slices from which areas CA1 and CA3 have been trimmed). Here, too, LTP is accompanied by a sustained increase in glutamate release (Bliss

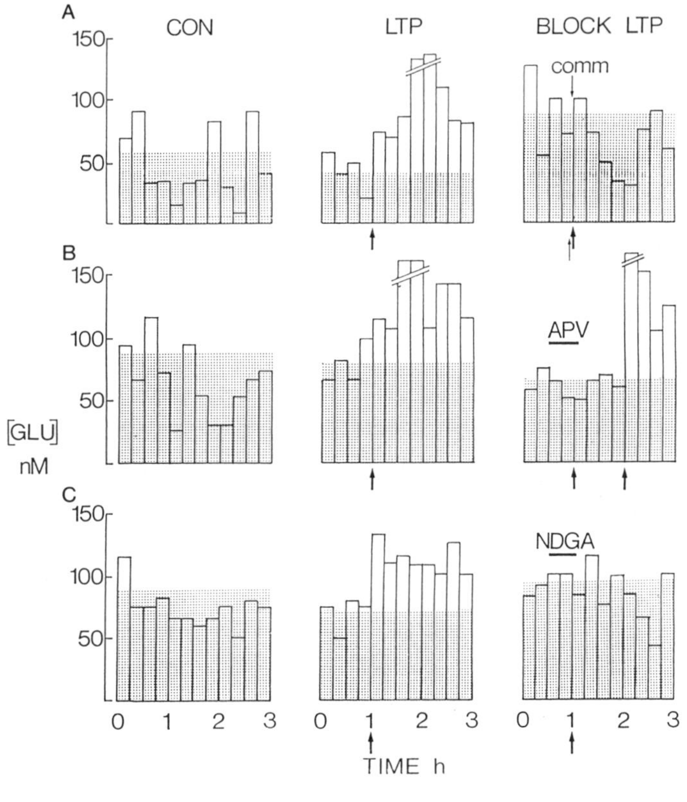

Figure 1.2 LTP in perforant path-granule cell synapses is associated with a sustained increase in the release of glutamate into push-pull perfusates. In each row (A–C) the release of glutamate, in 15-minute fractions, is shown for a single animal taken from a control group (CON), a group in which LTP was induced after 1 hour by tetanic stimulation of the perforant path (LTP), and a group in which the induction of LTP was blocked by (A) concurrent stimulation (arrows) of the perforant path and commissural input to the dentate gyrus; (B) inclusion in the perfusion medium of D(−)aminophosphonovaleric acid (D(−)APV; bar, 200 μM), or (C) the lipoxygenase and phospholipase A_2 inhibitor, nordihydroguaiaretic acid (NDGA; bar, 200 μM). An increase in glutamate concentration in the perfusate is seen only in the animals in which LTP was successfully induced. The stippling represents mean glutamate concentration in the perfusate during the first hour of the experiment. (See Bliss et al., 1986; Errington et al., 1987; Lynch et al., 1989b, by permission of *Neuroscience Letters* 30:693–701.)

et al., 1990b). In addition, as in the anesthetized preparation (Bliss et al., 1986), an activity-dependent increase in glutamate release can be demonstrated by increasing the stimulus rate from the test frequency of 1/30 Hz to 1 Hz, though the modest size of the increase (approximately 50% for a 30-fold increase in stimulus rate) suggests that much of the release at test rates of stimulation derives from an activity-independent pool. It is therefore likely that the increase in glutamate release following the induction of LTP is at least partly due to an increase in background release. The relative contributions of activity-dependent and activity-independent release to the extracellular glutamate concentration remain to be worked out in detail.

Ex vivo Studies

In another series of experiments we have used an ex vivo approach to the biochemical analysis of transmitter release (Bliss and Lynch, 1988). LTP is induced in the dentate gyrus unilaterally in the anesthetized animal, and, at a given time after induction, the dentate gyrus is removed. Control and potentiated tissues are incubated in radiolabeled glutamate and then exposed to a depolarizing stimulus (40 mM potassium) in the presence or absence of calcium. The proportion of total radioactivity released can then be compared in potentiated and control tissues. The calcium-dependent component of potassium-stimulated release is greater in the potentiated side than in the control side 2.5 minutes, 45 minutes, and 3 hours after induction (figure 1.3; Lynch et al., 1989c). An advantage of this technique is that measurements can be made from animals with chronically implanted electrodes in which LTP has been monitored for several days. In one such experiment we found an increase in calcium-dependent, potassium-stimulated release 72 hours after the induction of LTP (Bliss et al., 1987); no such increase was found in another group of animals examined 23 days after induction, by which time LTP of the excitatory postsynaptic potential (EPSP) had decayed to control values (Bliss et al., 1987). These ex vivo experiments on dentate slices, as well as similar unpublished experiments on synaptosomes, demonstrate that LTP is accompanied by an increase in the ability of potentiated tissue to release glutamate in response to a sustained depolarizing stimulus. Moreover, the effect can apparently last as long as LTP itself.

Interestingly, in all experiments with radiolabeled glutamate, increases were confined to the calcium-dependent component of potassium-stimulated release, a finding that suggests, in contrast to the endogenous release studies, that a vesicular pool was the principal contributor to the effect. Another finding was the absence of any change in accumulation of label, indicating that the increase in release was unlikely to be due to a decrease in the capacity of glutamate uptake carriers.

Considered together, these experiments demonstrate that LTP in the dentate gyrus is associated with a sustained increase in extracellular glutamate. The results could in principle be explained by increases in both

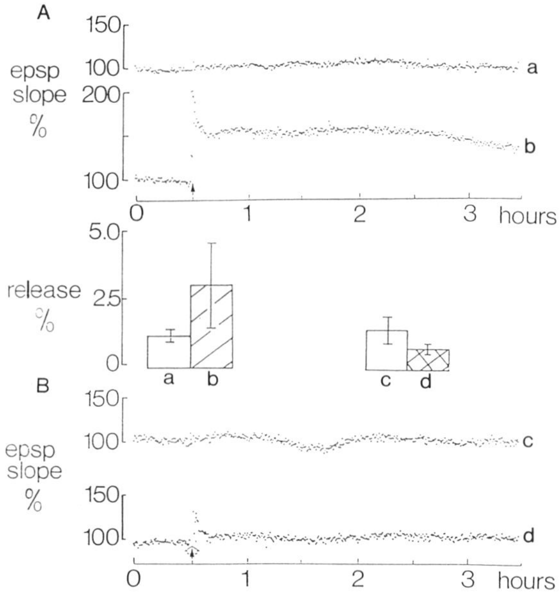

Figure 1.3 Ca^{2+}-dependent release of [^{3}H]glutamate is enhanced in potentiated tissue. (A) LTP was induced by unilateral tetanic stimulation of the perforant path in anesthetized animals (arrow). Plots of the population EPSP as a function of time are shown for the untetanized (a) and tetanized (b) sides in (A). After 45 minutes the dentate gyrus was removed from both sides, cross-chopped into slices, and incubated in [^{3}H]glutamate. The Ca^{2+}-dependent component of release elicited by exposure to 40 mM of K^+ is significantly greater in tissue from the potentiated side (hatched histogram, b) than from the untetanized control side (open histogram, a). (B) When the induction of LTP was blocked by simultaneous tetanization (arrows) of the perforant path and commissural inputs to the dentate gyrus (d), there was no difference in the release of labeled glutamate from the two sides (compare histograms c and d). Similar results were obtained 2.5 minutes and 3 hours after the induction of LTP. (Reprinted by permission from Lynch et al., 1989c, *Neuroscience Letters* 103:191–196.)

activity-dependent and activity-independent release from potentiated terminals, and/or by a change in the kinetics of uptake into presynaptic or postsynaptic neural elements or into glial cells. It seems safe to say, however, in view of the increased release of radiolabeled glutamate from "potentiated" synaptosomes, that the enhanced concentration of extracellular glutamate in LTP is unlikely to derive solely from glial cells or postsynaptic neuronal processes.

THE REQUIREMENT FOR A RETROGRADE MESSENGER

Evidence is compelling that LTP is triggered postsynaptically (Bliss and Lynch, 1988; Gustafsson and Wigström, 1990). As we have seen, the increase in glutamate associated with LTP is at least partly presynaptic in origin. How, then, does the presynaptic terminal learn about events occurring postsynaptically? In principle, information could be relayed through a monosynaptic or polysynaptic feedback loop, but this cannot explain the in vitro results where the anatomical basis for such hypothetical loops is absent. Two other possibilities are (1) a reduction in the concentration of calcium in the synaptic cleft as a result of the opening of voltage- and ligand-gated calcium channels, and (2) the release of a retrograde messenger from the postsynaptic cell (Bliss et al., 1986; Griffith, 1966; Sastry et al., 1988). The available evidence does not suggest that LTP is strongly correlated with changes in extracellular calcium (Bliss and Lynch, 1988; Mody and Heinemann, 1986; Taube and Schwartzkroin, 1985), and we have sought evidence for the second hypothesis. The possibility that the membrane lipid arachidonic acid, or one of its lipoxygenase metabolites (figure 1.4A), might be the putative transcellular messenger in LTP was first proposed in a study of the role of arachidonic acid and leukotrienes in mediating presynaptic inhibition in *Aplysia* sensory neurons (Piomelli et al., 1987). The idea received early support from the finding that activation of NMDA receptors stimulates the release of arachidonic acid from neurons in culture (Dumuis et al., 1988; Lazarewicz et al., 1988; Patel et al., 1990). It seems likely that the entry of calcium through NMDA-linked channels stimulates the production of arachidonic acid through activation of phospholipase A_2, a proposal supported by the finding that release of arachidonic acid is blocked by PLA_2 inhibitors (Dumuis et al., 1988; Patel et al., 1990). The arachidonic acid hypothesis allows a number of predictions to be made, which we have examined experimentally.

Prediction 1 Inhibitors of arachidonic acid production or of its metabolism through the lipoxygenase (but not cyclo-oxygenase) pathway will block the induction of LTP.

Test Nordihydroguaiaretic acid (NDGA), a lipoxygenase inhibitor that also suppresses the production of arachidonic acid from membrane phospholipids by inhibiting the activity of phospholipase A_2 (see figure 1.4A), blocks the induction of LTP in the dentate gyrus in vivo (Lynch et al., 1989b, figure 1.4B). In the dentate minislice, LTP is blocked by NDGA but not by the cyclo-oxygenase inhibitor indomethacin (Williams et al., 1991).

Prediction 2 LTP will be associated with a transient or sustained increase in the release of arachidonic acid into the extracellular compartment. (Note that the hypothesis as initially formulated does not distinguish between a triggering role for the retrograde messenger in which induction of LTP requires only a transient elevation in the signal, and a tonic role in which a sustained elevation is required.)

Test LTP in the perforant path is accompanied by a small but sustained increase in the concentration of arachidonic acid in perfusates obtained with a push-pull cannula from the dentate gyrus of anesthetized rats (figure 1.5). A similar persistent increase is seen in the extracellular

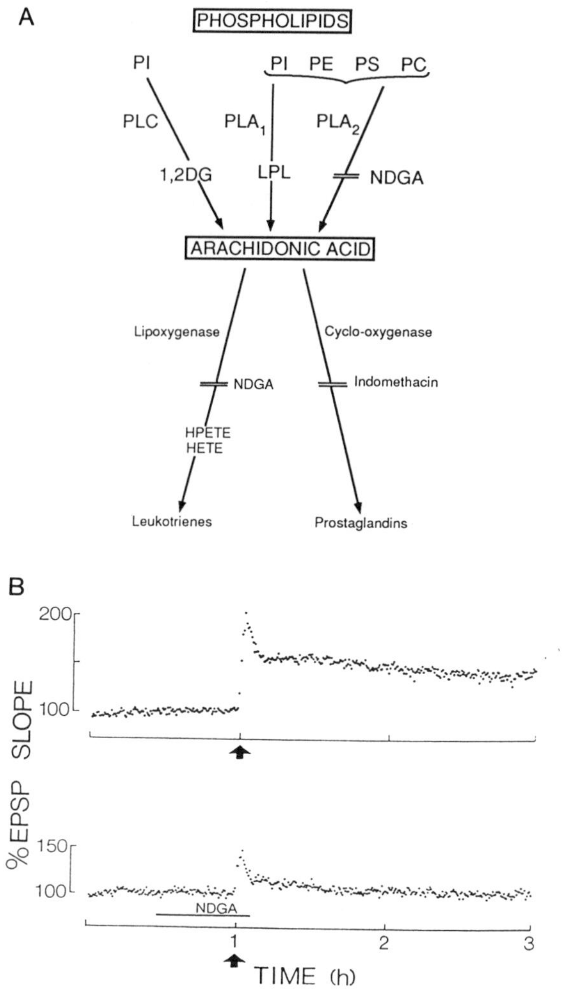

Figure 1.4 (A) Simplified scheme of the arachidonic acid metabolic cascade. NDGA and indomethacin are inhibitors of lipoxygenase/PLA_2 and cyclo-oxygenase respectively. (B) LTP of the population EPSP in the dentate gyrus of the anesthetized rat is blocked by NDGA. Means of six animals each in the control group (upper trace), and the group perfused with NDGA (200 μM, lower trace). Note that posttetanic potentiation is not affected. (PI = phosphatidylinositol; PC = phosphatidylcholine; PE = phosphatidylethanolamine; PS = phosphatidylserine; 1,2 DG = 1,2 diacylglycerol; LPL = lysophospholipase; NDGA = nordihydroguaiaretic acid; HPETE = 12-hydroperoxyeicosatetraenoic acid; HETE = 12-hydroxyeicosatetraenoic acid. (Reprinted by permission from Lynch et al., 1989b, *Neuroscience Letters* 30:693–701.)

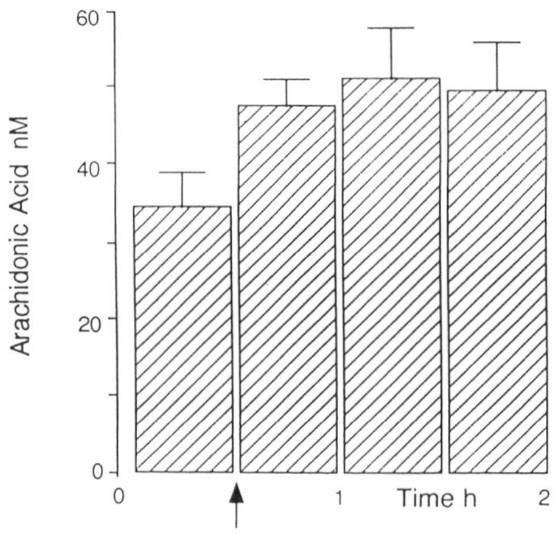

Figure 1.5 LTP in the dentate gyrus is associated with a sustained increase in the extracellular concentration of arachidonic acid. Histograms show the mean concentration (±SEM, n = 6) of arachidonic acid in push-pull perfusates collected before and after the induction of LTP (arrow). A second tetanus, given at 75 min, did not produce further potentiation.

content of the 12-lipoxygenase metabolite, 12-hydroxyeicosatetraenoic acid (12-HETE), together with a transient (approximately 1 hour) increase in its precursor, 12-hydroperoxyeicosatetraenoic acid (12-HPETE). There are no concomitant changes in the extracellular concentration of other membrane fatty acids (oleic, palmitic, linoleic, linolenic, stearic acids) measured by high performance liquid chromatography (HPLC) (M.A. Lynch, T.V.P. Bliss and C.R. Bramham, unpublished experiments; see Bliss et al., 1990b). This result suggests that the expression of LTP, at least in the first 1 to 2 hours, requires a persistent increase in the extracellular concentration of arachidonic acid.

Prediction 3 (1) Transient perfusion with arachidonic acid, in conjunction with transiently enhanced synaptic activation, will produce transient potentiation of synaptic transmission. (2) Perfusion with arachidonic acid alone will have no effect. (These are weak predictions in the sense that the hypothesis could survive their falsification. They are based on the assumptions that a continuous increase in the supply of arachidonic acid is required to maintain LTP and that arachidonic acid is only effective on recently active or "primed" terminals. The latter assumption was adopted to provide a simple explanation for the property of specificity which restricts LTP to activated synapses.)

Test The experiment to test this set of predictions led to an unexpected result. The second prediction was verified, but the potentiation produced in the dentate gyrus by the conjunction of arachidonic acid and low-intensity tetanic stimulation (by itself too weak to produce LTP) was slow in onset and could persist for many hours (Williams et al., 1989). Ar-

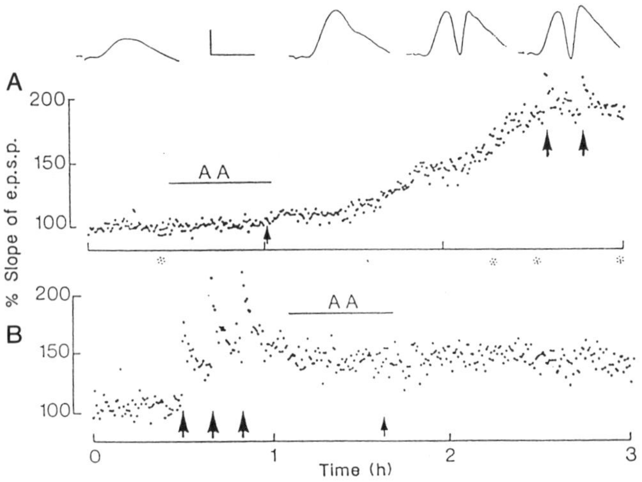

Figure 1.6 A delayed, activity-dependent enhancement of synaptic transmission is produced in the dentate gyrus when weak tetanic stimulation of the perforant path (small arrow) is combined with perfusion with arachidonic acid (200 μM). Neither procedure alone produces a long-lasting after-effect (not shown). Arachidonic acid–induced potentiation occludes tetanus-induced LTP (large arrows, top trace), and vice versa (lower trace). The sample traces in the top panel were collected at the times indicated by the asterisks. (Averages of five consecutive responses, calibration 4 mV, 5 milliseconds. From Williams et al. 1989. Reprinted by permission from *Nature* 341:739–742. Copyright © 1989 Macmillan Magazines Ltd.)

achidonic acid–induced potentiation was occluded by preceding tetanus–induced LTP, and vice versa, suggesting a convergence in the mechanisms mediating the two effects (figure 1.6).

Prediction 4 The hypothesis assumes that the release of arachidonic acid is stimulated by the opening of postsynaptic calcium-permeant channels linked to the NMDA receptor. This step is by-passed when arachidonic acid is supplied exogenously, and the hypothesis would therefore predict that NMDA antagonists would not block arachidonic acid–induced enhancement.

Test The NMDA antagonist D(−)aminophosphonovalerate (APV) does not block arachidonate-induced activity-dependent potentiation in the dentate gyrus in vivo (Williams et al., 1989).

Prediction 5 Arachidonic acid will stimulate transmitter release from primed (recently active) terminals.

Test Preliminary results suggest that this is the case. When transverse slices were perfused for 30 minutes with arachidonic acid while stimulating the perforant path and the Schaffer commissural projection at 0.25 Hz there was a delayed and persistent potentiation of the response in both projections which was accompanied by an increase in the release of glutamate into the perfusate (Williams et al., 1989). It is likely therefore that arachidonic acid–induced potentiation in the dentate and/or area CA1 is associated with an increase in transmitter release. In hippocampal slices preloaded with [^{3}H]glutamate and stimulated with 40 mM potassium, exposure to 5 μM arachidonic acid enhanced both the calcium-dependent and calcium-independent component of glutamate release. The 12-lipoxygenase metabolites 12-HPETE and 12-HETE induced an increase only in the calcium-dependent component of glutamate release, while a range of other fatty acids tested failed to increase either component (Lynch and Voss, 1990).

Prediction 6 LTP will be accompanied by an increase in the availability of free arachidonic acid at postsynaptic sites.

Test The arachidonic acid content of membrane fractions enriched in postsynaptic densities prepared from the hippocampus of potentiated animals was significantly higher than in control tissue. There was no difference between control and potentiated tissue in the arachidonic acid content of membranes from a synaptic terminal preparation (synaptosomes), or from a glial-enriched preparation (Lynch et al., 1989a).

While the present evidence cannot be regarded as conclusive, the results are generally consistent with the arachidonic acid hypothesis. The delayed onset of potentiation appears to disqualify arachidonic acid as a messenger in the initial phase of LTP, and raises the question of whether other messenger(s), perhaps operating in conjunction with arachidonic acid, are involved in generating the enhanced response during the first hour or so of LTP. There has been speculation that nitric oxide, which is released from cerebellar granule cells in culture by NMDA (Garthwaite et al., 1988), could perform such a role, but so far the evidence to support this hypothesis is lacking. Many other questions remain. Which is the more likely candidate, arachidonic acid or one of its 12-lipoxygenase metabolites? How much of the additional arachidonic acid released into the extracellular compartment following the induction of LTP derives from PLA_2 activity, and how much from phosphatidylinositol, via the activation of phospholipase C, and diacylglycerol lipase (see figure 1.4A), and do the relative proportions change with time? Does the messenger need to be continuously present to maintain the potentiated response, as suggested by the sustained increase in release of arachidonic acid, but apparently contraindicated by the fact that persistent potentiation can be produced by the transient conjunction of enhanced activity and exposure to arachidonic acid? How can the input specificity of LTP be reconciled with the notion of a retrograde messenger? With respect to the last question, the simplest explanation is that arachidonic acid is released only at synapses that have satisfied the criterion for the induction of LTP. At such synapses, the influx of calcium through postsynaptic NMDA receptor–linked channels could be expected to activate PLA_2, leading to an increase in free arachidonic acid available for release into the synaptic cleft. In addition, to explain the activity-dependence of arachidonic acid–induced potentiation, we postulate that presynaptic terminals need to be primed by recent activity. This provides a further safeguard against heterosynaptic activation arising from diffusion of arachidonic acid to neighboring inactive synapses. In our experiments, increased activity and exposure to arachidonic acid occurred simultaneously; the temporal relationship between these two events needs to be explored.

How does arachidonic acid produce its presynaptic effects? Experiments on synaptosomes prepared from dentate gyrus have established that arachidonic acid stimulates phosphatidylinositide hydrolysis, and leads to an elevation of cytosolic calcium (Voss et al., 1990). Similar increases are found in synaptosomes when potentiated tissue is compared with control tissue. A possible mode of action therefore is through stimulation of phosphoinositide turnover and the consequent production of the two second messengers diacylglycerol (DAG) and inositoltriphosphate (IP_3), the first acting to stimulate protein kinase C (PKC), and the second to release calcium from nonmitochondrial intracellular stores. PKC_γ, the predominant isoform of PKC in brain, is also directly activated by fatty acids, most potently by arachidonic acid (Sekiguchi et al., 1987). In this regard, it is intriguing to note that LTP induced in the presence of a PKC inhibitor persists for 1–2 hours (Lovinger et al., 1987; Reymann et al., 1988), suggesting that the PKC-dependent phase of LTP has a delayed onset, with a similar time course to that of arachidonic acid-induced potentiation. Both IP_3 and arachidonic acid increase the concentration of cytosolic calcium in synaptosomes from dentate gyrus (Lynch and Voss, 1991). The two effects are nonadditive, suggesting that arachidonic acid may produce its effect by stimulating the production of IP_3. An increase in exocytotic transmitter release can be expected from an elevation of cytosolic calcium in the presynaptic terminal, and may also be a consequence of the activation of PKC. A presynaptic role for PKC in the expression of LTP has been explored in an extensive series of experiments by Routtenberg and associates (1985), Linden and Routtenberg (1989), and Gispen and colleagues (1989). Correlations have been established between LTP and the translocation of PKC from cytoplasm to plasma membrane, and between LTP and the phosphorylation of a presynaptic substrate protein known variously as GAP43, F1 or B-50. The recent demonstration that the protein kinase inhibitor H7 blocks the expression of LTP in area CA1 when bath applied, but not when injected intracellularly into the postsynaptic neuron, also points to a presynaptic role for protein kinases in LTP (Malinow et al., 1989). The two bifurcating routes by which arachidonic acid could stimulate transmitter release, one by activation of PKC and the other through stimulation of IP_3 production, are incorporated in the scheme illustrated in figure 1.7.

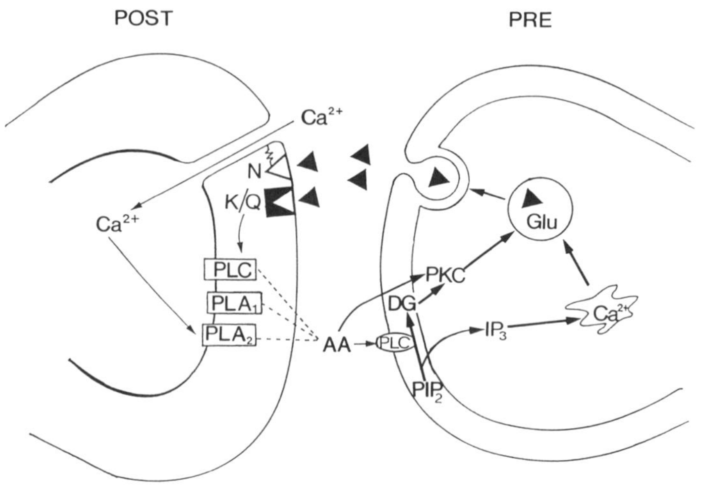

Figure 1.7 Hypothetical scheme illustrating the possible role of arachidonic acid or its metabolites as a retrograde messenger in LTP. The induction of LTP is triggered by permeation of calcium through the NMDA channel. The resulting rise in intradendritic calcium concentration activates PLA_2, with a consequent liberation of free arachidonic acid from phospholipids and diffusion into the synaptic cleft. At the presynaptic membrane, the increase in the extracellular concentration of arachidonic acid could act in a number of ways to stimulate an increase in transmitter release: for example, by stimulating PIP_2 hydrolysis, by activating PKC, or by exerting a direct effect on vesicular function. Increased transmitter release will activate PLC postsynaptically, via the metabotropic quisqualate receptor (K/Q), leading to the release of further arachidonic acid from diacylglycerol (see figure 1.4A). In this way, continued supplies of arachidonic acid could be provided after the initial calcium transient had declined. (AA = arachidonic acid; DG lipase = diacylglycerol lipase; IP_3 = inositol trisphosphate; Glu = glutamate; KQ = glutamate receptor of the kainate/quisqualate subtype; N = glutamate receptor of the NMDA subtype; PIP_2 = phosphatidylinositol-bisphosphate; PKC = protein kinase C; PLC = phospholipase C.

CONCLUSIONS

If the increase in glutamate concentration in the extracellular compartment associated with LTP cannot be attributed solely to an increase in activity-dependent release (i.e., to an increase in release per action potential), what is the source of the increase, and how is it related to LTP? An increase in activity-independent release could be due to changes in spontaneous quantal release, changes in nonquantal release, or changes in uptake. The possibility that changes in uptake play a role in LTP are strengthened by the recent finding that arachidonic acid inhibits glutamate uptake into retinal ganglion cells (Barbour et al., 1989). However, in the dentate gyrus arachidonic acid does not affect the capacity of the high affinity glutamate uptake system (Lynch and Voss, 1990). Moreover, perfusion with arachidonic acid alone, in the absence of increased synaptic activation, does not produce an enhancement of transmission (Williams et al., 1989). How would a change in steady-state concentration of glutamate in the synaptic cleft affect synaptic transmission? There is evidence that activation of glutamate receptors in CA1 pyramidal cells is a cooperative event, probably requiring that two molecules of ligand bind to the receptor (Mayer, 1989). If this is the case in the dentate gyrus, an increase in background glutamate levels could enhance synaptic transmission by priming a population of receptors that would not otherwise reach the level of receptor occupancy required for channel opening. An example of this kind of cooperativity at glycine-utilizing synapses is found in the goldfish Mauthner cell (Faber and Korn, 1988).

The hope that the presynaptic versus postsynaptic debate would be illuminated by a quantal analysis of minimal synaptic currents recorded in the whole cell patch clamp mode appeared to be realized by the recent publication of two independent studies which both concluded that there was a strong presynaptic component to the maintenance of LTP (Bekkers and Stevens, 1990; Malinow and Tsien, 1990). Unfortunately, if not in this field uncharacteristically, another quantal study has now come to the opposite conclusion (Foster and McNaughton, 1991). Our own less-than-daring prediction is that it will be some time before the matter is resolved, given the difficulty of arriving at unambiguous interpretations of synaptic variability in central neurons. Finally, we should remember that the mechanisms revealed by experiments in which LTP is followed for 1 to 2 hours are not necessarily the same as those that sustain LTP for 1 to 2 weeks or more.

REFERENCES

Aniksztejn, I., M. P. Roisin, R. Amsellem, and Y. Ben-Ari (1989). Long-term potentiation is not associated with a sustained enhanced release of endogenous excitatory amino acids. *Neuroscience* 28:387–392.

Barbour, B., M. Szatowski, N. Ingledew, and D. Attwell (1989). Arachidonic acid induces a prolonged inhibition of glutamate uptake into glial cells. *Nature* 342:918–920.

Bekkers, J. M., and C. F. Stevens (1990). Presynaptic mechanisms for long-term potentiation in the hippocampus. *Nature* 346:724–729.

Bliss, T. V. P., and T. Lømo (1973). Long-lasting potentiation of synaptic transmission in the dentate area of the anaesthetized rabbit following stimulation of the perforant path. *Journal of Physiology* 232:331–356.

Bliss, T. V. P., R. M. Douglas, M. L. Errington, and M. A. Lynch (1986). Correlation between long-term potentiation and release of endogenous amino acids from dentate gyrus of anaesthetized rats. *Journal of Physiology* 377:391–408.

Bliss, T. V. P., M. L. Errington, S. Laroche, and M. A. Lynch (1987). Increase in K^+-stimulated, Ca^{2+}-dependent release of [3H]glutamate from rat dentate gyrus three days after induction of long-term potentiation. *Neuroscience Letters* 83:107–112.

Bliss, T. V. P., and M. A. Lynch (1988). Long-term potentiation of synaptic transmission in the hippocampus: properties and mechanisms, in P. W. Landfield and S. A. Deadwyler (eds.), *Long-term Potentiation in the Hippocampus: From Biophysics to Behavior.* New York: Alan R. Liss, pp. 3–72.

Bliss, T. V. P., M. L. Errington, and M. A. Lynch (1990a). Long-term potentiation in the dentate gyrus in vivo is associated with a sustained increase in extracellular glutamate, in Y. Ben-Ari (ed.), *Excitatory Amino Acids and Neuronal Plasticity. Advances in Experimental Medicine and Biology.* New York: Plenum Press 268:269–278.

Bliss, T. V. P., M. L. Errington, M. A. Lynch, and J. H. Williams (1990b). Presynaptic mechanisms in hippocampal long-term potentiation, in E. R. Kandel, T. J. Sejnowski, and C. F. Stevens (eds.), *The Brain.* Cold Spring Harbor Symposia on Quantitative Biology, vol. 55 (in press).

Collingridge, G. L., S. J. Kehl, and H. McLennan (1983). Excitatory amino acids in synaptic transmission in the Schaffer collateral-commissural pathway of the rat hippocampus. *Journal of Physiology* 334:33–46.

Cotman, C. W., and J. V. Nadler (1981). Glutamate and aspartate as hippocampal transmitters: biochemical and pharmacological evidence, in J. Storm-Mathisen (ed.), *Glutamate: Transmitter in the Central Nervous System.* Chichester: Wiley, pp. 117–154.

Dolphin, A., M. L. Errington, and T. V. P. Bliss (1982). Long-term potentiation of the perforant path in vivo is associated with increased glutamate release. *Nature* 297:496–498.

Dumuis, A., et al. (1988). NMDA receptors activate the arachidonic acid cascade system in striatal neurons. *Nature* 336:68–70.

Errington, M. L., A. C. Dolphin, and T. V. P. Bliss (1983). A method for combining field potential recording with local perfusion in the hippocampus of the anaesthetized rat. *Journal of Neuroscience Methods* 7:353–357.

Errington, M. L., M. A. Lynch, and T. V. P. Bliss (1987). Long-term potentiation in the dentate gyrus: induction and increased glutamate release are blocked by D(−)aminophosphonovalerate. *Neuroscience* 20:279–284.

Faber D. S., and H. Korn (1988). Synergism at central synapses due to lateral diffusion of transmitter. *Proceedings of the National Academy of Science* 85:8708–8712.

Foster, T. C., and B. L. McNaughton (1991). Long-term enhancement of CA1 synaptic transmission is due to increased quantal size, not quantal content. *Hippocampus 1* (in press).

Garthwaite, J., S. L. Charles, and R. Chess-Williams (1988). Endothelium-derived relaxing factor release on activation of NMDA receptors suggests role as intercellular messenger in the brain. *Nature* 336:385–388.

Gispen, W. H., et al. (1989). The protein kinase C substrate protein B-50 in neural signal transduction and plasticity, in M. Ito and Y. Nishizuka (eds.), *Brain Signal Transduction and Memory.* Tokyo: Academic Press, pp. 110–116.

Griffith, J. S. (1966). A theory of the nature of memory. *Nature* 211:1160–1163.

Gustafsson, B., and H. Wigström (1990). Basic features of long-term potentiation in the hippocampus. *Seminars in Neuroscience* 2:321–333.

Lazarewicz, J. W., J. T. Wroblewski, M. E. Palmer, and E. Costa (1988). Activation of N-methyl-D-aspartate–sensitive glutamate receptors stimulates arachidonic acid release in primary cultures of cerebellar granule cells. *Neuropharmacology* 27:765–769.

Linden, D., and A. Routtenberg (1989). The role of protein kinase C in long-term potentiation: a testable model. *Brain Research Reviews* 14:279–296.

Lovinger, D. M., K. Wong, K. Murikami, and A. Routtenberg (1987). Protein kinase C inhibitors eliminate hippocampal long-term potentiation. *Brain Research* 436:177–183.

Lynch, M. A., M. P. Clements, K. L. Voss, and T. V. P. Bliss (1989a). Increased postsynaptic release and presynaptic actions of arachidonic acid suggest a retrograde messenger role in long-term potentiation. *Society for Neuroscience Abstracts* 15:86.

Lynch, M. A., M. L. Errington, and T. V. P. Bliss (1989b). Nordihydroguaiaretic acid blocks the synaptic component of long-term potentiation and the associated increases in release of glutamate and arachidonate: an in vivo study in the dentate gyrus of the rat. *Neuroscience* 30:693–701.

Lynch, M. A., M. L. Errington, and T. V. P. Bliss (1989c). The increase in [3H]glutamate release associated with long-term potentiation in the dentate gyrus is blocked by commissural stimulation. *Neuroscience Letters* 103:191–196.

Lynch, M. A., and K. Voss (1990). Arachidonic acid increases inositol phospholipid metabolism and glutamate release in synaptosomes prepared from hippocampal tissue. *Journal of Neurochemistry* 55:215–221.

Lynch, M. A., and K. Voss (1991). Presynaptic changes in long-term potentiation: elevated synaptosomal calcium concentration and basal phosphoinositide turnover in dentate gyrus. *Journal of Neurochemistry* 56:113–118.

Malinow, R., H. Schulman, and R. W. Tsien (1989). Inhibition of postsynaptic PKC or CaMKII blocks induction but not expression of LTP. *Science* 245:862–866.

Malinow, R., and R. Tsien (1990). Presynaptic changes revealed by whole cell recordings of long-term potentiation in rat hippocampal slices. *Nature* 346:177–180.

Mayer, M. (1989). Activation and desensitization of glutamate receptors in mammalian CNS, in D. Keeling and C. Benham (eds.), *Ion Transport*. London: Academic Press, pp. 183–196.

Mody, I., and U. Heinemann (1986). Laminar profiles of the changes in extracellular calcium concentration induced by repetitive stimulation and excitatory amino acids in the rat dentate gyrus. *Society for Neuroscience Abstracts* 11:782.

Nowak, I., et al., (1984). Magnesium gates glutamate-activated channels in mouse central neurones. *Nature* 307:462–465.

Patel, A. I., C. Sanfeliu, and A. Hunt (1990). Development and regulation of excitatory amino acid receptors involved in the release of arachidonic acid in cultured hippocampal neural cells. *Developmental Brain Research* 57:55–62.

Piomelli, D., et al. (1987). Lipoxygenase metabolites of arachidonic acid are second messengers for presynaptic inhibition of Aplysia sensory cells. *Nature* 328:38–43.

Reymann, K. G., U. Frey, R. Jork, and H. Matthies (1988). Polymixin B, an inhibitor of protein kinase C, prevents the maintenance of synaptic long-term potentiation in hippocampal CA1 neurons. *Brain Research* 440:305–314.

Routtenberg, A., D. Lovinger, and O. Steward (1985). Selective increase in phosphorylation of a 47 kDA protein (F1) directly related to long-term potentiation. *Behavioral and Neural Biology* 43:3–11.

Sastry, B. R., S. S. Chirwa, P. B. Y. May, and H. Maretic (1988). Substances released during tetanic stimulation of rabbit neocortex induce neurite growth in PC-12 cells and long-term potentiation in guinea pig hippocampus. *Neuroscience Letters* 91:101–105.

Sekiguchi, K., et al. (1987). Three distinct forms of rat brain protein kinase C: differential response to unsaturated fatty acids. *Biochemical and Biophysical Research Communications* 145:797–802.

Storm-Mathisen, J. (1981). Glutamate in hippocampal pathways, in G. Dichiara and G. L. Gessa (eds.), *Glutamate: Glutamate as a Neurotransmitter.* New York: Raven Press, pp. 43–45.

Taube, J. S., and P. A. Schwartzkroin (1985). Ineffectiveness of organic calcium channel blockers in antagonizing long-term potentiation. *Brain Research* 379:275–285.

Voss, K. L., M. P. Clements, and M. A. Lynch (1990). Increased intrasynaptosomal calcium concentration associated with long-term potentiation in the dentate gyrus may be triggered by arachidonic acid. *Neuroscience Letters Supplement* 38:S83.

Williams, J. H., M. L. Errington, M. A. Lynch, and T. V. P. Bliss (1989). Arachidonic acid induces a long-term activity-dependent enhancement of synaptic transmission in the hippocampus. *Nature* 341:739–742.

Williams, J. H., M. P. Clements, M. L. Errington, K. L. Voss, M. A. Lynch, and T. V. P. Bliss (1991). Retrograde messengers in long-term potentiation: a role for arachidonic acid? In B. Meldrum, F. Moroni and E. Costa (eds.), *Excitatory Amino Acids.* New York: Raven Press, pp. 487–493.

2 Trends in LTP Research

Laurent Aniksztejn, Marie-Paule Roisin, Alphonso Represa, and Yehzekel Ben-Ari

The mechanism of long-term potentiation (LTP) is being extensively investigated, particularly in three areas: the mechanisms of induction, the mechanisms of expression, and the morphological substrate of the potentiation. In the CA1 region of the hippocampus, induction of LTP is caused by a rise in $[Ca^{2+}]_i$ produced by the activation of *N*-methyl-D-aspartate (NMDA) receptors (Collingridge and Bliss, 1987; Malenka, et al., 1989), whereas in the mossy fibers synapse there is some evidence that the rise in $[Ca^{2+}]_i$ is produced by the activation of voltage-dependent Ca^{2+} channels (VDCC) (Williams and Johnston, 1989; Jaffe and Johnston, 1990, see also Zalutsky and Nicoll, 1990). Recent studies suggest that in the CA1 region, voltage-dependent Ca^{2+} channels may also be involved in the induction of LTP (Grover and Teyler, 1990; Regehr et al., 1989; Regehr and Tank, 1990; Westenbroek et al., 1990). In this chapter we first describe, in the CA1 region of the hippocampus, a similar Ca^{2+} dependent, NMDA-independent form of LTP produced by K^+ channel blockers (Aniksztejn and Ben-Ari, 1991).

Concerning the expression of LTP, the sequence of events responsible for the persistence of the potentiation has not clearly been determined. There are conflicting reports on whether the expression is associated (Bliss et al., 1986), or is not associated (Aniksztejn et al., 1989) with a sustained enhanced release of glutamate or aspartate. In the second part of this chapter, we provide, using a new method of in vitro local perfusion (Roisin et al., 1991), some evidence that the levels of the two excitatory amino acids are only transiently enhanced after the train of high-frequency electrical stimulation.

Finally, in the third part of this chapter, we discuss the possible morphological substrates of LTP. To this purpose we have centered our investigations on the hippocampal mossy fibers, which have a number of unique features enabling them to be readily identified, and we report that brief seizure episodes induce LTP in the CA3 region (Ben-Ari and Gho, 1988), and chronic models of epilepsy produce sprouting of mossy fibers and the establishment of new aberrant synapses (Ben-Ari and Represa, 1990).

TRANSIENT K^+ CHANNEL BLOCK PRODUCES A CA^{2+}-DEPENDENT NMDA-INDEPENDENT FORM OF LTP IN CA1

Potassium channels are important in modulating cellular excitability, notably by controlling the repolarization of the membrane potential after a single or a burst of action potential. They are therefore important in the integrative processes of the cell.

The consequence of the block of K^+ channels is the simultaneous activation of both presynaptic and postsynaptic elements by increasing the evoked transmitter release following each presynaptic action potential; this, in turn, augments the amplitude and the duration of the postsynaptic depolarization and facilitates the activation of the voltage-dependent calcium channels. Thus blockade of K^+ channels is useful to examine whether an increase of $[Ca^{2+}]_i$ by mechanisms other than the activation of the NMDA receptor can also generate LTP.

Ten K^+ channels (I_A, I_D, I_C, I_M, I_Q, I_{fIR}, I_K, I_{AHP}, I_{CT} and I_{KATP}) have been described in CA1 pyramidal cells of the hippocampus; they differ by their kinetics, threshold of activation and inactivation, and pharmacological sensitivity to various toxins (Brown et al., 1990; Storm, 1990).

Using intracellular and extracellular recordings in isolated CA1 hippocampal slices, we compared the effects of a variety of K^+ channel blockers on synaptic transmission. We found that a transient 10-minute application of tetraethylammonium (TEA) at a concentration (25 mM) that blocked I_C, I_M, and I_K produced a long-lasting (4-hour) enhancement of synaptic transmission. Similar application of a lower concentration of TEA (5 mM) that blocked only I_C and I_M produced only a transient increase of field excitatory postsynaptic potential (EPSP). Furthermore, a block of I_A and I_D by a large concentration of 4-AP (5 mM) produced a reversible increase in the field EPSP, which recovered after 60 to 80 minutes. The block of several other K^+ channels, including I_Q and I_{fIR} by Cs^+ (2 mM), I_{AHP} by norepinephrine (10 μM) and I_{KATP} by glyburide (10 μM), failed to produce a long-lasting effect. Intracellular recording indicated that the long-term effect produced by high concentrations of TEA (referred to here as LTP_K) was not due to a partial wash of the drug because 30 minutes after TEA there was a total recovery of the TEA sensitive fast after hyperpolarization (which was due to the activation of I_C). It also was not associated with an increase in input resistance or cell excitability, and it was not caused by a decrease of GABAergic inhibition because LTP_K can be produced in bicuculline-treated slices. LTP_K is due to a genuine increased synaptic efficacy. Induction of LTP_K was blocked by 6-cyano-7-nitroquinoxaline-2,3-dione (CNQX) (10 μM), the selective α-amino-3-hydroxy-5-methyl-4-isoxazole propionate (AMPA) antagonist but not by the selective NMDA antagonist, D-amino-5-phosphonovalerate (D-APV) (50 to 100 μM). This finding suggests that a release of glutamate acting on the quisqualate receptor is required to induce LTP_K (figure 2.1). We tested the

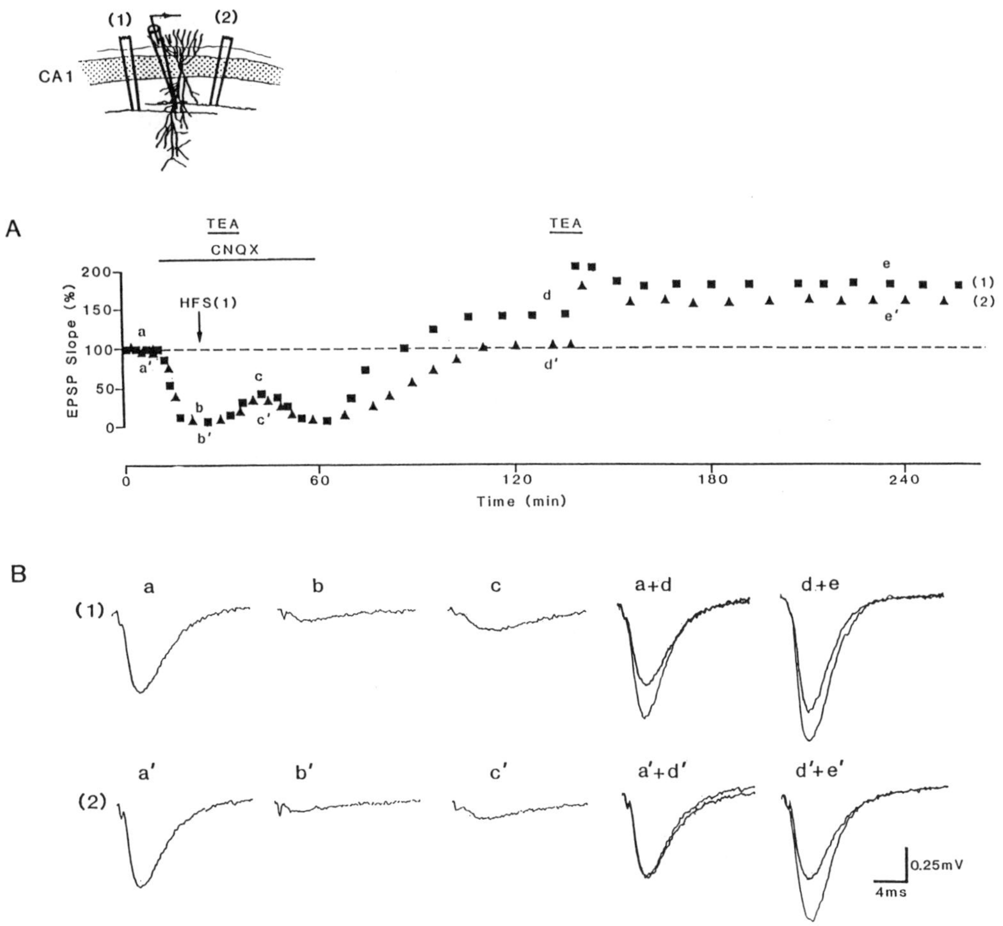

Figure 2.1 CNQX prevented the induction of TEA-induced LTP (LTP_K) but not the one produced by a train of high-frequency stimulation (LTP_E). Electrodes were positioned as shown in the diagram; two pathways were alternatively stimulated at 0.05 Hz. CNQX (10 μM) was applied 10 minutes before, and washout occurred 30 minutes after TEA. Electrical LTP was elicited by two tetani at 100 Hz for 1 second separated by 20 seconds, and was given at twice the control stimulation strength. The high-frequency stimulation (HFS) train was applied to one input (1) just before TEA application, the second input (2) serving as control. (A) CNQX, which blocked EPSP, prevented LTP_K (2) but not LTP_E (1). Eighty minutes after washing the first application of TEA, a second application of TEA produced a persistent potentiation of the untetanized pathway and increased the potentiation of the tetanized pathway. (B) Representative EPSPs recorded at a time marked by a letter.

effect of flunarizine (30 μM), a VDCC blocker, and found that it strongly reduced or blocked LTP_K.

Therefore, we conclude that the large increase in transmitter release induced by TEA will generate postsynaptic action potentials that do not repolarize over several milliseconds (due to the block of I_C, I_M, and I_K). This long-lasting depolarization will be associated with a large increase in Ca^{2+} influx via the activation of the voltage-dependent Ca^{2+} channels.

Recent observations also reflect the important role of the voltage-dependent Ca^{2+} channels in the induction of the LTP produced by electrical stimulation in the CA1 (see the introduction to this chapter). In keeping with this, we have now described a Ca^{2+}-dependent, NMDA-independent form of LTP, not requiring a tetanization of synaptic inputs. This suggests that in the CA1, two forms of LTP coexist. It is perhaps not surprising that the K^+ channels involved in LTP_K are those that are activated by a high level of depolarization and have a slow inactivation; they can therefore prevent or modulate activation of voltage-dependent Ca^{2+} channels.

Interestingly, induction of the two forms of LTP is prevented in physiological (low stimulation) conditions by inhibitory mechanisms. It may be pertinent to compare these mechanisms. Blockade of gamma-aminobutyric acid A ($GABA_A$) receptors by bicuculline facilitates the NMDA-dependent form of LTP, suggesting that the $GABA_A$ receptors provide an important inhibitory mechanism for the electrical LTP (LTP_E); the more sustained $GABA_B$ inhibition may also be involved in LTP_E. In contrast, blockade of repolarizing K^+ channels facilitates activation of voltage-dependent Ca^{2+} channels and induces LTP_K.

IS EXPRESSION OF LTP ASSOCIATED WITH A PERSISTENT ENHANCEMENT OF GLUTAMATE RELEASE?

To determine whether the expression (i.e., maintenance) of LTP is or is not caused by a persistent enhancement of transmitter release (i.e., presynaptic type of mechanism), some researchers have collected the material in vivo by push-pull cannulas and used high performance liquid chromatography (HPLC) to measure excitatory amino acids. Working in the fascia dentata Bliss and coworkers (1986) reported that a tetanic train of the perforant pathway evoked indeed a persistent (1–2 hours) enhanced release of glutamate. In the initial report, this conclusion was based on a comparison of one group of animals subjected to tetanic train and one that received only low-frequency stimulation. More recently, Lynch and coworkers (1989) reported a major increase in the release in a group of individual cases submitted to the same procedure.

In contrast, using a similar approach, we have found that the LTP induced by a tetanic train (Aniksztejn et al., 1989), phorbol esters (Aniksztejn et al., 1987) or mast cell degranulating peptide, a K^+ channel blocker (Aniksztejn et al., 1990) is not associated with a persistent increase in glutamate or aspartate release. More recently we have developed a more sensitive preparation in which the release of endogenous excitatory amino acids is locally measured in the slice by placing a collecting cannula above the CA1 region of the slice (Roisin et al., in press). This method enables researchers to combine the advantages of the slice technique, notably in terms of electrophysiology, with biochemical measures of the materials released during various conditions. We found that a train produced an LTP that was associated with a brief enhanced release of glutamate, which persisted for only 15 to 20 minutes (figure 2.2). Elsewhere we have discussed the possible reasons for the discrepancy between the results of Bliss and colleagues and ours (Roisin et al., 1990). It is possible that there are indeed differences between the Schaffer collaterals (in which most of our experiments were performed) and the perforant pathway, where most of the measures by the group of Bliss have been made. In chapter 1, Bliss suggests that in the CA1 region, the enhanced release of glutamate persists for 1 hour. In addition, Laroche and coworkers (1990), using an ex vivo approach in which the release of radioactive amino acids was studied in slices obtained from animals that had been trained in various learning paradigms, found a sustained enhanced release of glutamate in the fascia dentata but not in CA1. It is intriguing that patch clamp analysis has provided evidence in favor of the presynaptic hypothesis in CA1 (Malinow and Tsien, 1990; Bekkers and Stevens, 1990).

It bears stressing that the sensitivity of the method of collection (in vivo and in vitro) enables researchers to measure changes in glutamate release produced by trains of 10 Hz or more (figure 2.3). Electrical stimulation at lower frequencies (i.e., 0.033 Hz used as controls in most experimental conditions) does not produce major changes in glutamate or aspartate release. Therefore, if there is a persistent quasipermanent enhanced release of glutamate after a brief high-frequency train, as suggested by Bliss and colleagues, it will not originate from the activity-dependent evoked quantal release but from other sources including spontaneous quantal and nonquantal release and change in glial uptake (Brew and Attwell, 1987). It is not obvious that a massive increase in (ongoing) glutamate release will necessarily produce an increase in the signal-noise ratio. A large increase in extracellular glutamate may produce a depression of the EPSPs, and, at least in the hippocampus, intense tetanic stimulation produces LTP more readily than homosynaptic or heterosynaptic depressions of EPSPs, which is more consistently seen in the cerebellar or cerebral cortices (Ito, 1989).

IS LTP ASSOCIATED WITH SPROUTING AND NEOSYNAPTOGENESIS?

A mechanism that likely underlies the quasipermanent aspect of LTP and memory mechanisms is the establishment of new and more efficient synaptic connections. There is abundant literature on the increased den-

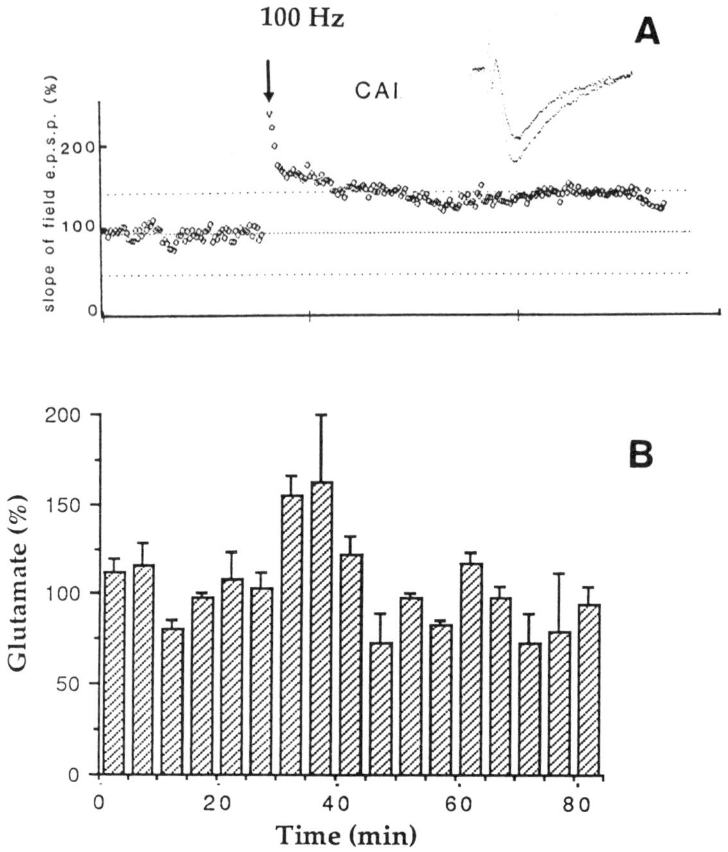

Figure 2.2 Relationship between LTP in the stratum radiatum of CA1 and in vitro release of glutamate. Hippocampal slices (500 μm) were placed in a fully submerged chamber and superfused with ACSF at a reduced flow rate of 0.5 ml/min. A cannula was placed in stratum radiatum of CA1, and 5-minute samples, collected at a rate of 25 μl/min during a 30-minute control period were used for HPLC analysis. The stimulating and recording electrodes were placed under visual control in the Schaffer collateral. (A) The slope of the field EPSP evoked by the Schaffer commissural stimulation (0.033 Hz, 0.05 millisecond duration) is expressed as a percentage of the 30-minute control level. The traces represent the field EPSP just before the high-frequency stimulation and the potentiated EPSP 30 minutes after the stimulation (100 Hz, 1 second). (B) Release of glutamate expressed as a percentage of the 30-minute control period (% mean ± SEM of mean). Note that the train produced transciently an increase (40%) of the release of glutamate (Student's *t*-test 0.05 compared to control).

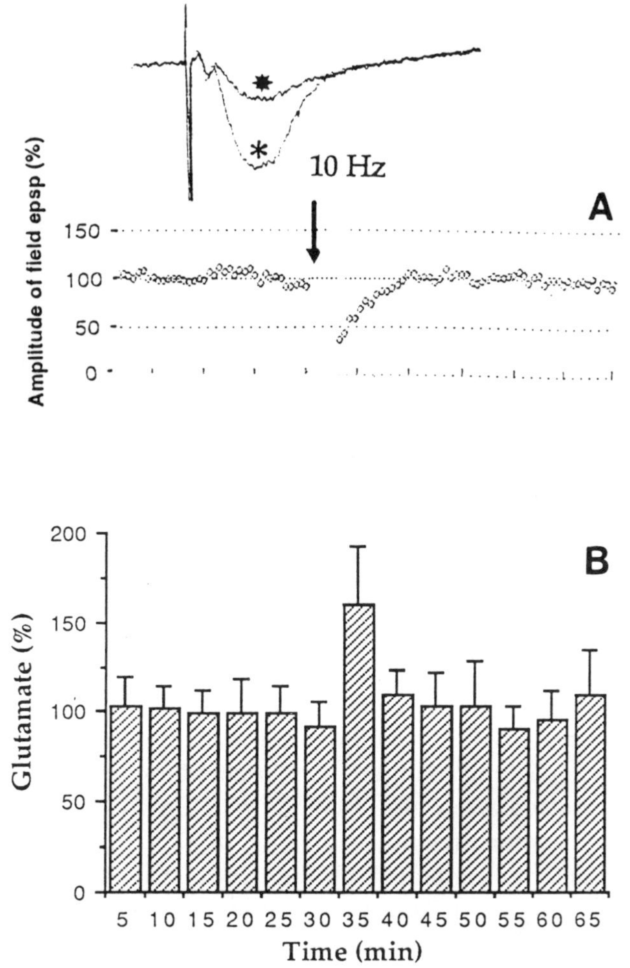

Figure 2.3 Relationship between the tetanic stimulation and the release of glutamate. The slices were perfused with ACSF, and 5-minute samples were collected from CA1 as described in figure 2.2. (A) The amplitude of the field EPSP evoked by the Schaffer commissural stimulation (0.033 Hz, 0.05-millisecond duration) is expressed as a percentage of the 30-minute control level. The traces represent the field EPSP just before (*) and during (★) the stimulation (10 Hz, 5 minutes). (B) Release of glutamate. The values were pooled from 10 independent experiments. Note that 10-Hz stimulation produced a transient increase in the release of glutamate (66%; Student's *t*-test 0.05 compared to control).

sity of synapses in various animal species subjected to enriched environments and other conditions thought to produce similar consequences. Thus a number of experimental procedures that increase electrical activity are in fact accompanied by changes in the form and shape of dentritic spines (Fifkova, 1985; Patel et al., 1988; Reeves and Steward, 1986; Glanzman et al., 1990).

In the hippocampus the axons of granule cells, the mossy fibers, have a number of unique features and markers that enable researchers to readily evaluate changes in the density of mossy fiber terminals, including zinc, dynorphin, and high-affinity kainate binding sites (see references in Ben-Ari and Represa, 1990). We have therefore examined recently whether hyperactivity produced use dependent changes in mossy fiber synapses.

In an earlier stage, we examined whether a brief episode of hyperactivity produced LTP in slice preparations (Ben-Ari and Gho, 1988). Using intracellular and extracellular recordings of CA3 pyramidal neurons, we found that bath application of kainate and other convulsive agents produced, as expected, recurrent ongoing interictal activity, which disappeared after washing the drugs. This brief (3–5 minutes) episode, however, was also associated with a long-lasting modification of the synaptic responses characterized by the fact that after the interictal episode, stimulation of various inputs produced an all-or-none giant EPSP instead of the graded EPSP recorded prior to the procedure. This change was not due to persistent change in cell excitability, or GABAergic inhibition, but reflected a genuine facilitation of synapse efficacy. Furthermore, NMDA receptor antagonists prevented the change without blocking the interictal activity generated by the convulsant agents. We conclude that a brief episode of interictal activity, such as the trains of high-frequency electrical stimulation, produced an NMDA-dependent LTP-like phenomenon. More recently (Gho and Ben-Ari, in preparation) we have directly shown that the EPSP generated by the excitatory recurrent collateral system is indeed potentiated by this procedure.

To examine whether hyperactivity in this system was associated with the establishment of novel synaptic connections, several laboratories have used various chronic models of epilepsy. Because seizures are associated with recurrent interictal activity, one would expect this type of enhanced activity to also produce permanent charges in the circuit. Kindling, an animal model of epilepsy in which subconvulsive electrical stimulations result in secondary generalized seizures (Goddard, 1967), has often been considered as an animal model of memory having many features in common with LTP. Thus NMDA seems to participate in the induction but not in the maintenance of kindling (Gilbert, 1988; Slater et al., 1985). Several studies have now shown that kindling induced mossy fiber sprouting in the hippocampus (Ben-Ari and Represa, 1990) and ectopic mossy fiber synaptogenesis in the fascia dentata (Sutula et al., 1988) and in CA3 (figure 2.4; Represa and Ben-Ari, 1990). It is tentative to suggest

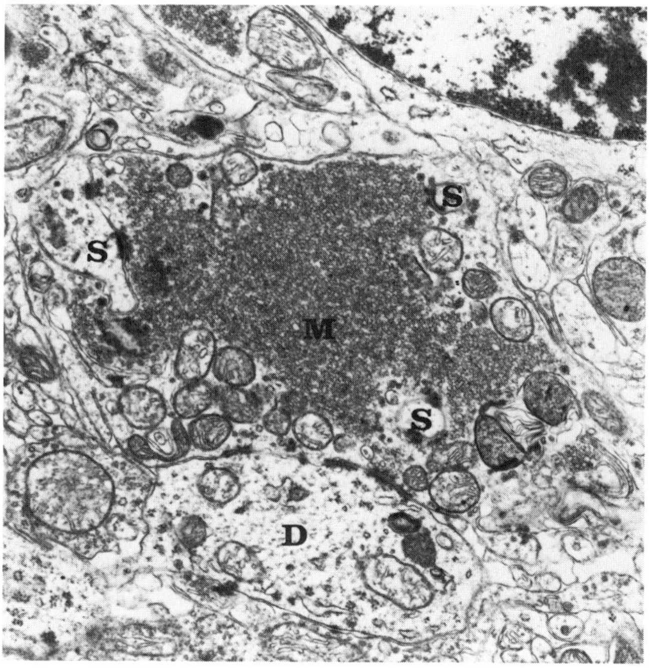

Figure 2.4 Electron micrograph of the stratum oriens of an amygdaloid kindled rat. Mossylike bouton (*M*) establish ectopic asymmetric synaptic contacts with dendritic spines (*S*) and symmetric junctions with the dendritic shafts (*D*) of pyramidal cells (8,200 ×).

that the increased excitability of kindled hippocampus is at least in part due to this synaptic remodeling.

Other models of epilepsy, including administration of kainate, also produce sprouting (Tauck and Nadler, 1985; Frotscher and Zimmer, 1983; Represa et al., 1987). Sprouting in these models is, however, complicated by the presence of lesions. Tauck and Nadler (1985) have also provided evidence that the novel synapses are indeed functional (see also Cronin and Dudek, 1988).

Aside from their interest as mechanisms of epileptogenesis, these observations are also of interest as a model to study the morphological substrate of plasticity. Indeed, it is now possible in this region to study the sequence of events leading from transient hyperactivity to neosynaptogenesis. Recent studies have already suggested several candidate mechanisms activated by seizures including (1) the rapid activation of immediate early genes as c-fos and c-jun, as well as their mRNA, on the granule cells (Dragunow and Robertson, 1987; Saffen et al., 1988; Morgan et al., 1987) and (2) the rise in the mRNA coding for nerve growth factor (Gall and Isackson, 1989) and brain derived neurotrophic factor (Zafra et al., 1990). Interestingly, the rise of mRNA produced by a parenteral administration of kainate is blocked by diazepam, which confirms the direct relationship between the seizure and mRNA activation. There is no doubt that exciting studies in the near future will enable researchers to precisely illustrate the mechanisms leading to sprouting in this model.

REFERENCES

Aniksztejn, L., M. P. Roisin, H. Gozlan, and Y. Ben-Ari (1987). Long-lasting potentiation produced by a phorbol ester in the hippocampus of the anaesthetized rat is not associated with a persistent enhanced release of excitatory amino acids. *Neuroscience Letter* 81:291–295.

Aniksztejn, L., M. P. Roisin, R. Amsellem, and Y. Ben-Ari (1989). Long-term potentiation in the hippocampus of the anaesthetized rat is not associated with a sustained enhanced release of endogenous excitatory amino acids. *Neuroscience* 28:387–392.

Aniksztejn, L., C. Charriaut-Marlangue, M. P. Roisin, and Y. Ben-Ari (1990). Long-term potentiation in the rat hippocampus induced by the mast cell degranulating peptide: analysis of the release of endogenous excitatory amino acids and proteins. *Neuroscience* 35:63–70.

Aniksztejn, L., and Y. Ben-Ari (1991). Novel form of long-term potentiation produced by a K^+ channel blocker in the hippocampus. *Nature* 349:67–69.

Bekkers, J. M., and C. F. Stevens (1990). Presynaptic mechanism for long-term potentiation in the hippocampus. *Nature* 346:724–729.

Ben-Ari, Y., and M. Gho (1988). Long-lasting modification of the synaptic properties of rat CA3 hippocampal neurones induced by kainic acid. *Journal of Physiology* 404:365–384.

Ben-Ari, Y., and A. Represa (1990). Brief seizure episodes induce long-term potentiation and mossy fiber sprouting in the hippocampus. *Trends in Neuroscience* 13:312–318.

Bliss, T. V. P., R. M. Douglas, M. L. Errington, and M. A. Lynch (1986). Correlation between long-term potentiation and release of endogenous excitatory amino acids from dentate gyrus of anaesthetized rats. *Journal of Physiology* (London) 377:391–408.

Brew, H., and D. Attwell (1987). Electrogenic glutamate uptake is a major current carrier in the membrane of axolotl retinal glial cells. *Nature* 327:707–709.

Brown, D. A., B. H. Gähwiler, W. Griffith, and J. V. Halliwell (1990). Membrane currents in hippocampal neurons. *Progress in Brain Research* 83:141–161.

Collingridge, G. L., and T. V. P. Bliss (1987). NMDA receptors—their role in long-term potentiation. *Trends in Neuroscience* 10:288–293.

Cronin, J., and F. E. Dudek (1988). Chronic seizures and collateral sprouting of dentate mossy fibers after kainic acid treatment in rats. *Brain Research* 474:181–184.

Dragunow, M., and H. A. Robertson (1987). Kindling stimulation induces c-fos protein(s) in granule cells of the rat dentate gyrus. *Nature* (London) 329:441–442.

Fifkova, E. (1985). A possible mechanism of morphometric changes in dendritic spines induced by stimulation. *Cellular and Molecular Neurobiology* 5:47–63.

Frotscher, M., and J. Zimmer (1983). Lesion induced mossy fibers to the molecular layer of the rat fascia dentata: identification of postsynaptic granule cells by the golgi-EM technique. *Journal Comparative Neurology* 215:299–311.

Gall, C. M., and P. J. Isackson (1989). Limbic seizures increase neuronal production of messenger RNA for nerve growth factor. *Science* 245:758–761.

Gilbert, M. E. (1988). The NMDA-receptor antagonist, MK801, suppress limbic kindling and kindled seizures. *Brain Research* 463:90–99.

Glanzman, D. L., E. R. Kandel, and S. Schachner (1990). Target-dependent structural changes accompanying long-term synaptic facilitation in aplysia neurons. *Science* 249: 799–801.

Goddard, G. V. (1967). Development of epileptic seizures through brain stimulation at low intensity. *Nature* 214:1020–1021.

Grover, L. M., and T. J. Teyler (1990). Two components of long-term potentiation induced by different patterns of afferent activation. *Nature* 347:477–479.

Ito, M. (1989). Long-term depression. *Annual Review of Neuroscience* 12:85–102.

Jaffe, D., and D. Johnston (1990). Induction of long-term potentiation at hippocampal mossy-fiber synapses follows a Hebbian rule. *Journal of Neurophysiology* 64:948–960.

Laroche, S., C. Redini-Del Negro, M. P. Clements, and M. A. Lynch (1990). Long-term activation of phosphoinositide turnover associated with increased release of amino acids in the dentate gyrus and hippocampus following classical conditioning in the rat. *European Journal of Neuroscience* 2:554–543.

Lynch, M. A., M. L. Errington, and T. V. P. Bliss (1989). Nordihydroguaiaretic acid blocks the synaptic component of long-term potentiation and the associated increases in release of glutamate and arachidonate: an in vivo study in the dentate gyrus of the rat. *Neuroscience* 30:693–701.

Malenka, R. C., J. Kauer, D. J. Perkel, and R. A. Nicoll (1989). The impact of postsynaptic calcium on synaptic transmission—its role in long-term potentiation. *Trends in Neuroscience* 12:444–450.

Malinow, R., and R. W. Tsien (1990). Presynaptic enhancement shown by whole cell recordings of long-term potentiation in hippocampal slices. *Nature* 346:177–180.

Morgan, J. I., D. R. Cohen, J. L. Hempstead, and T. Curran (1987). Mapping patterns of c-fos expression in the central nervous system after seizure. *Science* 237:192–197.

Patel, S. N., S. P. R. Rose, and M. G. Stewart (1988). Training induced dendritic spine density changes are specifically related to memory formation processes in the chick, gallus domesticus. *Brain Research* 463:168–173.

Reeves, T. M., and O. Steward (1986). Emergence of the capacity for LTP during reinnervation of the dentate gyrus: evidence that abnormally shaped spines can mediate LTP. *Experimental Brain Research* 65:167–175.

Regehr, W. G., J. A. Connor, and D. W. Tank (1989). Optical imaging of calcium accumulation in hippocampal pyramidal cells during synaptic activation. *Nature* 341:533–536.

Regehr, W. G., and D. W. Tank (1990). Postsynaptic NMDA receptor-mediated calcium accumulation in hippocampal CA1 pyramidal cell dendrites. *Nature* 345:807–810.

Represa, A., E. Tremblay, and Y. Ben-Ari (1987). Kainate binding sites in the hippocampal mossy fibers: localization and plasticity. *Neuroscience* 20:739–748.

Represa A., and Y. Ben-Ari (1990). Synaptic reorganization of hippocampal mossy fibers in epilepsy. *Médecine Sciences* 6:876–884.

Roisin, M. P., L. Aniksztejn, and Y. Ben-Ari (1990). Long-term potentiation is not associated with a sustained enhanced release of glutamate. In Y. Ben-Ari (ed.), *Excitatory Amino Acids and Neuronal Plasticity.* Advances in Experimental Medecine and Biology series, New York: Plenum Press, pp. 279–289.

Roisin, M. P., et al. (1991). A new method to measure endogenous transmitter release in localized regions of hippocampal slices. *Journal of Neuroscience Methods* (in press).

Saffen, D. W., A. J. Cole, P. F. Worley, B. A. Christy, K. Ryder, and J. M. Baraban (1988). Convulsant-induced increase in transcription factor messenger RNAs in rat brain. *Proceedings National Academic Science* USA 85:7795–7799.

Slater, N. T., A. Stelzer, and M. Galvan (1985). Kindling-like stimulus patterns induce epileptiform discharges in the guinea pig in vitro hippocampus. *Neuroscience Letters* 60: 25–31.

Storm, J. F. (1990). Potassium currents in hippocampal pyramidal cells. *Progress in Brain Research* 83:161–187.

Sutula, T., H. Xiao-Xian, J. Cavazos, and G. Scott (1988). Synaptic reorganization in the hippocampus induced by abnormal functional activity. *Science* 239:1147–1150.

Tauck, D. L., and J. V. Nadler (1985). Evidence for functional mossy fiber sprouting in hippocampal formation of kainic acid treated rats. *Journal of Neuroscience* 5:1016–1022.

Westenbroek, R. E., M. K. Ahlijanian, and W. A. Caterall (1990). Clustering of L-types Ca^{2+} channels at the base of major dendrites in hippocampal pyramidal neurons. *Nature* 347: 281–282.

Williams, S., and D. Johnston (1989). Long-term potentiation of hippocampal mossy fibers synapses is blocked by postsynaptic injection of calcium chelators. *Neuron* 3:583–588.

Zafra, F., B. Hengerer, J. Leibrock, H. Thoenen, and D. Lindholm (1990). Activity dependent regulation of BDNF and NGF mRNAs in the rat hippocampus is mediated by non-NMDA glutamate receptors. *The EMBO Journal* 9:3545–3550.

Zalutsky, R. A., and R. A. Nicoll (1990). Comparison of two forms of long-term potentiation in single hippocampal neurons. *Science* 248:1619–1624.

3 On the Locus of the Maintenance of Long-Term Potentiation in Area CA1 of Rat Hippocampus

Zafar I. Bashir, Simon T. Alford, Joanna F. Blake, Bruno G. Frenguelli, Stephen N. Davies, Klaus G. Reymann, and Graham L. Collingridge

There is a general consensus that in the Schaffer collateral-commissural pathway (SCCP), in the CA1 region of the hippocampus, the induction of long-term potentiation (LTP) involves processes located in the postsynaptic cell. The basis of the mechanism of induction of LTP has been established and is reviewed elsewhere (Collingridge and Lester, 1989; Collingridge and Singer, 1990). In brief, LTP is initiated by the transient activation of the postsynaptically located *N*-methyl-D-aspartate (NMDA) receptor system, which occurs, for example, during a brief period of synchronized high-frequency synaptic transmission. Ca^{2+} entering the cell by way of NMDA channels is believed to activate a cascade of biochemical events, which results in a localized, persistent increase in the size of the excitatory postsynaptic potential (EPSP). During low-frequency transmission, under standard experimental conditions, this EPSP is mediated predominantly through α-amino-3-hydroxy-5-methyl-4-isoxazolepropionate (AMPA) receptors.

An area of particular contention is the locus and nature of the modification that underlies this change in synaptic efficiency. In this chapter we first discuss some of our recently published data concerning this area of dispute (Davies et al., 1989; Reymann et al., 1990). We then present some results showing that the NMDA receptor–mediated component of synaptic transmission in the SCCP can also undergo LTP. These new results are discussed briefly in relation to the locus of maintenance of LTP.

SENSITIVITY EXPERIMENTS

Most work addressing the locus of the mechanisms responsible for the maintenance of LTP presents evidence either for a presynaptic change (e.g., increase in glutamate release) or for a postsynaptic change (e.g., increase in receptor number or alteration of channel properties). The alternative possibility that *both* loci are involved does not seem to have many supporters at the present time. The simplest interpretation of our experiments, which have addressed the issue of the locus of maintenance of this process, is that LTP in the SCCP is maintained by both presynaptic and postsynaptic changes. We have proposed that temporally distinct presynaptic and postsynaptic mechanisms maintain LTP; the relative importance of the postsynaptic contribution increasing with time (as the potentiation becomes more long term).

The experiments were based on the hypothesis that if LTP involves a postsynaptic change, then potentiated neurons should become more responsive to exogenously administered drugs that activate the synaptic receptors. An increase in agonist sensitivity should be largely independent of the nature of the postsynaptic change (e.g., increase in number of receptors, change in channel conductance properties, alteration in electrotonic properties of spines). However, for a postsynaptic change to be detected as an increase in sensitivity, then a number of experimental conditions have to be met. These include the following: (1) the agonist must be selective for the synaptic receptors that mediate the potentiated response; (2) the agonist application needs to be restricted predominantly to receptors at potentiated synapses; and (3) if the receptors are subject to pronounced desensitization, then the duration of application should mimic, as closely as possible, the kinetics of the synaptic release of the neurotransmitter. These conditions are considered in the following sections.

The Choice of Agonist

Sensitivity experiments were first performed using iontophoretically applied L-glutamate (Lynch et al., 1976; Mohan and Sastry, 1985; Taube and Schwartzkroin, 1988). In these earlier studies no evidence for an increase in sensitivity was found; indeed glutamate-induced excitation of CA1 cells often tended to decrease after the induction of LTP. With hindsight, however, it turns out that L-glutamate, although still the best candidate for the neurotransmitter in the SCCP, was probably an unfortunate choice of ligand to use. When applied exogenously in brain slices only a tiny fraction of the depolarizing action of L-glutamate is mediated via AMPA receptors (i.e., the receptors that mediate the EPSP that is modified in conventional LTP experiments). This point is illustrated in figure 3.1. These experiments used grease-gap recording methods applied to hippocampal slices (Blake et al., 1988), similar to those used extensively by Evans and Watkins for quantitative pharmacological analyses with hemisected spinal cord preparations (Evans et al., 1982). Figure 3.1 shows that 6-cyano-7-nitroquinoxaline-2,3-dione(CNQX), in a dose sufficient to abolish the AMPA receptor–mediated component of the synaptic response and practically abolish the response to bath-applied AMPA, had no effect on the response to bath-applied L-glutamate. The L-glutamate response was, however, slightly depressed (approximately ~15%) by a dose of D-2-amino-5-phosphonopentanoate (AP5) that abolished the residual synaptic responses and eliminated the response to bath-applied NMDA. In quantitative terms, the combination of 10 μM CNQX and 50 μM AP5 produced dose ratios of approximately 12 and 7 for antagonism of responses to NMDA and AMPA, respectively, but a dose ratio of only 1.5 for

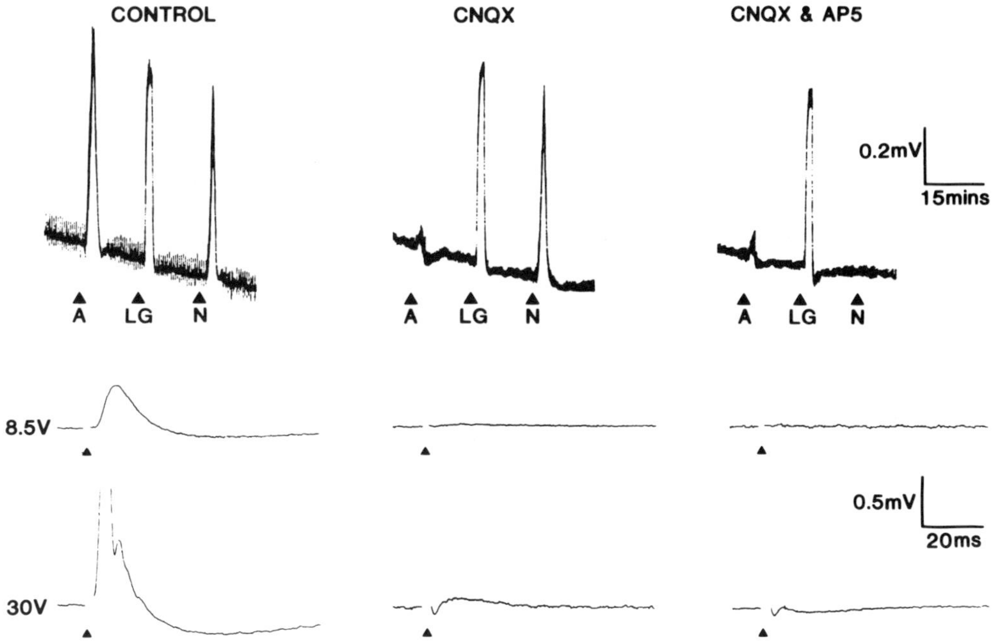

Figure 3.1 L-Glutamate–induced responses are fairly resistant to the actions of excitatory amino acid antagonists. The upper records are excerpts from a DC chart record measuring the potential across a grease barrier placed near the border between the stratum oriens and the alveus. The large deflections represent depolarizations of CA1 cells induced by agonists (A = AMPA, 7 μM; LG = L-glutamate, 3 mM; N = NMDA, 25 μM) added to the perfusate (for periods of approximately 90 seconds). The small deflections (in the control record) are filtered versions of synaptic responses evoked by low-frequency stimulation of the SCCP. The traces below are the synaptic responses evoked at two stimulus intensities. At 8.5 V the response mainly comprises a field EPSP; at 30 V a population spike is superimposed, and the response is truncated. CNQX (10 μM) greatly suppressed the synaptic responses and the depolarization induced by AMPA. Responses to NMDA and L-glutamate were unaffected. The further addition of AP5 (50 μM) eliminated the residual synaptic depolarization and the response to NMDA but only depressed responses to L-glutamate slightly. See Blake et al. (1988) for details of this grease-gap method.

antagonism of responses to L-glutamate (and L-aspartate). We believe that the depolarization elicited by L-glutamate in the presence of these antagonists and, therefore, the major depolarizing action of exogenously applied L-glutamate under control conditions is due to an electrogenic uptake process (Frenguelli et al., 1991). In other words, L-glutamate is avidly accumulated by neurons and glia such that synaptic receptors are largely protected from exogenously applied L-glutamate and in a manner that provides the depolarization that is recorded by the grease-gap technique (and presumably also that measured following iontophoretic applications). A hypothetical scheme summarizing the involvement of receptors and uptake processes in L-glutamate–induced depolarizations is presented in figure 3.2.

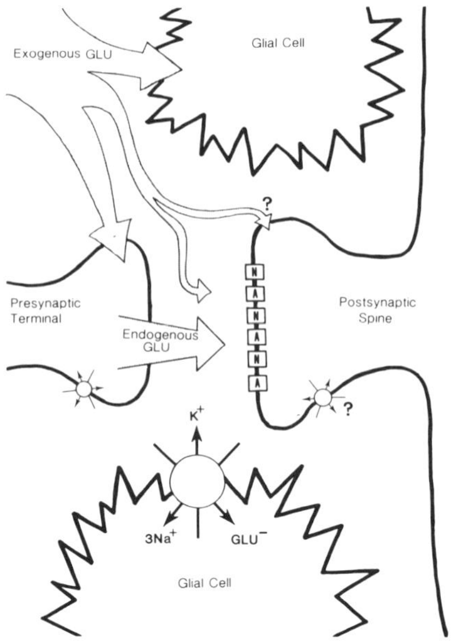

Figure 3.2 A Scheme to illustrate the differential ability of endogenous (i.e., synaptically-released) and exogenously applied L-glutamate to act on synaptic receptors. The postsynaptic complement of NMDA (N) and AMPA (A) receptors are placed on the spine. Uptake carriers will accumulate L-glutamate into glia and terminals (and possibly also postsynaptic cells). The carriers are shown accumulating 3 Na^+ with every 1 Glu in exchange for 1 K^+, as suggested from the studies of high-affinity uptake by Brew and Attwell (1987) and Barbour and colleagues (1988). This arrangement will depolarize carrier-bearing elements since there is a net inward movement of 1 +ve charge. The efflux of K^+ could also depolarize neighboring cells.

It seems that since the precise sources of the depolarization induced by L-glutamate are not known, and could vary according to the methods of application and recording, interpretation of results using L-glutamate is complex. We therefore decided to undertake sensitivity experiments using receptor-selective agonists. In this respect, we first used quisqualate in the belief that it was a selective ligand for what is now termed the AMPA receptor. However, quisqualate is now known to activate an excitatory amino acid receptor that is coupled to phospholipase C (the so-called metabotropic receptor; Sugiyama et al., 1987). In addition, quisqualate is probably a substrate for uptake processes (Lodge et al., 1980), and, when applied slowly so that only steady-state responses are measured, it appears to act like a partial agonist (Blake et al., 1988). Any of these properties of quisqualate could complicate interpretation of results, and, for these reasons, we changed to using AMPA itself as the probe for the AMPA receptor, which does not appear to have these complications.

The Method of Application

Because of the ease with which quantitative pharmacological information can be obtained, the low noise and stability of the recording system, and the observation that LTP can be followed for at least 24 hours (Blake et al., 1989), the grease-gap method would seem to be particularly useful for sensitivity experiments. Figure 3.3 shows one such experiment in which AMPA sensitivity slightly increased following the induction of LTP. On average, however, there was little if any change in sensitivity of agonist-induced responses with LTP. This could, of course, mean that there is no postsynaptic modification associated with LTP. Alternatively, the method of application could be inappropriate. Bath application would, of course, activate many AMPA receptors that were not associated with potentiated synapses; this would result in a large background signal against which changes were being sought. We believed, therefore, that if any change were to be reliably detected then the exogenously applied agonist would have to be restricted, as far as possible, to potentiated synapses. To achieve this localization we resorted to the iontophoretic method of administration, despite the many limitations with its quantification, so as to apply the agonist into stratum radiatum at the level of the stimulated SCC fibers. In our initial studies (using quisqualate), the agonist was applied for 1 to 2 seconds (at 30-second intervals) and responses recorded intracellularly. In our more recent studies (using AMPA), the agonist was

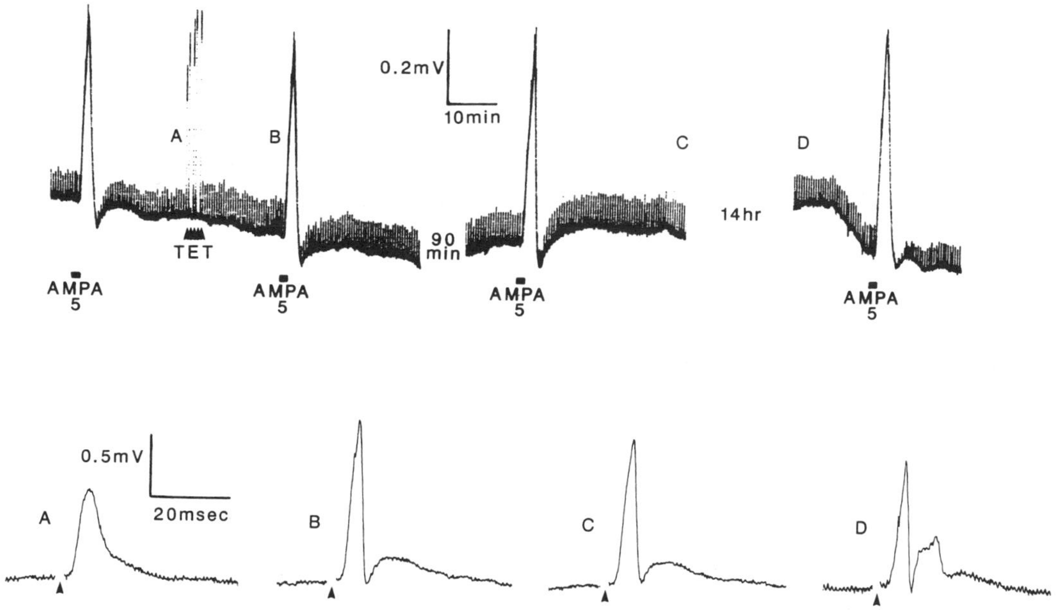

Figure 3.3 LTP and sensitivity to bath-applied AMPA. The chart recording measures DC potential recorded using the grease-gap method. The small upward deflections are filtered versions of synaptic responses, true representations of which are shown for the times indicated by A–D. (These records correspond to field EPSPs with, in B–D, a superimposed population spike). The large deflections are depolarizations to brief applications of 5 μM AMPA. LTP was induced at the time marked TET (5 trains each of 100 Hz for 0.5 seconds) and lasted for the duration of the experiment (a further 17 hours). In this example, the AMPA-induced depolarizations were increased slightly (approximately 15%) 17 hours after the tetanus. (From Blake et al., 1989.)

applied for 10 to 25 seconds (at 15-minute intervals) and responses recorded extracellularly. In both types of experiments the drug applications were the briefest possible commensurate with the maintenance of stable responses for the required periods. Both methods, however, involved slow drug applications with respect to the kinetics of neurotransmitter release. To be able to detect a change in receptor function underlying LTP assumes that the receptors behave similarly to transient (i.e., synaptic) activation as they do with prolonged (i.e., iontophoretic) administration. For example, if, as has been suggested (Trussell and Fischbach, 1989; Tang et al., 1989), desensitization of the synaptic receptors occurs, then this would have to be incomplete, and the desensitized state would have to express the increased receptor function.

Results

The intracellular studies using quisqualate detected an increase in sensitivity following the induction of LTP (Davies et al., 1989). This effect was not associated with any obvious changes in the passive properties of neurons. The increase in sensitivity could start within 15 minutes and continue to develop over the course of at least 30 minutes more. The slow nature of the effect made it difficult to quantify with intracellular recording; therefore, we turned to extracellular techniques to record agonist-induced "focal" potentials (Lambert et al., 1981) concomitantly with field EPSPs. This enabled experiments to be followed routinely for 3 hours after the induction of LTP. Using this approach, an increase in AMPA-induced responses was detected in most experiments where persistent (>1 hour) LTP was induced (Davies et al., 1989). Just as with the intracellular studies, the effect developed slowly; there was never any change in the first AMPA response, which was measured 5 to 10 minutes after conditioning the pathway, but the effect was often detected by the next response (measured 20 to 25 minutes after the tetani). The sensitivity increase continued to develop for approximately 30 minutes and invariably persisted throughout the recording period (figure 3.4).

That the generation of persistent LTP and the increase in AMPA sensitivity are causally related, rather than two independent consequences of tetanic stimulation, is indicated by three lines of evidence. (1) Under control conditions where tetanic stimulation did not result in persistent LTP, the increase in AMPA sensitivity was not seen. (2) If the tetanus was delivered in the presence of AP5, to block the induction of LTP, the increase in AMPA sensitivity did not occur. (3) If the kinase inhibitor K-252b was applied during, or immediately following, the tetanus, then only a transient LTP was generated and no increase in AMPA sensitivity developed. This latter experiment suggests that the increase in AMPA sensitivity is specifically related to the persistent, kinase-dependent component of LTP (Reymann et al., 1990).

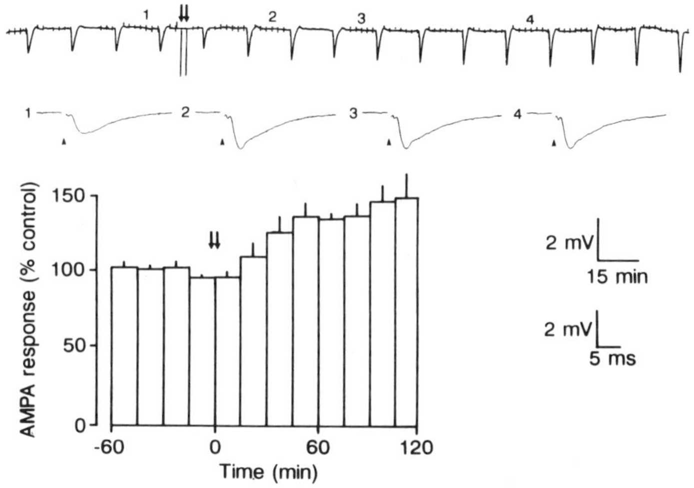

Figure 3.4 LTP and sensitivity to iontophoretically applied AMPA. The chart recording measures DC potential recorded using a microelectrode placed in stratum radiatum. The small deflections are filtered versions of synaptic responses, true representations of which are shown for the times indicated by 1–4. The large deflections are depolarizations to brief local applications of AMPA. LTP was induced at the time marked by arrows (2 trains each of 100 Hz for 1 second) and lasted for the duration of the experiment (a further 3 hours). The AMPA-induced responses increased slowly following the tetanus and remained potentiated for the remainder of the experiment. The histograms show the time-course of the change in AMPA responses for the 5 slices where, in this series of experiments, LTP that lasted for at least 2 hours was induced. (From Reymann et al., 1990.)

Discussion

The similarity of the results with both quisqualate and AMPA suggests that in both studies the same receptors (i.e., AMPA receptors) were being studied. Taken together, it can therefore be concluded that LTP is associated with a delayed increase in AMPA sensitivity of neurons, without associated changes in gross passive properties. Theoretically, this increase in sensitivity could be correlated with, but involve different mechanisms to, those that underlie persistent LTP. The simplest explanation of the results, however, is that persistent LTP is maintained by postsynaptic mechanisms that can be detected and studied using this iontophoretic method. The question remains as to what mediates the early phase of LTP. It could be argued that LTP is mediated early on by a postsynaptic change that is not detected by the iontophoretic method but then is replaced by a postsynaptic change that is detected. We prefer the possibility that LTP is mediated initially by a presynaptic change. Thus, our working hypothesis is that LTP is maintained by temporally distinct presynaptic and postsynaptic mechanisms. How does this relate to other lines of evidence concerning the maintenance of LTP in the CA1 region of the hippocampus?

RELEASE STUDIES

The possibility that LTP might be maintained by an increase in neurotransmitter release was provided by the demonstration that tetanic stimulation of the SCCP led to an enhanced spontaneous and stimulus-evoked efflux of [^{3}H]-D-aspartate from hippocampal slices (Skrede and Malthe-Sorenssen, 1981). Bliss and colleagues have presented considerable evidence that LTP is indeed associated with an enhanced release of L-glutamate, determined using radiotracer and endogenous release techniques. Although most of their evidence pertains to the dentate gyrus (see chapter 1), they also have evidence that LTP in area CA1 is accompanied by an increase in L-glutamate release (Bliss and Lynch, 1988). In this region, the increase in endogenous release is not as persistent as in the dentate gyrus, with a tendency to decline toward basal levels over a period of approximately 1 hour (Bliss, personal communication). Alternatively, Anikstejn and colleagues (1989) have presented evidence that L-glutamate release is not enhanced (for more than a few minutes) following the induction of LTP. Recently, however, this group has observed enhanced release for as much as 15 to 30 minutes in some slices (Roisin et al., 1990). Thus, a consensus seems to be emerging in which LTP in area CA1 is associated with an increase in L-glutamate release but that this is only evident for an early phase of LTP.

QUANTAL ANALYSES

Results from quantal analyses of LTP in area CA1 are currently controversial. Several studies have provided evidence for a change in one or the other of the "presynaptic" quantal parameters (n or p; Voronin, 1989; Malinow and Tsien, 1990; Bekkers and Stevens, 1990) whereas another study has presented evidence for a change in the postsynaptic quantal parameter q (Foster and McNaughton, 1991). However, as discussed elsewhere in this book (see chapters 7 and 9), the extent to which these parameters change with LTP may be dependent on the preparation (e.g., stage of development of the animal, method of inducing LTP). In addition, it is not certain whether the usual assumptions on which quantal analyses are based are valid for these synapes. Furthermore, it is by no means certain that the normal interpretations for the physical natures of n, p, and q are valid; for example, a change in q could be caused by alterations in transmitter content within vesicles rather than a postsynaptic change. Taken at face value, however, quantal analyses provide evidence for both presynaptic and postsynaptic changes. Relevant to our results from sensitivity experiments, in several of these studies (Voronin, 1989; Malinow and Tsien, 1990; Foster and McNaughton, 1991) there was a tendency for the postsynaptic component to increase and the presynaptic component to decrease with time, relative to the size of the LTP induced.

DIFFERENTIAL EXPRESSION OF AMPA- AND NMDA-RECEPTOR COMPONENTS

Two groups have presented evidence that LTP is mediated by postsynaptic mechanisms by comparing the ability of the NMDA and AMPA receptor–mediated components of synaptic transmission to undergo LTP. Muller and Lynch (1988) found preferential and Kauer et al. (1988) found selective LTP of the AMPA receptor component. Both groups reasoned that had LTP involved a presynaptic mechanism, then both components should have displayed similar LTP. This argument makes several assumptions, including a similar synaptic localization of the two sets of subsynaptic receptors and the absence of saturation of the NMDA receptors by the released transmitter under control conditions. These groups, however, were able to show posttetanic and paired-pulse potentiation of the NMDA receptor system. They therefore concluded that LTP was maintained exclusively by postsynaptic mechanisms, involving a selective modification of the AMPA receptor–mediated response. They supported this argument by attempting, without success, to demonstrate LTP of the pharmacologically isolated NMDA receptor–mediated response.

With respect to our sensitivity studies, the conclusion that LTP is maintained postsynaptically agrees with our findings for the mechanisms underlying persistent LTP but does not agree with our suggestion that initially LTP is maintained by presynaptic alterations. In view of this discrepancy we decided to undertake differential expression studies. There are a number of different ways in which the two receptor-mediated components of the EPSP can be recorded simultaneously, including in low Mg^{2+} (Coan and Collingridge, 1987), in cells depolarized by current injection outside of the range of voltage-dependent Mg^{2+} block (Collingridge et al., 1988; Wigström and Gustafsson, 1988), and by blocking the $GABA_A$ receptor–mediated (IPSP) (Herron et al., 1985; Dingledine et al., 1986). Müller and Lynch used the first, Nicoll's group the second, and we now report studies that have used the third method. Figure 3.5 shows the effects of tetanic stimulation on field EPSPs recorded in the presence of picrotoxin. The NMDA receptor–mediated component was defined before and after the induction of LTP using AP5. Note that both components of the synaptic response are increased following tetanic stimulation. The potentiation of the AP5-sensitive component was induced rapidly (<30 seconds) and persisted throughout the experiment (up to 2 hours). In these experiments we have never seen selective potentiation of the AMPA receptor component.

It could be argued that in these experiments potentiation of the NMDA receptor–mediated component was a secondary consequence of potentiation of the AMPA receptor–mediated component. We have, however, also demonstrated LTP of the NMDA receptor component under conditions where the AMPA receptor component has been blocked with CNQX (Bashir and Collingridge, 1990; Bashir et al., 1991). Under these condi-

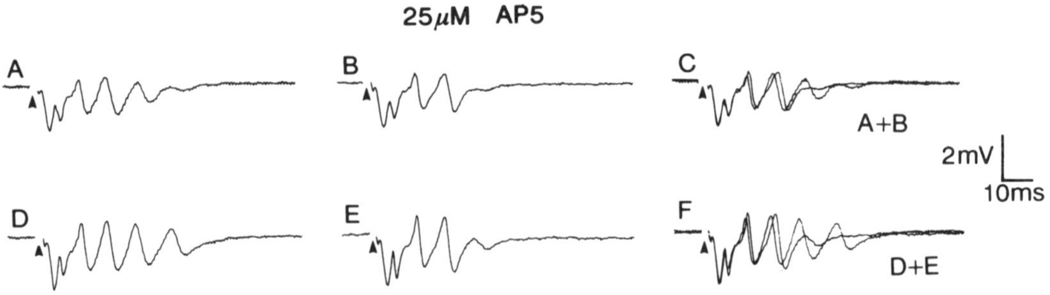

Figure 3.5 LTP of AMPA and NMDA receptor–mediated synaptic components. Responses are field EPSPs recorded in the presence of 50 μM picrotoxin, to block $GABA_A$ receptor–mediated inhibition. A shows a control, B a response in the presence of AP5, and C the superimposition of these two traces. D–F are the corresponding traces starting 30 minutes after the induction of LTP, induced by a tetanus (100 Hz, 1 second, test intensity). Note that LTP involved an increase in the entire waveform, especially the slower AP5-sensitive component.

tions (which include picrotoxin to block $GABA_A$ receptor–mediated IPSPs and 2-hydroxy-saclofen to block $GABA_B$ receptor–mediated IPSPs) the entire synaptic response is sensitive to AP5, both before and after the induction of LTP. LTP of NMDA receptor–mediated field EPSPs is induced rapidly (<30 seconds) and persists for the remainder of the experiment (up to 4 hours). It shares other properties with conventional LTP (i.e., of the AMPA receptor component) in that it is synapse-specific and its induction is blocked by AP5. Recently, we have also observed LTP of the NMDA receptor–mediated synaptic current directly (Bashir et al., 1991). An example of LTP of a pure NMDA receptor–mediated synaptic current is illustrated in figure 3.6. Other groups have since confirmed that the NMDA receptor–mediated EPSP in area CA1 can sustain LTP (unpublished observations from the laboratories of R. W. Tsien, T. H. Brown, S. N. Davies, and W. Francesconi).

LTP of the NMDA receptor–mediated synaptic conductance has important consequences for physiological and pathological functions, a discussion of which is outside the scope of this chapter. With respect to the locus of maintenance of LTP these results are not particularly helpful because the LTP could equally be expressed by presynaptic, or postsynaptic mechanisms (or both). These results do, however, substantially weaken the argument, based on differential expression studies, that LTP must be entirely postsynaptic in nature.

CONCLUDING REMARKS

Despite the considerable interest in LTP, the locus of the maintenance of this process is as contentious as ever. We believe that it is necessary to consider the results of several different approaches, including sensitivity experiments, release studies, quantal analyses, and differential expression studies. When we do this we see no reason to reject our working

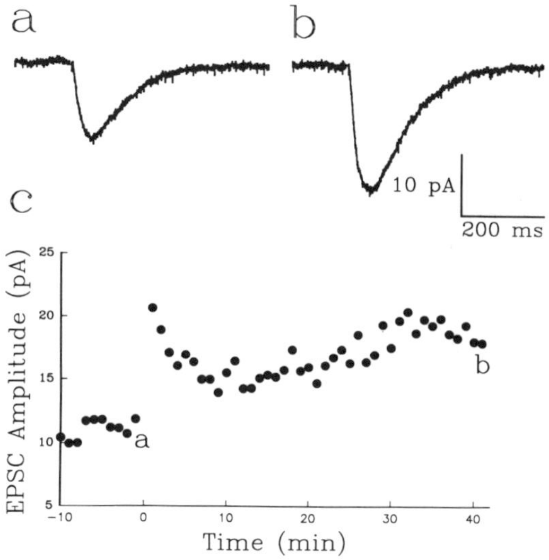

Figure 3.6 LTP of a pure NMDA receptor–mediated synaptic current. The current was recorded at −70 mV using the "perforated" patch-clamp method (Bekkers and Stevens, 1990) from a slice bathed in 10 μM CNQX, 50 μM picrotoxin, and 500 μM CGP 35348 to block AMPA, $GABA_A$, and $GABA_B$ receptor–mediated synaptic responses, respectively. Currents isolated in this manner can be eliminated with AP5 and increase in size with depolarization (to −50 mV). Traces show responses immediately before and 40 minutes after the induction of LTP (100 Hz, 200 milliseconds, test intensity). The graph shows the time-course of this LTP (each point is the average of 4 successive traces). See Bashir and associates (1991) for pooled data.

hypothesis that, in area CA1, LTP involves temporally distinct presynaptic and postsynaptic mechanisms. Like LTP, however, our scheme remains plastic and subject to modification should the appropriate stimulus arise.

At first sight it might seem odd to propose different loci at different times. Because LTP is induced within seconds and has the capacity to last weeks, however, it seems most unlikely that one mechanism accounts for the entire process. Indeed, several lines of evidence have already suggested that LTP comprises several serial processes. Our division into presynaptic and postsynaptic components correlates extremely well in time with what has been identified as kinase-resistant and kinase-dependent forms of potentiation, respectively (Lovinger et al., 1987; Reymann et al., 1988, 1990; Malinow et al., 1988, 1989; Malenka et al., 1989). It is thus tempting to speculate that the postsynaptic modification is brought about by one or more kinases that are activated directly or indirectly by the postsynaptic NMDA receptor–gated Ca^{2+} influx. Recently, it has been proposed that AMPA receptor subunits can exist in one of two forms, which are encoded by alternatively spliced mRNAs. One form, termed flip, produces a higher conductance channel than the other, termed flop (Sommer et al., 1990). Perhaps LTP involves the conversion of a floppy hippocampus into a flipping persistent structure.

ACKNOWLEDGMENTS

We are most grateful to Jeff Watkins for gifts of AMPA, AP5, and CNQX and to Mario Pozza for the gift of CGP 35348. Our work summarized here was supported by grants from The MRC, The Wellcome Trust, The Royal Society, and The University of Bristol. Bruno Frenguelli was supported by a GLAXO studentship. Dr. Reymann was supported in part by the German Academy of Sciences.

REFERENCES

Aniksztejn, L., M. P. Roisin, R. Amsellem, and Y. Ben-Ari (1989). Long-term potentiation in the hippocampus of the anaesthetized rat is not associated with a sustained enhanced release of endogenous excitatory amino acids. *Neuroscience* 28:387–392.

Barbour, B., H. Brew, and D. Attwell (1988). Electrogenic glutamate uptake in glial cells is activated by intracellular potassium. *Nature* 335:433–435.

Bashir, Z. I., and G. L. Collingridge (1990). Potentiation of an NMDA receptor-mediated EPSP in rat hippocampal slices in vitro. *Journal of Physiology* (London) 425:23P.

Bashir, Z. I., et al. (1991). Long-term potentiation of NMDA receptor–mediated synaptic transmission in the hippocampus. *Nature* 349:156–158.

Bekkers, J. M., and C. F. Stevens (1990). Presynaptic mechanism for long-term potentiation in the hippocampus. *Nature* 346:724–729.

Blake, J. F., M. W. Brown, and G. L. Collingridge (1988). A quantitative study of the actions of excitatory amino acids and antagonists in rat hippocampal slices. *British Journal of Pharmacology* 95:291–299.

Blake, J. F., M. W. Brown, and G. L. Collingridge (1989). A grease-gap method for studying LTP over long time periods in rat hippocampal slices. *British Journal of Pharmacology* 97:593P.

Bliss, T. V. P., and M. A. Lynch (1988). Long-term potentiation of synaptic transmission in the hippocampus—properties and mechanisms. *Neurology and Neurobiology* 35:3–72.

Brew, H., and D. Attwell (1987). Electrogenic glutamate uptake is a major current carrier in the membrane of axolotl retinal ganglion cells. *Nature* 327:707–709.

Coan, E. J., and G. L. Collingridge (1987). Characterization of an *N*-methyl-D-aspartate receptor component of synaptic transmission in rat hippocampal slices. *Neuroscience* 22:1–8.

Collingridge, G. L., C. E. Herron, and R. A. J. Lester (1988). Synaptic activation of *N*-methyl-D-aspartate receptors in the Schaffer collateral-commissural pathway of rat hippocampus. *Journal of Physiology* (London) 399:283–300.

Collingridge, G. L., and R. A. J. Lester (1989). Excitatory amino acid receptors in the vertebrate central nervous system. *Pharmacology Review* 41:143–210.

Collingridge, G. L., and W. Singer (1990). Excitatory amino acid receptors and synaptic plasticity. *Trends in Pharmacological Sciences* 11:290–296.

Davies, S. N., R. A. J. Lester, K. G. Reymann, and G. L. Collingridge (1989). Temporally distinct pre- and post-synaptic mechanisms maintain long-term potentiation. *Nature* 338:500–503.

Dingledine, R., M. A. Hynes, and G. L. King (1986). Involvement of *N*-methyl-D-aspartate receptors in epileptiform bursting in the rat hippocampal slice. *Journal of Physiology* (London) 380:175–189.

Evans, R. H., et al. (1982). The effects of a series of ω-phosphonic α-carboxylic amino acids on electrically evoked and excitant amino acid-induced responses in isolated spinal cord preparations. *British Journal of Pharmacology* 75:65–75.

Foster, T. C., and B. L. McNaughton (1991). Long-term synaptic enhancement in CA1 is due to increased quantal size, not quantal content. *Hippocampus* 1:79–91.

Frenguelli, B. G., J. F. Blake, M. W. Brown, and G. L. Collingridge (1991). Electrogenic uptake contributes a major component of the depolarising action of L-glutamate in rat hippocampal slices. *British Journal of Pharmacology* 102:355–362.

Herron, C. E., R. Williamson, and G. L. Collingridge (1985). A selective *N*-methyl-D-aspartate antagonist depresses epileptiform activity in rat hippocampal slices. *Neuroscience Letters* 61:255–260.

Kauer, J. A., R. C. Malenka, and R. A. Nicoll (1988). A persistent postsynaptic modification mediates long-term potentiation in the hippocampus. *Neuron* 1:911–917.

Lambert, J. D. C., J. A. Flatman, and H. Jahnsen (1981). Extracellular recordings of amino acid induced potential changes in hippocampal slices. *Journal of Neuroscience Methods* 3:311–315.

Lodge, D., D. R. Curtis, G. A. R. Johnston, and J. C. Bornstein (1980). In vivo inactivation of quisqualate: studies in the cat spinal cord. *Brain Research* 128:491–495.

Lovinger, D. M., K. L. Wong, K. Murakami, and A. Routtenberg (1987). Protein kinase C inhibitors eliminate hippocampal long-term potentiation. *Brain Research* 436:177–183.

Lynch, G., V. Gribkoff, and S. A. Deadwyler (1976). Long-term potentiation is accompanied by a reduction in dendritic responsiveness to glutamic acid. *Nature* 263:151–153.

Malenka, R. C., et al. (1989). An essential role for postsynaptic calmodulin and protein kinase activity in long-term potentiation. *Nature* 340:554–557.

Malinow, R., D. V. Madison, and R. W. Tsien (1988). Persistent protein kinase activity underlying long-term potentiation. *Nature* 335:821–824.

Malinow, R., H. Schulman, and R. W. Tsien (1989). Inhibition of postsynaptic PKC or CaMKII blocks induction but not expression of LTP. *Science* 245:862–866.

Malinow, R., and R. W. Tsien (1990). Presynaptic enhancement shown by whole-cell recordings of long-term potentiation in hippocampal slices. *Nature* 346:177–180.

Mohan, P. M., and B. R. Sastry (1985). Calcium and unit responses decrement to locally applied glutamate on rat hippocampal CA1 neurones. *European Journal of Pharmacology* 114:335–341.

Muller, D., and G. Lynch (1988). Long-term potentiation differentially affects two components of synaptic responses in hippocampus. *Proceedings of the National Academy of Sciences USA* 85:9346–9350.

Reymann, K. G., et al. (1990). Activation of a K-252b–sensitive protein kinase is necessary for a postsynaptic phase of long-term potentiation in area CA1 of rat hippocampus. *European Journal of Neuroscience* 2:481–486.

Reymann, K. G., U. Frey, R. Jork, and H. Matthies (1988). Polymyxin B, an inhibitor of protein kinase C, prevents the maintenance of synaptic long-term potentiation in hippocampal CA1 neurons. *Brain Research* 440:305–314.

Roisin, M. P., L. Aniksztejn, and Y. Ben-Ari (1990). Long-term potentiation is not associated with a sustained enhanced release of glutamate in the rat hippocampus in vivo and in vitro. In Y. Ben-Ari (ed.), *Excitatory Amino Acids and Neuronal Plasticity.* New York: Plenum Press, pp. 279–289.

Skrede, K., and D. Malthe-Sorenssen (1981). Increased resting and evoked release of transmitter following repetitive electrical stimulation of the hippocampus: a biochemical correlate to long-lasting synaptic potentiation. *Brain Research* 208:436–441.

Sommer, B., et al. (1990). Flip and flop: a cell-specific functional switch in glutamate-operated channels of the CNS. *Science* 249:1580–1585.

Sugiyama, H., I. Ito, and C. Hirono (1987). A new type of glutamate receptor linked to inositol phospholipid metabolism. *Nature* 325:531–533.

Tang, C.-M., M. Dichter, and M. Morad (1989). Quisqualate activates a rapidly inactivating high conductance ionic channel in hippocampal neurons. *Science* 243:1474–1477.

Taube, J. S., and P. A. Schwartzkroin (1988). Mechanisms of long-term potentiation: EPSP/spike dissociation, intradendritic recordings and glutamate sensitivity. *Journal of Neuroscience* 8:1632–1644.

Trussell, L. O., and G. D. Fischbach (1989). Glutamate receptor desensitization and its role in synaptic transmission. *Neuron* 3:209–218.

Voronin, L. L. (1989). Principles of long-term potentiation in mammalian brain. In H. Rahmann (ed.), *Fundamentals of Memory Formation: Neuronal Plasticity and Brain Function.* Stuttgart, New York: Gustav Fischer Verlag, pp. 175–188.

Wigström, H., and B. Gustafsson (1988). Presynaptic and postsynaptic interactions in the control of hippocampal long-term potentiation. *Neurology and Neurobiology* 35:73–107.

4 Increase in Endogenous Amino Acid Release in Long-Term Potentiation

Wim E. J. M. Ghijsen and Fernando H. Lopes Da Silva

Long-term potentiation (LTP) is a well-known model system to study basic mechanisms that are possibly related to memory formation. Since its discovery by Bliss and Lømo (1973), researchers in several laboratories have tried to unravel the cellular mechanisms underlying this phenomenon. Most studies have been performed in hippocampus tissue, where clearly defined monosynaptic pathways allow local electrical stimulation of afferent fibers and simultaneous recording of potentials in or near the stimulated postsynaptic cells. It is widely accepted that LTP is a synaptic phenomenon that is characterized by a persistent increase in the excitatory postsynaptic potential (EPSP) after a high-frequency tetanus train. At least in the *N*-methyl-D-aspartate (NMDA)–mediated pathways, LTP is induced in the postsynaptic cell by severe depolarization and subsequent entry of calcium through this receptor-gated channel (Collingridge, 1985). The resulting rise in free calcium concentration can trigger several messenger activities in the postsynaptic cell such as protein kinase C and calcium-calmodulin kinase II activity, which, in turn, can induce phosphorylation of certain (still unknown) substrate proteins (Malenka et al., 1989; Malinow et al., 1989).

In addition to these changes in postsynaptic events, evidence exists that after LTP induction presynaptic activity is required for its persistence. Especially Bliss and coworkers (1986; Lynch et al., 1985; Lynch and Bliss, 1986) have reported, both in in vivo (with push-pull cannulas) and in vitro (using slices and synaptosomes) studies that a prolonged enhancement of glutamate release takes place lasting at least 2 hours after the application of the tetanus. This enhanced release has been proposed to be triggered by a so-called retrograde messenger, possibly arachidonic acid, released from the postsynaptic cell by increased calcium-dependent phospholipase A_2 activity during LTP induction (Williams et al., 1989). In addition to this biochemical evidence for a presynaptic involvement in LTP, there are electrophysiological data (altered quantal release; Voronin, 1983; Malinow and Tsien, 1990; Bekkers and Stevens, 1990) and morphological data (increased number of synaptic vesicles; Meshul and Hopkins, 1990) in favor of a presynaptic mechanism in LTP. In contrast, Muller and Lynch (1989), using mainly electrophysiological criteria (paired-pulse facilitation) could not find evidence for such a presynaptic role during the persistent phase of LTP. Also, a prolonged increase of in vivo glutamate release during LTP could not be reproduced by Aniksztejn and colleagues (1989).

To get a better insight into whether presynaptic activity is altered during LTP we used a combination of electrophysiological and biochemical techniques. We stimulated in vivo Schaffer collaterals by a high-frequency tetanus (200 Hz, 200 milliseconds) in unanesthetized rats. After establishing LTP (30 minutes after tetanus application) in the CA1 stratum radiatum region, CA1 subslices were isolated from the stimulated tissue, and the endogenous release of the amino acid neurotransmitters glutamate and γ-aminobutyric acid (GABA) was determined 60 minutes after the tetanus and compared with the release from slices of non-tetanized control animals. In addition, by comparing the field potential amplitudes of paired conditioning and test stimuli in the stratum radiatum before and 30 minutes after tetanus application, we estimated whether paired-pulse facilitation was altered in this hippocampus region during LTP, which could be a measure for altered presynaptic activity (Zucker 1989; Muller and Lynch, 1989; Voronin and Kuhnt, 1990; Zalutsky and Nicoll, 1990).

Here we present evidence that potassium-induced, calcium-dependent release of both glutamate and GABA is clearly enhanced 60 minutes after tetanization in a time-dependent manner and that an upward shift in paired-pulse facilitation becomes apparent during LTP but only at high stimulation intensity levels.

ENDOGENOUS GLUTAMATE AND GABA RELEASE

It has been suggested that a change in presynaptic activity underlying the persistent phase of LTP would involve the enhancement of neurotransmitter (glutamate) release during at least 30 to 90 minutes after its induction (Bliss et al., 1986). For that reason we studied the amino acid neurotransmitter release at about 60 minutes after in vivo application of the tetanus.

Methods

LTP was induced by tetanic stimulation of the Schaffer collateral fibers; male Wistar rats (weight: 200–250 gr) were used. Under anesthesia, electrode bundles were implanted for stimulation of the Schaffer collaterals and recording from the CA1 area using the same procedure as Kamphuis and associates (1990). The stimulus intensity at which the rats were tetanized was 40% to 50% of the intensity just under that giving the maximal field potential amplitude recorded in the stratum radiatum. Test stimuli were applied at this intensity, using a paired-pulse protocol (20-millisecond time interval) every 2.5 minutes during 30 minutes before and 30 minutes after the tetanus. Input-output curves were made just before application of the tetanus and 25 minutes after the tetanus, and both input-output curves were compared. This procedure was repeated once or twice until a clear leftward shift could be observed in the input-output curve, which was taken as criterion for LTP. On basis of these criteria, 14 rats showed LTP with an increase of 35 ($\pm$5%) in field potential amplitude compared with the level before tetanus. For the biochemical experiments, data from 12 LTP animals were compared with data from 5 control animals with implanted electrodes but that received either a stimulus train at 1/8 Hz at 40% to 50% of maximal stimulus intensity for 320 seconds (2 rats) or no stimulus at all (3 rats). No systematic difference in slice amino acid release occurred between the stimulated and unstimulated controls.

Thirty minutes after the (last) tetanus or low-frequency stimulus train in case of controls, rats were decapitated and three hippocampus CA1 subslices around the stimulated region were selected for use in the release experiments. After incubation of these subslices for 15 minutes at 34° C in calcium-containing Krebs-Ringer buffer (2 mM) they were transferred to wells containing 500 μl of this medium. Release was measured in samples taken from media exposed to the subslices just after transfer of the slices to the next well (Kamphuis et al., 1990). Using this method the subslices were subsequently exposed to calcium-containing buffer for two 4-minute periods (basal release), to buffer containing 2 mM of ethylene glycolbis (amino ethyl ether) tetra-acetate (EGTA) instead of calcium and 50 mM of potassium chloride for three 1-minute periods (potassium-induced, calcium-independent release) and, after repolarization for 6 minutes in 3.5 mM of potassium chloride medium, to buffer containing 2 mM of calcium and 50 mM of potassium chloride for three 1-minute periods (total release). Potassium-induced, calcium-dependent release was estimated by subtracting the potassium-induced, calcium-independent release values from the corresponding total release values. Finally, the subslices were homogenized for estimation of the total amino acid content. The latter was determined in the samples by means of reversed-phase high performance liquid chromatography (HPLC) after precolumn derivatization with o-phtalaldehyde using the same procedure as Verhage and associates (1989).

Results

Using this approach, no difference in basal release between LTP and control slices could be observed. In figure 4.1A the potassium-induced, calcium-*in*dependent release of glutamate and GABA during the first minute (initial) and third minute (plateau) of potassium chloride elevation is shown. Although the initial release of both amino acids tended to be higher in the LTP subslices, no significant differences were found between the two groups at both times. The tendency for an initial larger release during LTP could reflect an enhanced availability of cytosolic amino acids to be extruded by reversal of the respective uptake carriers driven by the severe (50 mM) potassium-depolarization applied in these experiments.

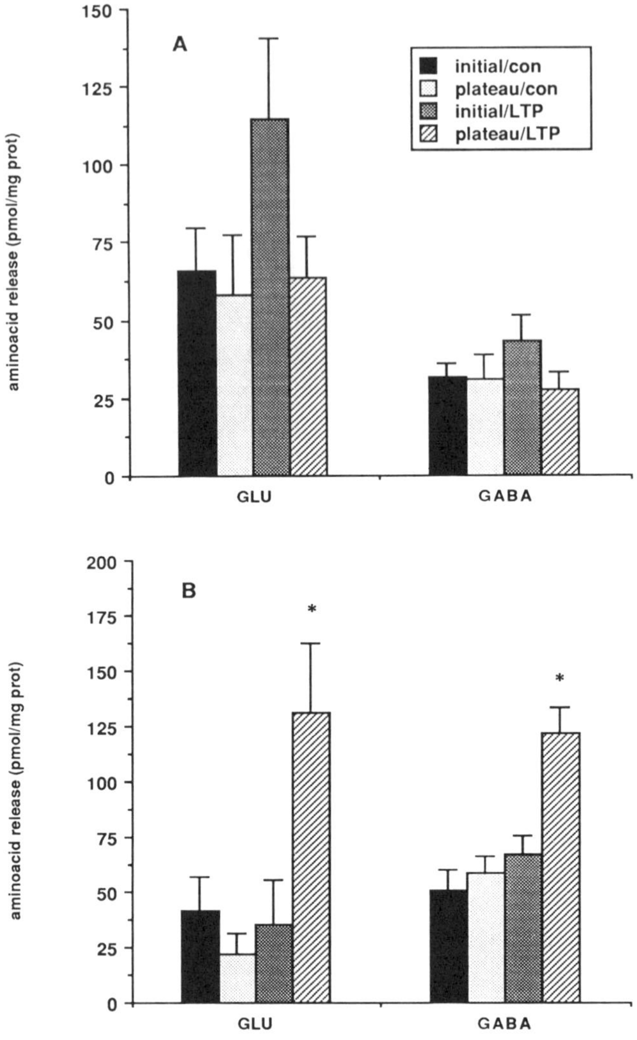

Figure 4.1 Effect of LTP on (A) endogenous potassium-induced calcium-independent and (B) potassium-induced, calcium-dependent release of glutamate and GABA. The results are presented as mean ± SEM separately for the first minute of potassium depolarization (initial) and after 3 minutes of potassium depolarization (plateau). The asterisks indicate significant differences compared to control values ($p < .05$).

Estimation of the potassium-induced, calcium-*de*pendent component of release at both incubation times gives a different picture (figure 4.1B). Whereas after 1 minute of potassium chloride elevation, glutamate and GABA release was about the same for both groups, a further increase of release of both amino acids was observed only in the LTP subslices, that reached a highly significant level at the plateau phase (3 minutes). Apparently, during LTP there are additional amounts of amino acid neurotransmitter recruitable for release by means of long depolarization periods, whereas in the control situation the maximal release was already reached 1 minute after potassium chloride elevation. In controls even a slight depletion of glutamate for release tends to occur after 3 minutes of potassium depolarization.

Discussion

These findings suggest the following mechanisms for release during the maintenance of LTP:

1. No clear differences in basal or carrier-mediated release of glutamate and GABA could be observed between LTP and control subslices. This observation is in agreement with the absence of any difference between both groups in total contents of these amino acids. Nevertheless, the direct accessible cytosolic pools of glutamate tended to increase in the subslices after induction of LTP, leading to an initial burst of carrier-mediated release during potassium depolarization.

2. The main differences were observed in the potassium-induced, calcium-*de*pendent component of release. Initially, at 1 minute of potassium chloride depolarization, no increase in release occurred above the control level. However, in LTP subslices the release dynamics were clearly changed. The rise in amino acid release after 3 minutes of potassium depolarization suggests an enhanced recruitment and/or activation of the vesicular neurotransmitter pool, causing a higher efficiency of release on (prolonged) stimulation.

3. The finding of an enhancement of endogenous potassium-induced, calcium-*de*pendent glutamate release confirms the in vitro observations of Lynch and coworkers (1985, 1986) studying release in slices and synaptosomes. Moreover, the present results permit us to extend their conclusions because we found an increase in glutamate release of the endogenous component, whereas those authors studied only the isotope-labeled glutamate release. In addition, these results indicate a change in release dynamics during LTP. Such an increase still existing 60 minutes after tetanic stimulation can exert a direct effect in establishing long-term enhancement of excitation of the postsynaptic cell, typical for LTP.

4. The observed increase in GABA release during LTP is robust. To our knowledge such an effect has not been reported before in studies on LTP. In a study by Bliss and coworkers (1986), in vivo GABA release did not clearly change during LTP. The increased release of GABA during LTP

may cause a decrease in GABA-receptor sensitivity. The decrease in paired-pulse depression, reported in the next section, might be explained by such a mechanism. It was suggested that blocking postsynaptic GABA-receptor activity may facilitate induction of LTP without influencing the maximal amount of potentiation (Wigström and Gustafsson, 1985).

PAIRED-PULSE RESPONSES (PPR)

Most studies in which paired-pulse responses were studied in LTP were carried out, in vitro, at a fixed intensity of paired-pulse stimulation. It is known, however, that the amount of paired-pulse facilitation (PPF) changes with stimulus intensity for a given interpulse interval (de Jonge and Racine, 1987; Kamphuis et al., 1987), such that the ratio between the response to the test stimulus (E_2) and that to the conditioning stimulus (E_1) can switch from facilitation (PPF) at relatively low stimulus intensities to depression (PPD) at stronger intensities. This PPD has been interpreted as being caused by the effect of recurrent inhibitory synapses that would be activated only at relatively high stimulus intensities. Therefore, it was of interest to investigate whether changes in the E_2/E_1 ratio occur in CA_1 LTP in vivo, as a function of stimulus intensity. This could indicate whether (1) a change in PPF at low stimulus intensity may occur during CA_1 in in vivo LTP, in contrast to what has been found in hippocampal slices in vitro, and (2) a change in PPD at strong stimulus intensity may take place that could indicate that recurrent inhibition may be affected in LTP.

Results

The effects of stimulus intensity on the amplitude of E_2 and E_1 and on the E_2/E_1 ratio for an interstimulus interval of 20 milliseconds in the control period (pretetanus) and during LTP (20–30′ posttetanus) were determined. In all these experiments in the control period, the saturation level of the E_1 amplitude was determined by stimulating at increasing stimulus intensities. The value of E_1 just under the saturation level was normalized as 100% and the corresponding stimulus intensity was also set to 100%. For each rat, all the other amplitude values, both for E_1 and E_2, were referred to this normalized value. The same was done for the stimulus intensities.

The increases in the amplitude of E_1 and of E_2 as function of stimulus intensity have different slopes particularly for intensities at or above the level of 50%; that of E_2 is steeper than that of E_1. Figure 4.2 shows that there was a tendency for PPF to decrease during LTP at low stimulation intensities, whereas with strong stimulations (100%), the tendency was in the opposite direction. These differences, however, did not reach a significant level.

To determine whether the E_2/E_1 ratio differed between the control and LTP periods, it is important to analyse these ratios independently of

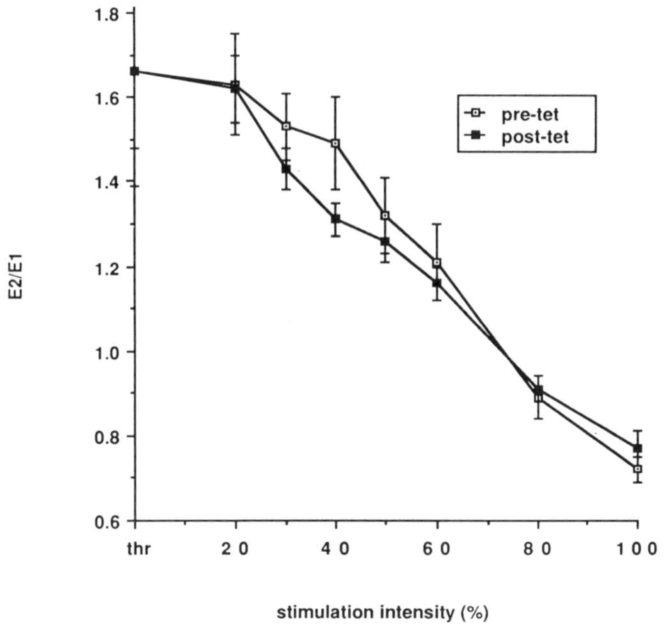

Figure 4.2 Effect of LTP on paired-pulse response, given in terms of the excitability ratio, calculated as the ratio between the amplitude of the test response (E_2) divided by that of the conditioned response (E_1). Stimulation intensity is expressed as percentage of the intensity giving maximal pretetanus E_1 level, starting with the threshold (thr) value.

stimulus intensity. We therefore plotted the mean values of E_2 versus those of E_1 in the control period and during LTP for all stimulus intensities and for all rats, as shown in figure 4.3. A comparison between these plots of E_1 versus E_2 showed two remarkable features:

1. For the lower range of values of E_1 (<50%), the relationships were approximately linear and similar for both periods.
2. The distribution of values corresponding to the higher range of E_1 (>50%) differed considerably from linearity and differed also between the control and LTP periods. In the plots of figure 4.3, the line along which E_2 equals E_1 is indicated. In this way, it can readily be seen that in the low range ($E_1 < 60\%$) PPF is clearly dominant for both periods, whereas in the high range ($E_1 > 60\%$), it appears that both PPF and PPD may be found.

To analyze whether the relationship between E_1 and E_2 differed between the two periods for the low range of values ($E_1 < 60\%$), we applied regression analysis. Linear regression yields lines that did not differ in slopes: $b = 1.2 \pm 0.1$ for the control period and 1.4 ± 0.1 for the LTP period, the coefficient of correlation being 0.86 for the former and 0.94 for the latter.

Figure 4.3 shows that the plot of E_2 versus E_1 crosses the line ($E_2 = E_1$) at a higher E_1 value for the LTP than for the control group. This fact indicates that during LTP, PPF persists for larger values of E_1 than in controls. We

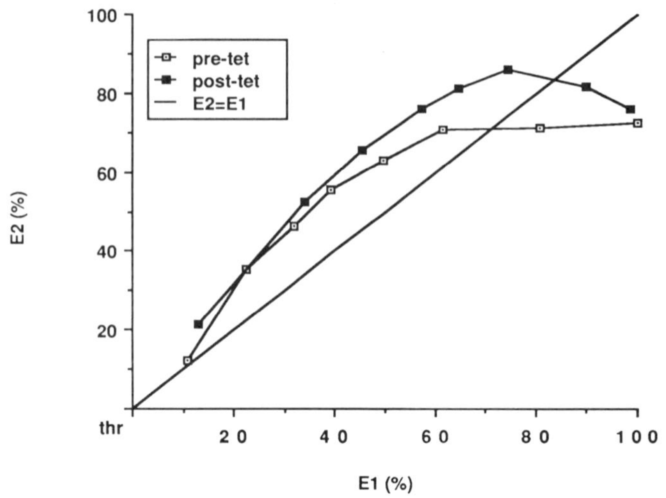

Figure 4.3 Effect of LTP on the relationship between E_1 and E_2 for control and LTP animals. The straight line represents the values $E_2 = E_1$. Note that for low values of E_1, there is facilitation ($E_2 > E_1$), but for larger values, there is depression ($E_2 < E_1$). The amplitude of E_1 at which the transition from facilitation to depression occurs is lower for controls than for the LTP group. E_1 and E_2 values are expressed as percentages of the pretetanus maximal E_1 level, starting with the threshold (thr) value.

tested, statistically, whether the values of E_1 at which the switch between PPF and PPD was first observed, along the input-output curves, differed between the two groups: the corresponding mean ($\pm$ SEM) values were 79 $\pm$ 5% for the control and 93 $\pm$ 4% for the LTP group of 14 rats. In this respect the difference between the two groups was significant at $p < .001$ (Wilcoxon signed rank test).

Therefore, we may draw the conclusion that the switch from PPF to PPD was found at larger E_1 values, indicating a relative decrease in the tendency for PPD to occur. To the best of our knowledge, such an effect was not previously reported to occur during CA_1 LTP, whether in vivo or in vitro.

The implication of this new finding is that during LTP of CA_1, in vivo, there is a tendency for *dis*inhibition to occur, but this can only be seen at relatively high stimulus intensities.

Discussion

The mechanism underlying this disinhibition is not yet clear. It should be noted that the disinhibition only becomes evident at high stimulus intensities. This means that the underlying process probably has a relatively high threshold. It is therefore not likely that an enhancement of the mechanisms underlying the PPF, which is found at low stimulation range, can be responsible for this disinhibition encountered at high ranges. This implies that other mechanisms play the most important role in this phenomenon of disinhibition.

Two possibilities can be considered because both are related to high threshold phenomena: (1) a decrease in recurrent inhibition, in an afterhyperpolarizing potential or in both and (2) an enhancement of a depolarizing potential that has a different sensitivity than the usual EPSP.

Evidence for the possibility of reduced GABA inhibition, either feedforward or recurrent, was not found by Haas and Rose (1984) in the CA_1 subarea although these authors suggest that some form of intrinsic (K^+ currents) disinhibition may occur during LTP. Miles and Wong (1987) showed that after tetanic stimulation of afferents to CA_3 pyramidal cells, recurrent inhibition was reduced by more than 20%, but it is not yet known whether the same applies to the CA_1 subarea. In another hippocampal subarea, the fascia dentata, Maru and coworkers (1989) reported a long-lasting reduction of PPD during LTP of the perforant path. These results were extended by Kanda and colleagues (1989), who showed, in vivo, a strong reduction in the relative strength of PPD after the tetanus. This PPD was enhanced by diazepam, and its reduction was interpreted as a result of a reduction in sensitivity of the granule cells to GABA. These results are strikingly similar to our present findings, although they were obtained in another area of the hippocampus and using a somewhat different protocol. It is likely that the changes reported here for the CA1 area and by Maru and coworkers (1989) for the fascia dentata may be due to a common mechanism, namely a prolonged decrease in GABA-receptor sensitivity, such as has been also observed during and after the application of a tetanus (Wong and Watkins, 1982; Stelzer et al., 1987; Chen et al., 1990).

An alternative possibility is that an enhancement of a depolarization component with high threshold may also take place, but this question needs further investigation at the microphysiological level.

It should be stressed that it is not simple to combine the electrophysiological findings reported here with the biochemical findings described in the previous section. Nevertheless, we consider that the most likely working hypothesis is that the decrease in PPD we found could be caused by desensitization of GABA receptors induced by the increase in GABA release. In addition, we should note that applications of GABA can cause an enhancement of NMDA-induced depolarizations (Walden et al., 1989). This process might also contribute to the decrease in PPD.

REFERENCES

Aniksztejn, L., M. P. Roisin, R. Amsellem, and Y. Ben-Ari (1989). Long-term potentiation in the hippocampus of the anaesthetized rat is not associated with a sustained enhanced release of endogenous excitatory amino acids. *Neuroscience* 28:387–392.

Bekkers, J. M., and C. F. Stevens (1990). Presynaptic mechanism for long-term potentiation in the hippocampus. *Nature* 346:724–729.

Bliss, T. V. P., R. M. Douglas, M. L. Errington, and M. A. Lynch (1986). Correlation between long-term potentiation and release of endogenous amino acids from dentate gyrus of anaesthetized rats. *Journal of Physiology* (London) 377:391–408.

Bliss, T. V. P., and T. Lømo (1973). Long-lasting potentiation of synaptic transmission in the dentate area of the anaesthetized rabbit following stimulation of the perforant path. *Journal of Physiology* (London) 232:331–356.

Chen, Q. X., A. Stelzer, A. R. Kay, and R. K. S. Wong (1990). $GABA_A$ receptor function is regulated by phosphorylation in acutely dissociated guinea-pig hippocampal neurones. *Journal of Physiology* (London) 420:207–221.

Collingridge, G. L. (1985). Long-term potentiation in the hippocampus: mechanisms of initiation and modulation by neurotransmitters. *Trends in Pharmacological Sciences* 6:407–411.

Haas, H. L., and G. Rose (1984). The role of inhibitory mechanisms in hippocampal long-term potentiation. *Neuroscience Letters* 47:301–306.

de Jonge, M., and R. J. Racine (1987). The development and decay of kindling-induced increases in paired-pulse depression in the dentate gyrus. *Brain Research* 412:318–328.

Kamphuis, W., et al. (1990). Kindling increases the K^+-evoked Ca^{2+}-dependent release of endogenous GABA in area CA1 of rat hippocampus. *Brain Research* 511:63–70.

Kamphuis, W., W. J. Wadman, and F. H. Lopes Da Silva (1987). Changes in local evoked potentials in the rat hippocampus (CA1) during kindling epileptogenesis. *Brain Research* 440:433–446.

Kanda, M., et al. (1989). Effects of LTP-inducing tetanic stimulations of the perforant path on the commissural inhibition and facilitation of dentate granule cell discharge. *Brain Research* 484:325–332.

Lynch, M. A., and T. V. P. Bliss (1986). Long-term potentiation of synaptic transmission in the hippocampus of the rat; effect of calmodulin and oleoyl-acetyl-glycerol on release of [^{3}H]glutamate. *Neuroscience Letters* 65:171–176.

Lynch, M. A., M. L. Errington, and T. V. P. Bliss (1985). Long-term potentiation of synaptic transmission in the dentate gyrus: increased release of [^{14}C]glutamate without increase in receptor binding. *Neuroscience Letters* 62:123–129.

Malenka, R. C., et al. (1989). An essential role for synaptic calmodulin and protein kinase activity in long-term potentiation. *Nature* 340:554–557.

Malinow, R., H. Shulman, and R. W. Tsien (1989). Inhibition of postsynaptic PKC or CaMKII blocks induction but not expression of LTP. *Science* 245:862–865.

Malinow, R., and R. W. Tsien (1990). Presynaptic enhancement shown by whole-cell recordings of long-term potentiation in hippocampal slices. *Nature* 346:177–180.

Maru, E., H. Ashida, and J. Tatsuno (1989). Long-lasting reduction of dentate paired-pulse depression following LTP-inducing tetanic stimulations of perforant path. *Brain Research* 478:112–120.

Meshul, C. K., and W. F. Hopkins (1990). Presynaptic ultrastructural correlates of long-term potentiation in the CA1 subfield of the hippocampus. *Brain Research* 514:310–319.

Miles R., and R. K. Wong (1987). Inhibitory control of local excitatory circuits in the guinea-pig hippocampus. *Journal of Physiology* 388:611–629.

Muller, D., and G. Lynch (1989). Evidence that changes in presynaptic calcium currents are not responsible for long-term potentiation in hippocampus. *Brain Research* 479:290–299.

Stelzer, A., N. T. Slater, and G. Bruggencate (1987). Activation of NMDA receptors blocks GABAergic inhibition in an in vitro model of epilepsy. *Nature* (London) 326:698–701.

Verhage, M., E. Besselsen, F. H. Lopes da Silva, and W. E. J. M. Ghijsen (1989). Ca^{2+}-dependent regulation of presynaptic stimulus-secretion coupling. *Journal of Neurochemistry* 53:1188–1194.

Voronin, L. L. (1983). Long-term potentiation in the hippocampus. *Neuroscience* 10:1051–1069.

Voronin, L. L., and U. Kuhnt (1990). Long-term potentiation affects facilitation ratio of EPSPs recorded from CA1 pyramidal cells in the guinea pig hippocampal slice. *Neuroscience Research Communications* 6:149–155.

Walden, J., E.-J. Speckmann, and D. Bingmann (1989). Augmentation of glutamate responses by GABA in the rat's motorcortex in vivo. *Neuroscience Letters* 101:209–213.

Wigström, H., and B. Gustafsson (1985). Facilitation of hippocampal long-lasting potentiation by GABA antagonists. *Acta Physiologica Scandinavia* 125:159–172.

Williams, J. H., M. L. Errington, M. A. Lynch, and T. V. P.Bliss (1989). Arachidonic acid induces a long-term activity-dependent enhancement of synaptic transmission in the hippocampus. *Nature* 341:739–742.

Wong, R. K. S., and D. J. Watkins (1982). Cellular factors influencing GABA response in hippocampal pyramidal cells. *Journal of Neurophysiology* 48:938–951.

Zalutsky, R. A., and R. A. Nicoll (1990). Comparison of two forms of long-term potentiation in single hippocampal neurons. *Science* 248:1619–1624.

Zucker, R. S. (1989). Short-term synaptic plasticity. *Annual Review of Neuroscience* 12:13–31.

5 Presynaptic Versus Postsynaptic Changes in Long-Term Potentiation

Françis Crepel

In 1973, Bliss and Lømo discovered long-term potentiation (LTP) of synaptic transmission using excitatory amino acids (EAAs) as neurotransmitters. Since then, understanding the underlying cellular mechanisms as well as evaluating its possible role in learning and memory has been the object of intensive studies. Because conventional synapses have only two sides—presynaptic and postsynaptic—efforts have been devoted to determine which side (or sides) is involved in the observed use-dependent change in synaptic strength.

Researchers generally agree that, at least in the dentate gyrus and in the CA1 subfield of the hippocampus, LTP does have two components, namely induction and maintenance (Bliss and Lynch, 1988); maintenance probably includes several subcomponents (see chapters 11 and 15). They also generally agree that, at these synapses, LTP is induced postsynaptically by the conjunction of a strong depolarization of the postsynaptic cell (owing to a tetanization of the afferents) and activation of its *N*-methyl-D-aspartate (NMDA) receptors by EAAs released by presynaptic fibers, thus allowing an entry of calcium through NMDA receptor–gated channels (Collingridge et al., 1983; see also the review in Bliss and Lynch, 1988).

The debate is therefore focused on the maintenance of LTP, with, in theory, three possibilities: maintenance of LTP is exclusively postsynaptic, exclusively presynaptic, or involves both sides of the synapse. As we discuss, the present state of the art is that the latter hypothesis is the most likely to be true. But first we'll have a brief overview of four aspects of this debate.

In chapter 1, Bliss reviews the experimental evidences of his group showing that, in the dentate gyrus and in CA1, induction of LTP by tetanization of the afferents is followed by a prolonged enhancement of glutamate release during in vivo, in vitro, and ex vivo experiments. These results were obtained by the use of several techniques including measurements of glutamate content and calcium-dependent release in potentiated versus control tissues (push-pull cannulation in vivo and glutamate release from slices and synaptosomes in in vitro experiments). The enhancement of glutamate release was significant for at least 2 hours after induction of LTP in the dentate gyrus, for at least 1 hour in CA1 (with, however, more variability), and up to 3 days in ex vivo experiments (Bliss et al., 1987). Some decline, however, in glutamate release seemed to occur in almost all presented data after, say, 1 hour. As expected, the increase in glutamate release no longer occurred when induction of LTP was prevented by treatments such as blockade of NMDA receptors by D-2-aminophosphono-5-valeric acid (APV).

Because these experiments clearly support the presence of a presynaptic component in the maintenance of LTP (but see chapter 2), Bliss also discusses the identification of the retrograde messenger released from the postsynaptic cell and acting on presynaptic endings to enhance glutamate release. Because calcium increase in the postsynaptic cell during induction of LTP is likely to activate phospholipase A_2, arachidonic acid might be a good candidate. Indeed, Bliss presents evidence for a small but significant increase of arachidonic acid release in the dentate gyrus after induction of LTP, and he also shows that substances such as nordihydroguaiaretic acid (NDGA), which block arachidonic acid metabolism, also block LTP of excitatory postsynaptic potentials (EPSPs) in CA1 and in the dentate gyrus. Furthermore, by fractionation experiments, the increase in arachidonic acid after LTP was only found in the postsynaptic fraction, and finally, he reports that in vivo as well as in vitro (dentate gyrus and CA1), subthreshold tetanus plus arachidonic acid application, leads to a slow development of LTP whereas arachidonic acid alone has no effect. Therefore, these data are altogether consistent with the hypothesis that arachidonic acid acts as a retrograde messenger during the late phase of LTP, leaving open what happens during the first 30 minutes. A possible role of other fatty acids such as oleic acid also remains to be determined (see chapter 11).

Bliss's findings, which clearly support the view that a presynaptic component participates in the maintenance of LTP, is strongly challenged by Ben-Ari. His group found only transient increase of glutamate release in CA1 in vivo or in vitro after LTP when using apparently the same protocol as in the Bliss experiments (Aniksztejn et al., 1989). The increase in glutamate release, however, could last up to 40 minutes, which is not far from the results of Bliss's group in CA1 (see above).

In fact, the main part of Ben-Ari's findings have related use-dependent modifications of synaptic strength with establishment of new connections, which indeed would be a fairly good example of presynaptic and postsynaptic changes! The study was conducted on a different model, namely synapses between mossy fibers and pyramidal cells in the CA3 subfield of the hippocampus. Contrary to synapses in the dentate gyrus and in CA1, postsynaptic receptors of these synapses are only of the non-NMDA type, but they can nevertheless exhibit LTP (see, for instance, Zalutsky and Nicoll, 1990).

The first question was: What happens when epileptic seizures affect this structure? This question was tackled by the use of two different models of experimental epilepsy, induced respectively by kainate injection or kindling of the amygdala in the rat. In both cases, mossy fiber sprouting was observed in the dentate gyrus (after kainate injections) and in CA3 (kindled animals). The important issue is that in kindled animals, sprouting was observed without any visible brain damage and, indeed, after only a few epileptic episodes. Furthermore, mossy fiber sprouting was also observed in human epileptic patients, as revealed by kainate binding of mossy fibers. The next question was: Is there any relationship between sprouting and LTP?

In in vitro experiments on CA3 pyramidal cells, bath application of kainate induces the appearance of giant bursts, which are entirely blocked by the non-NMDA receptor antagonist 6-cyano-7-nitroquinoxaline-2,3 dione (CNQX), but are insensitive to APV. After washout of kainate, EPSPs recorded in CA3 neurons appear durably potentiated, an effect that is APV sensitive and therefore resembles LTP. Thus, these results altogether show that epileptiform activities can induce a polysynaptic LTP-like event in CA3 neurons and also induce mossy fiber sprouting in CA3: the possible causal relationships between the two phenomena remain to be analyzed in detail. Because, however, granule cells do not express GAP-43 as stated by Routtenberg, the cellular mechanism underlying mossy fiber sprouting remains to be elucidated. Moreover, as has also been pointed out, a remote possibility remains that no sprouting of mossy fibers occurs in kindled animals, but that the level of detection of already existing "aberrant" connections is increased for some unknown reason in these animals.

Collingridge (see chapter 3) advocates that maintenance of LTP in CA1 involves both a presynaptic and a postsynaptic component ("sitting on the fence," as he says). He first presents an analysis of the pharmacology of the non-NMDA receptors of CA1 cells, as studied by the grease-gap method. This showed that α-amino-3-hydroxy-5-methylisoxazole-4-propionic acid (AMPA) leads to dose-dependent depolarizations of CA1 neurons, which are readily antagonized by CNQX, whereas glutamate-induced responses are only partly CNQX sensitive. In addition, because quisqualate can also activate phospholipase C, he used AMPA in experiments aiming to test the evolution of AMPA receptors of pyramidal cells after induction of LTP. The latter experiments were done in conventional slices, and AMPA was applied to CA1 pyramidal cells by iontophoresis. A first series of experiments showed that the potentiated response after induction of LTP is as sensitive to CNQX as the control one, indicating that the AMPA component of the EPSP is potentiated after tetanization of the afferents. A second series of experiments tested the sensitivity of CA1 neurons to AMPA before and after induction of LTP. The results are clearcut because they show that AMPA-mediated responses start to gradually increase over time—approximately 30 minutes after induction of LTP. As expected, if the tetanus is applied in the presence of APV, no LTP occurs and no change in sensitivity of pyramidal cells to AMPA is detected. Moreover, as also shown by others (see chapters 10 and 11), Collingridge shows that in the presence of protein kinase inhibitors such as K-252 b, LTP induced by tetanization of the afferents decays within 1 hour, indicating the presence of early (kinase insensitive) and late (kinase sensitive) phases of LTP. Interestingly, K-252 b also blocks the increase of the sensitivity of CA1 cells to AMPA but does not reverse it once it is established. From these data, Collingridge suggests that the early (decremental) phase of the maintenance of LTP is entirely presynaptic, whereas the late phase involves a postsynaptic component consisting of an increase in the sensitivity of postsynaptic cells to glutamate. Of course, these results fit well with those of Baudry and Lynch (see chapter 12) and are also in agreement with the release experiments of both Bliss and Ben-Ari's groups (see before). Latter results, however, are more in favor of a persistent increase of glutamate release after LTP than of a transient one, because Collingridge shows that the NMDA component of the synaptic response is also durably potentiated after tetanization of the afferents, which is, of course, simple to understand if glutamate release is permanently increased. To be fair, such an increase of the NMDA component of synaptic responses has not been found by Larson in similar experiments (see chapter 9), which raises a slight question. Furthermore, Collingridge's results also have technical limitations. In particular, it has been stressed that measuring sensitivity of postsynaptic cells to AMPA with the use of field potentials may be tricky, because of, for example, changes in the distribution of AMPA receptors over time on these neurons after LTP. Finally, the question of a possible desensitization of AMPA receptors after repetitive applications of AMPA, several seconds each, has also to be considered, although it should in principle lead to underestimation rather than overestimation of the evolution of AMPA sensitivity of CA1 neurons after LTP. Nonetheless, these results as they are already strongly support the view that postsynaptic modifications of AMPA receptors of postsynaptic neurons occur during a relatively late phase of LTP.

In chapter 4, Lopes da Silva evaluates the participation of the presynaptic side to LTP by both biochemical and electrophysiological methods. By studies of endogenous glutamate and GABA release in CA1 subslices after LTP induced in vivo, this group was able to demonstrate a significant enhancement of the potassium-induced, calcium-dependent release of both substances 1 hour after tetanus, thus confirming previous observations by Bliss and coworkers on glutamate release (see above). Moreover, Lopes da Silva shows that this increase in glutamate release involves the endogenous component, and not only the isotope-labeled glutamate release. The unexpected increase of GABA release after induction of LTP might cause a decreased GABA receptor sensitivity at potentiated synapses as well as a decrease in paired-pulse depression (PPD) (see below).

Indeed, electrophysiological studies performed in vivo attempted to compare the field potential amplitudes of paired conditioning and test stimuli in stratum radiatum before and 30 minutes after tetanus application, to estimate whether paired-pulse facilitation (PPF) was altered in the hippocampus during LTP, which could be a measure for altered presynaptic activity (see chapter 4). These experiments were performed with various intensities of paired-pulse stimulation, thus allowing a switch from PPF at relatively low-stimulus intensities to PPD at stronger intensities, the latter effect being currently interpreted as a result of recurrent inhibitory synapses. As previously reported by Lynch and coworkers (Muller and Lynch, 1989), no change of PPF was observed after LTP, which suggests that no presynaptic change occurs during LTP, or that these changes involve different steps from those accounting for PPF. In contrast, PPD was decreased in potentiated tissues, suggesting some "disinhibition," possibly from a desensitization of GABA receptors induced by the increase in GABA release (see above), other mechanisms (see chapter 4), or both.

It has been generally emphasized that LTP at synapses using non-NMDA receptors (for instance, at mossy fiber synapses with CA3 pyramidal cells as well as at synapses between parallel fibers and Purkinje cells in the cerebellum) raises the question of other mechanisms operating both for induction and maintenance of use-dependent synaptic changes. Another question still open is the possible role of glial cells and of uptake processes in LTP. Finally, there is not yet any hard data on the problem of the saturation of receptors prior to or during LTP, which, of course, is also a limitation for our understanding of what is really happening on the postsynaptic side of synapses.

What conclusions can be drawn from this discussion? At presynaptic level, it seems reasonable to believe that there is a sizeable enhancement of glutamate release, which contributes to the maintenance of LTP for at least 1 hour in CA1 and certainly for longer in the dentate gyrus (see chapters 1 and 4). This fits well with data on quantal analysis in LTP, even though this methodology also has uncertainties of its own (see chapter 6). The presynaptic increase of glutamate release during LTP is also supported by the enhancement of both NMDA and non-NMDA components of EPSPs during LTP, even though there is not yet a firm consensus on this point (see above), and more generally, a presynaptic change during LTP is also pointed out by the phosphorylation of presynaptic proteins such as F1 (see chapter 11). On this basis, the search for a retrograde messenger is legitimate, and arachidonic acid is certainly our best candidate so far. However, the increase of glutamate release may well be somehow decremental after 1 hour, and in this respect, the late increase in AMPA sensitivity of postsynaptic cells (see above) is certainly an important factor that allows this relatively late phase of LTP to be nondecremental, thus in keeping with the "Calpain hypothesis" (see chapter 12). Finally, the possibility of structural changes (see chapters 2 and 14) during the maintenance of LTP is certainly an additional factor, the importance of which has to be more precisely delineated, especially during the early, intermediate, and late phases of LTP. However, given the numerous uncertainties and contradictions that exist today, these conclusions should be considered as the present state of the art in a rapidly moving field.

REFERENCES

Aniksztejn, L., M. P. Roisin, R. Amsellem, and Y. Ben-Ari (1989). Long-term potentiation in the hippocampus of the anaesthetized rat is not associated with a sustained enhanced release of endogenous excitatory amino acids. *Neuroscience* 28:387–392.

Bliss, T. V. P., M. L. Errington, S. Laroche, and M. A. Lynch (1987). Increase in potassium stimulated, calcium dependent release of H^3-glutamate from rat dentate gyrus 3 days after induction of long-term potentiation. *Neuroscience Letter* 83:107–112.

Bliss, T. V. P., and M. A. Lynch (1988). Long-term potentiation of synaptic transmission in the hippocampus: properties and mechanisms. In P. W. Landfield and S. A. Deadwyler (eds.), *Long-term Potentiation, from Biophysics to Behavior.* New York: Alan R. Liss, pp. 3–72.

Bliss, T. V. P., and T. Lomo (1973). Long-lasting potentiation of synaptic transmission in the area dentata of the anesthetized rabbit following stimulation of the perforant path. *Journal of Physiology* (Lond.) 232:331–356.

Collingridge, G. L., S. J. Kehl, and H. McLellan (1983). Excitatory amino acids in synaptic transmission in the Schaeffer collateral-commissural pathway of the rat hippocampus. *Journal of Physiology* (Lond.) 334:33–46.

Muller, D., and G. Lynch (1989). Evidence that changes in presynaptic calcium currents are not responsible for long-term potentiation in the hippocampus. *Brain Research* 479:290–299.

Zalutsky, R. A., and R. A. Nicoll (1990). Comparison of two forms of long-term potentiation in single hippocampal neurons. *Science* 248:1619–1624.

6 Application of Quantal Analysis to the Study of Long-Term Potentiation: Errors, Assumptions, and Precautions

John M. Bekkers and Charles F. Stevens

Recently, we (Bekkers and Stevens, 1990a) and others (Voronin, 1988; Malinow and Tsien, 1990; Foster and McNaughton, 1991) have applied the method of quantal analysis to answer the question, what is the site of expression of long-term potentiation (LTP) in the hippocampus? Quantal analysis is long-established at the neuromuscular junction as the method of choice for distinguishing presynaptic and postsynaptic loci of synaptic plasticity (Del Castillo and Katz, 1954; McLachlan, 1978); quantal analysis therefore seems to be the natural tool to use at hippocampal synapses when addressing questions concerning expression of LTP. Unfortunately, central synapses are in general more complex, from the point of view of quantal analysis, than the neuromuscular junction, and one must be careful not to adopt the method uncritically. Our purpose in this chapter is to discuss some of the assumptions and complications behind quantal analysis, as used by us in the study of synaptic plasticity in both hippocampal slices and cultures.

This chapter is divided into four parts. First, we give a brief description of the most idealized kind of quantal analysis, to establish the basic ideas and vocabulary. Some of the formal assumptions of the method are discussed in this part. Second, we generalize the simple quantal analysis so that it accounts for complications that we have observed in both our culture and slice systems. Third, we discuss some assumptions about synaptic homogeneity that must be made to apply the analysis. Finally, we outline some future strategies that may overcome some of the problems discussed here.

SIMPLE FORM OF THE QUANTAL THEORY

This section briefly describes the basic theory and a simple physical interpretation. For more complete accounts, consult original papers (Del Castillo and Katz, 1954; Katz and Miledi, 1965) and reviews (Steinbach and Stevens, 1976; Martin, 1977; McLachlan, 1978; Redman, 1990).

Formulation of the Basic Quantal Theory

The basic quantal theory views the synapse as follows: The presynaptic terminal contains N release sites, at each of which a single neurotransmitter-loaded vesicle, or "quantum" of neurotransmitter, is available to be released into the synaptic cleft. When an action potential arrives in the presynaptic terminal, each of the N vesicles has, for a short time, an enhanced probability p of being released. It is assumed that p is the same for each releasable vesicle and does not depend on whether any other vesicle is or has been released. When the contents of any one vesicle are dumped into the cleft, the neurotransmitter binds to receptors in the postsynaptic membrane, giving rise to a synaptic current in the postsynaptic cell (if the postsynaptic cell is voltage clamped; otherwise, a synaptic potential) of amplitude a. It is assumed that a is the same following the release of any one of the N presynaptic vesicles. The simplest way for this to be the case is to assume that every vesicle delivers the same amount of neurotransmitter to a constant subpopulation of postsynaptic receptors. Amplitude a is often called the quantal size, or unitary event, because it is the smallest synaptic response that can be elicited at the synapse; all other responses are integer multiples of this unit. (Hereafter we assume for convenience that one is measuring excitatory postsynaptic currents, EPSCs, while voltage clamping the postsynaptic cell. The theory applies equally well to synaptic potentials.)

Because the release of quanta of transmitter is a probabilistic process, the exact number released fluctuates from trial to trial, where a "trial" means the arrival of a (constant) action potential in the presynaptic terminal. It can be shown from simple statistical theory that the trial-to-trial variability in the number of vesicles released follows a binomial distribution; that is, the probability p_n of finding just n vesicles released is

$$p_n = N!/(n!(N - n)!)p^N(1 - p)^{N-n} \tag{6.1}$$

Of course, experimentally one measures an EPSC, the amplitude of which is just a times the number of vesicles released. A histogram of the amplitudes will look like a series of bars centered on $0, a, 2a, 3a \ldots$ with their relative heights given by equation (6.1). The mean of this histogram (the mean size of the measured EPSCs averaged over many trials) is

$$m = aNp \tag{6.2}$$

The variance of this response is given by

$$v = a^2Np(1 - p) \tag{6.3}$$

An example of data for a quantal analysis is shown in figure 6.1. This figure shows records made in a pair of hippocampal neurons maintained in culture for 12 days. At the top are superimposed six action potentials elicited consecutively in the presynaptic cell; below are shown the corresponding EPSCs measured in the postsynaptic cell. In some of the traces (e.g., the first and last) an isolated miniature EPSC is visible after the

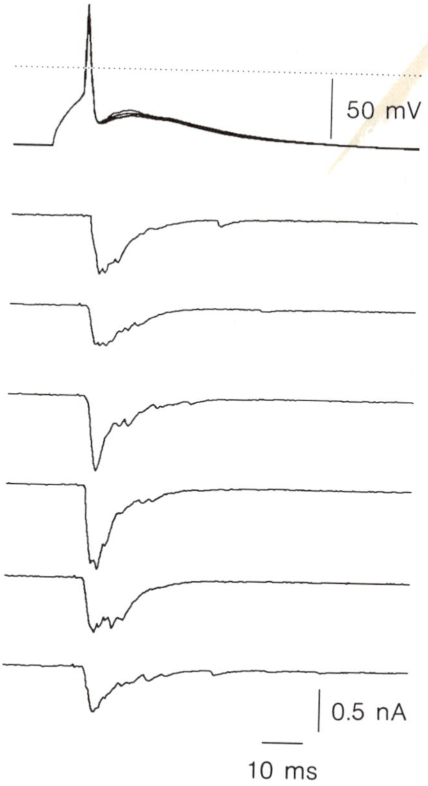

Figure 6.1 Quantal fluctuations in monosynaptic EPSCs recorded in a pair of hippocampal neurons in cell culture. Upper traces show superimposed action potentials fired consecutively in the presynaptic cell by injecting 0.8 nA for 10 milliseconds at 1-second intervals; lower traces show the corresponding EPSCs recorded in the postsynaptic cell while voltage clamping at −60 mV. The whole-cell patch clamp method was used to record from both cells. The external solution contained 10 mM of magnesium and .75 mM of calcium; the patch solution contained potassium methylsulfate.

evoked EPSC. These EPSCs have a ragged appearance because of variation in the exact time at which individual packets of neurotransmitter are exocytosed ("latency jitter"; Barrett and Stevens, 1972). Therefore, it is not meaningful to use the peak amplitude as a measure of synaptic transmission, and instead one takes the time integral of the currents to obtain a charge. Charge is insensitive to latency jitter. The quantal analysis applies equally well to synaptic charge.

It should be noted in passing that, for the purposes of the theory, the N release sites need not necessarily reside in the same presynaptic bouton; rather, they may be distributed across any number of boutons, provided these are all identical. For example, it has been suggested (Korn et al., 1981) that inhibitory boutons onto Mauthner's cell have just one release site apiece. In this case, therefore, N also corresponds to the number of boutons.

Application of the Basic Theory to Analysis of LTP

How is this formulation of use in answering the question of the site of expression of LTP? Reframing the question in terms of the parameters of quantal analysis, the mean postsynaptic response can increase after LTP if a, N, or p increases (equation (6.2)). According to the above physical interpretation of the quantal hypothesis, N and p are parameters dealing with the presynaptic neuron, whereas a originates in the postsynaptic cell. Thus, if one can show that N or p (or both) increases after LTP, a site of presynaptic expression is implicated, whereas an increase in a suggests expression at a postsynaptic site.

How could one extract the quantal parameters a, N, and p before and after LTP? One way is the following. As just mentioned, in this ideal case a histogram of amplitudes of evoked EPSCs would consist of discrete peaks spaced at constant intervals a in size; thus, one could directly read off this quantity from the histogram. Alternatively, one can often observe in the postsynaptic cell occasional spontaneous miniature EPSCs (mEPSCs). Each of these is thought to arise in the spontaneous release from the presynaptic terminal of a single vesicle of neurotransmitter; the mEPSCs amount to a background level of synaptic transmission owing to leakage of transmitter from the presynaptic terminal, even in the absence of a presynaptic action potential. By this interpretation, a can be directly measured from the amplitude of an mEPSC. With a in hand, one now calculates the mean and variance of the histogram of evoked EPSCs, yielding numbers for the left-hand sides of equations (6.2) and (6.3). These two equations now contain just two unknowns, N and p, which can be solved for. This procedure can be applied both before and after LTP.

As an extension, having a, N, and p, one can calculate from equation (6.1) the expected relative heights of the peaks in the amplitude histogram and compare these with the experimental histogram. The three quantal parameters may then be varied slightly to maximize the agreement between theoretical and experimental histograms.

The approach just described, in which all three quantal parameters are extracted from the amplitude histograms, is often referred to as a "full" quantal analysis. However, for the purposes of simply distinguishing presynaptic (N and p) and postsynaptic (a) mechanisms of synaptic plasticity, a simpler approach is sometimes adopted. This involves calculating from the amplitude histogram a quantity called the coefficient of variation (CV), defined as

$$CV = \sqrt{v/m^2} = \sqrt{(1 - p)/Np} \qquad (6.4)$$

using the definitions in equations (6.2) and (6.3). The utility of the CV is that the postsynaptic parameter, a, cancels, leaving only a dependence on the presynaptic parameters. Thus, if the CV before and after LTP is found to be the same, a change in a is implicated; a changed CV points to a change in N and p, and thus a presynaptic expression of LTP.

Ambiguities in Conclusions About LTP Expression Based on the Simple Theory

Even supposing that the simple quantal analysis theory provides an accurate description of synaptic transmission, it possesses a number of shortcomings that can potentially mislead one about the site of expression of LTP.

First, an observed change in the postsynaptic parameter a does not necessarily imply that the change is postsynaptic. A larger response to the exocytosis of a single vesicle of transmitter could, as just stated, be a result of a modification of postsynaptic receptors to make them more sensitive; but it could also be a result of a systematic increase in the amount of transmitter contained within all presynaptic vesicles, or of a change in the mechanisms that remove transmitter from the cleft on the time scale of synaptic transmission. Thus, in principle a change in a is compatible with either presynaptic or postsynaptic expression of LTP.

Second, in principle it is possible at any one synapse that the number N of release sites becomes extremely large, while the release probability p of each vesicle becomes extremely small. Under these conditions, one can show by algebraic manipulation of equation (6.1) that the predicted amplitude distribution changes, becoming a Poisson distribution.

$$p_n = \lambda^n e^{-\lambda}/n! \tag{6.5}$$

where

$$\lambda = Np \tag{6.6}$$

is the mean number of vesicles released, averaged over many trials. Under these conditions, the expressions for the mean and variance of the measured amplitude histogram become (compare equations [6.2] and [6.3])

$$m = a\lambda \tag{6.7}$$

$$v = a^2\lambda \tag{6.8}$$

Note that the parameters N and p no longer appear separately, but only as the product Np; that is, the two presynaptic parameters are now lumped together. How might this lead to ambiguity of conclusions regarding expression of LTP? Suppose that, prior to LTP, a normally functioning synapse is accompanied by a silent synapse at which transmitter release is normal but all the postsynaptic receptors are switched off. After induction of LTP, these silent receptors are switched on, clearly a postsynaptic mechanism; however, this switch will appear to quantal analysis like a doubling in the number of release sites, N. Thus, if one finds from the analysis that N increases after LTP, one could not be certain that LTP was really presynaptic; only a clear increase in p would allow one to unambiguously posit a presynaptic mechanism. Unfortunately, in the Poisson limit, when N and p are lumped together, one cannot know which of these two parameters has changed: the conclusion regarding presynaptic or postsynaptic expression of LTP remains uncertain.

It is indeed fortuitous that, following LTP in culture, (1) the Poisson limit is often not approached, and (2) p increases. This allows one to disregard the above two precautions, and to state unambiguously that expression of LTP in this system is primarily presynaptic. Unfortunately, the situation in the slice is not so clearcut (Bekkers and Stevens, 1990a).

GENERALIZED FORM OF QUANTAL ANALYSIS FOR USE IN HIPPOCAMPAL SLICES AND CULTURES

This section discusses a number of problems that arise in applying quantal analysis to the hippocampal system. Ways in which these problems may be circumvented, by generalizing the simple theory given in the previous section, are described.

The Problem of Baseline Noise

Baseline, or instrument, noise is included in the variance calculated from the evoked synaptic currents. Thus, another term, the noise variance, must be added to equations (6.3) and (6.8) for the expected variance. Furthermore, baseline noise must also be incorporated in the calculated distribution to superimpose on the experimental histogram of EPSC sizes. Assuming that the baseline noise has a constant distribution and is independent of synaptic transmission, it may be incorporated by forming a convolution of the noise distribution with the noise-free theoretical distribution. The noise distribution can be directly measured from event-free regions of the current traces recorded in the postsynaptic cell. The definition and formal rationale of convolution can be found elsewhere (Redman, 1990); intuitively, it can be thought of as a way of linearly folding one distribution into another.

In practice, the measured baseline noise is rather small in whole-cell patch clamped neurons, compared with the sizes of evoked EPSCs, and does not contribute much to the analysis.

The Problem of Distribution in Quantal Size a

The simple theory just discussed assumes that the unit postsynaptic response elicited by a single quantum of neurotransmitter, the unitary event, has a fixed size, a. We have found, however, in our culture and slice systems that the unitary events measured at a single or a few synapses have a broad, skewed distribution (Bekkers et al., 1990). This finding means that the observed fluctuation in the evoked synaptic response is, in terms of the quantal hypothesis, a mixture of both presynaptic fluctuation in the number of quanta of transmitter released and postsynaptic fluctuation in the size of the current elicited by each quantum. This additional source of fluctuation must be incorporated in the theory.

One can show that, when allowing for a distribution in a, equations (6.2) and (6.3) for the mean and variance of evoked synaptic responses become

$$m' = \alpha Np \tag{6.9}$$

$$v' = v + \alpha^2 Npc_m{}^2 \tag{6.10}$$

where c_m is the CV for the size distribution of mEPSCs, given by $c_m = \sqrt{v_m/\alpha^2}$

Here α and v_m are the measured mean and variance, respectively, of the distribution of unitary events (or mEPSCs), and v is given by equation (6.3) except with α replacing a. It can be seen that the modified mean, m', is basically the same as before (compare equation [6.2]), with the mean α in place of a; but the modified variance, v', now contains an additional term to account for the extra variability introduced by the unitary events. With these new equations, one can follow a similar procedure as for the simple theory: measure α and v_m from the distribution of mEPSCs recorded in the postsynaptic cell, calculate m' and v' from the histogram of evoked synaptic currents, and then solve for the two unknowns, N and p.

As in the simple case of quantal analysis, it is prudent to superimpose the theoretical distribution on the observed histogram of evoked EPSCs, then adjust the quantal parameters for best fit. This theoretical distribution can be calculated as follows. First, one needs a function to describe the measured distribution of mEPSC amplitudes. Empirically, a gamma function provides a good description (McLachlan, 1978), as does a function we have derived elsewhere (Bekkers et al., 1990). Second, one calculates the probability distribution for finding an amplitude x from the release of exactly k vesicles of transmitter,

$$P_k(x) = p_k C^k(x) \tag{6.11}$$

Here p_k is the binomial probability of k releases, calculated from equation (6.1), and $C^k(x)$ is the kth-order convolution of the function describing the mEPSC amplitude distribution, which in general would be calculated numerically. Finally, the distribution for any number of releases is found by summing equation (6.11) over all possible values of k (0 to N). Although this procedure is complicated, it does not introduce any more free parameters; the distribution in a is measured experimentally, and so only N and p need to be optimized by curve-fitting.

The Problem of Cable Attenuation

Synapses on a central neuron are often distributed across the cell's dendritic tree, electrically remote from the soma where, in the typical experiment, the recording electrode is placed. This may cause problems for quantal analysis. Consider the situation in which active synapses are uniformly scattered across the dendrites of a neuron, some far from the soma so their current is heavily filtered before reaching the recording electrode, some close to the soma. Suppose that spontaneous mEPSCs arise with equal frequency from all of these synapses; the measured distribution of mEPSC amplitudes will then appear broader than from a single synapse, because it will contain a wider range of currents from large (proximal synapses) to small (remote distal synapses). Again, assuming that proximal or distal synapses are not favored when an action potential arrives in the presynaptic terminals, the histogram of evoked EPSCs will also appear broader than from a single synapse, simply reflecting the increased broadness of the underlying mEPSC distribution. Thus, provided the synapses are in every other respect identical, the generalized quantal analysis applied to this case is formally identical to that in which all synapses are proximal. N and p will be correctly extracted; only α will be underestimated, because it is an average that now includes the more severely attenuated distal contributions.

The situation is more complicated if, for example, there are many synapses on a neuron but only a subset of these are activated by an action potential in the presynaptic fiber. Suppose the active synapses are all located very close to the soma and subject to little cable attenuation. The mEPSC distribution, on the other hand, is formed by accumulating mEPSCs originating in all of the synapses, both proximal and distal, and not just the proximal ones that are actually active. The whole-cell mEPSC distribution is inappropriate for use in the quantal analysis of a subset of synapses with different α. Since this may actually be the situation in a hippocampal neuron, it is important to consider ways in which the possibility for error may be reduced.

We have recently done a cable analysis of hippocampal neurons in cell culture using a method of eliciting mEPSCs at known places on a dendrite by applying hypertonic solution (Bekkers and Stevens, 1990b). We concluded that the mean amplitude, as seen from the soma, of mEPSCs originating at a synapse located x μm from the soma falls off with x approximately as $exp(-x/170)$. This assumes a dendritic diameter of 1 μm. On the other hand, the mean charge carried by the mEPSCs (found by averaging the time integrals of individual mEPSCs) declines much more slowly with distance, approximately as $exp(-x/1000)$. In practical terms, this means one can substantially reduce the effect of cable attenuation by using histograms of charge carried by synaptic currents, rather than histograms of just the amplitudes of the currents. (Recall that another reason for using the time integrals of currents was given earlier, namely, to remove the problem of latency jitter).

Typically, the dendrites of cultured hippocampal neurons used in our studies have diameters extending for several hundred microns with diameters tapering from 1 to 2 μm near the soma down to less than 0.1 μm at the tips. Thus, even when synaptic charge is being considered, substantial cable attenuation of the most distal synapses may occur.

Application of the Generalized Quantal Analysis

The foregoing generalized theory has been applied to pairs of synaptically connected hippocampal neurons grown in cell culture. (Some preliminary examples are shown in Bekkers and Stevens, 1989, figure 3.) The theory provides a very good fit to histograms of charge carried by EPSCs in three different calcium concentrations. The fitted quantal parameters behave as expected.

It should be noted that a popular shortcut approach to quantal analysis is the so-called method of failures. The starting point for this method is the assumption that the Poisson limit obtains (equations [6.5]–[6.8]). One then counts the number of trials for which a presynaptic spike failed to elicit an EPSC; this gives a value for p_0, the probability of zero releases. Equation (6.5) for the Poisson case gives $p_0 = e^{-\lambda}$, allowing one to solve for λ ($= Np$). The practical difficulty with this method, in the light of the generalized quantal analysis just given, is that a "failure" is now ambiguously defined. Because of the distribution in a, one observes a continuum in the sizes of EPSCs; one therefore may have to adopt an arbitrary threshold as to what does or does not constitute a failure. This difficulty is avoided by fitting a continuous curve to the measured continuous distribution of synaptic responses.

ASSUMPTIONS CONCERNING SYNAPTIC HOMOGENEITY IN APPLYING QUANTAL ANALYSIS TO HIPPOCAMPAL CULTURES AND SLICES

This section will describe some additional difficulties that may affect a quantal analysis in the hippocampus. These problems are more difficult to deal with effectively than those listed in the previous section. However, under some conditions they may be ameliorated, as we discuss.

Heterogeneity of a, N, and p Between Different Synapses

The theory so far has assumed that one is dealing with just one synapse or, at least, that all synapses are identical. Hippocampal neurons are known to receive many synaptic inputs; one must therefore address possible heterogeneity in the contributions of different synapses. We discuss two possible kinds of heterogeneity: presynaptic (differences in N and p) and postsynaptic (differences in α).

Presynaptic Heterogeneity Presynaptic heterogeneity may arise in several ways. One way is for heterogeneity to be inherent to individual presynaptic terminals, perhaps owing to random variability in synaptic architecture. Another way is for the heterogeneity to reside in the different collaterals of the afferent axons: some collaterals may be intermittently silent, causing the synapses attached to those collaterals to have a lower apparent p than terminals that are reliably invaded by action potentials. A variant on this situation, which almost certainly occurs in the typical slice experiment, is that distinct axonal tracts are only intermittently activated. This arises because one normally uses extracellular stimulation to fire *en passant* fibers, which is unlikely to activate exactly the same axons from trial to trial. The end result is that one is recording from a fluctuating population of synapses. This problem is avoided in culture and in slice experiments where only a single presynaptic cell is excited (Sayer et al., 1989; see chapter 8). A third possibility, which is a further variant on the previous one, is that polysynaptic activation occurs sporadically. Sporadic polysynaptic activation means that stimulation of the presynaptic cell sometimes activates pathways that lead first to other excitatory neuron(s), and thence to the postsynaptic cell being recorded from. This, too, would tend to cause intertrial variability in the number of contributing synapses. A final possibility is that, after an LTP-inducing tetanus, only a subset of synapses modify their release properties; thus, the heterogeneity may arise only after LTP. This last possibility is plausible in view of the suggestion that LTP in culture may be expressed inhomogeneously across synapses (Bekkers and Stevens, 1990a).

One can imagine a hierarchy of increasingly general heterogeneity in the release process. At the lowest level, each synapse may possess the same number N of release sites, and release is still independent, but the probability of release p may differ from one synapse to the next. Thus, the release process is still binomially distributed at individual synapses, but the overall distribution measured for all synapses is a sum of binomial distributions. At a more general level, even the Ns may differ between synapses. Some workers use a multivariate fitting process to fit general statistical models to their amplitude histograms (Sayer et al., 1989); however, these require high quality data to be convincing.

Postsynaptic Heterogeneity Postsynaptic heterogeneity may arise by intersynapse variation in the density or sensitivity of postsynaptic receptors. In this case, a naive quantal analysis of the sort just described would yield some kind of average a, with no information about the distribution of quantal sizes between synapses.

A Theory to Circumvent the Effect of Synaptic Heterogeneity In applying quantal analysis to the slice preparation, we developed an argument to test the significance of synaptic heterogeneity. The argument goes as follows: Suppose there are n synapses on a particular neuron. Each of these $k = 1, 2 \ldots n$ synapses will, in general, have its own quantal size a_k, release probability p_k, and number of release sites N_k; after a tetanus, the kth input will be potentiated by a factor f_k. A complete quantal analysis would have to estimate $3n$ parameters and n potentiation factors.

For this multisynapse case, the mean EPSC size would be

$$m = \sum_k m_k \tag{6.12}$$

in the unpotentiated state, and

$$m_P = \sum_k m_k f_k \tag{6.13}$$

in the potentiated state, where m_k is the mean contribution of the kth synapse, given by $m_k = a_k N_k p_k$ using equation (6.2). The overall potentiation factor f is defined to be $f = m_P/m$.

The total variance v of unpotentiated synapses is, assuming all synapses behave independently,

$$v = \sum_k v_k \tag{6.14}$$

where v_k is the variance for the kth synapse. We now restrict our attention to the Poisson limit in which p is small; this appears to be valid for the slice preparation (Bekkers and Stevens, 1990a). For the potentiated synapses, using the result that LTP is expressed presynaptically (Bekkers and Stevens, 1990a; Malinow and Tsien, 1990),

$$v_P = \sum_k f_k v_k \tag{6.15}$$

This result follows from equations (6.6) and (6.8) by multiplying release probability p by the potentiation factor f appropriate to each synapse. Now consider the quantity r, defined as $r = h/h_P$, where h is the squared value of the coefficient of variation (CV) of EPSCs before a tetanus and h_P is the corresponding quantity in the potentiated slice. Using the definition of the CV (equation [6.4]) and substituting equations (6.12) through (6.15), one obtains

$$r = \frac{\sum_k v_k}{\sum_k f_k v_k} \frac{\left(\sum_k f_k m_k\right)^2}{\left(\sum_k m_k\right)^2} \tag{6.16}$$

If all synapses were identical, this would simplify to $r = f$; a plot of the quantity r, calculated for each LTP experiment, versus the measured potentiation factor f for that experiment, would yield points that lie along a diagonal line. In general, however, if the subscripted quantities in equation (6.16) were very different from each other, then this nonuniformity in synaptic properties could lead to values for r and f that lie anywhere on the r/f plot. Although any one cell might fortuitously possess synapses with just the right combination of f_k, m_k, and v_k that its r value lies on the diagonal, it is unlikely that this would be the case for many different cells. However, as seen in figure 4 of Bekkers and Stevens (1990a), the results from 10 different slice experiments do, in fact, lie close to the diagonal. This finding suggests that individual synapses studied under these conditions are not greatly heterogeneous in their properties. We cannot, however, place limits on their homogeneity.

FUTURE STRATEGIES FOR THE APPLICATION OF QUANTAL ANALYSIS IN THE HIPPOCAMPUS

The goal of this chapter is to discuss the problems and assumptions of quantal analysis applied to our hippocampal slice and culture systems, so as to judge the strength of our conclusion, based on quantal analysis, concerning the expression of LTP. The conclusion of this chapter is that, provided one applies a generalized form of quantal analysis that takes into account such factors as baseline noise, cable attenuation, and distribution of mEPSC amplitudes, the analysis is self-consistent and accurately describes the data. Thus, we feel confident in our conclusion, based on the generalized analysis and, in particular, on the data from culture, that the expression of LTP is primarily presynaptic.

Despite the success of the generalized quantal analysis, it does not address the problem of possible heterogeneity of synapses. In the previous section an argument was presented that suggests that this problem may be minor in the slice; however, it is difficult to know how to address it rigorously. In the ideal experiment, one would stimulate just one afferent fiber and record from just one synapse. This may be possible in the culture system. Synaptogenesis in culture occurs over a rather stereotyped time course (Bartlett and Banker, 1984): synapses first appear after 4 or 5 days, then increase in density. Therefore, it should be possible to find cell pairs that have only one synaptic contact. This likelihood could be increased by growing cell pairs in isolation from other cells, for instance, by plating at very low density, or by restricting pairs to small areas by using nonpermissive substrates elsewhere (Segal and Furshpan, 1990). In the ideal experiment, therefore, one would apply quantal analysis to the study of LTP at just one synapse.

The recent introduction of the patch clamp slice technique has reinvigorated the application of quantal analysis to the hippocampal slice preparation. For example, Jack and coworkers (1990) and Andersen and coworkers (1990) have reported the existence, under particular stimulus paradigms, of peaks in their histograms of evoked synaptic currents. Such peaks are not observed in culture, as expected from the broadness of the distribution of amplitudes of unitary events. Explanations for the origin of these peaks in slices are keenly awaited. It will also be interesting to study synaptic fluctuations in the slice when only a single presynaptic cell is stimulated, rather than a population of afferent fibers, as is usually the case (see chapter 8). This situation would remove possible complications from stimulus fluctuations.

It is refreshing that even so venerable a method as quantal analysis is still capable of generating much interest.

REFERENCES

Andersen, P., O. Hvalby, M. Raastad, and J. F. Storm (1990). Synaptic integration in hippocampal CA1 neurons. *Cold Spring Harbor Symposium of Quantitative Biology* 55 (in press).

Barrett, E. F., and C. F. Stevens (1972). Quantal independence and uniformity of presynaptic release kinetics at the frog neuromuscular junction. *Journal of Physiology* (London) 227:665–689.

Bartlett, W. P., and G. B. Banker (1984). An electron microscopic study of the development of axons and dendrites by hippocampal neurons in culture. II. Synaptic relationships. *Journal of Neuroscience* 4:1954–1965.

Bekkers, J. M., G. B. Richerson, and C. F. Stevens (1990). Origin of variability in quantal size in cultured hippocampal neurons and hippocampal slices. *Proceedings of the National Academy of Science USA* 87:5359–5362.

Bekkers, J. M., and C. F. Stevens (1989). NMDA and non-NMDA receptors are co-localized at individual excitatory synapses in cultured rat hippocampus. *Nature* 341:230–233.

Bekkers, J. M., and C. F. Stevens (1990a). Presynaptic mechanism for long-term potentiation in the hippocampus. *Nature* 346:724–729.

Bekkers, J. M., and C. F. Stevens (1990b). Cable analysis of rat hippocampal neurons in culture: a novel approach. *Society for Neuroscience Abstracts* 16:674.

Del Castillo, J., and B. Katz (1954). Quantal components of the endplate potential. *Journal of Physiology* (London) 124:560–573.

Foster, T. C., and B. L. McNaughton (1991). Long-term enhancement of CA1 synaptic transmission is due to increased quantal size, not quantal content. *Hippocampus* 1:79–91.

Jack, J. J. B., et al. (1990). Quantal analysis and nerve cell modelling in the mammalian central nervous system. *Cold Spring Harbor Symposium of Quantitative Biology* 55 (in press).

Katz, B., and R. Miledi (1965). The measurement of synaptic delay, and the time course of acetylcholine release at the neuromuscular junction. *Proceedings of the Royal Society* (London) B 161:483–495.

Korn, H., A. Triller, A. Mallet and D. S. Faber (1981). Fluctuating responses at a central synapse: *n* of binomial fit predicts number of stained presynaptic boutons. *Science* 213:898–901.

Malinow, R., and R. W. Tsien (1990). Presynaptic enhancement shown by whole-cell recordings of long-term potentiation in hippocampal slices. *Nature* 346:177–180.

Martin, A. R. (1977). Junctional transmission. II. Presynaptic mechanisms. In E. R. Kandel (ed.), *Handbook of Physiology. The Nervous System, Vol. 1.* Bethesda: American Physiological Society, pp. 329–355.

McLachlan, E. M. (1978). The statistics of transmitter release at chemical synapses. In R. Porter (ed.), *International Review of Physiology, Neurophysiology III, Vol. 17.* Baltimore: University Park Press, pp. 49–117.

Redman, S. J. (1990). Quantal analysis of synaptic potentials in neurons of the central nervous system. *Physiological Reviews* 70:165–198.

Sayer, R. J., S. J. Redman, and P. Andersen (1989). Amplitude fluctuations in small EPSPs recorded from CA1 pyramidal cells in the guinea pig hippocampal slice. *Journal of Neuroscience* 9:840–850.

Segal, M. M., and E. J. Furshpan (1990). Epileptiform activity in microcultures containing small numbers of hippocampal neurons. *Society for Neuroscience Abstracts* 16:21.

Steinbach, J. H., and C. F. Stevens (1976). Neuromuscular transmission. In R. Llinas and W. Precht (eds.), *Frog Neurobiology,* Heidelberg: Springer-Verlag, pp. 33–92.

Voronin, L. L. (1988). In H. L. Haas and G. Buzsaki (eds.), *Synaptic Plasticity in the Hippocampus,* Berlin: Springer, pp. 27–30.

7 The Mechanisms of Expression of Long-Term Synaptic Enhancement: Thesis, Antithesis, Synthesis

Bruce L. McNaughton

INTRODUCTION: PRESYNAPTICISTS VERSUS POSTSYNAPTICISTS (ONE MORE ROUND)

The study of long-term enhancement (LTE/LTP) of neurotransmission in the hippocampus is at a critical phase in its history. It is generally agreed that cooperative, "Hebbian" mechanisms underlie its *induction* at most terminals (McNaughton et al., 1978), as a result of postsynaptic integration of afferent activity (Harris et al., 1984; Collingridge et al., 1983; Gustafsson et al., 1987). A remarkable body of apparently contradictory evidence, however, is amassing favoring both presynaptic (Bliss and Lynch, 1988) and postsynaptic (e.g., Davies et al., 1989; Douglas et al., 1982; Kauer et al., 1988; Muller and Lynch, 1988) mechanisms of *expression*. Recently a new dimension was added to this controversy when results from this laboratory (Foster and McNaughton, 1990, 1991) suggested that LTE is due to increased quantal size, and a report by Malinow and Tsien (1990), who concluded the opposite (i.e., an increase in quantal content of the excitatory postsynaptic potentials [EPSP]). In this chapter, the evidence and assumptions underlying both conclusions are critically evaluated and hypotheses are proposed that we hope will help to resolve the issue. The principle suggestion is that *both sets of conclusions are essentially correct*. As the detailed reports of both groups have been published, they are reviewed only briefly here. (In the following discussion, MT refers to the Malinow and Tsien study and FM refers to our own.)

The FM study was conducted in two phases. First, we used the method of simultaneous recording from synaptically coupled cells, using conventional sharp-electrode intracellular recording in current clamp mode. The presynaptic member cell was located in CA3, and the postsynaptic one in CA1. Such studies are technically difficult, and the yield of successful dual impalements held long enough to complete the LTE protocol was too low for any statistically reliable conclusion to be drawn; however, these studies did provide an essential control for the techniques employed in phase 2. In this technique, finely controlled, very weak electrical stimulation was applied to the afferent fibers. At first, the stimulus was set below threshold for any response, as determined by an on-line average of 30 or more responses. The stimulus was then adjusted in small steps to the point at which a very small EPSP was detected in the on-line average. Earlier studies on the dentate gyrus (McNaughton et al., 1981) had shown that a steplike transition from no response to a small average response could be detected in this manner, at which point it was assumed that a single fiber projecting to the recorded cell was being activated. In the present studies, very close correspondence was obtained between the average unitary EPSPs using dual recording, and those obtained with minimal stimulation on a substantially larger population of cells (table 7.1). Thus, we are confident that multifiber responses contributed negligibly to our results.

To ensure that the methods of quantal analysis were sensitive and reliable enough to discriminate changes in the quantal content of the EPSP from changes in quantal size, FM used pairs of test stimuli separated by 50 milliseconds, delivered once every 5 seconds. At this interval, there is an increase in the statistical probability (p) of quantal release from those release sites that are in a "loaded" or releasable state (n). Under conditions of low resting release probability, in which few loaded sites are actually used up on a given trial, this results in an average increase in EPSP quantal content on the second response of a pair; a process known as presynaptic facilitation. As p increases, the relative facilitation becomes masked by a net depression due to the slow recovery of the full complement of loaded sites. It had previously been shown that, whereas depression increases during post-tetanic potentiation (PTP), there is no change during LTE. Thus, LTE does not involve a change in the formal probability parameter (McNaughton, 1982). It remained possible, however, that the number of release sites was increased following LTE induction. The strategy was thus to show first that the methods could detect the expected increase in mean quantal content (i.e., the np product) during facilitation, and then determine whether EPSP changes of comparable magnitude during LTE would also be associated with increased quantal content.

To induce LTE, FM used the "cooperativity" method (McNaughton et al., 1978), in which large numbers of afferents are synchronously activated at high frequency. The FM studies were carried out on fully adult rats, and all data sets were accepted for analysis for which LTE was observed in the population response to multifiber stimulation. Three relatively independent methods were used to estimate quantal parameters: the method of failures, the coefficient of variation, and noise deconvolution using the assumption that transmitter release conforms approximately to a binomial process. These methods are discussed at length in the following sections. All led to the same general conclusions.

We found that during paired-pulse facilitation quantal content (m) significantly increased. Afer LTE induction, however, there was no significant change in m. Quantal size (q) was significantly increased.

The MT study employed the same minimal stimulation technique to attempt to activate single afferent fibers, and the recently developed

Table 7.1 Summary of the quantal analysis results of Foster and McNaughton (1990). Column 1 shows the quantal parameters obtained from the dual impalement method using CA3–CA1 cell pairs. The subsequent three pairs of columns (i.e., 2–3, 4–5, 6–7) give parameters for "minimal stimulation" paired-pulse studies (50-millisecond pulse interval) for the baseline period, 5–20 minutes post-LTE and 20–40 minutes post-LTE respectively. Note the close agreement between the parameters for cell pairs and minimal stimulation, as well as that measures related to quantal release increase during facilitation (t_0 vs. t_{50}), whereas measures related to quantal size increase following LTE (columns 2–3 vs. 4–5 and 6–7). Complete statistical details can be found in Foster and McNaughton (1991).

	1 CA3–CA1 Pairs	2 Minimal Stim Baseline t_0	3 Minimal Stim Baseline t_{50}	4 Minimal Stim LTE 20 min t_0	5 Minimal Stim LTE 20 min t_{50}	6 Minimal Stim LTE 40 min t_0	7 Minimal Stim LTE 40 min t_{50}
EPSP (μV)	264 (60) 72–674	290 (32) 101–751	474 (38) 198–1181	371 (33) 81–1004	580 (62) 136–1833	386 (37) 67–760	586 (67) 135–1529
q opt (μV)	220 (18) 141–350	245 (15) 88–398	258 (15) 77–407	301 (20) 98–553	298 (18) 122–512	323 (23) 98–560	326 (23) 120–580
m_{opt}	1.18 (0.17) 0.51–2.04	1.30 (0.09) 0.43–2.70	1.96 (0.12) 0.68–3.9	1.36 (0.09) 0.36–2.70	1.99 (0.14) 0.75–4.65	1.25 (0.10) 0.32–2.92	1.86 (0.14) 0.68–3.68
n_{opt}	3.8 (0.29) 2–5	5.28 (0.3) 2–9	6.03 (0.39) 3–11	5.47 (0.46) 2–12	4.49 (0.22) 2–8	5.28 (0.47) 2–11	4.62 (0.21) 2–7
p_{opt}	0.29 (0.03) 0.17–0.46	0.24 (0.01) 0.09–0.43	0.34 (0.02) 0.15–0.61	0.26 (0.02) 0.11–0.60	0.42 (0.02) 0.23–0.61	0.26 (0.03) 0.09–0.66	0.38 (0.10) 0.21–0.60
q fall (μV)	227 (33) 136–485	231 (27) 71–460	216 (17) 71–460	265 (17) 99–544	248 (18) 115–447	301 (27) 88–583	307 (37) 125–565
m_{fall}	1.09 (0.16) 0.52–2.08	1.38 (0.11) 0.45–2.57	2.04 (0.12) 0.69–2.92	1.40 (0.11) 0.29–2.93	2.01 (0.13) 0.75–2.94	1.37 (0.15) 0.25–2.94	1.79 (0.15) 0.96–2.96
q_{cv} (μV)	183 (19) 89–296	161 (16) 8–390	126 (14) 26–380	230 (38) 27–1261	208 (53) 27–1791	255 (44) 45–1112	211 (35) 11–813
m_{cv}	1.38 (0.22) 0.49–2.58	2.83 (0.51) 0.56–16.31	4.66 (0.39) 0.73–10.25	2.62 (0.45) 0.13–14.65	5.07 (0.66) 0.10–17.27	2.31 (0.33) 0.38–6.25	3.95 (0.60) 1.14–13.10

technique of whole-cell patch clamping. Because of the low resistance electrodes and tight seal between cell and electrode, this method substantially reduces recording noise, and permits large currents to be applied in voltage clamp mode. Malinow and Tsien exploited the latter property to induce LTE without convergent input by pairing single fiber stimulation with intense postsynaptic depolarization. Their experiments were conducted on infant rats, 3 to 5 weeks old. For analysis, they used only the coefficient of variation method. Their main result was that there was a large increase in estimated mean quantal content; however, this increase only accounted for about one-half of their average EPSP growth. They suggested that the residual change might be postsynaptic.

QUANTAL ANALYSIS: METHODS, ASSUMPTIONS, PROBLEMS, AND UTILITY

As with most synapses, hippocampal neurotransmission fluctuates in apparently discrete steps (del Castillo and Katz, 1954; Kuno, 1971; McNaughton et al., 1981; Sayer et al., 1989; Friedlander et al., 1990). In many systems this fluctuation is adequately characterized by the stochastic equation:

$$V = qm = q(np)$$

where V is the average synaptic potential, q is the postsynaptic potential generated by a single quantum, and m is the mean number of quantal units observed per response. The variable m can be further broken down into the product of n, the number of "sites" or statistically independent, equivalent physical entities that *could* possibly contribute to the composite response, and p, the probability that an individual entity *will* contribute on any given trial. The physical bases of these phenomenological parameters are not completely understood, and indeed, there clearly are cases in which more complex expressions must be assumed. It is generally agreed, however, that n and p are expressions of presynaptic processes controlling the release of neurotransmitter, whereas q is a composite presynaptic and postsynaptic parameter reflecting how much transmitter is released per quantum as well as the sensitivity of the postsynaptic membrane and various other postsynaptic biophysical parameters.

Whereas there is little question that evoked release of neurotransmitter occurs from discrete sites on the nerve terminal in the form of packets or "quanta" of (more or less) the same amplitude, the physical bases of these empirical observations and the resulting statistics of the observed response distributions have been subjects of intense experimental and theoretical effort for many years. Much of this effort has concentrated on determining whether the release process is adequately described by a simple binomial distribution in which there are n release sites, each with the same independent probability of releasing a quantum of a fixed amount of transmitter, each of which interacts with the postsynaptic membrane independently with the same effectiveness q. If all of these assumptions were correct, and if recording technology permitted noiseless collection of data in sufficient quantity, the issue over the mechanism of LTE expression might have been resolved years ago. Unfortunately, the assumptions are almost certainly incorrect to some generally unknown degree, recording is inherently noisy, and experimental preparations drift, thus precluding easy collection of very large stationary samples. Herein lies at least one major source of the controversy. These assumptions are fulfilled to a close approximation at preparations such as neuromuscular junctions or squid giant synapses, which have the additional advantage of sufficiently low noise that spontaneous quantal release events (miniature endplate potentials, or MEPPs) can be measured with sufficient accuracy to show unambiguously the distribution of quantal sizes. At such synapses, release is approximately binomial. (See Korn and Faber, 1987, for an overview of these and other pertinent issues.) All that is generally available in experiments on central neurons, however, is a noisy distribution of observed EPSP sizes, in which individual peaks are seldom obvious, and a distribution of noise in the absence of evoked signal.

Noise Deconvolution

A powerful statistical technique known as "noise deconvolution" has been developed for removing the effects of background noise (Edwards et al., 1976; Korn et al., 1982), thus permitting an assessment of whether this simple statistical model adequately accounts for the observed response variation, and what the values of the individual parameters are.

Let the observed distribution of response sizes be $r(v)$ and the noise distribution be $n(v)$. One is interested in recovering the distribution of actual EPSP or "signal" sizes $s(v)$, and, from this distribution, making inferences about the underlying probability distribution, $p(v)$, that would be obtained with an infinite sample. The response distribution is a convolution of the signal and noise distributions. Mathematical convolution of two functions is equivalent to flipping one function about the zero axis, sliding the flipped function past the other in small steps, and taking the product of the two functions at each step. This series of operations can be thought of as a "blurring" of the image $s(v)$ by a blurring function, $n(v)$, to produce a blurred image, $r(v)$. Thus, the presumably discrete peaks of the probability distribution are smeared out so that the final observed distribution represents a sum of Gaussians whose standard deviations all equal the noise SD (assuming no intrinsic variance in q), and whose amplitudes are approximately proportional to the respective probabilities.

A number of related methods have been developed in an attempt to deconvolve $n(v)$ (which can be measured reasonably accurately and is usually approximately Gaussian) from $r(v)$ to obtain $s(v)$ (Edwards et al., 1976; Wong and Redman, 1980; Jack et al., 1981; Korn et al., 1982; Redman and Walmsley, 1983). All of these methods to date involve some assumptions about the nature of $s(v)$. In particular, $s(v)$ is always assumed to be discrete (meaning that there is no variance in quantal size at a given site), quanta are assumed not to interact, the number of sites and their release probabilities are assumed to be constant, and it is assumed that the noise, $n(v)$, does not affect the size of the EPSP itself, but only adds linearly to the measurement. To the extent that the foregoing assumptions are correct, it has been possible in a few cases to obtain reasonably reliable estimates of the (assumed) discrete probability distributions which underlie the response histograms (Sayer et al., 1989, 1990), without making the additional strong assumption of a binomial process (i.e., one with uniformity of release probability and quantal size across release sites). In these cases, the deconvolved distributions do not differ substantially from the predictions of a simple binomial model. A similar conclusion was obtained using the unconstrained deconvolution at another vertebrate central synapse (Korn and Faber, 1987). It should also be pointed out that, even if quantal sizes and release probabilities were not *exactly* uniform across release sites, the final distribution would approximate a binomial distribution, provided that the variance in these parameters was relatively small compared to the mean across sites. Note, however, that there are cases in which the binomial assumption is clearly inappropriate. This situation can occur, for example, if either the postsynaptic receptors or the membrane potential is saturated by single quanta (Edwards et al., 1976; Jack et al., 1981; Hirst et al., 1981), or if there were spatial or temporal fluctuations in release probabilities or number of sites (Brown et al., 1976). In the former case, neither changes in number of quanta released, nor changes in the amount of transmitter contained in a quantum would increase the EPSP. However, changes in release probabilities or number of sites would lead to a decrease in failure rate in either case. As discussed in the following section, hippocampal synapses appear to exhibit substantial numbers of failures, and the failure rate goes down under conditions known to increase m, whereas it does not change after LTE induction.

The foregoing provides reasonable justification for the a priori assumption, which FM and others have made, that release follows approximately binomial statistics at these synapses, at least in the adult. The advantage of making this assumption is that there are substantially fewer free parameters in the statistical model (especially if p is fairly small so that the Poisson approximation is applicable). Hence *reasonably* reliable estimates of the parameters can be obtained using a substantially smaller sample size. The word "reasonably" is emphasized because there is an important sense in which the reliability of the parameter estimates for a single experiment is irrelevant to the question at hand (although it clearly is relevant for other questions). In a sufficiently large sample, the means of the noisy estimates of quantal size q and mean quantal content m from individual cases will converge on the *population mean* of these parameters. The FM minimal stimulation results indicate that the errors of the estimates, although clearly substantial, nevertheless are small enough to resolve statistically significant changes in these parameters in a sample of approximately 30 experiments. We find that m increases significantly during facilitation, by an amount sufficient to account for the increase of the EPSP. On the contrary, during LTE, we find no change in the average m, but a significant change in the mean of the estimate of q, sufficient to account for the observed long-term EPSP enhancement. We make no assumptions concerning the reliability of the estimates for individual cases, which, incidentally, is why we have declined to draw any conclusions from the outcome of the few successful dual impalement experiments in which LTE was attempted. Such conclusions would have been unreliable without substantially larger samples, which were unobtainable for technical reasons.

The Method of Failures

Irrespective of the form of the underlying probability distribution, there exists, by definition, a finite probability that on some trials there will be failures of release. In the case of the binomial distribution this is $(1 - p)^n$. If p is small and n is large, the Poisson approximation holds, in which case the probability of failure is e^{-m}. Thus, in principle, by counting failures one should be able to determine whether the np product m has changed. The same *general* consideration applies for *any arbitrary discrete probability distribution*. Any change in the failure rate implies a change in either the number of sites or one or more of the associated probabilities. Two problems arise. First, when the probability of failures is relatively small, large samples are needed for the observed failure rate to approximate the theoretical value. Several independent analyses suggest that p is small enough for the observation of substantial numbers of failures at hippocampal synapses (McNaughton et al., 1981; McNaughton, 1982; Sayer et al., 1990). Second, when noise is introduced, the proportion of *actual* release events associated with negative or zero amplitude measurements increases with the standard deviation of the noise, and decreases with quantal size. Thus, noise causes the mean quantal content to be underestimated because some release events will be counted as failures. Therefore, reductions in the apparent failure rate do not, in themselves, provide unambiguous evidence for an increase in m, because increases in q will inevitably reduce the number of spuriously counted failures. This is particularly true if the ratio of quantal size to noise standard deviation is low. On the other hand, if the mean unitary EPSP increases significantly in a set of experiments, with no significant reduction in apparent failures, this can be taken as good prima facie evidence both that q has in fact increased and that the ratio of quantal size to noise variance is actually large enough that spurious failures make up a relatively small proportion of actual failures. FM observed a significant change in mean EPSP during LTE, with no change in apparent failures (counted as twice the total of responses less than or equal to zero). In contrast, during facilitation, failures decreased significantly.

Assuming that binomial conditions hold, and that p is quite small, the mean quantal content can be estimated from the proportion of failures using the Poisson approximation; however, this measure, called m_f, increasingly overestimates m as p increases. The error is about 40% at $p = 0.5$, and becomes infinite as p approaches 1. Sayer and associates (1990) found a p of approximately 0.27 for their successful unconstrained deconvolution case. Our average from binomial deconvolution was 0.23, and the individual np products were highly consistent with the results from the failures method. During facilitation, m_f increased significantly, although proportionally less than the increase in the EPSP, as would be expected if the binomial p were on the order of approximately 0.3 or less and *some* of the apparent failures were spurious effects of the added recording noise.

Coefficient of Variation Method

For the Poisson approximation to the binomial distribution (valid for small p), the mean $m = np$ and variance s^2 are equal. If one first subtracts the variance due to recording noise from the EPSP variance, the residual variance should estimate the product of the variance of the probability distribution and the square of the quantal size. The observed mean EPSP (V) estimates the product of the quantal size and m. Squaring and dividing by the residual variance one obtains:

$$V^2/S^2 = m^2q^2/s^2q^2 = m^2/s^2 = m \text{ (since } m = s^2\text{)}$$

This estimate of mean quantal content is commonly designated m_{cv} because it is based on the squared reciprocal of the coefficient of variation (S/V). For a binomial process, m_{cv} substantially overestimates m for low n and large p. For p, the overestimate is nonlinear, accelerating with increased p. At perforant path synapses, synaptic depression during repetitive activation as well as reduced responses in low calcium media are both associated with reductions in m_{cv} values (McNaughton et al., 1981). In the FM study, there was a large and significant increase in m_{cv} during facilitation. Indeed, as expected from the nonlinear relation effect of increased p, the increase in m_{cv} was appreciably greater than the actual facilitation of the EPSP. This resulted in a spurious *decrease* in the corresponding estimate of quantal size during facilitation. During LTE, however, there was no increase in m_{cv}, the EPSP growth being adequately accounted for by increased q.

MT found a substantial increase in m_{cv} after LTE induction; however, this accounted for only about one-half of the average EPSP growth. The possibility that the residual increase was a result of increased quantal size was acknowledged by MT. They also carried out an important control experiment in which they applied a dose of the glutamate receptor antagonist CNQX and showed that the reduced EPSP that resulted was not associated with a reduction of m_{cv}. Thus, a presumably purely postsynaptic manipulation had no effect on this measure. The inference was that their increased m_{cv} must therefore be a presynaptic effect.

CAVEATS AND QUIBBLES

Throwing Out the Baby with the Bathwater

In both MT and an earlier study by Voronin (1988), a questionable procedure was used to select the data for inclusion in the overall analysis. Only those cases were analyzed for which the mean unitary EPSP exhibited an increase after the LTE induction treatment. At first this selection procedure might seem reasonable: in an experiment designed to elucidate the mechanism of LTE expression, why would one want to include data in which there is *apparently* no LTE? The logical flaw resides in there being essentially two factors that control synaptic efficacy, m and q. Suppose that, for whatever reason, the measure that does *not* underlie LTE is subject to large, random fluctuations during the experiment. Some of these fluctuations may be large enough to obscure the more moderate effect of LTE induction on the other parameter, so that the net EPSP appears smaller, or unchanged. This selection procedure will result in a spurious conclusion that the fluctuating parameter underlies LTE. Indeed, when FM reanalyzed their data using this procedure, a significant increase in m was observed. Suspiciously, however, the same reduced data set also showed a reduction in paired-pulse facilitation during LTE, much as occurs during PTP. This effect does not occur in population studies (McNaughton, 1982; Zalutsky and Nicoll, 1990), which suggests that fluctuations in resting release probability are the major source of the spontaneous variation in m during such experiments.

According to their report, MT excluded only 4 of 18 experiments in this fashion. It thus seems unlikely that this selection bias could have accounted for the entire effect; however, it has already been pointed out that only about one-half of the EPSP growth was accounted for by increased m_{cv} in the first place. Inclusion of the rejected data could conceivably tilt the balance of the predominant effect to an increase in q.

Is Anybody Listening?

At face value, an increase in m_{cv} appears to lead to the conclusion that presynaptic mechanisms are at work. The validity of such a conclusion based on m_{cv}, however, depends rather heavily on at least one component of the binomial assumption (or its Poisson approximation): that quantal size is roughly constant across release sites. Consider the extreme case in which the postsynaptic membrane opposite some release sites contains no receptors in the naive state: the release sites merely dump transmitter vainly into an empty cleft. Addition of receptors during LTE induction would lead to an apparent increase in m by all three analysis methods. The same general spurious result would be obtained if the distribution of quantal sizes across different release sites were highly skewed before LTE induction, and became more Gaussian following induction. The reduction in variance would cause m_{cv} to increase. This factor may be of considerable importance given the observation by Bekkers and coworkers (1990) that, *in developing tissue*, quantal sizes at a single release site appear to be highly variable, with a highly positively skewed distribution. Judging from the noise deconvolution results of Sayer and associates (1989), the distribution of quantal sizes appears to be more normal in adult tissue.

Garbage In, Garbage Out?

A simple (minded) resolution to the controversy would be to conclude that one or the other of the conclusions of MT and FM is simply incorrect. One can invent reasons why this might be the case. For example, it is clear that noise is a severe problem with the conventional recording technique used by FM, and one might be inclined to favor MT's results for this reason; however, the price of such a conclusion would be the necessity of formulating some rather ad hoc arguments as to why the methods appear to give the correct answer in the case of facilitation.

On the other hand, the whole-cell recording method is not without its problems, not the least of which is the introduction of foreign substances into the postsynaptic neuron. In fact, MT do comment on LTE induction's being only possible for a short period after patch formation, even though LTE that is induced during this time is apparently maintained. The argument in this case would have to be that the foreign substances induce the expression of a mechanism that does not occur under normal conditions. Indeed, one aspect of MT's data does appear to be rather unusual: the magnitude of the reported LTE is far in excess, by a factor of about five, of that usually reported from either in vitro or in vivo experiments. Actually, this extreme enhancement is one of the most exciting components of MT's results, because it suggests that a much wider dynamic range of synaptic efficacy is possible than hitherto suspected. Thus, recourse to the strong version of the "artifact" argument would appear to be both risky and theoretically unattractive; however, the possibility that a weaker version might contribute to the discrepancy is considered in the following section.

Which Came First, the Chicken or the Egg?

I have already alluded to the possibility that, under some circumstances, "receptor-free" transmitter release sites might exist. The activity-induced addition of receptors to these sites under some conditions, but not others, might account for part of the apparent discrepancy. Let us now inquire as to what these conditions might be. In my own view, there are two prime candidates. The first possible reason for the discrepancy arises because MT used neonatal (3- to 5-week-old) rat pups, whereas FM used fully adult animals. The second possibility arises because the whole-cell recording technique may enable sufficient currents to be passed to permit much more effective depolarization of the immediate postsynaptic sites than is obtained with the "cooperativity" method and conventional recording, particularly in the absence of GABA blockers. First I discuss the developmental hypothesis.

The postnatal period around 3 weeks of age is critical in the development of the hippocampus. Except for the fascia dentata, in which neurogenesis continues well beyond this period (Altman and Das, 1965), most hippocampal neurons are in place at this time. Synaptogenesis, however, is still actively in progress (Crain et al., 1973; Loy, 1980; Schwartzkroin, 1982), and the expression of some form of electrically induced LTE is, in fact, supernormal, with a peak somewhere in the interval between 2 and approximately 5 weeks (Harris and Teyler, 1984). The behavioral data also strongly attest to the importance of this developmental epoch for hippocampally dependent behaviors such as exploration (File, 1978) and spatial learning capacity (Rudy et al., 1987). Thus, it might come as no surprise if there were differences in LTE expression mechanisms that were specially suited to this critical developmental window.

Concerning the role of depolarization, most theories of distributed information storage have called for economical use of modifiable synapses (Marr, 1971; McNaughton and Nadel, 1990). Thus, it should also not be surprising if the full expression of the LTE process required the intense depolarization that may be experimentally achievable only with the whole-cell technique.

THESIS, ANTITHESIS, SYNTHESIS: A TWO-COMPONENT PROCESS

What the foregoing has been leading to is the proposal, by no means a novel one (Davies et al., 1989; Racine et al., 1983), that there are two mechanisms of LTE expression. The current debate may have clarified the nature of these mechanisms, and lead one to the suggestion that the appropriate definition of these processes should be LTE_n and LTE_q. The former process hypothetically involves the addition of new transmitter release sites to the presynaptic membrane, and the latter involves the addition of postsynaptic receptors. Possibly, LTE_n may have both a different developmental time course from LTE_q, as well as a different "cooperativity" threshold for activation. A possible scenario is illustrated in figures 7.1 and 7.2.

The hypothesis of a two-component process involving independently variable presynaptic and postsynaptic components has several attractive properties from the perspective of neural computation and memory formation. A number of models call for "fast" and "slow" weight changes with a multiplicative relationship, which is embodied in the present hypothesis. As pointed out elsewhere (McNaughton and Nadel, 1990), the ability to form new release sites between cells where none existed means that the hypothetical distributed memory network is effectively much less sparsely connected than one must assume on the basis of existing morphological synapses. This would solve a serious information storage capacity limitation, which is otherwise difficult to avoid in present models. It is also likely that other regions of the nervous system might

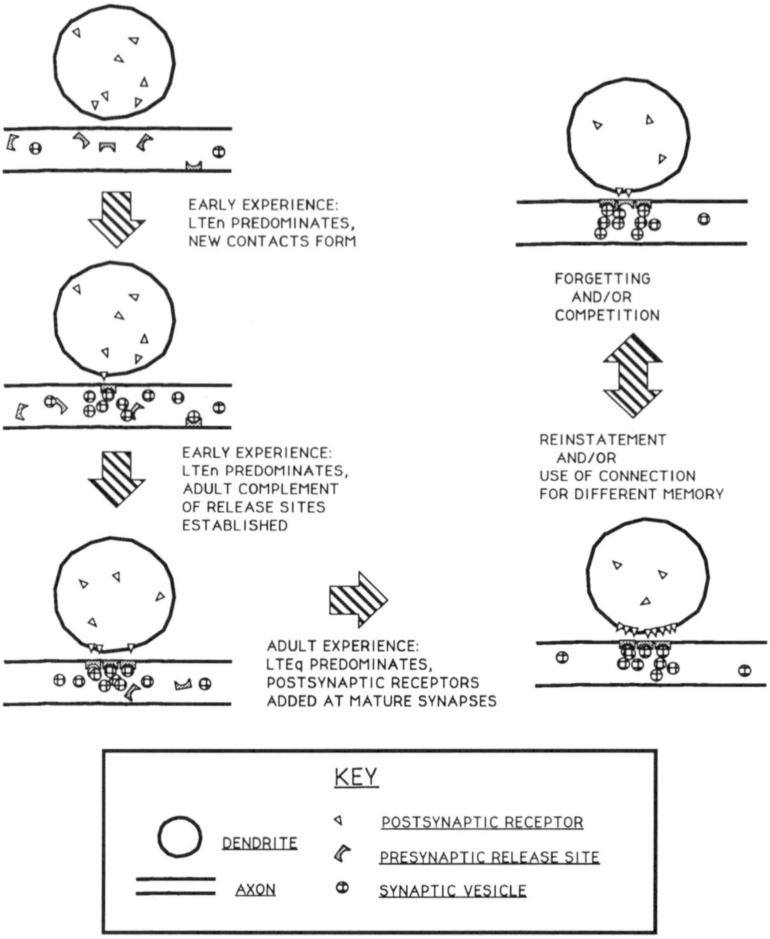

Figure 7.1 Two hypothetical mechanisms for LTE expression, LTE_n and LTE_q. Presumably, synaptogenesis in early postnatal development requires both the addition of new release sites (LTE_n) as well as the addition of new receptors (LTE_q). After development is complete, which may take several months, it is assumed that the capacity for LTE_n expression subsides, whereas that for LTE_q reaches asymptote and persists.

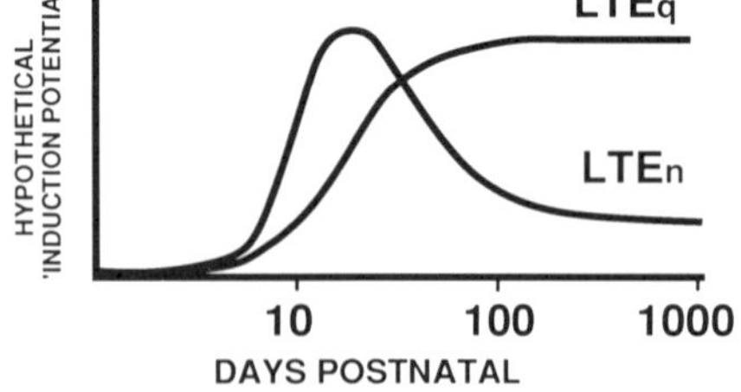

Figure 7.2 Hypothetical developmental timecourse for LTE_n and LTE_q. Note logarithmic time scale.

exploit different balances of these two processes for different purposes, such as the activity-dependent establishment of terminal segregation in visual and other cortical systems. Finally, the possibility has yet to be ruled out that some of the increase in m_{cv} observed by MT is due to long-lasting changes in the formal release parameter p, which may be inducible early but not late in development, possibly through changes in presynaptic calcium dynamics. Unfortunately, the necessary paired-pulse tests were not included in the MT design. These considerations, in conjunction with the recent fascinating results of Zalutsky and Nicoll (1990) on the mossy fiber system, suggest that we must keep open the possibilities that there may be not only an LTE_n and an LTE_q, but also an LTP.

ACKNOWLEDGMENTS

This work was supported by a grant from the National Science Foundation.

REFERENCES

Altman, J., and G. Das (1965). Autoradiographic and histological evidence of post-natal hippocampal neurogenesis in rats. *Journal of Comparative Neurology* 124:319–336.

Bekkers, J. M., G. B. Richerson, and C. F. Stevens (1990). Origin of variability in quantal size in cultured hippocampal neurons and hippocampal slices. *Proceedings of the National Academy of Science USA* 87:5359–5362.

Bliss, T. V. P., and M. A. Lynch (1988). Long-term potentiation of synaptic transmission in the hippocampus: Properties and mechanisms. In P. Landfield and S. Deadwyler (eds.), *Long-Term Potentiation: From Biophysics to Behavior.* New York: Alan R. Liss, pp. 3–72.

Brown, T. H., D. H. Perkel, and M. W. Feldman (1976). Evoked neurotransmitter release: statistical effects of nonuniformity and nonstationarity. *Proceedings of the National Academy of Science USA* 73:2913–2917.

Collingridge, G. L., S. J. Kehil, and H. McLennan (1983). Excitatory amino acids in synaptic transmission in the Schaffer collateral-commissural pathway of the rat hippocampus. *Journal of Physiology* (London) 334:33–46.

Crain, B., C. W. Cotman, D. Taylor, and G. Lynch (1973). A quantitative electron microscopic study of synaptogenesis in the dentate gyrus of the rat. *Brain Research* 63:195–204.

Davies, S. N., R. A. J. Lester, K. G. Reymann, and G. L. Collingridge (1989). Temporally distinct pre- and postsynaptic mechanisms maintain long-term potentiation. *Nature* 338:500–503.

del Castillo, J., and B. Katz (1954). Statistical factors involved in neuromuscular facilitation and depression. *Journal of Physiology* (London) 124:574–585.

Douglas, R. M., G. V. Goddard, and M. Riives (1982). Inhibitory modulation of long-term potentiation: evidence for a postsynaptic locus of control. *Brain Research* 240:259–272.

Edwards, F. R., S. J. Redman, and B. Walmsley (1976). Statistical fluctuations in charge transfer at 1a synapses on spinal motorneurons. *Journal of Physiology* (London) 259:665–688.

File, S. E. (1978). The ontogeny of exploration in the rat; habituation and effects of handling. *Developmental Psychobiology* 11:321–328.

Foster, T. C., and B. L. McNaughton (1990). LTE in CA1 is associated with an increase in apparent quantal size. In L. R. Squire (ed.), *Symposium Medicum Hoechst 23: The Biology of Memory.* New York: Schattauer Verlag (in press).

Foster, T. C., and B. L. McNaughton (1991). Long-term synaptic enhancement in hippocampal field CA1 is due to increased quantal size, not quantal content. *Hippocampus* 1:79–91.

Friedlander, M. J., R. J. Sayer, and S. J. Redman (1990). Evaluation of long-term potentiation of small compound and unitary EPSPs at the hippocampal CA3–CA1 synapse. *Journal of Neuroscience* 10:814–825.

Gustafsson, B., H. Wigström, W. C. Abraham, and Y.-Y. Huang (1987). Long-term potentiation in the hippocampus using depolarizing current pulses as the conditioning stimulus for single volley synaptic potentials. *Journal of Neuroscience* 7:774–780.

Harris, E. W., A. H. Ganong, and C. W. Cotman (1984). Long-term potentiation in the hippocampus involves activation of *N*-methyl-D-aspartate receptors. *Brain Research* 323:132–137.

Harris, K. M., and T. J. Teyler (1984). Developmental onset of long-term potentiation in area CA1 of the rat hippocampus. *Journal of Physiology* (London) 346:27–48.

Hirst, G. D. S., S. J. Redman, and K. Wong (1981). Post-tetanic potentiation and facilitation of synaptic potentials evoked in cat spinal motorneurones. *Journal of Physiology* (London) 321:97–109.

Jack, J. J. B., S. J. Redman, and K. Wong (1981). The components of synaptic potentials evoked in cat spinal motoneurons by impulses in single group 1a afferents. *Journal of Physiology* (London) 321:65–96.

Kauer, J. A., R. C. Malenka, and R. A. Nicoll (1988). A persistent postsynaptic modification mediates long-term potentiation in the hippocampus. *Neuron* 1:911–917.

Korn, H., and D. S. Faber (1987). Regulation and significance of probabilistic release mechanisms at a central synapse. In G. E. Edelman, W. E. Gall, and W. M. Cowan (eds.), *Synaptic Function.* New York: Wiley and Sons, pp. 57–108.

Korn, H., A. Mallet, A. Triller, and D. S. Faber (1982). Transmission at a central synapse. II. Quantal description of release with a physical correlate of *n*. *Journal of Neurophysiology* 48:679–707.

Kuno, M. (1971). Quantum aspects of central and ganglionic synaptic transmission in vertebrates. *Physiology Review* 51:647–678.

Loy, R. (1980). Development of afferent lamination in Ammon's horn of the rat. *Anatomy and Embryology* 159:257–275.

Malinow, R., and R. W. Tsien (1990). Presynaptic changes revealed by whole-cell recordings of long-term potentiation in rat hippocampal slices. *Nature* 346:177–180.

Marr, D. (1971). Simple memory: a theory for archicortex. *Philosophical Transactions of the Royal Society of London B* 262:23–81.

McNaughton, B. L. (1982). Long-term synaptic enhancement and short-term potentiation in rat fascia dentata act through different mechanisms. *Journal of Physiology* (London) 324:249–262.

McNaughton, B. L., C. A. Barnes, and P. Andersen (1981). Synaptic efficacy and EPSP summation in granule cells of rat fascia dentata studied in vitro. *Journal of Neurophysiology* 46:952–966.

McNaughton, B. L., R. M. Douglas, and G. V. Goddard (1978). Synaptic enhancement in fascia dentata: cooperativity among coactive afferents. *Brain Research* 157:277–293.

McNaughton, B. L., and L. Nadel (1990). Hebb-Marr networks and the neurobiological representation of action in space. In M. A. Gluck and D. E. Rumelhart (eds.), *Neuroscience and Connectionist Theory.* New York: Lawrence Erlbaum, pp. 1–63.

Muller, D., and G. Lynch (1988). Long-term potentiation differentially affects two components of synaptic responses in hippocampus. *Proceedings of the National Academy of Science USA* 85:9346–9350.

Racine, R. J., N. W. Milgram, and S. Hafner (1983). Long-term potentiation phenomena in the rat limbic forebrain. *Brain Research* 260:217–231.

Redman, S., and B. Walmsley (1983). Amplitude fluctuations in synaptic potentials evoked in cat spinal motoneurones at identified group 1a synapses. *Journal of Physiology* 343:135–145.

Rudy, J. W., S. Stadler-Morris, and P. Albert (1987). Ontogeny of spatial navigation behaviors in the rat: dissociation of "proximal" and "distal" cue based behaviors. *Behavioral Neuroscience* 101:62–73.

Sayer, R. J., M. J. Friedlander, and S. J. Redman (1990). The time course and amplitude of EPSPs evoked at synapses between pairs of CA3/CA1 neurons in the hippocampal slice. *Journal of Neuroscience* 10:826–836.

Sayer, R. J., S. J. Redman, and P. Andersen (1989). Amplitude fluctuations in small EPSPs recorded from CA1 pyramidal cells in the guinea pig hippocampal slice. *Journal of Neuroscience* 9:840–850.

Schwartzkroin, P. A. (1982). Development of rabbit hippocampus physiology. *Developmental Brain Research* 2:469–486.

Voronin, L. L. (1988). Quantal analysis of long-term potentiation. In H. L. Haas and G. Buzsaki (eds.), *Synaptic Plasticity in the Hippocampus.* Berlin: Springer-Verlag, pp. 27–30.

Wong, K., and S. J. Redman (1980). The recovery of a random variable from a noisy record with application to the study of fluctuations in synaptic potentials. *Journal of Neuroscience Methods* 2:389–409.

Zalutsky, R. A., and R. A. Nicoll (1990). Comparison of two forms of long-term potentiation in single hippocampal neurons. *Science* 248:1619–1624.

8 Long-Term Potentiation: Biophysical and Biochemical Mechanisms

Roberto Malinow and Richard W. Tsien

It is widely believed that long-lasting changes in synaptic function provide the cellular basis for learning and memory in both vertebrates and invertebrates (Hebb, 1949; Eccles, 1953; Goelet et al., 1985; Alkon and Nelson, 1990). The most thoroughly characterized example of such synaptic plasticity in the mammalian nervous system is long-term potentiation (LTP). The remarkable feature of LTP is that a short burst of synaptic activity can trigger persistent enhancement of synaptic transmission lasting at least several hours, and possibly weeks or longer (Bliss and Gardner-Medwin, 1973). First found in the hippocampus (Lømo, 1966; Bliss and Lømo, 1973), this phenomenon has recently been described in areas of the mammalian CNS including the visual cortex (Artola and Singer, 1987) and motor cortex (Iriki et al., 1989). There is intense interest in understanding the cellular and molecular basis for this form of synaptic plasticity (Lynch and Baudry, 1984; Collingridge and Bliss, 1987; Bliss and Lynch, 1988; Nicoll et al., 1988; Stevens, 1989; Brown et al., 1988; Cotman et al., 1989; Kennedy, 1989; Malenka et al., 1989a).

Most studies on mechanisms of LTP have focused on synaptic transmission in the CA1 field of the hippocampus, at synapses between Schaffer collaterals and CA1 pyramidal cells, an area rich in *N*-methyl-D-aspartate (NMDA) receptors (Cotman et al., 1989) and Ca^{2+}-dependent protein kinases (Nishizuka, 1988; Kennedy, 1989). Induction of LTP requires a temporal conjunction of presynaptic transmitter release and postsynaptic depolarization (Gustafsson et al., 1987; Malinow and Miller, 1986; Collingridge and Bliss, 1987; Brown et al., 1988), a combination of events resembling that envisioned by Hebb (1949). It is generally agreed that these factors work together: glutamate to activate the NMDA-receptor channel and postsynaptic depolarization to free the channel from block by extracellular Mg^{2+} (Ascher and Nowak, 1988; Mayer and Westbrook, 1987). The NMDA receptor allows a significant Ca^{2+} influx (MacDermott et al., 1986) and increases $[Ca^{2+}]_i$ in postsynaptic spines (Regehr and Tank, 1990); the rise in $[Ca^{2+}]_i$ is necessary for LTP (Lynch et al., 1983; Malenka et al., 1988).

Many questions remain about what happens next. What is the mechanism of the long-lasting synaptic modification and its relationship to Ca^{2+}

signaling? Our work has been directed toward understanding the role of Ca^{2+}-dependent protein kinases and elucidating the nature of the persistent change. A key question is whether synaptic transmission is strengthened by increased transmitter release or enhanced postsynaptic receptivity. There is considerable controversy about this issue. Evidence in favor of a strictly postsynaptic mechanism for the expression of LTP has come from the groups of Gary Lynch (Müller et al., 1988) and Roger Nicoll (Kauer et al., 1988). Their results indicated that the expression of LTP was associated with a selective enhancement of the response of AMPA α-amino-3-hydroxy-5-methyl-4-isoxazole proprionate receptors, but not NMDA receptors. Thus, they concluded that the locus of expression must be postsynaptic. This conclusion is appealingly simple: if induction and expression of LTP are both localized within the postsynaptic spine, they could be linked by purely intracellular signaling mechanisms.

On the other hand, early evidence from Timothy Bliss and colleagues and others has provided support for enhancement of presynaptic release. Using a push-pull cannula system in vivo, Dolphin, Errington, and Bliss (1982) found evidence for increased release of ^{3}H-glutamate in the dentate gyrus in association with LTP, and proposed that presynaptic release was elevated (see also Skrede and Malthe-Sorenssen, 1981). However, Bliss and coworkers (1986) were careful to point out that some questions remain unanswered. Which type of cell is the source of the increase? Could the increased concentration of glutamate in the perfusate be due to decreased uptake? If presynaptic glutamate release is truly increased, is this evoked by action potentials or merely an increase in nonquantal leakage? What is the nature of the retrograde communication across the synaptic cleft that must be postulated to link postsynaptic induction and presynaptic expression? Having discussed these questions, Bliss and Lynch (1988), concluded that the available evidence provided "plausible though not conclusive reasons for attributing the enhanced release to an increase in the amount of transmitter released per action potential from potentiated terminals; it is probable that only a rigorous quantal analysis, not presently available, will finally settle the issue."

This chapter describes progress toward such analysis. A major obstacle to statistical analysis of synaptic variability has been the poor signal-to-noise ratio of conventional intracellular recordings (see Redman, 1990, for review). We have overcome this problem by applying the whole-cell voltage clamp technique to study synaptic transmission in conventional hippocampal slices (Malinow and Tsien, 1990a). We find that robust LTP can be recorded with much improved signal resolution and biochemical access to the postsynaptic cell. Prolonged dialysis of the postsynaptic cell blocks the triggering of LTP, with no effect on expression of LTP. The improved signal resolution unmasks a large trial-to-trial variability, reflecting the probabilistic nature of transmitter release. Changes in the synaptic variability and a decrease in the proportion of synaptic failures during LTP provide two lines of evidence to demonstrate that transmitter release is significantly enhanced (Malinow and Tsien, 1990a). These biophysical approaches are complemented by studies in which we explored mechanisms of LTP induction and expression and their localization by direct intracellular injection of protein kinase inhibitors into individual postsynaptic cells (Malinow et al., 1989).

EXPERIMENTAL STRATEGY AND METHODS

Transverse hippocampal slices (400–500 μm) were obtained from 3- to 5-week-old rats by standard methods (Alger and Nicoll, 1982). Slices were submerged and superfused continuously with a modified Earle's solution containing NaCl, 119 mM; KCl, 2.5 mM; $MgCl_2$, 1.3 mM; $CaCl_2$, 2.5 mM; NaH_2PO_4, 1.0 mM; $NaHCO_3$, 26.2 mM; glucose, 11 mM; and gassed with 95% O_2/5% CO_2 (pH 7.4) at room temperature (22°C). Picrotoxin (20 μM) was used to block inhibitory transmission; a cut was made between regions CA3 and CA1 to prevent epileptiform activity. Synaptic transmission was elicited with bipolar stainless steel stimulating electrodes at two locations; each electrode delivered a stimulus every 4 seconds; stimuli from the two electrodes were separated by 2 seconds. Excitatory postsynaptic potentials (EPSCs) were recorded with a patch electrode (3–7 MΩ tip resistance, no fire polishing or Sylgard coating) in the whole-cell mode (Axopatch 1D). Pipette solution contained Cs-gluconate, 100 mM; Ethylene glycol-bis(β-aminoethyl ether)N,N,N′,N′-tetraacetic acid (EGTA), 0.6 mM; $MgCl_2$, 5 mM; adenosine triphosphate (ATP), 2 mM; guanosine triphosphate (GTP), 0.3 mM; and 4-[2-Hydroxyethyl]-1-piperazine ethanesulfonic acid (HEPES), 40 mM (pH 7.2 with CsOH). Holding potential was kept constant at a level between −60 and −70 mV. EPSCs were amplified 50-fold to 500-fold, filtered at 1 KHz, digitized at 10 KHz, and stored. For a given experiment, EPSC amplitudes were determined by averaging the current over a 10- to 20-millisecond window at the peak response and subtracting a baseline estimate from the same record. A similar procedure was used to measure the background noise before the synaptic stimulation (Sayer et al., 1989).

RESULTS

Whole-Cell Recordings from Hippocampal Slices

We were able to make whole-cell voltage-clamp recordings from CA1 neurons in rat hippocampal slices without special procedures for exposing or cleaning the neurons (see also Barnes and Werblin, 1987; Coleman and Miller, 1989; Blanton et al., 1989). Positive pressure was applied to the recording pipette during penetration of the slice; high-resistance (1–5 GΩ) seals on cell bodies 2 to 3 cell diameters below the surface were then obtained by suction. After breaking into the cell, synaptic currents were elicited with bipolar stimulation electrodes placed in the stratum radiatum of CA1. Stable synaptic recordings could be maintained for as long as 10 hours. The input resistance was typically 100 to 200 MΩ in whole-cell recordings.

Whole-cell current recording offers better resolution than even the most favorable microelectrode recordings (Sayer et al., 1989; Redman, 1990; Foster and McNaughton, 1991). The low background noise of whole-cell recordings facilitated the study of small synaptic responses. In most experiments, we used minimal stimulation, only slightly stronger than the highest stimulus that gave only failures. Under these conditions, activation is thought to be restricted to a single synapse onto the monitored neuron (McNaughton et al., 1981; Foster and McNaughton, 1991). (This was supported by experiments in which a single CA3 neuron was directly stimulated by an intracellular microelectrode while simultaneously recording from a CA1 neuron [Malinow and Tsien, 1990b]). The resulting synaptic currents showed a large intertrial variability that was much greater than the background noise, but similar time courses (figures 8.1A,B), supporting the view that they originated from the same synapse. There were occasional clear failures (see figures 8.1A, 8.4A,B), and sporadic spontaneous events that resembled the elicited response, ranging in amplitude from less than 1 pA up to approximately 10 pA (see figure 8.1B, inset).

The average synaptic current for minimal stimulation was 6.7 pA in a representative series of 17 experiments. This is in reasonable agreement with estimates of synaptic current from minimal EPSPs recorded with high resistance microelectrodes if one allows for the measured input resistance in those experiments (Sayer et al., 1990; Foster and McNaughton, 1991).

Whole-Cell Recordings of LTP

To optimize the chances of obtaining LTP under whole-cell recording conditions, we used internal solutions with minimal Ca^{2+} buffering to avoid block of LTP, and with Cs^{+} as the main cation to enhance voltage control of the postsynaptic membrane. We also included ATP and GTP in the internal solution to allow activity of protein kinases or GTP-binding proteins. Following a stable baseline period of 10 to 15 minutes, we were able to induce LTP by pairing a steady postsynaptic depolarization to around 0 mV with continued activation of the test pathway (40 stimuli at 2 Hz). This pairing procedure resulted in LTP in 14 of 18 experiments (figures 8.1C, 8.3A, 8.4C). In contrast, no potentiation was found in transmission through a simultaneously monitored control pathway that did not receive presynaptic stimuli during the postsynaptic depolarization (see figures 8.1D, 8.3B). Furthermore, synaptic stimulation at 2 Hz without postsynaptic depolarization did not give synaptic enhancement ($n = 5$). Thus, the potentiation was synapse-specific and required a combination of presynaptic activity and postsynaptic depolarization, just as seen in conventional recordings of LTP.

To investigate whether diffusible cytoplasmic factors are involved in

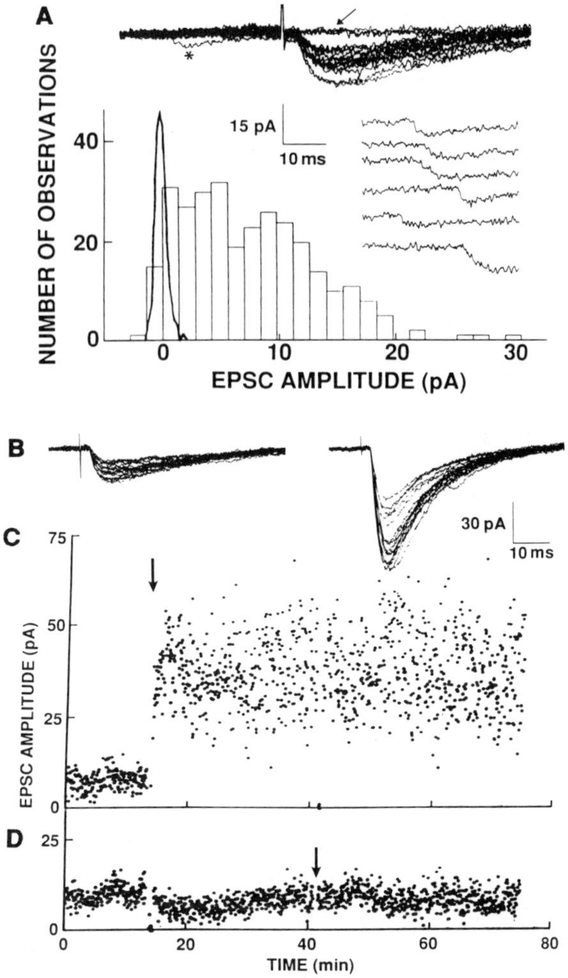

Figure 8.1 Whole-cell recordings of synaptic transmission in conventional hippocampal slices show large intertrial variability, synapse-specific LTP, and loss of induction but not expression with prolonged dialysis. (A) Sixteen consecutive records of synaptic currents, superimposed. Note spontaneous event in baseline period (*) and synaptic failures (arrow). (B) Amplitude distribution histograms for 200 consecutive synaptic currents (bars) and baseline noise (smooth curve). Bin sizes were 1.4 pA for EPSC and 0.14 pA for baseline noise. Inset: representative spontaneous synaptic currents. Note the variability in amplitude and time course but general similarity to evoked responses. (C,D) Plots of synaptic responses against time in a postsynaptic cell receiving two independent inputs. In C, LTP was selectively induced in one pathway by a pairing procedure 15 minutes following break-in (arrow); in the other pathway (D), the pairing procedure was applied 25 minutes later, but failed to induce LTP, in contrast to the maintenance of LTP in C. In the pairing procedure, the cell was depolarized from −70 mV to ~0 mV while the paired (conditioned) pathway was stimulated 40 times at 2 Hz with no change in stimulus strength. Nonconditioned pathway received no stimuli during the postsynaptic depolarization. Inset: families of consecutive current records showing EPSCs of conditioned pathway, collected before (left) and 30 minutes after pairing (right). (Reprinted by permission from R. Malinow and R. W. Tsien, *Nature*, vol. 346, pp. 177–180. Copyright © 1990 Macmillan Magazines Ltd.)

potentiation, we attempted to trigger LTP at different times after gaining whole-cell access (see figure 8.1C,D). Pairing soon after beginning whole-cell recording (approximately 20 minutes or less) consistently resulted in LTP lasting more than 1 hour (see figures 8.1, 8.3, 8.4). However, no potentiation was found with pairing more than 30 minutes after whole-cell access (6 of 7 experiments). One possibility is that some diffusible postsynaptic component is needed to trigger LTP, but not to maintain the potentiation.

Analysis of Presynaptic and Postsynaptic Factors

To understand the basis of the synaptic variability and its possible relation to fluctuations in transmitter release, we modified presynaptic or postsynaptic functions by changing the bathing medium (figure 8.2). Elevating $[Ca^{2+}]_o$ to increase presynaptic release enhanced the synaptic currents (see figure 8.2A). The amplitude histogram changed from a highly skewed distribution (see figure 8.2B) to a nearly symmetrical bell shape (see figure 8.2C). In contrast, when we added low concentrations of the glutamate receptor antagonist 6-cyano-7-nitroquinoxaline-2,3-dione (CNQX) to modify postsynaptic responsiveness, the average synaptic current was dramatically reduced but the shape of the distribution remained unchanged (see figure 8.2A,E). Thus, the distributions before and after CNQX matched closely when normalized by their means (see figure 8.2D). Similar results were obtained with CNQX at lower $[Ca^{2+}]_o$ (not shown).

To obtain a simple and revealing index of synaptic variability, we computed $CV^{-2} = M^2/\sigma^2$ where CV is the coefficient of variation, M is the mean synaptic current, and σ^2 is the variance about M, for a given epoch of consecutive responses from t to $t + \tau$. This kind of analysis has been applied to synaptic transmission in other systems (e.g., del Castillo and Katz, 1954; Martin, 1977). We can compute the expected behavior of M^2/σ^2 if we make assumptions regarding the mechanisms underlying synaptic transmission. In the simplified case of a binomial distribution of transmitter release, where p is the probability of release for each of N available quanta, v is the vesicular content, and z is the postsynaptic response to a fixed amount of transmitter,

$$M^2/\sigma^2 = (Npvz)^2/Np(1 - p)(vz)^2 = Np/(1 - p)$$

Thus, M^2/σ^2 is independent of changes in z and is a useful measure of some changes in presynaptic function, but not all factors (e.g., v). It increases in proportion to N, and at least linearly with p, as experimentally confirmed at the neuromuscular junction (del Castillo and Katz, 1954). The lack of dependence of M^2/σ^2 on the postsynaptic responsiveness (z), holds for more general cases as long as z does not vary from trial to trial within a given epoch (see Malinow and Tsien, 1990a).

Assuming that z is constant for an epoch, the theory predicts that changes in M^2/σ^2 between epochs will result from changes in release

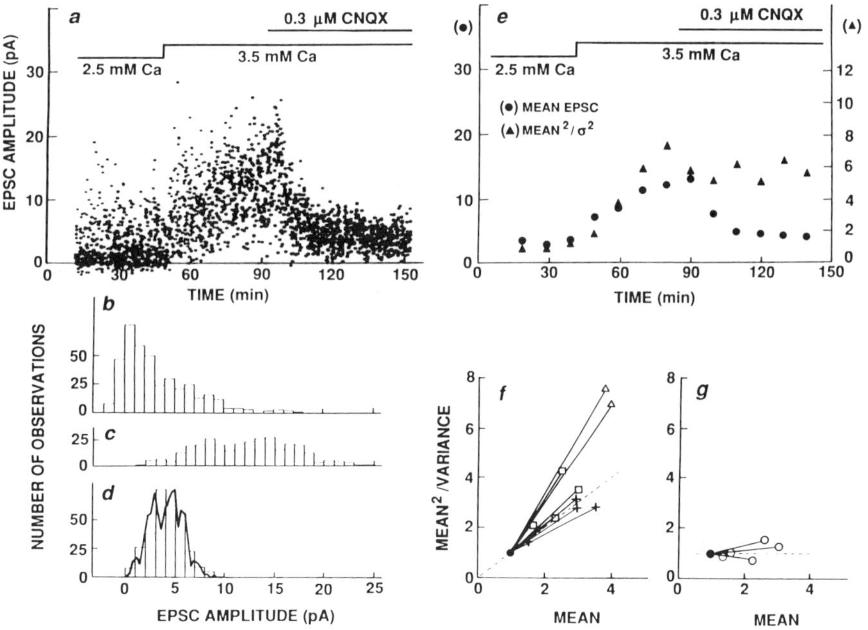

Figure 8.2 Selective changes in presynaptic and postsynaptic function produce expected changes in mean and variance of synaptic currents. Agents acting through presynaptic mechanisms affect shape of distribution histograms and M^2/σ^2 whereas inhibition of postsynaptic receptors does not. (A) EPSC amplitude plotted against time. Bathing calcium was elevated from 2.5 mM to 3.5 mM and 0.3 μM of CNQX was applied where shown. (B,C,D) Amplitude distribution histograms for (B) 300 EPSCs before manipulation, (C) after elevation of calcium, and (D) after subsequent addition of CNQX. Continuous line in D shows data from C, normalized to mean EPSC amplitude in D. Note close agreement of normalized histograms. (E) Plot of mean EPSC amplitude, M (circles), and M^2/σ^2 (triangles) for the experiment shown in A, with τ = 10 minutes (150 trials). (F) Plot of M^2/σ^2 against M for several presynaptic manipulations: calcium increased from 2.5 to 3.5 mM (triangles); magnesium decreased from 1.3 to 0.65 mM in the presence of 50 μM APV (squares); 10 μM 4-aminopyridine (diamonds); increased stimulus strength to recruit more fibers (cross). (G) Plot of M^2/σ^2 against M for experiments in which CNQX (0.2–0.3 μM) was bath applied. For each experiment in F and G, lines connect points obtained before and after manipulation; M and M^2/σ^2 were computed for 300 trials prior to the manipulation, and 300 trials at the peak of the effect, and normalized by the values corresponding to the smaller M for that experiment. Note that presynaptic manipulations that are thought to increase p affect M^2/σ^2 more than the mean, whereas increasing stimulus strength, which increases N, affects M^2/σ^2 as much as M. These findings are expected for a binomial release process, as explained in the text. (Reprinted by permission from R. Malinow and R. W. Tsien, *Nature*, vol. 346, pp. 177–180. Copyright © 1990 Macmillan Magazines Ltd.)

characteristics but not postsynaptic modifications. This was tested by examining changes in M^2/σ^2 following interventions known to affect presynaptic or postsynaptic mechanisms. As figure 8.2E illustrates, raising extracellular calcium dramatically increased M^2/σ^2. This was found for all experimental maneuvers expected to affect presynaptic release: lowering magnesium, application of 4-aminopyridine (not shown), or increasing the stimulus strength to recruit more afferent fibres (see figure 8.2F, n = 10). In general, M^2/σ^2 increased at least as much as the mean synaptic current. In contrast, addition of CNQX produced no significant change in M^2/σ^2, despite its large effect on synaptic transmission (n = 5; see figures 8.2E,G).

Changes During LTP

Does M^2/σ^2 change with LTP? Figure 8.3B compares M^2/σ^2 of the test pathway with that of the control (unpaired) pathway, for the 14 experiments showing potentiation of mean synaptic current (see figure 8.3A). Following pairing, M^2/σ^2 increased significantly in the test pathway, with no change in the control pathway. The increase in M^2/σ^2 with LTP could

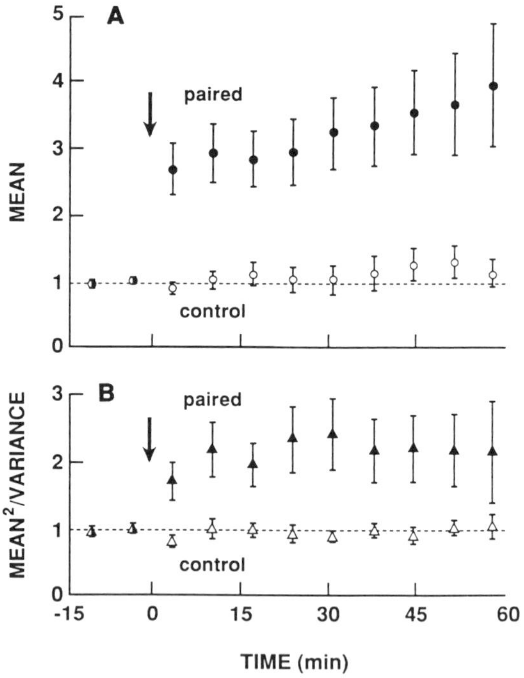

Figure 8.3 A synapse-specific increase in M^2/σ^2 associated with LTP. Results from the 14 of 18 experiments that showed LTP with pairing (in the other 4 experiments with no LTP, M^2/σ^2 remained unchanged; not shown). (A) Ensemble averages and SEMs of M for the paired pathway (filled circles) and the control pathway (open circles, n = 10; in 4 experiments this pathway was not monitored). Arrow marks time of pairing procedure (as in figures 8.1, 8.2). (B) Ensemble averages of M^2/σ^2 for paired (filled triangles) and nonpaired (open triangles) pathways for the same experiments as in A. (Reprinted by permission from R. Malinow and R. W. Tsien, *Nature*, vol. 346, pp. 177–180. Copyright © 1990 Macmillan Magazines Ltd.)

arise from various presynaptic mechanisms: an increase in the number of available vesicles; an increase in the probability of release of some or all vesicles; or changes in nonvesicular release. It would not be expected from uniform changes in the number, sensitivity, or conductance of glutamate receptor channels, or in the effectiveness of charge transfer from spines to dendrites.

If the expression of LTP involves an increased probability of release or a greater number of available quanta, one would expect fewer failures of transmission during LTP. Figure 8.4 illustrates an experiment in which failures and responses were clearly resolvable. The amplitude distribution histogram displayed a distinct peak at zero amplitude, which matched the amplitude distribution of the noise (figure 8.4, inset). The area under the zero amplitude peak was used to estimate the percentage of failures. In this experiment, the proportion of failures was 27% prior to pairing (see figure 8.4D), falling to 11% between 5 and 22 minutes after pairing (see figure 8.4E). This change accompanied a 2.8-fold increase in mean synaptic current from figure 8.4D to figure 8.4E. During a later epoch (from t = 40 to t = 57 minutes), the synaptic enhancement was 2.1-fold relative to control, and the proportion of failures was 15% (see figure 8.4F).

This decrease in the proportion of failures was a consistent finding. Figure 8.5 shows collected results from five experiments in which failures could be clearly resolved. Three of the recordings were obtained with minimal stimulation and two with intracellular microelectrode stimulation of a CA3 neuron (Malinow and Tsien, 1990b). The collected data from all five experiments showed a mean (±SEM) decrease in failures from 63 ± 11% in control to 17 ± 8% after pairing, consistent with a greater likelihood of transmitter release during LTP. This conclusion is supported by the overall amplitude distribution, which changes from a skewed shape in control (see figure 8.4D) to a bell shape during LTP (see figure 8.4E), as with increasing extracellular calcium (see figure 8.2B,C).

Changes in NMDA Receptor–Mediated Transmission Can Be Detected

If presynaptic transmitter release is enhanced, one might expect to find an increase in both the kainate/quisqualate–sensitive (KQ) and NMDA-sensitive components of the EPSP. The available evidence is not consistent. On one hand, Kauer and coworkers (1988) and Müller and Lynch (1988) found no significant increase in the NMDA component under conditions that normally produce LTP; thus, they concluded that the expression of LTP must be purely postsynaptic. On the other hand, Bashir and Collingridge (1990) have reported a significant potentiation of NMDA-mediated transmission under similar conditions.

We have looked for changes in the NMDA-sensitive component under conditions similar to those in our other experiments. To reveal the NMDA receptor component, the external $[Mg^{2+}]_o$ was lowered to 0.65 mM, the membrane potential was held near −60 mV, and KQ receptors were

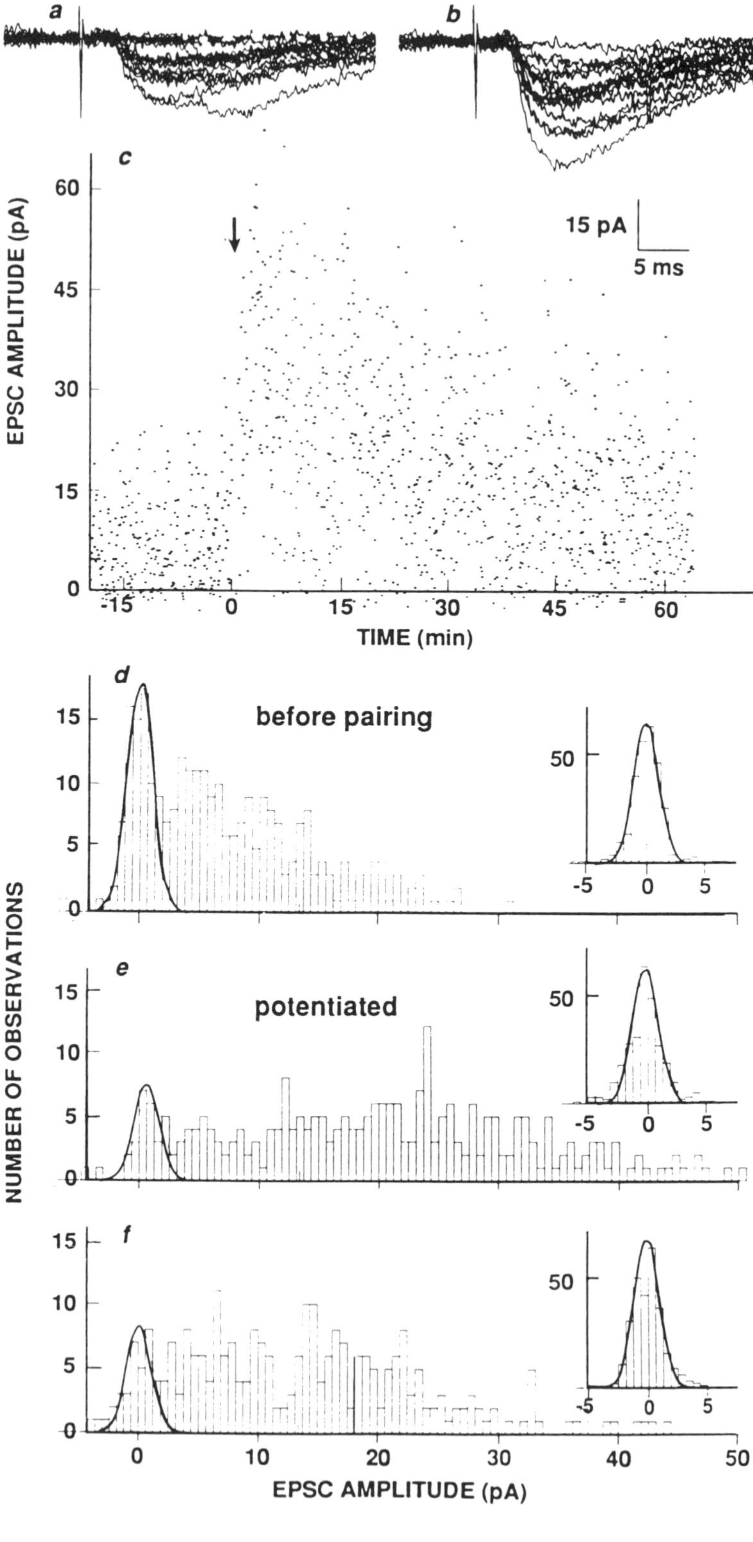
a
b
c
15 pA
5 ms
EPSC AMPLITUDE (pA)
60
45
30
15
0
-15
0
15
30
45
60
TIME (min)
d
before pairing
e
potentiated
f
NUMBER OF OBSERVATIONS
EPSC AMPLITUDE (pA)
0
10
20
30
40
50
-5
0
5

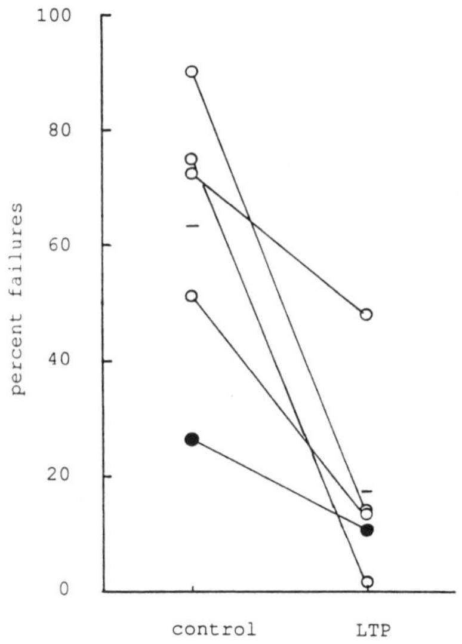

Figure 8.5 Consistent decrease in proportion of synaptic failures during LTP. Collected results from five experiments. Horizontal lines show mean percentage of failures (63 ± 11% in control before pairing, 17 ± 8% during LTP after pairing). Filled symbols show results from experiment illustrated in figure 8.4. The two experiments with the highest percentage of failures in control were recordings of one-to-one transmission from presynaptic CA3 neurons, stimulated with an intracellular microelectrode. (Data from Malinow and Tsien, 1990a.)

Figure 8.4 Decreases in the proportion of synaptic failures associated with LTP. (A,B) Groups of 16 consecutive EPSCs taken (A) before and (B) 40 minutes after a pairing procedure to induce LTP. (C) Amplitude of EPSCs elicited by minimal stimulation plotted against time. Arrow marks pairing procedure (see figure 8.1). (D,E) Amplitude distribution histograms for 17-minute epochs prior to pairing (D, from $t = -17$ to $t = 0$) and after pairing (E, from $t = 5$ to $t = 22$ minutes; F, from $t = 40$ to $t = 57$ minutes). Smooth curves are gaussians whose height was adjusted to fit the first peak in the amplitude distribution. The half-width of the gaussians, 2.5 pA, was obtained by fitting amplitude histograms of the baseline noise during the same epochs (insets). The proportion of failures was estimated as the area under the gaussian curve. (Reprinted by permission from R. Malinow and R. W. Tsien, *Nature,* vol. 346, pp. 177–180. Copyright © 1990 Macmillan Magazines Ltd.)

blocked by including 1 to 10 μM of CNQX in the superfusing solutions. Figure 8.6 shows a representative experiment (A) and collected results from nine recordings, obtained in the presence of 1 μM of CNQX (B). The results show a clear and significant increase in the NMDA component during LTP in the test pathway (B), but not in the control pathways (not shown). The potentiated EPSPs were completely blocked by the NMDA receptor blocker 2-amino-5-phosphonovalerate (APV). Thus, our findings show that an enhancement of the NMDA-receptor component can be detected.

Further work is needed to understand how our results and those of Bashir and Collingridge (1990) may be reconciled with the results of Kauer and associates (1988) and Muller and Lynch (1988). We find that the NMDA response is quite sensitive to membrane potential—even a few millivolts hyperpolarization (which can occur after a tetanus) can reduce the NMDA response by 50%. Thus in all our experiments, the NMDA-mediated transmission in the control pathway was monitored and found to be unchanged. Similarly, ambient glycine concentration can affect NMDA responses (Johnson and Ascher, 1987; Thompson et al., 1989), and this action can be modulated by CNQX (Lester et al., 1989). To allow for such complications, we looked for LTP of the NMDA component under a variety of conditions: with 1 μM of CNQX, with 10 μM of CNQX, and with 10 μM of CNQX plus exogenous glycine. In all cases, there was clear and significant potentiation of an APV-sensitive EPSP. If anything, the potentiation was more pronounced with 1 μM of CNQX or with 10 μM of CNQX and 300 μM of glycine than with 10 μM of CNQX alone, but the differences were not dramatic enough to be statistically significant.

In addition to the experimental considerations just mentioned, another possibility is that the NMDA receptor was closer to saturation in the earlier experiments. In our opinion, the possibility of NMDA saturation was not excluded by previous arguments based on the demonstration of synaptic potentiation with paired pulses (Muller and Lynch, 1988) or after tetani (Kauer et al., 1988); these forms of potentiation can take place by recruitment of silent boutons as well as previously active boutons, so some enhancement would be seen regardless of NMDA receptor saturation at previously active boutons. In contrast, during LTP, enhancement of transmission is thought to be restricted to previously active synapses because local transmitter release must occur to induce LTP. NMDA receptor saturation would thus impose a more stringent limitation during LTP than with paired-pulse facilitation or posttetanic potentiation.

Signal Transduction Between Postsynaptic Induction and Presynaptic Expression: Role of Ca^{2+}-Dependent Protein Kinases

A key question at this point is how a rise in postsynaptic $[Ca^{2+}]_i$ can lead to a long-lasting enhancement of presynaptic function. A generic working hypothesis, favored by many investigators, is that Ca^{2+} acts through a signal transduction pathway that involves a Ca^{2+}-dependent protein

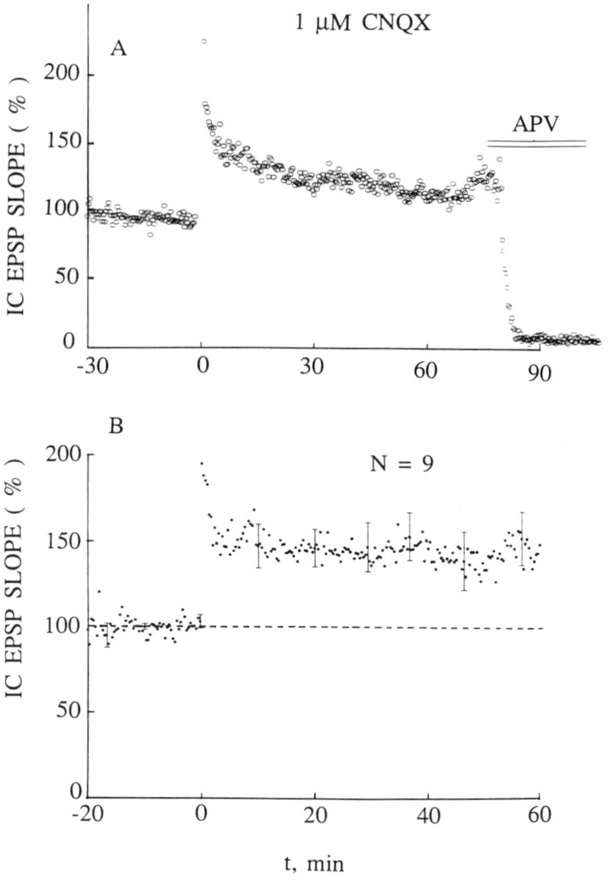

Figure 8.6 Enhancement of NMDA-receptor response during LTP. (A) Representative experiment in the presence of 1 μM of CNQX to block KQ receptors. Relative amplitude of EPSP, recorded with an intracellular microelectrode plotted against time. Tetanic stimulation was applied at t = 0. Abolition of EPSPs by 50 μM of APV demonstrates that EPSP was mediated by NMDA receptors. For further experimental details, see Malinow and coworkers (1989). (B) Collected results from similar experiments in a total of nine slices. EPSPs amplitudes were normalized to control values before tetanic stimulation, then ensemble averaged. Bars indicate SEM. Note significant and long-lasting potentiation of the NMDA receptor–mediated response.

kinase such as protein kinase C (PKC) or multifunctional calcium/calmodulin/dependent protein kinase (CaMKII; see Malinow et al., 1988; Cotman et al., 1989; Kennedy, 1989; Malenka et al., 1989b). We have tested these ideas by postsynaptic intracellular injection of peptides that are potent and selective inhibitors of either PKC or CaMKII (Malinow et al., 1989). PKC(19-31) or PKC(19-36) are peptide fragments forming the pseudosubstrate region of the PKC regulatory domain (House and Kemp, 1987). They are more than 600-fold more potent as blockers of PKC (IC50 ~0.1 μM) than as blockers of CaMKII. In contrast, the glu^{27} derivative of PKC(19-31) is relatively inactive against either kinase and serves as a useful control against nonspecific effects.

The results of intracellular injection of peptides are illustrated in figure 8.7A–D. PKC(19-31) and PKC(19-36) blocked LTP when delivered to the postsynaptic cell with the recording intracellular microelectrode; they had no significant effect on transmission to a group of neighboring cells, monitored extracellularly; $[Glu^{27}]$PKC(19-31), the control peptide, failed to block LTP. These results are compatible with effects of injecting PKC (Hu et al., 1987), or PKC inhibitory peptides (Andersen et al., 1990).

To investigate the role of postsynaptic CaMKII, we used the peptide fragment CaMKII(273-302), which inhibits CaMKII at much lower concentrations than PKC. A control was provided by CaMKII(284-302), a shorter peptide that is much less effective in blocking CaMKII. When delivered to postsynaptic cells through the recording microelectrode, CaMKII (273-302) blocks LTP (see figure 8.7E–F), while CaMKII(284-302) does not.

Figure 8.7 Selective postsynaptic block of PKC or CaMKII prevents LTP. Diagram shows stimulation and recording conditions (see text). (A) Extracellular recordings of transmission show persistent potentiation following a tetanus (arrow). (B) Simultaneous monitoring of synaptic potentials using an intracellular microelectrode whose tip is filled with 3 mM of PKC(19-31); ($n = 8$). Following the tetanus there is no persistent potentiation. (C) Transmission in a nontetanized pathway, monitored through the same PKC(19-31)–containing electrode, is constant throughout the experiment, indicating no nonspecific depressant effect on basal synaptic transmission. (D) Transmission monitored in a different set of slices with 3 mM of $[Glu^{27}]$PKC(19-31) in the intracellular electrode shows LTP after a conditioning tetanus ($n = 6$ pathways from three slices). (E–H) Recordings of transmission in experiments testing the involvement of CaMKII. (E) Extracellular monitoring shows LTP after tetanic stimulation. (F) Simultaneous monitoring of synaptic potentials with intracellular electrode containing 1.1 mM of CaMKII(273-302) shows no persistent potentiation after tetanic conditioning. (G) Transmission in a nontetanized pathway, monitored with the CaMKII(273-302)–containing electrode, is constant throughout the experiment. (H) Transmission monitored in a different set of slices, using 1.1 mM of CaMKII(284-302) in the intracellular electrode shows LTP after a tetanus ($n = 5$ pathways from three slices). Error bars indicate SEMs for representative time points. Insets: average of 10 consecutive potentials obtained at the times designated on time axis. Scale bars for A and E: 0.33 mV, 12.5 milliseconds; for B,D,F, and H: 5 mV and 12.5 milliseconds. Peptides PKC(19-31), PKC(19-36) were generously provided by Dr. John J. Nestor, Jr. and Dr. Bruce Kemp, respectively. (From Malinow et al., 1989. Copyright 1989 by the AAAS.)

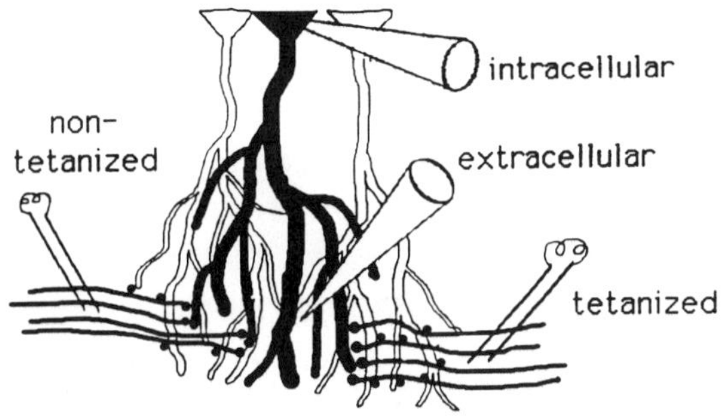
intracellular
non-
tetanized
extracellular
tetanized

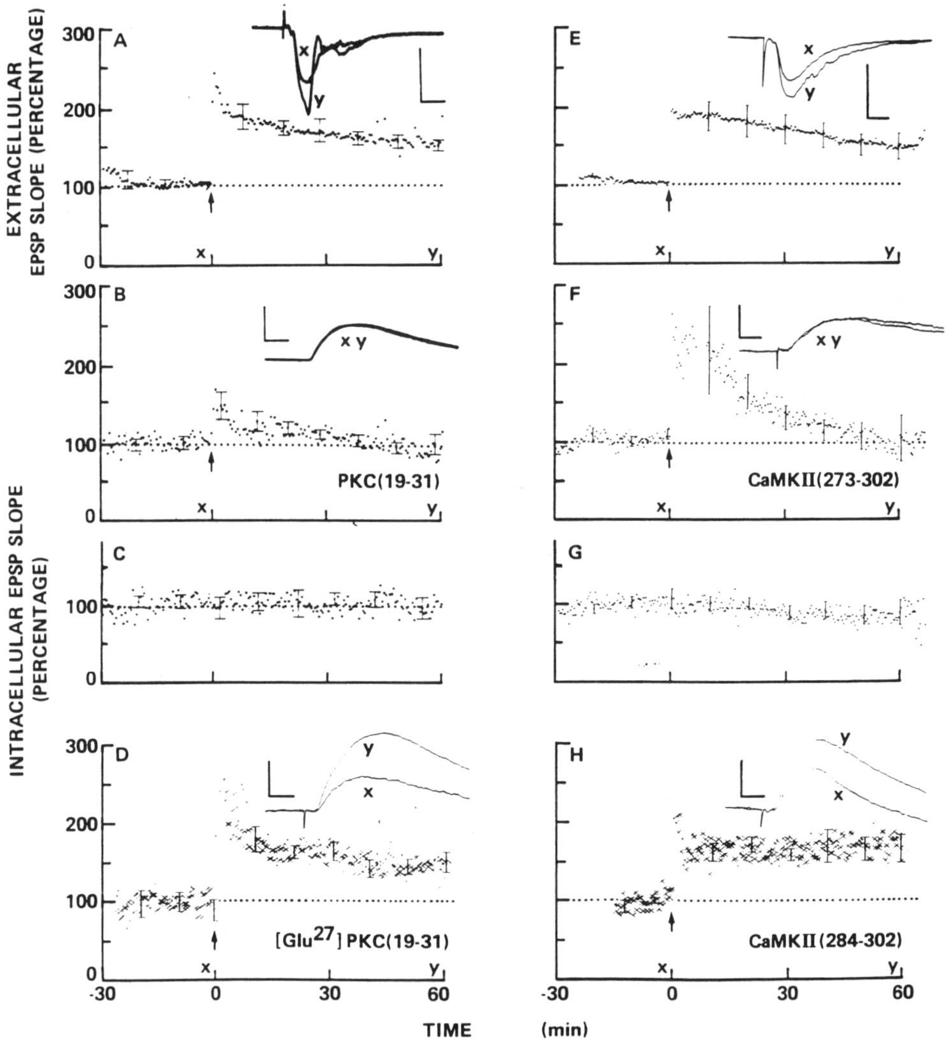
EXTRACELLULAR
EPSP SLOPE (PERCENTAGE)
INTRACELLULAR EPSP SLOPE
(PERCENTAGE)
A
B
C
D
E
F
G
H
PKC(19-31)
[Glu27] PKC(19-31)
CaMKII(273-302)
CaMKII(284-302)
TIME (min)

We obtained similar results with a calmodulin-blocking peptide (not shown; see also Malenka et al., 1989b). The effects of the CaMKII fragments are almost certainly not explained by block of PKC, since CaMKII(284-302) is more effective than CaMKII(273-302) in blocking PKC but much less effective in preventing LTP (Malinow et al., 1989). We thus conclude that postsynaptic PKC and CaMKII are *both* required for the establishment of LTP.

Persistent Signaling Outside the Postsynaptic Cell?

To determine if the postsynaptic kinases are involved in the *expression* of LTP, we impaled cells with microelectrodes containing protein kinase inhibitors *after* the high-frequency stimulation had already established potentiated transmission (see insets, figure 8.8). To our surprise, we found that established LTP was *not* suppressed by intracellular postsynaptic 1-(5-isoquinolinylsulfonyl)-2-methyl-piperazine H-7. Delayed introduction of a combination of PKC(19-31) and CaMKII(273-302) was similarly ineffective (Tsien et al., 1990). Control procedures showed that the agents were successfully delivered (see figure 8.8D) and that LTP had indeed been established before the impalement (see figures 8.8E,F). Thus, once established, the persistent signal is inaccessible to postsynaptic injection of H-7 (or to the kinase-blocking peptides). Interestingly, established LTP remains sensitive to bath application of H-7 (figures 8.8E, 8.9). The effect of bath-applied H-7 is selective for the potentiated path-

Figure 8.8 Expression of LTP is insensitive to postsynaptic H-7 application. Insets indicate recording configurations before and after delayed impalement with H-7–containing microelectrode. (A) Synaptic potentials are monitored extracellularly (no microelectrode) in response to alternate stimulation of two independent pathways (unconnected points: stim 1; and connected points: stim 2). Tetanic conditioning is delivered to stim 1 (arrow, 1). After the establishment of stable LTP an intracellular recording with an H-7–containing electrode is obtained (B) and monitoring of synaptic potentials begins within 2 minutes of penetration (at $t = 0$ on lower axis). As monitored by the H-7–containing intracellular electrode, synaptic transmission from the potentiated pathway (stim 1, *) does not decay during the observation period and parallels transmission from the unpotentiated pathway (stim 2; $n = 13$). In this panel, synaptic strength in each pathway is normalized relative to average data for the first 5 minutes of transmission in the untetanized pathway. (C,D) To determine if H-7 from the intracellular electrode has reached the synaptic zone, the previously unpotentiated pathway (stim 2) is tested for the ability to generate LTP (7 slices). Delivery of a tetanus to stim 2 results in slowly decaying potentiation but no LTP as monitored with the intracellular electrode (D), despite a large persistent potentiation seen with the extracellular electrode (C). (E,F) In eight slices, H-7 is subsequently bath applied and a comparable synaptic diminution of pathway 1 is seen with both extracellular monitoring and with the H-7–filled intracellular microelectrode. Occlusion or reduction of the effect of externally applied H-7 would have been expected if postsynaptic H-7 had already inhibited the potentiated transmission. (From Malinow et al., 1989. Copyright 1989 by AAAS.)

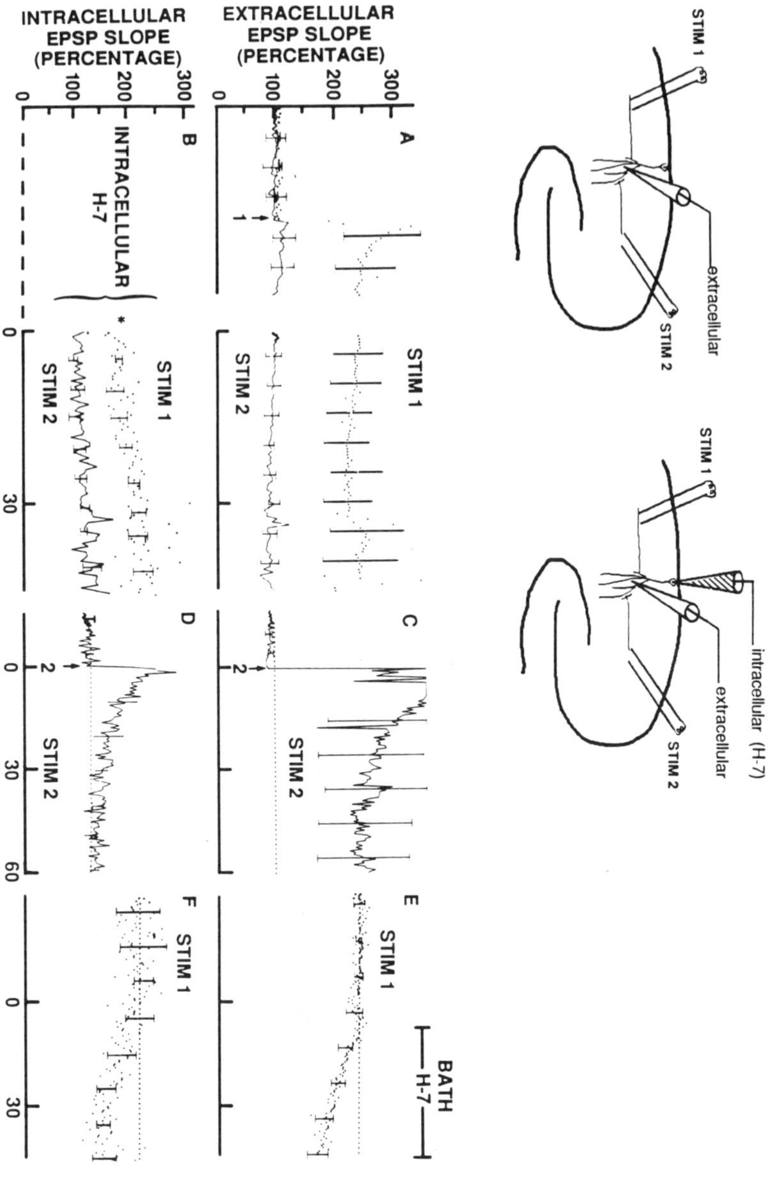
STIM 1
extracellular
STIM 2
intracellular (H-7)
EXTRACELLULAR EPSP SLOPE (PERCENTAGE)
INTRACELLULAR EPSP SLOPE (PERCENTAGE)
A
B
C
D
E
F
INTRACELLULAR H-7
BATH H-7
TIME (min.)

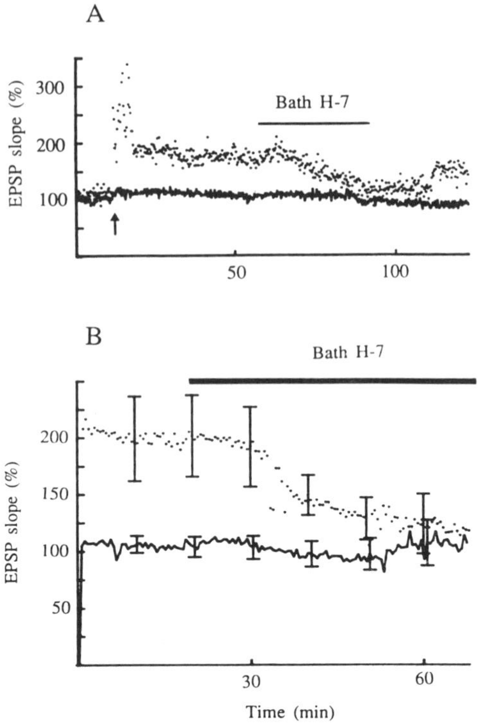

Figure 8.9 Expression of LTP is reversibly inhibited by bath applied H-7. (A) Representative experiment. Arrow marks tetanic stimulation. (For experimental details, see Malinow et al., 1988.) (B) Ensemble average of EPSP amplitudes in 20 experiments, plotted against time. Transmission from two different pathways is monitored with an extracellular electrode. One pathway (unconnected dots) was previously potentiated by delivery of a high-frequency stimulus, whereas the other pathway (connected dots) was not conditioned. H-7 (50–300 μM) was applied to the bath as indicated. Note that the drug acts relatively selectively in suppressing the potentiation in the conditioned pathway while leaving transmission in the control pathway essentially unaffected.

way (figure 8.9). Thus, we conclude that the maintenance of LTP depends on H-7–sensitive persistent signaling somewhere outside the postsynaptic cell, possibly in the presynaptic terminal.

Is There LTP Between Individual Neurons?

Although the induction of LTP is widely believed to require a coactive population of input cells to activate postsynaptic NMDA receptors, it has generally been assumed that established LTP is a property of individual synapses. The most complete study to date, however, suggests that populations of neurons are required to express LTP. LTP between individual neurons in hippocampal slices was studied by impaling a presynaptic CA3 neuron intracellularly and monitoring a postsynaptic CA1 neuron with a whole-cell pipette (figure 8.10). Five such pairs were obtained. Synaptic currents were quite small (mean = 0.57 ± 0.2 pA) and variance measurements did not reveal an obvious probabilistic event (figure 8.11).

Generating amplitude distribution density estimates with a gaussian kernel did, however, display events whose amplitude was outside the range of the noise (see figure 8.11). Pairing continued presynaptic activity with postsynaptic depolarization induced a persistent potentiation of synaptic transmission, which revealed a clear variance greater than the background noise. This potentiation was associated with a marked change in the density estimate (figure 8.11) showing a decline of failures and a shift in responses from a skewed distribution to a more symmetric pattern.

DISCUSSION AND CONCLUSIONS

The main conclusions of our studies are as follows:

1. Whole-cell recordings can be used to study synaptic transmission in neurons well below the surface of conventional brain slices over many hours. This method allows access to deeper cells that are more likely to retain intact dendritic structures and functional properties. The approach is an alternative to methods that require cleaning of the surface of slices (Edwards et al., 1989).

2. Whole-cell recordings offer a much better signal-to-noise ratio than conventional intracellular recordings, facilitating statistical analysis of

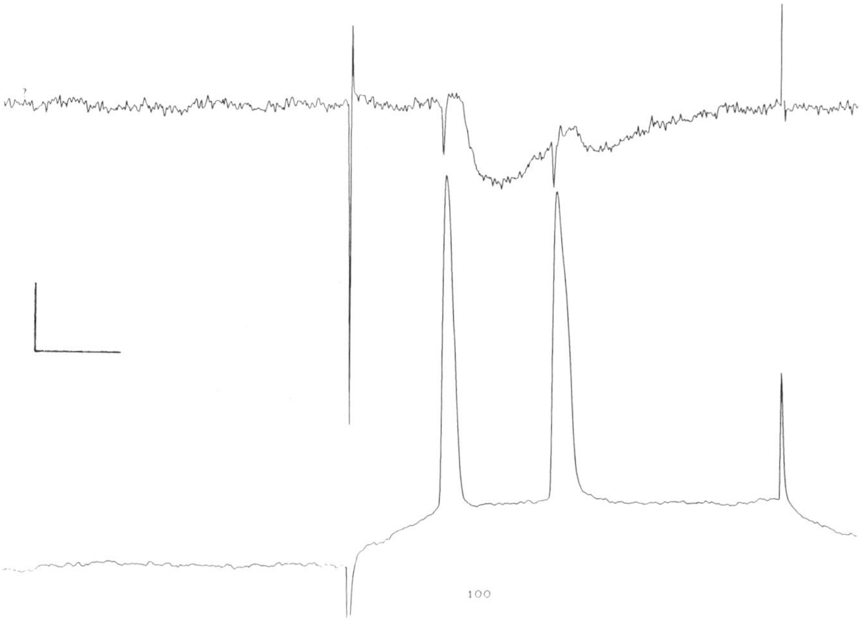

Figure 8.10 Simultaneous monitoring of presynaptic CA3 cell with intracellular electrode (lower trace) and CA1 cell with whole-cell patch pipette (upper trace). Note postsynaptic currents time locked to presynaptic action potentials. Calibration bars: 20 milliseconds; 20 mV (lower); 15 pA (upper).

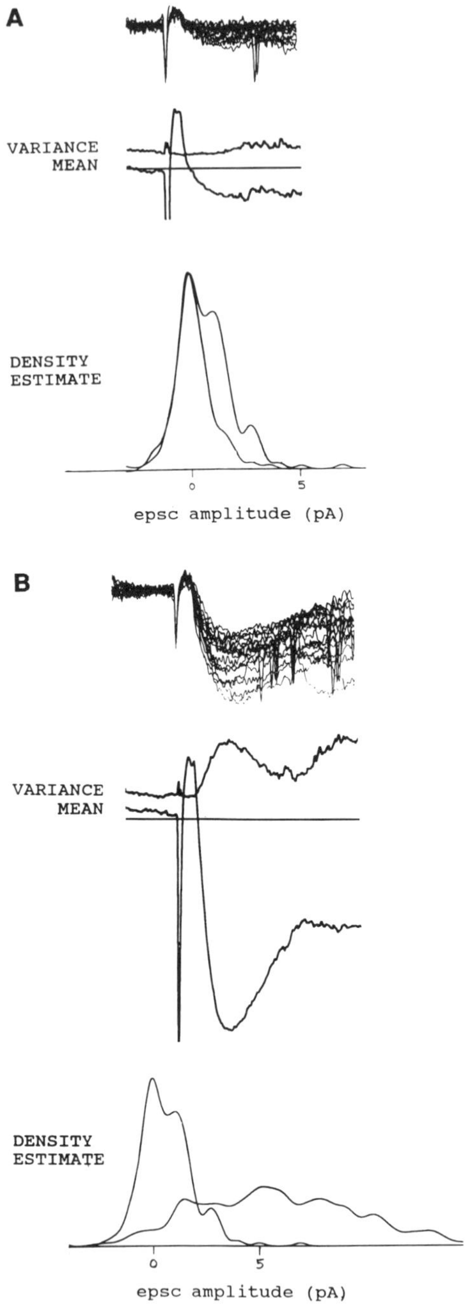

Figure 8.11 LTP of synaptic transmission between individual CA3 and CA1 neurons in hippocampal slice. (A) Sixteen consecutive traces obtained prior to potentiation; mean (MEAN) and variance (VARIANCE) for 50 consecutive traces; amplitude density estimates of noise and signal. (B) Same measurements obtained 45 minutes later.

small synaptic signals. Under favorable circumstances, quantal responses can be distinguished from synaptic failures (see figures 8.1 and 8.4).

3. Experiments conform with theory in supporting M^2/σ^2 as a simple measure of changes in presynaptic function in hippocampal slices. This approach might be useful in characterizing neuroactive drugs whose locus of action is unknown.

4. Synapses can display LTP even after the postsynaptic cell has been accessed by a whole-cell recording pipette. This opens up the possibility of probing the postsynaptic mechanisms of LTP with a wide range of biochemical compounds that could not be reliably delivered with intracellular microelectrodes. Some obvious possibilities include large proteins or even nucleic acids.

5. Interestingly, the ability to undergo LTP was lost after longer periods of whole-cell recording, as if some key cytoplasmic constituent were washed out, even though LTP established earlier during the recording did not decay. This contrast supports the idea that induction and persistence of LTP involve different molecular events, possibly in different locations (Malinow et al., 1989; Goh and Pennefather, 1989; Segal and Patchornik, 1989).

6. When LTP was induced relatively soon after break-in, the degree of potentiation was large, ranging up to tenfold and averaging more than threefold. The magnitude of the enhancement is considerably greater than seen with other recording methods. The difference was not due to depressed levels of basal transmission in whole-cell recordings; the number or frequency of presynaptic action potentials (40 stimuli at 2 Hz) was certainly not excessive. One possibility is that whole-cell recordings are particularly effective in achieving strong depolarizations of postsynaptic spines (particularly with cesium as the main internal cation). Whatever the explanation, the whole-cell experiments provide a measure of the inherent power of the mechanisms underlying LTP. A large degree of persistent synaptic plasticity is of obvious interest for neural modeling (e.g., McNaughton and Morris, 1987).

7. LTP of up to tenfold was seen with intracellular stimulation of single CA3 neurons (Malinow and Tsien, 1990b). This result provides the first direct evidence that LTP is a property of one-to-one connections between presynaptic and postsynaptic neurons, rather than an emergent property of a large number of converging presynaptic inputs (compare Friedlander et al., 1990).

8. Biophysical analysis and biochemical approaches provide three complementary lines of evidence for an enhancement of presynaptic function during LTP, as suggested previously by other approaches (Skrede and Malthe-Sorenssen, 1981; Dolphin et al., 1982; Routtenberg, 1985; Malenka et al., 1986; Malinow et al., 1989).

9. The analysis of M^2/σ^2 is relatively model independent, and does not require failures. M^2/σ^2 increased significantly and remained elevated dur-

ing LTP; it was unchanged in pathways not undergoing potentiation (figure 8.3B). LTP was associated with a clear change in M^2/σ^2, and the shape of the amplitude histogram was similar to that seen with elevated $[Ca^{2+}]_o$.

10. An analysis based on failures gives a more direct view of presynaptic function. This method does not require that a single synapse be activated, an issue for analyses based on changes in M^2/σ^2. In all cases in which unitary events were large relative to the background noise so that failures were clearly resolved, the occurrence of failures was greatly diminished; the proportion of failures fell by about fivefold during LTP (e.g., figure 8.4E). In some experiments, failures were common during the control run and completely disappeared with LTP.

11. Although all the biophysical results support an increase in the likelihood of transmitter release, they do not exclude some change in postsynaptic responsivity. We found that M increased more than M^2/σ^2, particularly 30 to 60 minutes after pairing; the late change in M might reflect a delayed increase in postsynaptic responsivity as suggested by iontophoretic application of AMPA (Davies et al., 1989). This possibility might be in line with a recent report of minimal EPSPs in which an increase in quantal size but no clear change in quantal content was detected in association with a 30% potentiation (Foster and McNaughton, 1991). The enhancement of transmitter release may have been more pronounced in our experiments simply because the potentiation was much larger.

12. A third and rather different line of evidence is based on postsynaptic injection of inhibitors of protein kinases, H-7, or peptide inhibitors of Ca^{2+}-dependent kinases. After its establishment, LTP appears unresponsive to postsynaptic H-7 or to delivery of both peptides in combination, although it remains sensitive to externally applied H-7 (figure 8.8). These results suggest that LTP is maintained by a signaling pathway not entirely contained within the postsynaptic cell. One possibility is that the pathway includes a presynaptic protein kinase such as PKC.

13. Our evidence supporting presynaptic changes with LTP is striking in light of previous studies showing that induction is postsynaptic (Wigström et al., 1986; Malinow and Miller, 1986; Sastry et al., 1986; Kelso et al., 1986; Lynch et al., 1983; Malenka et al., 1988; Malinow et al., 1989). The combination of results makes it difficult to escape the conclusion that a retrograde message must travel from the conditioned postsynaptic cell to modify presynaptic function (see Bliss and Lynch, 1988). Because the proportion of failures decreases and M^2/σ^2 increases soon after pairing, the retrograde signaling must occur promptly.

14. A retrograde message might act jointly with a presynaptic signal (e.g., elevated $[Ca^{2+}]_i$). This would constitute a presynaptic *and* function, somewhat similar to the *and* operation of glutamate + depolarization at the postsynaptic NMDA receptor. In principle, the retrograde signal could

spread laterally along the presynaptic afferent to modify synaptic boutons onto other postsynaptic cells (Bonhoeffer et al., 1989).

15. An enhancement of presynaptic function effectively increases the signal-to-noise ratio of evoked synaptic release relative to "background noise" produced by the ambient level of glutamate within brain tissue. For signal processing, this is a more robust and efficient mechanism than an elevated postsynaptic receptivity, which would increase both signal and noise together.

ACKNOWLEDGMENTS

We are grateful to Dr. Daniel Madison for contributing some of the H-7 experiments illustrated in figure 8.8. We thank Drs. D. D. Friel, J. A. Kauer, D. V. Madison, and R. S. Zucker for helpful discussion. This work was supported by the Javits Investigator award NS24067 to R.W.T.

REFERENCES

Andersen, P., et al. (1990). Injection of a peptide inhibitor of protein kinase C blocks the induction of long-term potentiation in rat hippocampal cells *in vitro. Journal of Physiology* 429:25P.

Alger, B. E., and R. A. Nicoll (1982). Feed-forward dendritic inhibition of rat hippocampal pyramidal cells studied *in vitro. Journal of Physiology* 328:105–123.

Alkon, D. L., and T. J. Nelson (1990). Specificity of molecular changes in neurons involved in memory storage. *Federation of American Societies for Experimental Biology* 4:1567–1576.

Artola, A., and W. Singer (1987). Long-term potentiation and NMDA receptors in rat visual cortex. *Nature* 330:649–652.

Ascher, P., and L. Nowak (1988). Electrophysiological studies of NMDA receptors. *Trends in Neuroscience* 10:284–288.

Barnes, S., and F. Werblin (1987). Gated currents generate single spike activity in amacrine cells of the tiger salamander retina. *Proceedings of the National Academy of Sciences USA* 83:1509–1512.

Bashir, Z. I., and G. L. Collingridge (1990). Potentiation of an NMDA receptor-mediated EPSP in rat hippocampal slices *in vitro. Journal of Physiology* 425:23P.

Bekkers, J. M., and C. F. Stevens (1989). NMDA and non-NMDA receptors are co-localized at individual excitatory synapses in cultured rat hippocampus. *Nature* 241:230–233.

Blanton, M. G., J. J. Lo Turco, and A. R. Kriegstein (1989). Whole cell recording from neurons in slices of reptilian and mammalian cerebral cortex. *Journal of Neuroscience Methods* 30:203–210.

Bliss, T. V. P., R. M. Douglas, M. L. Errington, and M. A. Lynch (1986). Correlation between long-term potentiation and release of endogenous amino acids from dentate gyrus of anaesthetized rats. *Journal of Physiology* 377:391–408.

Bliss, T. V. P., and A. Gardner-Medwin (1973). Long-lasting potentiation of synaptic transmission in the dentate area of the unanaesthetized rabbit following stimulation of the perforant path. *Journal of Physiology* 232:357–374.

Bliss, T. V. P., and T. Lømo (1973). Long-lasting potentiation of synaptic transmission in the dentate area of the anaesthetized rabbit following stimulation of the perforant path. *Journal of Physiology* (London) 232:331–356.

Bliss, T. V. P., and M. Lynch (1988). Long-term potentiation of synaptic transmission in the hippocampus: properties and mechanisms. In P. W. Landfield and S. A. Deadwyler (eds.), *Long-term Potentiation: From Biophysics to Behavior.* New York: Alan R. Liss, pp. 3–72.

Bonhoeffer, T., V. Staiger, and A. Aertsen (1989). Synaptic plasticity in rat hippocampal slice cultures: local "Hebbian" conjunction of pre- and postsynaptic stimulation leads to distributed synaptic enhancement. *Proceedings of the National Academy of Sciences USA* 86:8113–8117.

Brown, T. H., P. F. Chapman, E. W. Kairiss, and C. L. Keenan (1988). Long-term synaptic potentiation. *Science* 242:724–728.

Chang, F., and W. T. Greenough (1984). Transient and enduring morphological correlates of synaptic activity and efficacy change in the rat hippocampal slice. *Brain Research* 309:35–46.

Coleman, P. A., and R. F. Miller (1989). Measurement of passive membrane parameters with whole-cell recordings from neurons in the intact amphibian retina. *Journal of Neurophysiology* 61:218–230.

Collingridge, G. L., and T. V. P. Bliss (1987). NMDA receptors—their role in long-term potentiation. *Trends in Neurosciences* 10:288–293.

Cotman, C. W., et al. (1989). The role of the NMDA receptor in central nervous system plasticity and pathology. *Journal of the National Institutes of Health Research* 1(2):65–74.

Davies, S. N., R. A. J. Lester, K. G. Reymann, and G. L. Collingridge (1989). Temporally distinct pre- and post-synaptic mechanisms maintain long-term potentiation. *Nature* 330:500.

del Castillo, J., and B. Katz (1954). Quantal components of the end-plate potential. *Journal of Physiology* 124:560–573.

Dolphin, A. C., M. L. Errington, and T. V. P. Bliss (1982). Long-term potentiation of the perforant path *in vivo* is associated with increased glutamate release. *Nature* 297:496.

Eccles, J. C. (1953). *The Neurophysiological Basis of Mind.* Oxford: Clarendon Press.

Edwards, F. A., A. Konnerth, and T. Sakmann (1989). A thin slice preparation for patch clamp recordings from synaptically connected neurones of the mammalian central nervous system. *Pfluegers Archives* 414:600.

Foster, T. C., and B. L. McNaughton (1991). Long-term synaptic enhancement in CA1 is due to increased quantal size, not quantal content. *Hippocampus* 1:79–91.

Friedlander, J. J., R. J. Sayer, and S. J. Redman (1990). Evaluation of long-term potentiation of small compound and unitary EPSPs at the hippocampal CA3–CA1 synapse. *Journal of Neuroscience* 10:814–825.

Goelet, P., V. F. Castellucci, S. Schacher, and E. R. Kandel (1985). The long and short of long-term memory—a molecular framework. *Nature* 322:419–422.

Goh, J. W., and P. A. Pennefather (1989). Pertussis toxin–sensitive G protein in hippocampal long-term potentiation. *Science* 244:980–983.

Gustafsson, B., H. Wigström, W. C. Abraham, and Y. Y. Huang (1987). Long-term potentiation in the hippocampus using depolarizing current pulses as the conditioning stimulus to single volley synaptic potentials. *Journal of Neuroscience* 7:774–780.

Hebb, D. O. (1949). *Organization of Behavior.* New York: John Wiley.

House, C., and B. E. Kemp (1987). Protein kinase C contains a pseudosubstrate prototype in its regulatory domain. *Science* 238:1726–1728.

Hu, G. Y., et al. (1987). Protein kinase C injection into hippocampal pyramidal cells elicits features of long-term potentiation. *Nature* 328:426–429.

Iriki, A., C. Pavlides, A. Keller, and H. Asanuma (1989). Long-term potentiation in the motor cortex. *Science* 246:1385–1387.

Johnson, J. W., and P. Ascher (1987). Glycine potentiates the NMDA response in cultured mouse brain neurons. *Nature* 325:529–531.

Kauer, J. A., R. C. Malenka, and R. A. Nicoll (1988). A persistent postsynaptic modification mediates long-term potentiation in the hippocampus. *Neuron* 1:911–917.

Kelso, S. R., A. H. Ganong, and T. H. Brown (1986). *Proceedings of the National Academy of Sciences USA* 83:5326–5330.

Kennedy, M. B. (1989). Regulation of synaptic transmission in the central nervous system: long-term potentiation. *Cell* 59:777–787.

Lester, A. J. R., et al. (1989). Interaction of 6-cyano-7-nitroquinoxaline-2,3-dione with the *N*-methyl-D-aspartate receptor–associated glycine binding site. *Molecular Pharmacology* 35:565–570.

Lømo T. (1966). Frequency potentiation of excitatory synaptic activity in the dentate area of the hippocampal formation. *Acta Physiologica Scandinavica Supplement* 277:128.

Lynch, G., and M. Baudry (1984). The biochemistry of memory: a new and specific hypothesis. *Science* 224:1057–1063.

Lynch, G., et al. (1983). Intracellular injections of EGTA block induction of hippocampal long-term potentiation. *Nature* 305:719–721.

MacDermott, A. B., et al. (1986). NMDA-receptor activation increases cytoplasmic calcium concentration in cultured spinal cord neurones. *Nature* 321:519–522.

McNaughton, B. L., C. A. Barnes, and P. Andersen (1981). Synaptic efficiacy and EPSP summation in granule cells of rat fascia dentat studied in vitro. *Journal of Neurophysiology* 46:952–966.

McNaughton, B. L., and R. G. M. Morris (1987). Hippocampal synaptic enhancement and information storage within a distributed memory system. *Trends in Neuroscience* 10:408–415.

Malenka, R. C., J. A. Kauer, D. J. Perkel, and R. A. Nicoll (1989a). The impact of postsynaptic calcium on synaptic transmission—its role in long-term potentiation. *Trends in Neuroscience* 12:444–450.

Malenka, R. C., et al. (1989b). *Nature* 340:554–557.

Malenka, R. C., J. A. Kauer, R. S. Zucker, and R. A. Nicoll (1988). Postsynaptic calcium is sufficient for potentiation of hippocampal synaptic transmission. *Science* 242:81–84.

Malenka, R. C., D. V. Madison, and R. A. Nicoll (1986). Potentiation of synaptic transmission in the hippocampus by phorbol esters. *Nature* 321:695–697.

Malinow, R., D. V. Madison, and R. W. Tsien (1988). Persistent protein kinase activity underlying long-term potentiation. *Nature* 335:820–824.

Malinow, R., and J. P. Miller (1986). Postsynaptic hyperpolarization during conditioning reversibly blocks induction of long-term potentiation. *Nature* 321:529–530.

Malinow, R., H. Schulman, and R. W. Tsien (1989). Inhibition of postsynaptic PKC or CaMKII blocks induction but not expression of LTP. *Science* 245:862–866.

Malinow, R., and R. W. Tsien (1990a). Presynaptic enhancement revealed by whole-cell recordings of long-term potentiation in rat hippocampal slices. *Nature* 346:177–180.

Malinow, R., and R. W. Tsien (1990b). Long-term potentiation of synaptic transmission between individual CA3 and CA1 neurons in rat hippocampal slices. *Society for Neuroscience Abstracts* 16:145.

Martin, A. R. (1977). Junctional transmission. II. Presynaptic mechanisms. In J. M. Brookhart and V. B. Mountcastle (eds.), *Handbook of Physiology: The Nervous System*. American Physiological Society, Sect. 1, vol. I, Chap. 10, pp. 329–355.

Mayer, M. L., and G. L. Westbrook (1987). The physiology of excitatory amino acids in the vertebrate central nervous system. *Progress in Neurobiology* 28:197–276.

Muller, D., M. Joly, and G. Lynch (1988). Contributions of quisqualate and NMDA receptors to the induction and expression of LTP. *Science* 242:1694.

Muller, D., and G. Lynch (1988). Long-term potentiation differentially affects two components of synaptic responses in hippocampus. *Proceedings of the National Academy of Sciences USA* 85:9346–9350.

Nicoll, R. A., J. A. Kauer, and R. C. Malenka (1988). The current excitement in long-term potentiation. *Neuron* 1:97–103.

Nishizuka, Y. (1988). The molecular heterogeneity of protein kinase C and its implications for cellular regulation. *Nature* 334:661–665.

Redman, S. J. (1990). Quantal analysis of synaptic potentials in neurons of the central nervous system. *Physiology Review* 70:165–198.

Regehr, W. G., and D. W. Tank (1990). Postsynaptic NMDA-receptor mediated calcium accumulation in hippocampal CA1 pyramidal cell dendrites. *Nature* 345:807–810.

Routtenberg, A. (1985). Protein kinase C activation leading to protein F1 phosphorylation may regulate synaptic plasticity by presynaptic terminal growth. *Behavioral and Neural Biology* 44:186–200.

Sastry, B. R., J. W. Goh, and A. Auyeung (1986). Associative induction of posttetanic and long-term potentiation in CA1 neurons of rat hippocampus. *Science* 232:988.

Sayer, R. J., M. J. Friedlander, and S. J. Redman (1990). The time course and amplitude of EPSPs evoked at synapses between pairs of CA3/CA1 neurons in the hippocampal slice. *Journal of Neuroscience* 10:826–836.

Sayer, R. J., S. J. Redman, and P. Andersen (1989). Amplitude fluctuations in small EPSPs recorded from CA1 pyramidal cells in the guinea-pig hippocampal slice. *Journal of Neuroscience* 9:840–850.

Segal, M., and A. Patchornik (1989). Modulation of $(Ca)_i$ by a caged EGTA affects neuronal plasticity in the rat hippocampus. *Society for Neuroscience Abstracts* 15:166.

Skrede, K. K., and D. Malthe-Sorenssen (1981). Increased resting and evoked release of transmitter following repetitive electrical tetanization in hippocampus: a biochemical correlate to long-lasting synaptic potentiation. *Brain Research* 208:436.

Stevens, C. F. (1989). Strengthening the synapses. *Nature* 338:460–461.

Thompson, A. M., V. E. Walker, and D. M. Flynn (1989). Glycine enhances NMDA-receptor mediated synaptic potentials in neocortical slices. *Nature* 338:422–424.

Tsien, R. W., H. Schulman, and R. Malinow (1990). Peptide inhibitors of PKC and CaMK block induction but not expression of long-term potentiation. In Y. Nishizuka, M. Endo, and C. Tanaka (eds.), *The Biology and Medicine of Signal Transduction.* Advances in Second Messenger and Phosphoprotein Research. New York: Raven Press, vol. 24, pp. 101–107.

Wigström, H., B. Gustafsson, Y. Y. Huang, and W. C. Abraham (1986). Hippocampal long-term potentiation is induced by pairing single afferent volleys with intracellularly injected depolarizing pulses. *Acta Physiologica Scandinavia* 126:317–319.

9 Sites and Mechanisms for Expression of Long-Term Potentiation

John Larson, José Ambros-Ingerson, and Gary Lynch

Long-term potentiation (LTP) has become a subject of intense interest in neuroscience both because it is an intriguing physiological phenomenon and because it represents a plausible encoding mechanism for certain kinds of memory. The cellular processes responsible for LTP can be divided into three sets of events: induction, expression, and stabilization. This chapter is concerned with the second of these points and, in particular, whether expression involves presynaptic or postsynaptic modifications. This issue has become intertwined with questions about induction and stabilization, and it is necessary to consider these relationships before discussing work on expression itself.

There is general agreement that induction of LTP involves stimulation of NMDA receptors (Collingridge et al., 1983; Harris et al., 1984) under depolarizing conditions that unblock their voltage-sensitive ionophores (Nowak et al., 1984; Mayer et al., 1984) followed by a change in postsynaptic calcium levels (Lynch et al., 1983; Malenka et al., 1988). Expression and stabilization are only rarely distinguished in discussions of LTP, and this is a possible source of confusion in the literature. LTP in field CA1 can persist with little evident decrement for as long (weeks) as recording arrangements are stable (Staubli and Lynch, 1987), and indeed this is a property that suggests a role for the potentiation effect in memory. It is possible that a single modification increases synaptic strength (i.e., expresses LTP) by changing some aspect of the junction that is extraordinarily stable but there is no reason to assume this a priori and indeed it seems unlikely. Many of the changes hypothesized to express LTP (e.g., receptor or ion channel modifications, enzyme activation) would not be expected to last for anything like the duration of LTP if for no other reason than protein turnover. (Notable exceptions are a decrease in spine resistance due to structural modifications or synaptogenesis [or both]; however, recent studies argue against the first of these ideas.) If LTP expression does involve changes in the conformational or functional states of specific species of proteins, then it would seem necessary to assume that further modifications ("stabilization") would be needed to ensure that replacement proteins would be likely to find their way into the same states. Note that the idea of stabilization is distinct from that of maintenance; the latter term has been used to indicate an active process that continues to support the expression mechanism long after the induction event. A maintenance process would be constrained by the same problems of protein turnover just mentioned, whereas stabilization is a process that reorganizes the synapse, perhaps structurally, such that expression persists much longer than the stabilization event itself.

Failure to recognize that qualitatively different effects may be responsible for expression versus stabilization has confounded the interpretation of pharmacological and biochemical studies on LTP. The experiments of Gustafsson and Wigström (1988), which suggest that expression of LTP requires about 20 seconds to develop, are of interest in this regard. It is not at all apparent that many and perhaps most of the drugs reported to block LTP have significant effects on the potentiation found in the first minute after high-frequency stimulation. Thus, it is possible that LTP is fully expressed initially under these conditions but the drugs prevent the potentiation from being stabilized. This point has been made explicit in experiments using inhibitors of calcium-activated proteases (del Cerro et al., 1990a) and antagonists of the receptor for the platelet activating factor (del Cerro et al., 1990b). Also noteworthy in this context is the finding that the potentiation present between 15 and 30 seconds after high-frequency stimulation is reversed by episodes of hypoxia beginning within 60 to 120 seconds (but not later) of the stimulation (Arai et al., 1990). This implies that the stabilization process requires more time to go to completion than the changes associated with expression. These points will be developed more fully elsewhere (Lynch et al., 1991).

The possible existence of distinctly different expression versus stabilization mechanisms has direct relevance for the debate concerning the presynaptic versus postsynaptic nature of LTP. One might well imagine, for example, that coordinated presynaptic and postsynaptic changes are required to stabilize an expression device that exists purely in one or the other locus. From this perspective, experimental manipulations that affect the degree of LTP found tens of minutes after high-frequency stimulation cannot by themselves be used to form arguments about whether expression involves presynaptic or postsynaptic changes (see, e.g., Malinow et al., 1989; Linden and Routtenberg, 1989). The following review of the locus and nature of the expression mechanisms reflects these arguments. The extensive literature on the chemistries involved in producing expression are not discussed in any detail because, in most cases, these results do not discriminate between stabilization and expression; instead, work directed at the sites and mechanisms of the modifications underlying fully developed potentiation are emphasized.

FORMS OF LTP

The first issue arising in a discussion of LTP substrates concerns the relationships among the different forms of potentiation described in various synaptic systems and preparations. Do these represent variations on a single mechanism or do synapses possess multiple mechanisms for changing strength in a lasting fashion? The traditional physiological approach to synaptic plasticity is to identify and characterize mechanisms that can change synaptic strength, and early work on neuromuscular and spinal cord synapses identified facilitation and posttetanic potentiation (PTP) as short-lasting forms of plasticity. The discovery of LTP arose from extensions of this research to hippocampus (Bliss and Lømo, 1973). It has become popular to label as LTP any potentiation effect persisting beyond the duration of PTP, and such effects have now been described at a number of peripheral and central synapses. It is also becoming clear, however, that "LTP" effects vary in their induction and expression mechanisms as well as in their duration. The induction mechanism for LTP has been best characterized for synapses in the CA1 field of hippocampus where, as previously noted, it requires activation of *N*-methyl-D-aspartate (NMDA) receptors (Collingridge et al., 1983; Harris et al., 1984) under conditions of strong postsynaptic depolarization normally provided by the cooperative action of many synapses stimulated at high frequency (Kelso and Brown, 1986; Kelso et al., 1986). NMDA receptor activation results in an increase in postsynaptic calcium concentration that is necessary for LTP induction (Lynch et al., 1983; Malenka et al., 1988).

LTP effects in other synaptic systems have been described that have clearly different induction mechanisms, and it is likely that different expression mechanisms are also involved. For example, NMDA receptor–independent potentiation is observed in invertebrate neuromuscular junctions (Baxter et al., 1985) and vertebrate sympathetic ganglia (Brown and McAfee, 1982; Briggs et al., 1985; Koyano et al., 1985). There seems to be no reason to believe that LTP-like effects differing in induction mechanisms would share similar expression mechanisms and, indeed, the decay rate of the potentiation effects found in the periphery call into question the wisdom of labeling these as "LTP." This issue is also brought out by recent studies of hippocampal mossy fiber synapses showing a potentiation that differs from CA1 LTP in both induction and expression mechanisms. Thus, mossy fiber potentiation is not dependent on NMDA receptors (Harris and Cotman, 1986) or postsynaptic calcium (Zalutsky and Nicoll, 1990), and expression is accompanied by a decrease in paired-pulse facilitation (Staubli et al., 1990b; Zalutsky and Nicoll, 1990) in contrast to CA1 LTP (Muller and Lynch, 1989a). This last result suggests that mossy fiber potentiation is due to enhanced transmitter release whereas the CA1 results do not favor enhanced release. It appears that multiple mechanisms exist for inducing and expressing long-term changes in synaptic transmission and that qualitatively different forms of potentiation coexist even within the hippocampus. The possibility exists that progress in the field is being hindered by labeling disparate effects as "LTP."

Research on LTP can be seen not only as an extension of an historical line of physiological experimentation on forms of synaptic plasticity but also as a new approach to the long-studied question of how the brain encodes memory. Although there is extensive contact between the behavioral and physiological traditions in the study of LTP, there are also points of departure. A physiological emphasis will lead to experimental paradigms that increase the opportunity for observing interactions between the components of synaptic transmission or for isolating the contributions of one of these to the subsequent operation of the synapses; work that is concerned with LTP from a psychological perspective will necessarily favor experimental designs that reflect circumstances that could occur in behaving animals. The plausibility of any form of synaptic plasticity, be it a variant of LTP or not, as a memory substrate is of paramount importance to the behavioral tradition. This latter consideration led us to begin studying LTP using short bursts of stimulation pulses designed to mimic the bursts of action potentials generated by hippocampal pyramidal cells in freely moving rats (Ranck, 1973; Fox and Ranck, 1981). A single burst (4 pulses at 100 Hz) to the Schaffer commissural (SC) inputs to CA1 cells elicited only short-term potentiation (STP) lasting a few seconds, but repeated bursts could induce both a decremental STP (10–15 minutes) and nondecremental LTP. Maximal LTP occurred when bursts were repeated at 5 Hz (i.e., in the frequency range of the endogenous hippocampal EEG theta rhythm [Larson et al., 1986]). Saturation of LTP occurred after only 10 bursts at this frequency. Similar results have also been obtained at perforant path synapses in dentate gyrus (Greenstein et al., 1988). The optimal interburst interval was found to be due to a property of the network such that stimulation of any input to a postsynaptic cell 200 milliseconds before a burst would prime the cell by suppressing feedforward inhibition and allow the excitatory postsynaptic potentials (EPSPs) evoked by the burst to summate temporally in a more effective way and activate NMDA receptor currents (Larson and Lynch, 1986, 1988, 1989; Lynch et al., 1987; see also Diamond et al., 1988; Pacelli et al., 1989). Moreover, NMDA receptor antagonists completely eliminated both STP and LTP effects induced by this "theta-burst" pattern of stimulation (Larson and Lynch, 1988), suggesting that it only induces effects that are triggered postsynaptically. Finally, chronic recording studies indicate that the LTP induced by theta-burst stimulation remains stable without decrement for weeks or until stimulation-recording conditions can no longer be maintained (Staubli and Lynch, 1987).

Several important results arose from these studies. First, they established the minimal conditions for inducing LTP in CA1 by synaptic stimulation alone in the absence of pharmacological manipulation of synaptic inhibition. Notable LTP can be induced by a single four-pulse burst to a primed cell; maximal LTP can be induced by as few as 40 pulses given in a theta-burst pattern. Second, the burst stimulation paradigm has provided a simple assay for drug treatment effects on the physiological events antecedent to LTP induction. Theta-burst stimulation evokes a stereotyped postsynaptic response pattern that contains a significant NMDA receptor–mediated component (Larson and Lynch, 1988); this response can be used to evaluate nonspecific effects of pharmacological treatments that impair LTP (Arai et al., 1990; del Cerro et al., 1990a and b; Muller et al., 1990). Third, they provided an intriguing link between the limbic system theta rhythm and the induction of LTP. Because hippocampal theta is pronounced during exploration (Vanderwolf, 1969) and some forms of learning (Eichenbaum et al., 1987), one function of the rhythm may be to gate neuronal activity at the optimal frequency for inducing LTP. Indeed, Otto and colleagues (1991) have found evidence that hippocampal pyramidal cells do fire in repetitive bursts similar to those used in the LTP experiments when rats are sampling odors in an olfactory discrimination task. Fourth, the correspondence between naturally occurring activity patterns and LTP induction increases the likelihood that LTP occurs during behavior and that timing rules based on these relationships may prove useful in explorations of memory functions in simulations of hippocampal and cortical neural networks. This last point is discussed elsewhere (Larson and Lynch, 1989; Lynch et al., 1990b).

The following discussion is mainly restricted to studies of the CA1 field because, as previously argued, LTP in this region has induction properties and persistence consistent with a role for the effect in long-term memory.

LOCUS OF LTP EXPRESSION

Determination of the substrate of LTP expression involves two issues: the site of expression and its underlying mechanism. The locus of LTP expression is meant to refer to the type of synapse that exhibits potentiation; mechanism refers to the biochemical and structural modification that enhances transmission. This section considers evidence regarding the locus of expression; the nature of the mechanism will be dealt with below.

There are three possible sites for LTP expression in field CA1: (1) extant synapses—potentiation is expressed by changes in efficacy at the same synapses recorded during baseline conditions; (2) silent synapses—LTP is expressed by enhanced transmission at synapses that do not contribute notably to control responses but are activated after LTP induction; and (3) new synapses—LTP expression is due to synaptogenesis. Two types of studies could, in principle, distinguish among these alternatives. First, electron microscopic studies have found changes in the proportions of certain synapse types after LTP (Lee et al., 1980, 1981; Chang and Greenough, 1984). It is not clear, however, whether these changes represent formation of new connections or the transformation of synapses from one configuration to another. Second, the technique of quantal analysis could unambiguously rule out new or silent synapses if it is found that the quantal parameter, m or quantal content, does not change after LTP. Both activation of silent synapses and formation of new synapses would increase the number of sites at which responses are recorded and hence increase quantal content (*m*). Unfortunately, the results of quantal analysis in the CA1 field are conflicting and subject to several interpretations. These problems are now considered.

According to the quantal hypothesis (del Castillo and Katz, 1954), the mean postsynaptic response ($\overline{X}$) to stimulation of a single synaptic input is equal to the product of the quantal postsynaptic response (*a*) and the mean quantal content (*m*), which is further composed of the product of the release probability for a quantum (*p*) and the number of available quanta or release sites (*n*). A change in *a* is traditionally interpreted as a postsynaptic effect; changes in *m*, *p*, or *n* are considered presynaptic. Table 9.1 presents some alternative interpretations of results from quantal analysis. It can be seen that almost any change in quantal parameters after LTP could be attributed to either presynaptic or postsynaptic effects or both. It bears repeating, however, that activation of silent synapses or growth of new synapses should be accompanied by a change in quantal content and therefore that a negative result from quantal analysis would argue strongly against these interpretations of LTP.

It has not yet been possible to apply the most direct method of quantal analysis to CNS synapses because this analysis requires that spontaneous quantal events (mEPSPs or mEPSCs) be measured at the same synapses from which evoked responses are measured. Three recent studies have relied on two indirect methods to determine whether changes in transmission before and after LTP can be attributed to presynaptic or postsynaptic changes. Foster and McNaughton (1991) used conventional intracellular recordings and noise deconvolution techniques to extract quantal parameters from distributions of postsynaptic response sizes. They conclude that LTP is due to an increase in *a*, with no change in *m*. As expected, paired-pulse facilitation was found to result from an increase in *m*, in particular, an increase in release probability, *p*. However, the re-

Table 9-1 Ambiguities in Site of Change Resulting from an Unambiguous Quantal Analysis Outcome

Explanation of outcome	Outcome of Analysis: Δa	Δm	Δn	Δp
Presynaptic	Δ Vesicle content	Δ Release Δ Number of synapses (silent or new)	Δ Release sites Δ Number of synapses (silent or new)	Δ Release probability
Postsynaptic	Δ Receptors (number, affinity, or conductance) Δ Spine resistance	Δ Number of synapses (silent or new)	Δ Number of synapses (silent or new)	Δp of high conductance receptor state

liability of noise deconvolution to resolve quantal components of responses in hippocampal synapses, particularly with small sample sizes, has been called into question (Sayer et al., 1989). The main problem here is that the signal-to-noise ratio is too small to observe discrete peaks representing quantal increments in the evoked response histograms so assumptions must be made a priori regarding the nature of the underlying distributions. Two other laboratories have used the newly developed method of whole-cell patch-clamp recordings from neurons in hippocampal slices to analyze fluctuations in transmission at higher signal-to-noise ratios than are possible using high-resistance microelectrodes. Unfortunately, even under these conditions distinct quantal peaks are rarely seen in distributions of evoked response amplitudes. Malinow and Tsien (1990) simply measured the mean and variance of EPSC distributions before and after LTP. If transmission follows binomial statistics, it follows that the mean response size ($\overline{X}$) is given by $\overline{X} = a \cdot n \cdot p$, and the variance ($s^2$) is given by $s^2 = a^2 \cdot n \cdot p \cdot (1 - p)$. From these relations, it can be seen that if LTP is due to an increase in quantal size (a), then the response variance should increase much more than the mean. What was found, however, was that the variance increased linearly with the mean. Similar findings were described by Bekkers and Stevens (1990) using similar techniques. It can be noted from the binomial equations that variance scales linearly with the mean only for changes in n or for changes in p when the initial value of p is very low.

Bekkers and Stevens (1990) noted that p may in fact be low because the distributions can be fit to Poisson functions. However, it is difficult to reconcile this with the high levels of extracellular calcium in the slice experiments, and previous work that has established that transmitter release in hippocampus can be described by the same equations that govern release at neuromuscular junctions (Rahamimoff, 1968; Muller and Lynch, 1989b). Indeed, it may be more reasonable to conclude that LTP in the patch-clamp experiments is due to an increase in the statistical parameter, n. This leads to some interesting and provocative interpretations.

Figure 9.1 shows several possible interpretations of an increase in n. The top part of the diagram depicts the conventional interpretation of an increase in number of synaptic vesicles or release sites at an extant synapse as the mechanism of LTP expression. The bottom part illustrates three mechanisms by which silent synapses could be activated after LTP induction. A synapse might be silent because there is normally no transmitter release, no postsynaptic receptors, or there is a high-resistance spine neck that chokes off current flow from the spine into the dendrite. It is important to emphasize that any mechanism for activating silent synapses would be detected in quantal analysis as an increase in n.

The possible existence of multiple synapse connections between CA3 and CA1 cells can introduce further complications into the equations of quantal analysis. If we admit the possibility that individual synapses can differ in the quantal size parameter a, situations can arise in which the

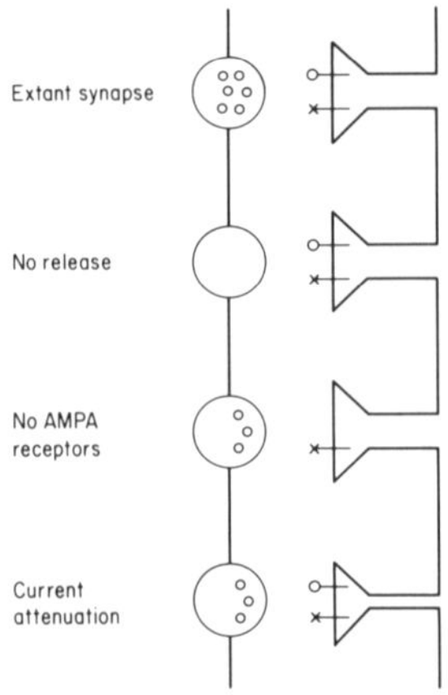

Figure 9.1 Potential mechanisms for an increase in the number of recorded release sites after LTP. The diagram illustrates a single presynaptic axon making four synaptic connections with a single postsynaptic cell. The top synapse illustrates LTP being accompanied by an increase in release sites at an extant synapse. The lower synapses illustrate weak or silent synapses that could be activated after LTP because they now release transmitter or express AMPA receptors, or the postsynaptic spine no longer attenuates synaptic current flow into the dendrite.

assumptions about mean and variance of evoked response distributions for a simple binomial or Poisson distribution are no longer valid. This point can be best illustrated by results of numerical calculations based on mathematical analysis of the multiple synapse case (figure 9.2). In this case, one axon makes five synaptic contacts onto a single postsynaptic cell. One synapse is relatively strong but nonplastic whereas the others are weak (relatively silent) before LTP but can express potentiation. The analysis assumes that both release parameters (n and p) are constant between synapses and not subject to change with LTP. Under these conditions, response variance can be shown to scale almost linearly with potentiation, reproducing the result of quantal analysis obtained in the whole-cell recording experiments. This example serves only to illustrate the complexities of the analysis when multiple synapses are involved.

In summary, the published results of quantal analysis of LTP in CA1 are conflicting and subject to alternative interpretations. It seems premature at this point to rely on existing methods of quantal analysis to decide the questions of locus and mechanism of LTP expression. There are, however, other experimental data pertinent to the three hypotheses just outlined (release, spine resistance, and receptors) that apply both to the silent synapse and extant synapse cases. These data provide constraints on mechanisms by which these hypotheses can account for LTP expression, and these constraints are discussed in the following sections.

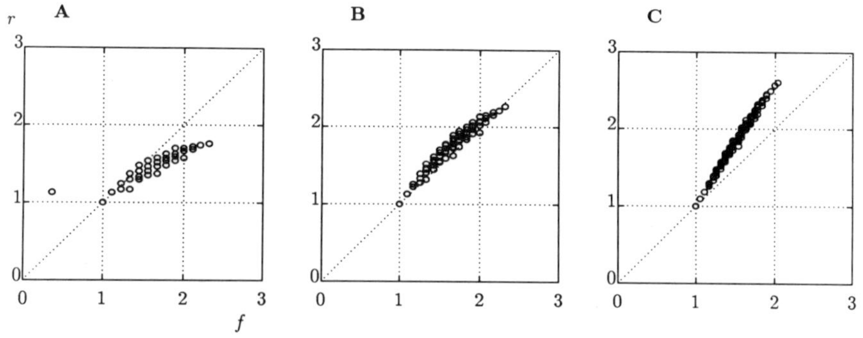

Figure 9.2 The plots show the effects of variations in the quantal size parameter (QSP) a for a multisynaptic system when other factors are held constant. Analysis reveals that in a probabilistic release system (e.g., binomially distributed) with k synapses the potentiation factor f—the ratio of the potentiated to control response—is given by $[\Sigma_{i=1}^{k} \bar{a}_i]/[\Sigma_{i=1}^{k} a_i]$ where a_i and $\bar{a}_i$ are the QSP of synapse i before and after potentiation. The ratio of coefficients of variation squared r measures the degree with which potentiation is accompanied by a change in response variability. In this system, r is given by $[(\Sigma_{i=1}^{k} a^2_i)(\Sigma_{i=1}^{k} \bar{a}_i)^2]/[(\Sigma_{i=1}^{k} a_i)^2(\Sigma_{i=1}^{k} \bar{a}^2_i)]$.

These figures show the results of numerical calculations for a system with five synapses: four are weak and plastic and one is strong and nonplastic. In panel A the control values are $a_1 = 5$, $a_{2,3,4,5} = 1$ while the potentiated value for $\bar{a}_1$ is fixed and the rest are allowed to vary in the range from 1 to 4. In panel B the control values are $a_1 = 8$, $a_{2,3,4,5} = 1$ while the potentiated value for $\bar{a}_1$ is fixed and the rest vary from 1 to 5. In panel C the control values are $a_1 = 15$, $a_{2,3,4,5} = 1$ while the potentiated value for $\bar{a}_1$ is fixed and the rest range from 1 to 6.

THE "RELEASE" HYPOTHESIS

Bliss and coworkers (see Bliss and Lynch, 1988, for review) have strongly argued that LTP expression is due to increased glutamate release. Constraints on the release hypothesis are provided by three lines of evidence. First, experimental manipulations thought to affect release probability do not interact with LTP although they do interact with each other. For example, paired-pulse facilitation is thought to reflect increased release probability (Magelby, 1973; Zucker, 1973), but control and potentiated synapses display identical paired-pulse facilitation (McNaughton, 1982; Muller and Lynch, 1989a). Similarly, increases in extracellular calcium concentrations (Mulkeen et al., 1988; Muller and Lynch, 1989a) or application of 4-aminopyridine (Haas and Greene, 1985; Muller and Lynch, 1989a) have identical effects on potentiated and control synapses, although both manipulations reduce paired-pulse facilitation (Muller and Lynch, 1989a). 4-Aminopyridine also has smaller effects as the extracellular calcium is raised, indicating that these two manipulations also interact with each other. Finally, phorbol esters increase transmission without affecting potentiated synapses differentially but, at the same time, do reduce paired-pulse facilitation (Muller et al., 1990). Together these results make it unlikely that LTP is expressed as an increase in release probability at extant synapses.

Studies of the CA3 region indicate that there is a form of long-lasting potentiation that does affect paired-pulse facilitation. High-frequency stimulation of the mossy fibers induces potentiation in the CA3 field that is accompanied by a dramatic reduction in paired-pulse facilitation (Staubli et al., 1990b; Zalutsky and Nicoll, 1990). Mossy fiber potentiation, as just noted, also differs in its induction mechanism as it is insensitive to NMDA receptor antagonists (Harris and Cotman, 1986) and postsynaptic injections of calcium chelators (Zalutsky and Nicoll, 1990). Thus, in terms of both induction and expression mechanisms mossy fiber potentiation is clearly distinct from CA1 LTP. It appears likely that mossy fiber potentiation may be purely a presynaptic effect whose expression is due to enhanced release probability. It is important to note that these experiments demonstrate that it is possible to detect effects of potentiation on paired-pulse facilitation when a presynaptic mechanism is indicated. The lack of interaction between presynaptic manipulations and LTP in CA1 provides severe constraints on release probability mechanisms, although an increase in number of release sites or a presynaptic change in quantal size are not ruled out.

Second, attempts to measure increases in stimulation-evoked, calcium-dependent glutamate release after LTP in CA1 have not been successful (Aniksztejn et al., 1989). Of course, this is not conclusive evidence against a release hypothesis because one cannot be certain that what is measured is transmitter released from presynaptic terminals.

Third, synapses in the CA1 field contain two types of postsynaptic glutamate receptors, α-amino-3-hydroxy-5-methylisoxazole-4-propionic acid (AMPA) and NMDA receptors, and it would be expected that increased release should affect responses mediated by both receptor types equivalently. Normal synaptic transmission is mediated almost exclusively by the AMPA receptors (Collingridge et al., 1983), so it is clear that these receptors normally express LTP. NMDA receptor–mediated responses evoked by transmitter release can be recorded under conditions of low extracellular magnesium ions (Muller and Lynch, 1988b; Coan and Collingridge, 1985) or high-frequency stimulation (Herron et al., 1986; Larson and Lynch,1988); when this is done, the NMDA responses show much smaller changes after LTP than do the AMPA receptor–mediated responses (Muller and Lynch, 1988a; Muller et al., 1988, 1989; Kauer et al., 1988). The possibility that NMDA receptors cannot express LTP because they are saturated under control conditions is unlikely since they do express robust posttetanic potentiation (Kauer et al., 1988) and paired-pulse facilitation (Muller et al., 1988); furthermore, NMDA responses also increase as extracellular calcium is raised (Muller and Lynch, 1990). Thus, increased release affects NMDA receptors at least to the same degree as AMPA receptors, yet LTP has a much greater effect on AMPA than NMDA responses. Demonstrations that NMDA responses can show persistent potentiation effects under certain conditions (Muller et al., 1988; Bashir and Collingridge, 1990) do not refute the argument that LTP is expressed selectively by AMPA receptors.

This issue has also been tested at synapses in the piriform cortex. Synapses between the afferent lateral olfactory tract (LOT) and piriform cells as well as the synapses of the intrinsic associational (ASSN) system both contain AMPA and NMDA receptors that behave similarly to those in CA1 (Jung et al., 1990a). Both systems also exhibit NMDA receptor–dependent LTP (Jung et al., 1990b; Kanter and Haberly, 1990). Measurements of NMDA receptor–mediated responses evoked by either LOT or ASSN fiber stimulation in low magnesium medium before and after LTP induction using theta-burst stimulation indicated that these components express much less LTP than the AMPA receptor–mediated components (Jung et al., 1990b). These results are thus in accord with results obtained in CA1.

THE "SPINE" HYPOTHESIS

A second hypothesis holds that changes in the morphology of dendritic spines might have biophysical consequences that increase postsynaptic currents evoked by constant amounts of transmitter release. Computer simulations of dendritic spines indicate that decreases in the longitudinal electrical resistance of the spine neck can enhance synaptic currents under certain conditions (Rall, 1978; Coss and Perkel, 1985). When the neck resistance is large, a transient synaptic conductance change produces a large depolarization in the spine head that attenuates the synaptic current evoked by the conductance change (Koch and Poggio, 1983; Wilson, 1984; Brown et al., 1988). Thus a large spine neck resistance results in a nonlinear relation between synaptic current and synaptic conductance. Under these conditions, a morphological change in the spine neck that reduces its longitudinal resistance (widening or shortening) can reduce the current-attenuation effect by making the current-conductance relation more linear; such a change could explain LTP. Electron microscopic studies in the CA1 region suggest that such changes may accompany LTP. Specifically, the number of synapses in which the postsynaptic element is a short, wide-necked, "sessile" spine is increased in potentiated tissue (Chang and Greenough, 1984; Schottler, 1990) as is the number of synapses lacking spines altogether (Lee et al., 1980, 1981; Chang and Greenough, 1984).

A potential problem for the spine resistance hypothesis is raised by the finding (just described) that LTP is expressed by postsynaptic responses mediated by AMPA receptors with only small changes in those mediated by NMDA receptors. Spine simulations suggest, however, that the current-attenuation effect of spines is more severe for fast conductances than slow conductances (Wilson, 1984). For slow currents, the spine head depolarization is more evenly spread throughout the dendrite; thus, the current-attenuation effect of the spine is reduced. Because NMDA currents are much slower than AMPA currents (Forsythe and Westbrook, 1988; Collingridge et al., 1988; Muller et al., 1988), it remains possible that the spine resistance hypothesis could explain LTP expression.

A testable prediction of the spine resistance hypothesis is that manipulations of synaptic conductance should have proportionately greater effects on potentiated versus control spines because the curves relating current to conductance will be steeper (more linear) for potentiated spines. Provided that LTP involves no change in the true synaptic conductance, it follows that marked reductions in synaptic conductance should remove most of the difference between control and potentiated connections (i.e., the potentiated response should be reduced more by experimental manipulations that reduce conductance). We have recently conducted experiments to test this idea (Jung et al., 1991). Two separate sets of inputs converging on a common population of postsynaptic CA1 cells were used; one of which was given theta-burst stimulation to induce LTP and the other served as a control. Effects of two different conductance-decreasing treatments—lowering of extracellular calcium and partial blockade of postsynaptic receptors—were compared for potentiated and control responses. We found that reductions of synaptic conductance by 50% to 75% using either method did not have any differential effects on potentiated versus control responses.

A second prediction of the spine hypothesis is that slowing of AMPA responses until they resemble NMDA currents should render them incapable of expressing LTP. When this was achieved by reducing the temperature, slow AMPA responses did express LTP (Larson and Lynch, 1991). Thus, the spine resistance hypothesis does not account for the differential expression of LTP by the two receptor types.

THE "RECEPTOR" HYPOTHESIS

The simplest interpretation of the selective expression of LTP by AMPA receptor–mediated responses is that potentiation is due to a modification of the ligand binding or conductance properties of these receptors. However, direct experimental evidence in favor of the receptor hypothesis is lacking. Attempts to detect enhanced AMPA binding using synaptic membrane fractions or autoradiographic techniques in our laboratory have not yet proven successful (Lynch et al., 1990a). Recent experiments using ionophoresis of quisqualate and AMPA have shown increases in receptor sensitivity after LTP (Davies et al., 1989), but the effect develops much more slowly than does LTP and hence its relationship to LTP expression is uncertain.

Although the direct evidence concerning the receptor hypothesis is largely negative, there are reasons to hypothesize that AMPA receptors may be modifiable in situ. Ligand binding studies indicate that AMPA receptors can change their binding affinities in response to sulfhydryl blocking agents (Terramani et al., 1988) and phospholipases (Massicotte et al., 1990; Massicotte and Baudry, 1990). Interestingly, phospholipase inhibitors interfere with LTP formation (Williams and Bliss, 1989; Massicotte et al., 1991; Okada et al., 1989). These results suggest that conformational changes in the AMPA receptor (these treatments do not alter NMDA binding properties) could regulate agonist affinity.

Recent studies of rat brain AMPA receptors expressed in oocytes also suggest that these receptors may be subject to modifiability. Specifically, it was found that the nootropic compound aniracetam increases the conductance of AMPA but not NMDA or GABA receptors; moreover, infusion of this drug into slices of hippocampus causes a rapid and reversible increase in the size of EPSPs (Ito et al., 1990). These results suggest a relatively direct test of the hypothesis that LTP changes the properties of the AMPA receptor since such an effect might be expected to interact with a second manipulation (i.e., aniracetam) that also acts on the receptors. This result has been obtained: the percent increases in synaptic responses produced by aniracetam were reduced by almost 50% by prior induction of LTP (Staubli et al., 1990a).

CONCLUSIONS

The sites and mechanisms of expression of LTP are far from settled. This chapter concentrates on expression of LTP at hippocampal CA1 synapses because this variant of LTP has induction and persistence properties attractive for a memory encoding mechanism. Electron microscopic surveys and application of quantal analysis techniques have failed to convincingly resolve the issue of the site of LTP expression. One point that has not been addressed in detail is the possibility that LTP is due to synaptogenesis; some indications exist that this possibility may be the case. Obviously, construction of new synapses would require both presynaptic and postsynaptic modifications. The possibility has been raised that different forms of LTP manifested after different stimulation conditions, different brain regions, or at different developmental periods may account for some of the discrepant findings in the literature. The experimental data pertinent to hypotheses about mechanisms of LTP expression have been discussed to constrain the types of mechanisms that could be involved at CA1 synapses. Several lines of evidence suggest that the hypothesis that LTP results from an increase in transmitter release at extant synapses is unlikely; tests of the spine resistance hypothesis have not provided positive results. A receptor-based expression mechanism appears attractive and has now received experimental support. It is anticipated that further experimental studies will increase the constraints on expression mechanisms and that continued work on AMPA receptor subtypes may yield new insights into how synapses can change their efficacy for indefinite periods.

REFERENCES

Aniksztejn, L., M. P. Roisin, R. Amsellem, and Y. Ben-Ari (1989). Long-term potentiation in the hippocampus of the anesthetized rat is not associated with a sustained enhanced release of endogenous excitatory amino acids. *Neuroscience* 28:387–392.

Arai, A., J. Larson, and G. Lynch (1990). Anoxia reveals a vulnerable period in the development of long-term potentiation. *Brain Research* 511:353–357.

Bashir, Z. I., and G. L. Collingridge (1990). Potentiation of an NMDA receptor–mediated EPSP in rat hippocampal slices in vitro. *Journal of Physiology* (London) 425:23P.

Baxter, D. A., G. D. Bittner, and T. H. Brown (1985). Quantal mechanism of long-term synaptic potentiation. *Proceedings of the National Academy of Sciences USA* 82:5978–5982.

Bekkers, J. M., and C. F. Stevens (1990). Presynaptic mechanism for long-term potentiation in the hippocampus. *Nature* 346:724–729.

Bliss, T. V. P., and T. Lømo (1973). Long-lasting potentiation of synaptic transmission in the dentate area of the anaesthetized rabbit following stimulation of the perforant path. *Journal of Physiology* (London) 232:334–356.

Bliss, T. V. P., and M. A. Lynch (1988). Long-term potentiation of synaptic transmission in the hippocampus: Properties and mechanisms. In P. W. Landfield and S. A. Deadwyler (eds.), *Long-Term Potentiation: From Biophysics to Behavior.* New York: Alan R. Liss, pp. 3–72.

Briggs, C. A., T. H. Brown, and D. A. McAfee (1985). Neurophysiology and pharmacology of long-term potentiation in the rat sympathetic ganglion. *Journal of Physiology* (London) 359:503–521.

Brown, T. H., et al. (1988). Biophysical properties of dendrites and spines that may control the induction and expression of long-term synaptic potentiation. In P. W. Landfield and S. A. Deadwyler (eds.), *Long-Term Potentiation: From Biophysics to Behavior.* New York: Alan R. Liss, pp. 201–264.

Brown, T. H., and D. A. McAfee (1982). Long-term synaptic potentiation in the superior cervical ganglion. *Science* 215:1411–1413.

Chang, F.-L. F., and W. T. Greenough (1984). Transient and enduring morphological correlates of synaptic activity and efficacy change in the rat hippocampal slice. *Brain Research* 309:35–46.

Coan, E. J., and G. L. Collingridge (1985). Magnesium ions block an *N*-methyl-D-aspartate receptor–mediated component of synaptic transmission in rat hippocampus. *Neuroscience Letters* 53:21–26.

Collingridge, G. L., C. E. Herron, and R. A. J. Lester (1988). Synaptic activation of *N*-methyl-D-aspartate receptors in the Schaffer collateral–commissural pathway of rat hippocampus. *Journal of Physiology* (London) 399:283–300.

Collingridge, G. L., S. J. Kehl, and H. McLennan (1983). Excitatory amino acids in synaptic transmission in the Schaffer-commissural pathway of the rat hippocampus. *Journal of Physiology* (London) 334:33–46.

Coss, R. G., and D. H. Perkel (1985). The function of dendritic spines: a review of theoretical issues. *Behavioral and Neural Biology* 44:151–185.

Davies, S. N., R. A. J. Lester, K. G. Reymann, and G. L. Collingridge (1989). Temporally distinct pre- and post-synaptic mechanisms maintain long-term potentiation. *Nature* 338:500–503.

del Castillo, J., and B. Katz (1954). Quantal components of the end-plate potential. *Journal of Physiology* (London) 124:560–573.

del Cerro, S., A. Arai, and G. Lynch (1990b). Inhibition of long-term potentiation by an antagonist of platelet-activating factor receptors. *Behavioral and Neural Biology* 54:213–217.

del Cerro, S., J. Larson, M. W. Oliver, and G. Lynch (1990a). Development of hippocampal long-term potentiation is reduced by recently introduced calpain inhibitors. *Brain Research* 530:91–95.

Diamond, D. M., T. V. Dunwiddie, and G. M. Rose (1988). Characteristics of hippocampal primed burst potentiation in vitro and in the awake rat. *Journal of Neuroscience* 8:4079–4088.

Eichenbaum, H., M. Kuperstein, A. Fagan, and J. Nagode (1987). Cue-sampling and goal-approach correlates of hippocampal unit activity in rats performing an odor-discrimination task. *Journal of Neuroscience* 7:716–732.

Forsythe, I. D., and G. L. Westbrook (1988). Slow excitatory postsynaptic currents mediated by *N*-methyl-D-aspartate receptors on cultured mouse central neurones. *Journal of Physiology* (London) 396:515–533.

Foster, T. C., and B. L. McNaughton (1990). Long-term synaptic enhancement in CA1 is due to increased quantal size, not quantal content. *Hippocampus* 1:79–91.

Fox, S. E., and J. B. Ranck, Jr. (1981). Electrophysiological characteristics of hippocampal complex-spike cells and theta cells. *Experimental Brain Research* 41:399–410.

Greenstein, Y. J., C. Pavlides, and J. Winson (1988). Long-term potentiation in the dentate gyrus is preferentially induced at theta rhythm periodicity. *Brain Research* 438:331–334.

Gustafsson, B., and H. Wigström (1988). Physiological mechanisms underlying long-term potentiation. *Trends in Neuroscience* 11:156–162.

Haas, H. L., and R. W. Greene (1985). Long-term potentiation and 4-aminopyridine. *Cellular and Molecular Neurobiology* 5:297–301.

Harris, E. W., and C. W. Cotman (1986). Long-term potentiation of guinea pig mossy fiber responses is not blocked by *N*-methyl-D-aspartate antagonists. *Neuroscience Letters* 70:132–137.

Harris, E. W., A. H. Ganong, and C. W. Cotman (1984). Long-term potentiation in the hippocampus involves activation of *N*-methyl-D-aspartate receptors. *Brain Research* 323:132–137.

Herron, C. E., R. A. J. Lester, E. J. Coan, and G. L. Collingridge (1986). Frequency-dependent involvement of NMDA receptors in the hippocampus: a novel synaptic mechanism. *Nature* 322:265–268.

Ito, I., S. Tanabe, A. Kohda, and H. Sugiyama (1990). Allosteric potentiation of quisqualate receptors by a nootropic drug aniracetam. *Journal of Physiology* (London) 424:533–543.

Jung, M. W., J. Larson, and G. Lynch (1990a). Role of NMDA and non-NMDA receptors in synaptic transmission in rat piriform cortex. *Experimental Brain Research* 82:451–455.

Jung, M. W., J. Larson, and G. Lynch (1990b). Long-term potentiation of monosynaptic EPSPs in rat piriform cortex in vitro. *Synapse* 6:279–283.

Jung, M. W., J. Larson, and G. Lynch (1991). Evidence that changes in spine neck resistance are not responsible for expression of LTP. *Synapse* 7:216–220.

Kanter, E. D., and L. B. Haberly (1990). NMDA-dependent induction of long-term potentiation in afferent and association fiber systems of piriform cortex in vitro. *Brain Research* 525:175–179.

Kauer, J. A., R. C. Malenka, and R. A. Nicoll (1988). A persistent postsynaptic modification mediates long-term potentiation in the hippocampus. *Neuron* 1:911–917.

Kelso, S. R., and T. H. Brown (1986). Differential conditioning of associative synaptic enhancement in hippocampal brain slices. *Science*, 232:85–87.

Kelso, S. R., A. H. Ganong, and T. H. Brown (1986). Hebbian synapses in hippocampus. *Proceedings of the National Academy of Sciences USA* 83:5326–5330.

Koch, C., and T. Poggio (1983). A theoretical analysis of electrical properties of spines. *Proceedings of the Royal Society of London* B218:455–477.

Koyano, K., K. Kuba, and S. Minota (1985). Long-term potentiation of transmitter release induced by repetitive presynaptic activities in bull-frog sympathetic ganglia. *Journal of Physiology* (London) 359:219–233.

Larson, J., and G. Lynch (1986). Induction of synaptic potentiation in hippocampus by patterned stimulation involves two events. *Science* 232:985–988.

Larson, J., and G. Lynch (1988). Role of *N*-methyl-D-aspartate receptors in the induction of synaptic potentiation by burst stimulation patterned after the hippocampal theta rhythm. *Brain Research* 441:111–118.

Larson, J., and G. Lynch (1989). Theta pattern stimulation and the induction of LTP: the sequence in which synapses are stimulated determines the degree to which they potentiate. *Brain Research* 489:49–58.

Larson, J., and G. Lynch (1991). A test of the spine resistance hypothesis for LTP expression. *Brain Research* 538:347–350.

Larson, J., D. Wong, and G. Lynch (1986). Patterned stimulation at the theta frequency is optimal for the induction of hippocampal long-term potentiation. *Brain Research* 368:347–350.

Lee, K., M. Oliver, F. Schottler, and G. Lynch (1981). Electron microscopic studies of brain slices: the effects of high frequency stimulation on dendritic ultrastructure. In G. Kerkut and H. V. Wheal (eds.), *Electrical Activity in Isolated Mammalian C.N.S. Preparations*. New York: Academic Press, pp. 189–212.

Lee, K., F. Schottler, M. Oliver, and G. Lynch (1980). Brief bursts of high frequency stimulation produce two types of structural changes in rat hippocampus. *Journal of Neurophysiology* 44:247–258.

Linden, D. J., and A. Routtenberg (1989). The role of protein kinase C in long-term potentiation: a testable model. *Brain Research Reviews* 14:279–296.

Lynch, G., et al. (1983). Intracellular injections of EGTA block induction of hippocampal long-term potentiation. *Nature* 305:719–721.

Lynch, G., B. A. Bahr, and P. W. Vanderklish (1991). Induction and stabilization of long-term potentiation. In G. Snoek (ed.), *Glutamate, Cell Death, and Memory,* Heidelberg: Springer–Verlag (in press).

Lynch, G., M. Kessler, A. Arai, and J. Larson (1990a). The nature and causes of hippocampal long-term potentiation. *Progress in Brain Research* 83:233–250.

Lynch, G., J. Larson, D. Muller, and R. Granger (1990b). Neural networks and networks of neurons. In J. L. McGaugh, N. M. Weinberger, and G. Lynch (eds.), *Brain Organization and Memory: Cells, Systems, and Circuits,* New York: Oxford, pp. 390–400.

Lynch, G., J. Larson, U. Staubli, and M. Baudry (1987). New perspectives on the physiology, pharmacology, and chemistry of memory. *Drug Development Research* 10:295–315.

Magelby, K. L. (1973). The effect of repetitive stimulation on facilitation of transmitter release at the frog neuromuscular junction. *Journal of Physiology* (London) 234:327–352.

Malenka, R. C., J. A. Kauer, R. S. Zucker, and R. A. Nicoll (1988). Postsynaptic calcium is sufficient for potentiation of hippocampal synaptic transmission. *Science* 242:81–84.

Malinow, R., H. Schulman, and R. W. Tsien (1989). Inhibition of postsynaptic PKC or CaMKII blocks induction but not expression of LTP. *Science* 245:862–866.

Malinow, R., and R. W. Tsien (1990). Presynaptic enhancement shown by whole-cell recordings of long-term potentiation in hippocampal slices. *Nature* 346:177–180.

Massicotte, G., and M. Baudry (1990). Modulation of AMPA/quisqualate receptors by phospholipase A_2 treatment. *Neuroscience Letters* 118:245–248.

Massicotte, G., M. Kessler, G. Lynch, and M. Baudry (1990). *N*-methyl-D-aspartate and quisqualate/DL-α-amino-3-hydroxy-5-methylisoxazole-4-propionic acid receptors: differential regulation by phospholipase C treatment. *Molecular Pharmacology* 37:278–285.

Massicotte, G., M. W. Oliver, G. Lynch, and M. Baudry (1991). Effect of bromophenacylbromide, a phospholipase A_2 inhibitor, on the induction and maintenance of LTP in hippocampal slices. *Brain Research* 538:49–53.

Mayer, M. L., G. L. Westbrook, and P. B. Guthrie (1984). Voltage-dependent block by Mg^{2+} of NMDA responses in spinal cord neurons. *Nature* 309:261–263.

McNaughton, B. L. (1982). Long-term synaptic enhancement and short-term potentiation in rat fascia dentata act through different mechanisms. *Journal of Physiology* (London) 324:249–262.

Mulkeen, D., R. Anwyl, and M. Rowan (1988). The effects of external calcium on long-term potentiation in the rat hippocampal slice. *Brain Research* 447:234–238.

Muller, D., P.-A. Buchs, Y. Dunant, and G. Lynch (1990). Protein kinase C activity is not responsible for the expression of long-term potentiation in hippocampus. *Proceedings of the National Academy of Sciences USA* 87:4073–4077.

Muller, D., M. Joly, and G. Lynch (1988). Contributions of quisqualate and NMDA receptors to the induction and expression of LTP. *Science* 242:1694–1697.

Muller, D., J. Larson, and G. Lynch (1989). The NMDA receptor–mediated components of responses evoked by patterned stimulation are not increased by long-term potentiation. *Brain Research* 477:369–399.

Muller, D., and G. Lynch (1988a). Long-term potentiation differentially affects two components of synaptic responses in hippocampus. *Proceedings of the National Academy of Sciences USA* 85:9346–9350.

Muller, D., and G. Lynch (1988b). *N*-methyl-D-aspartate receptor-mediated component of synaptic responses to single-pulse stimulation in rat hippocampal slices. *Synapse* 2:666–668.

Muller, D., and G. Lynch (1989a). Evidence that changes in presynaptic calcium currents are not responsible for long-term potentiation in the hippocampus. *Brain Research* 479:290–299.

Muller, D., and G. Lynch (1989b). Rate-limiting step for transmission at excitatory synapses in hippocampus. *Synapse* 3:67–73.

Muller, D., and G. Lynch (1990). Synaptic modulation of *N*-methyl-D-aspartate receptor–mediated responses in hippocampus. *Synapse* 5:94–103.

Nowak, L., et al. (1984). Magnesium gates glutamate-activated channels in mouse central neurones. *Nature* 307:462–465.

Okada, D., S. Yamagishi, and H. Sugiyama (1989). Differential effects of phospholipase inhibitors in long-term potentiation in the rat hippocampal mossy fiber synapses and Schaffer/commissural synapses. *Neuroscience Letters* 100:141–146.

Otto, T., H. Eichenbaum, S. I. Wiener, and C. G. Wible (1991). Learning-related patterns of CA1 spike trains parallel stimulation parameters optimal for inducing hippocampal long-term potentiation. *Hippocampus* (in press).

Pacelli, G. J., S. Wei, and S. R. Kelso (1989). Activity-induced depression of synaptic inhibition during LTP-inducing patterned stimulation. *Brain Research* 486:26–32.

Rahamimoff, R. (1968). A dual action of calcium on neuromuscular facilitation. *Journal of Physiology* (London) 195:471–481.

Rall, W. (1978). Dendritic spines and synaptic potency. In R. Porter (ed.), *Studies in Neurophysiology*. Cambridge: Cambridge University Press, pp. 203–209.

Ranck, J. B., Jr. (1973). Studies on single neurons in dorsal hippocampal formation and septum in unrestrained rats. Part I. Behavioral correlates and firing repertoires. *Experiments in Neurology* 41:462–531.

Sayer, R. J., S. J. Redman, and P. Andersen (1989). Amplitude fluctuations in small EPSPs recorded from CA1 pyramidal cells in the guinea-pig hippocampal slice. *Journal of Neuroscience* 9:840–850.

Schottler, F. E. (1990). The nature and role of structural changes in long-term potentiation. Ph.D. thesis, Univ. California, Irvine.

Staubli, U., M. Kessler, and G. Lynch (1990a). Aniracetam has proportionately smaller effects on synapses expressing long-term potentiation: evidence that receptor changes subserve LTP. *Psychobiology* 18:377–381.

Staubli, U., J. Larson, and G. Lynch (1990b). Mossy fiber potentiation and long-term potentiation involve different expression mechanisms. *Synapse* 5:333–335.

Staubli, U., and G. Lynch (1987). Stable hippocampal long-term potentiation elicited by "theta" pattern stimulation. *Brain Research* 435:227–234.

Terramani, T., M. Kessler, G. Lynch, and M. Baudry (1988). Effects of thiol reagents on ^{3}H-AMPA binding to rat telencephalic membranes. *Molecular Pharmacology* 34:117–123.

Vanderwolf, C. H. (1969). Hippocampal electrical activity and voluntary movement in the rat. *Electroencephalography and Clinical Neurophysiology* 26:407–418.

Williams, J. H., and T. V. P. Bliss (1989). An in vitro study of the effect of lipoxygenase and cyclo-oxygenase inhibitors of arachidonic acid on the induction and maintenance of long-term potentiation in the hippocampus. *Neuroscience Letters* 107:301–306.

Wilson, C. J. (1984). Passive cable properties of dendritic spines and spiny neurons. *Journal of Neuroscience* 4:281–297.

Zalutsky, R. A., and R. A. Nicoll (1990). Comparison of two forms of long-term potentiation in single hippocampal neurons. *Science* 248:1619–1624.

Zucker, R. S. (1973). Changes in the statistics of transmitter release during facilitation. *Journal of Physiology* (London) 229:787–810.

II Role of Calcium-Dependent Enzymes in Long-Term Potentiation

10 The Role of Protein Kinase Activity in Long-Term Potentiation

David J. Perkel and Roger A. Nicoll

The early steps in the generation of long-term potentiation (LTP) of synaptic transmission in the CA1 region of the hippocampus now appear to be relatively clear (Bliss and Lynch, 1988; Gustafsson and Wigström, 1988; Malenka et al., 1989). Presynaptic transmitter release coincident with postsynaptic depolarization permits entry of calcium ions through postsynaptic *N*-methyl-D-aspartate (NMDA) receptors. The resulting rise in intracellular calcium concentration is thought to trigger a biochemical cascade that causes enhanced synaptic transmission. Although these latter mechanisms are still unclear, the classes of mediators proposed to follow the rise in intracellular calcium include the calcium-activated proteases known as calpains (Lynch and Baudry, 1984), protein kinases (Linden and Routtenberg, 1989), and protein synthetic machinery (Frey et al., 1988; Otani et al., 1989; Stanton and Sarvey, 1984). In this chapter, we discuss experiments addressing the role of protein kinases in LTP.

Much evidence has accumulated concerning the role of protein kinase activity in LTP (Linden and Routtenberg, 1989). Studies using a number of experimental approaches have demonstrated that phosphorylation of certain proteins by kinases is enhanced after tetanic stimulation and can influence LTP, possibly at multiple stages in the biochemical cascade. Progress has been made toward identifying which kinases may be involved, their cellular localization, and their major substrates. Nonetheless, a number of questions remain concerning the role of kinases, not only in synaptic plasticity, but also in basal synaptic transmission.

It is possible to distinguish three basic classes of evidence that have been used to test the notion that protein kinase activity plays a role in LTP. First, biochemical studies can examine whether any changes in rate or extent of protein phosphorylation accompany LTP. This approach provides the most direct evidence for kinase (and/or phosphatase) action in that it is possible to use assays that measure protein phosphorylation. The conclusions that can be drawn, however, are limited to correlations (Linden and Routtenberg, 1989); it is difficult to determine whether changes in phosphorylation are a cause or a consequence of LTP or some unrelated epiphenomenon. In addition, because of the practical requirement of homogenizing tissue for this type of experiment, it is difficult to address the question of cellular localization of any kinase(s) and substrate(s) that may be involved.

Second, the effects of compounds that activate kinases can be compared with the effects of LTP. If a particular kinase is sufficient to generate LTP, activators of that kinase should at least cause an enhancement of synaptic transmission. In addition, if the activator and LTP operate through the same mechanism, it should be possible to demonstrate occlusion between maximal activation of the kinase and LTP. This kind of experiment should, assuming that a highly selective kinase-activating compound is available, provide evidence that kinases can trigger LTP. It is difficult, however, to establish absolute mimicry. Although initial results may suggest mimicry, more extensive investigations might differentiate the compound's actions from the effects of LTP. One must also consider the possibility, when performing occlusion experiments, that measured responses could become saturated and not reveal real enhancement of synaptic transmission. There is the additional problem that LTP might induce kinase activity in only a subset of those subcellular compartments where a particular kinase is present, and gross application of a kinase activator might thus be expected to have actions in addition to those caused by LTP.

Third, pharmacological agents that prevent the activation of kinases or block protein phosphorylation can be tested to determine whether they interfere with LTP. This type of experiment is the most commonly used approach that has the possibility of establishing a necessary role for kinase activity in LTP. As is the case for any pharmacological manipulation, however, the conclusions that can be drawn are severely limited by the degree of selectivity of the compounds involved. In addition, it is difficult to distinguish between antagonism of a permissive process and antagonism of one that is selectively activated by the LTP-inducing stimulus.

Each class of evidence just outlined thus has its own strengths and limitations. We discuss each in detail in the following sections, with particular emphasis on electrophysiological experiments. By combining evidence from a variety of complementary approaches, one can begin to elucidate the role played by various protein-kinase pathways in the generation of LTP.

PROTEIN PHOSPHORYLATION ASSOCIATED WITH LTP

The first strategy just outlined, that of examining protein phosphorylation, has allowed the demonstration that increased kinase activity is associated with LTP. Early evidence of this type came from post-hoc phosphorylation assays; when homogenates of hippocampi that had been subjected to high-frequency, LTP-inducing stimulation were incubated with ^{32}P-ATP, a 47 kD protein called F1 exhibited increased phosphorylation (Routtenberg and Lovinger, 1985). This protein was subsequently found to be the same protein that several other groups had studied and given the names GAP-43, B50, and P-57 (Skene, 1989). In addition, there was a translocation of phospholipid-induced kinase activity from the cytosolic to the membrane fraction of the homogenate (Akers et al., 1986), consistent with previous findings that activation of protein kinase C (PKC) is related to attachment to the membrane (Kraft and Anderson, 1983). Tissue from animals in which induction of LTP had been blocked by application of the NMDA receptor antagonist 2-amino-5-phosphono valeric acid (APV) (Collingridge et al., 1983) did not show the increased ability to phosphorylate F1 (Linden et al., 1988). Because F1 is a substrate of the calcium- and phospholipid-dependent PKC (Akers and Routtenberg, 1985; Nishizuka, 1984), it was suggested that PKC activity might mediate LTP. It has apparently not been possible thus far to demonstrate increased in situ phosphorylation of F1 after LTP.

ACTIVATION OF PKC ENHANCES SYNAPTIC TRANSMISSION

Early experiments utilizing the mimicry approach also suggested a role for PKC in LTP. Application of phorbol esters, which potently and selectively activate PKC at the diacylglycerol-binding site (Nishizuka, 1984), caused a prolonged increase in synaptic efficacy in hippocampal slices maintained in vitro; a phorbol ester that is inactive with respect to PKC activation did not affect synaptic transmission (Malenka et al., 1986). This increase in synaptic strength persisted long after removal of the phorbol ester, although the possibility could not be excluded that the hydrophobic phorbol ester remained in the tissue and bound to PKC. Furthermore, in the presence of phorbol ester, tetanic stimulation of afferent fibers did not produce further potentiation. Because phorbol ester application apparently mimicked the effects of LTP, these results led to the suggestion that phorbol ester activated PKC and saturated the LTP mechanism. An alternative interpretation is that phorbol ester had two separate effects: increase of the excitatory postsynaptic potential (EPSP) by a mechanism independent of LTP and blockade of the LTP-inducing mechanism.

Subsequent studies confirmed the strong potentiating effects of phorbol esters, but also revealed a number of differences between their effects and the consequences of LTP. It was found that if the less hydrophobic ester phorbol-12, 13-diacetate (PDAc) was used at lower concentrations, prolonged washing after removing the compound caused the EPSP to return to baseline levels, indicating that the LTP mechanism is not irreversibly activated by phorbol esters (Gustafsson et al., 1988; Muller et al., 1988b). In both studies it was noted that the increase of the EPSP caused by phorbol ester application was accompanied by a reduction in the degree of paired-pulse facilitation, an effect that was not observed with LTP (Gustafsson et al., 1988; McNaughton, 1982; Muller and Lynch, 1988; Muller and Lynch, 1989).

Another difference between the effects of phorbol esters and LTP is observed when the NMDA component of the excitatory postsynaptic current (EPSC) is examined. Using whole-cell voltage-clamp recording from pyramidal cells in hippocampal slices (Edwards et al., 1989; Hestrin et al., 1990), it is possible to distinguish components of the EPSC that are mediated by the NMDA and non-NMDA classes of glutamate receptor. When the cell is held at depolarized potentials, both components can be recorded. Application of PDAc (1 μM) caused a large increase in the NMDA component as well as the non-NMDA component of the EPSC (figure 10.1). This observation serves to contrast the effect of the phorbol ester with previous findings that after LTP, the enhancement of synaptic transmission occurs primarily in the non-NMDA component of the EPSP (Kauer et al., 1988b; Muller et al., 1988a). Because it has been shown that phorbol esters increase transmitter release in hippocampal slices (Malenka et al., 1987), one simple way to interpret these results is to suppose that the additional transmitter released in the presence of phorbol ester has access to both types of receptors.

A number of studies have also questioned whether LTP is occluded by the presence of PKC activators. Application of lower concentrations of phorbol ester induced a substantial increase in synaptic efficacy, but did not affect the magnitude of tetanus-induced potentiation (Gustafsson et al., 1988; Muller et al., 1988b). Similarly, the magnitude of phorbol ester–induced potentiation after LTP is comparable to that induced in naive synapses (Gustafsson et al., 1988; Muller et al., 1990).

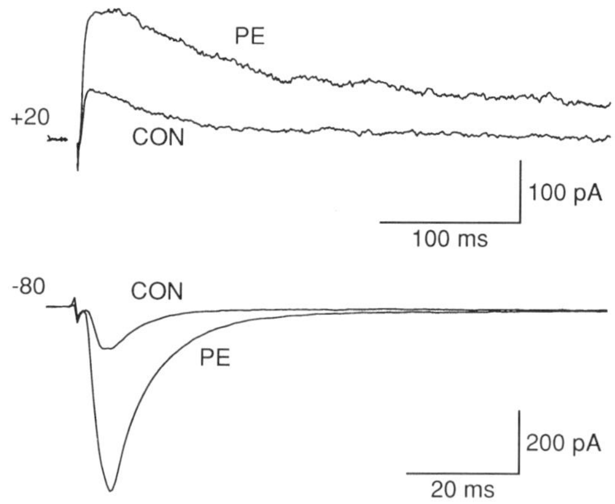

Figure 10.1 Phorbol ester application causes enhancement of both NMDA and non-NMDA components of the EPSC. Whole-cell voltage-clamp recording of a CA1 pyramidal cell in a 250-μm thick rat hippocampal slice. With the cell clamped at −80 mV (lower traces), 1 μM of PDAc caused a substantial increase in the EPSC mediated by non-NMDA receptors. At +20 mV (upper traces), the EPSC was outward and exhibited the characteristic slow decay of NMDA receptors. PDAc caused a substantial increase of the NMDA component. Ringer solution contained (in mM): NaCl, 119; KCl, 2.5; $MgSO_4$, 1.3; $CaCl_2$, 2.5; NaH_2PO_4, 1; $NaHCO_3$, 26.2; glucose, 11; Na-HEPES, 10; picrotoxin, 0.1; glycine 0.001; pH 7.2. Whole-cell pipette solution consisted of (in mM): CsF, 130; NaCl, 10; Na-EGTA, 10; Na-HEPES, 10; pH 7.2 (From Hestrin et al., 1990.)

On the surface, these results might be interpreted as an argument against the involvement of PKC in LTP because the application of phorbol esters caused an increase in the EPSP (presumably through its action on PKC), but did not interfere with LTP. However, careful examination of EPSPs within 10 minutes of a tetanus reveals that a low concentration of PDAc reduces the rate of decay of potentiation following a brief tetanus (Asztely et al., 1990). It has also been shown that application of the phorbol ester 12-O-tetradecanoyl-phorbol-13-acetate (TPA) in vivo has no effect on basal synaptic transmission, but prolongs tetanus-induced potentiation (Lovinger and Routtenberg, 1988; Routtenberg et al., 1986). It thus appears that phorbol esters may have actions that can interact with LTP.

It is also possible that LTP has consequences that are not mimicked by low concentrations of phorbol esters. Despite the partial mismatch of effects of LTP and PKC, we cannot conclude that PKC plays no role in LTP. It appears likely, however, that at lower concentrations, phorbol ester is acting presynaptically because it increases transmitter release, reduces paired-pulse facilitation, and increases both non-NMDA and NMDA receptor–mediated components of the EPSC. Because LTP does not appear to share some of these effects, a role for presynaptic PKC in LTP seems uncertain.

In one of the most direct tests of whether postsynaptic PKC could affect synaptic transmission, purified PKC was introduced into hippocampal pyramidal cells through the recording microelectrode (Hu et al., 1987). Although no manipulation was performed to activate the kinase, a gradual increase was observed in the EPSP and probability of eliciting an action potential. Heat-inactivated kinase did not have this effect. The PKC-induced enhancement of synaptic transmission resembled LTP, but that study did not address whether EPSPs that had grown in the presence of PKC were capable of exhibiting LTP.

Another class of PKC activator is the cis-unsaturated fatty acid oleate, which renders the kinase active even in the absence of calcium (Murakami et al., 1986). Not only is this compound active, but it is possible that similar molecules could be generated endogenously through the phospholipase A_2 pathway. In the dentate gyrus in vivo, application of oleate did not affect baseline transmission but prolonged tetanus-induced potentiation (Linden et al., 1987).

A role for kinases other than PKC has not been demonstrated using the approach of applying activators. Among the potential candidates are cyclic adenosine monophosphate (cAMP)–dependent protein kinase (PKA), cyclic guanosine monophosphate (cGMP)–dependent protein kinase (PKG) and calcium-calmodulin–dependent protein kinase type II (CaMKII). One reason for the relative paucity of evidence is the lack of selective activators of these kinases. Generation of multiple calcium-mediated action potentials in the absence of presynaptic stimulation does not cause LTP (Malenka et al., 1989), but it is not known whether such activity causes a sufficient rise in intracellular calcium concentration in dendritic spines to activate CaMKII. There are membrane-permeant analogs of cyclic nucleotides, however, which would presumably have among their actions the activation of cAMP-dependent protein kinase and cGMP-dependent protein kinase. At present, it is not known whether such kinases interact with excitatory synaptic transmission, LTP, or both.

KINASE INHIBITORS AFFECT THE TIME-COURSE OF LTP

Experiments using the approach of applying pharmacological tools to block kinase activity have been numerous, and they provide the strongest evidence that protein kinase activity is necessary for the establishment of the full complement of LTP effects. We discuss three aspects of kinase involvement: temporal requirements for kinase activity, cellular localization of kinase activity, and type of kinase involved.

The clearest result from a number of studies is that application of kinase inhibitors before giving high-frequency stimulation results in a potentiation whose initial magnitude is similar to that seen in normal conditions, but which subsequently decays back to baseline levels over a time-course that lasts between 20 and 60 minutes. Such findings have been obtained with extracellular application of several kinase inhibitors: polymyxin B, mellitin, sphingosine, H-7, and K-252b (Kauer et al., 1988a; Lovinger et al., 1987; Malinow et al., 1988; Reymann et al., 1988; Reymann et al., 1990; Reymann et al., 1988). Each of these kinase inhibitors has its own characteristic profile of specificity against different kinases and against other cellular processes unrelated to kinases; however, they overlap in their antagonism of PKC. Taken together, these results point strongly toward an obligatory role for a protein kinase, possibly PKC, in LTP.

Similarly, inhibitors of calmodulin, which would be expected to block activation of CaMKII, interfere with the potentiation after a tetanus; there is some discrepancy, however, about the time-course of this effect (Finn et al., 1980; Reymann et al., 1988). In addition, the two primary calmodulin inhibitors used, trifluoperazine and calmidazolium, may have other actions in addition to their calmodulin antagonism. Nonetheless, these experiments suggest that a calmodulin-dependent process is a necessary step in LTP.

In addition, postsynaptic application of H-7, calmidazolium, or potent and selective peptide inhibitors of calmodulin (CaMKII or PKC; see the following) reduces the duration of tetanus-induced potentiation in a manner strongly resembling those obtained with bath application (Malenka et al., 1989; Malinow et al., 1989). These results are consistent with a necessary role for postsynaptic kinase activity in LTP.

There is some question about the effects of kinase inhibitors if they are applied after the establishment of LTP. Malinow and colleagues (1988) reported that bath application of H-7 after establishment of LTP resulted in the return of the EPSP to baseline levels, although it had no effect on unpotentiated pathways in the same slices. They concluded that persistent protein kinase activity was necessary for the long-lasting enhancement of the EPSP. However, Muller and colleagues (1990) have performed essentially the same experiment as Malinow and colleagues (1988) and found different results. Although H-7 caused a depression of the potentiated EPSP, it also reduced the EPSP in the unpotentiated pathway by a similar amount. They concluded that their results did not support a role for an H-7–sensitive kinase in the persistent enhancement of synaptic transmission following induction of LTP.

Similarly, Reymann and coworkers (1990) reported that K-252b, a kinase inhibitor that is more potent than H-7 (Kase et al., 1987), did not affect unpotentiated EPSPs, but tetanization in the presence of the inhibitor resulted in a decremental form of potentiation. When the compound was applied 60 minutes after the tetanus, there was no effect on potentiated EPSPs, but when it was applied immediately after the tetanus, the potentiation decayed to baseline levels over a period of approximately 60 minutes.

We have performed similar experiments using H-7, and our results are illustrated in figure 10.2. We were unable to demonstrate a selective action of H-7 on potentiated EPSPs as compared with unpotentiated EPSPs. While these results do not necessarily rule out a role for kinase activity in maintaining enhanced EPSPs, they point out one of the difficulties associated with pharmacological tools that may not be completely selective. It

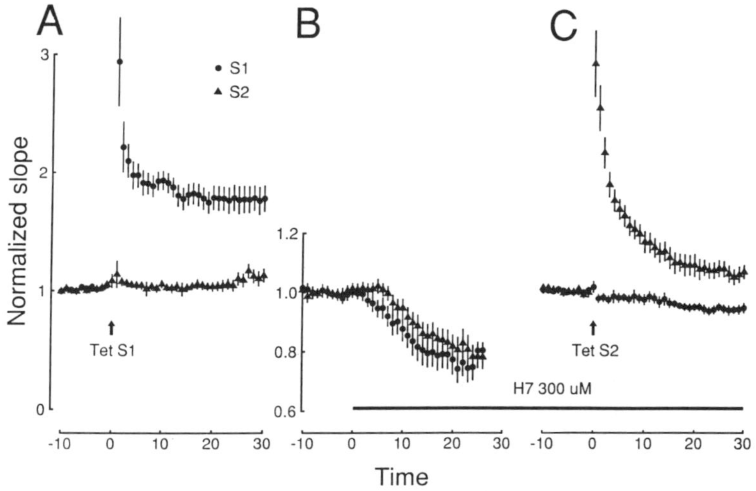

Figure 10.2 H-7 reduces the EPSP by a similar amount in potentiated and nonpotentiated pathways. (A) LTP was elicited in one of two independent pathways converging on a region recorded by a single field electrode. After approximately 30 minutes, the stimulus strengths of the two pathways were adjusted to give similar size EPSPs. (B) A new baseline was established, and H-7 (300 μM) was applied in the perfusion medium. (C) A subsequent tetanus applied to the control pathway resulted in a decremental form of potentiation, consistent with previous findings.

is possible, however, that this depressant action of H-7 on EPSPs reflects a role for kinase activity in regulating synaptic transmission (Llinás et al., 1985), and as such is a potentially interesting finding with respect to the basic mechanisms of transmitter release. However, K-252b has been reported not to have an effect on synaptic transmission (Kase et al., 1987; Reymann et al., 1990).

The site of action of kinase or calmodulin inhibitors when they are applied extracellularly is unknown. Presumably, the lipophilic nature of these compounds, which allows them to cross the cell membrane, would give them access to both presynaptic and postsynaptic sides of the synapse. By applying them to the postsynaptic cell through an intracellular recording pipette, it is possible to address the cellular localization of the

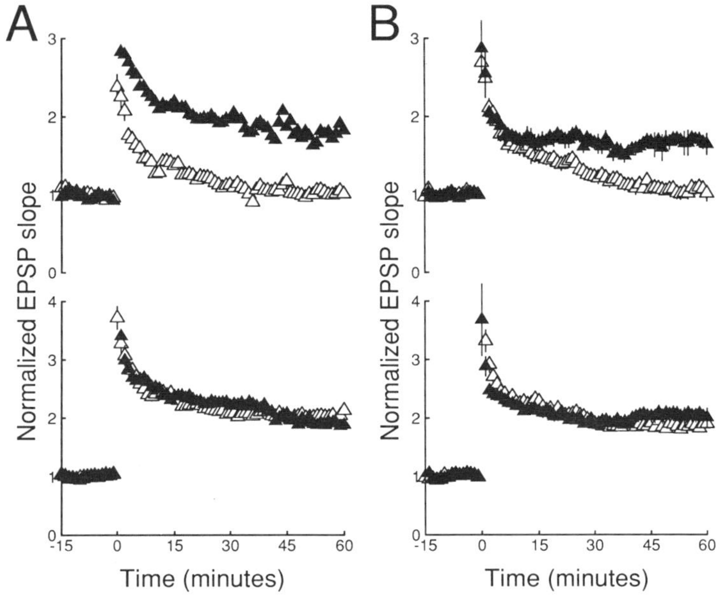

Figure 10.3 Postsynaptic calmodulin and protein kinase activity are necessary for generating LTP. Conventional intracellular recordings were made from CA1 pyramidal cells in rat hippocampal slices using standard techniques. EPSPs were elicited every 10 seconds, and the average initial slope is plotted in 1-minute bins through the course of the experiment. (A) Calmodulin-binding peptide (CBP; open symbols) or a similar but inactive peptide (CTP_2; filled symbols) was present in the recording pipette (190 μM in 3 M CsCl). Upper panel illustrates intracellular EPSP slope, and lower panel shows extracellular field EPSP slope recorded simultaneously in the same slices. Cells containing CBP (n = 11) showed a decremental potentiation following tetanus, while those containing CTP_2 (n = 8) showed normal LTP. (B) When recording pipettes contained H-7 (20 mM in 1% DMSO and the normal electrolyte, 3 M CsCl), tetanization resulted in a decremental potentiation that returned to baseline levels after approximately 45 minutes (open symbols; n = 8). In another population recorded with pipettes containing 3 M CsCl and 1% DMSO, normal, nondecremental LTP was observed (filled symbols; n = 6). Simultaneously recorded field potentials in the two populations of slices exhibited similar degrees of stable LTP. (Redrawn after Malenka et al., 1989, by permission from *Nature* 340:554–557. Copyright 1989 Macmillan Magazines Ltd.)

necessary kinase activity. Postsynaptic application of H-7, calmidazolium, or peptide inhibitors of calmodulin (CaMKII or PKC) results in decremental potentiation that returns to baseline levels in 20 to 40 minutes (Malenka et al., 1989; Malinow et al., 1989). An example of this effect is illustrated in figure 10.3A, in which cells were recorded using pipettes filled with a calmodulin-binding peptide (CBP) derived from the sequence of the calmodulin-binding domain of CaMKII (Kelly et al., 1988). Figure 10.3B shows the decremental potentiation found in cells in which H-7 had been applied through the recording pipette. Malinow and colleagues (1989) have used specific antagonist peptides against PKC and CaMKII, and they provided evidence that both kinases are necessary for generating nondecremental LTP. By using peptide inhibitors of cellular processes, it may be possible to attain degrees of specificity that have heretofore been impossible.

CONCLUSION

There is now very strong evidence that we must include the phenomenon of LTP among the vast array of cellular processes that are regulated by protein kinase activity. By combining the strengths of the various biochemical, electrophysiological, and pharmacological approaches that are now available, it will be possible to elucidate in greater detail the mechanisms by which kinases are involved by LTP-inducing stimuli, the roles played by the relevant substrates, and the mechanisms linking protein phosphorylation to enhanced synaptic transmission.

REFERENCES

Akers, R. E., et al. (1986). Translocation of protein kinase C activity may mediate hippocampal long-term potentiation. *Science* 231:587–589.

Akers, R. F., and A. Routtenberg (1985). Protein kinase C phosphorylates a 47 Mr protein (F1) directly related to synaptic plasticity. *Brain Research* 334:147–151.

Asztely, F., E. Hanse, and B. Gustafsson (1990). The early decay of long-term potentiation in the hippocampal CA1 region in vitro is reduced by activators of protein kinase C. *Brain Research* 521:355–358.

Bliss, T. V. P., and M. A. Lynch (1988). Long-term potentiation of synaptic transmission in the hippocampus: properties and mechanisms. In P. W. Landfield and S. A. Deadwyler (eds.), *Long-Term Potentiation: From Biophysics to Behavior.* New York: Alan R. Liss.

Collingridge, G. L., S. J. Kehl, and H. McLennan (1983). Excitatory amino acids in synaptic transmission in the Schaffer collateral—commissural pathway of the rat hippocampus. *Journal of Physiology* 334:33–46.

Edwards, F. A., A. Konnerth, B. Sakmann, and T. Takahashi (1989). A thin slice preparation for patch clamp recordings from neurones of the mammalian central nervous system. *Pflügers Archives* 414:600–612.

Finn, R. C., M. Browning, and G. Lynch (1980). Trifluoperazine inhibits long-term potentiation and the phosphorylation of a 40,000 dalton protein. *Neuroscience Letters* 19:103–108.

Frey, U., M. Krug, K. G. Reymann, and H. Matthies (1988). Anisomycin, an inhibitor of protein synthesis, blocks late phases of LTP phenomena in the hippocampal CA1 region. *Brain Research* 452:57–65.

Gustafsson, B., Y.-Y. Huang, and H. Wigström (1988). Phorbol ester–induced potentiation differs from long-term potentiation in the guinea pig hippocampus in vitro. *Neuroscience Letters* 85:77–81.

Gustafsson, B., and H. Wigström (1988). Physiological mechanisms underlying long-term potentiation. *Trends in Neuroscience* 11:156–162.

Hestrin, S., R. A. Nicoll, D. J. Perkel, and P. Sah (1990). Analysis of excitatory synaptic action in the rat hippocampus using whole cell recording from thin slices. *Journal of Physiology* 422:203–225.

Hu, G. Y., et al. (1987). Protein kinase C injection into hippocampal pyramidal cells elicits features of long-term potentiation. *Nature* 328:426–429.

Kase, H., et al. (1987). K-252 compounds, novel and potent inhibitors of protein kinase C and cyclic nucleotide-dependent protein kinases. *Biochemical and Biophysical Research Communications* 142:436–440.

Kauer, J. A., R. C. Malenka, and R. A. Nicoll (1988a). NMDA application potentiates synaptic transmission in the hippocampus. *Nature* 334:250–252.

Kauer, J. A., R. C. Malenka, and R. A. Nicoll (1988b). A persistent postsynaptic modification mediates long-term potentiation in the hippocampus. *Neuron* 1:911–917.

Kelly, P. T., R. P. Weinberger, and M. N. Waxham (1988). Active site-directed inhibition of Ca^{2+}/calmodulin–dependent protein kinase type II by a bifunctional calmodulin binding peptide. *Proceedings of the National Academy of Sciences USA* 85:4991–4995.

Kraft, A. S., and W. B. Anderson (1983). Phorbol esters increase the amount of Ca^{2+}/phospholipid-dependent protein kinase associated with plasma membrane. *Nature* 301:621–623.

Linden, D. J., and A. Routtenberg (1989). The role of protein kinase C in long-term potentiation: a testable model. *Brain Research. Brain Research Reviews* 14:279–296.

Linden, D. J., F. S. Sheu, K. Murakami, and A. Routtenberg (1987). Enhancement of long-term potentiation by cis-unsaturated fatty acid: relation to protein kinase C and phospholipase A_2. *Journal of Neuroscience* 7:3783–3792.

Linden, D. J., K. L. Wong, F. S. Sheu, and A. Routtenberg (1988). NMDA receptor blockade prevents the increase in protein kinase C substrate (protein F1) phosphorylation produced by long-term potentiation. *Brain Research* 458:142–146.

Llinás, R., et al. (1985). Intraterminal injection of synapsin I or calcium/calmodulin–dependent protein kinase II alters neurotransmitter release at the squid giant synapse. *Proceedings of the National Academy of Sciences USA* 82:3035–3039.

Lovinger, D. M., and A. Routtenberg (1988). Synapse-specific protein kinase C activation enhances maintenance of long-term potentiation in rat hippocampus. *Journal of Physiology* (London) 400:321–333.

Lovinger, D. M., K. Wong, K. Murakami, and A. Routtenberg (1987). Protein kinase C inhibitors eliminate hippocampal long-term potentiation (LTP). *Brain Research* 436:177–183.

Lynch, G., and M. Baudry (1984). The biochemistry of memory: a new and specific hypothesis. *Science* 224:1057–1063.

Malenka, R. C., G. S. Ayoub, and R. A. Nicoll (1987). Phorbol esters enhance transmitter release in rat hippocampal slices. *Brain Research* 403:198–203.

Malenka, R. C., et al. (1989). An essential role for postsynaptic calmodulin and protein kinase activity in long-term potentiation. *Nature* 340:554–557.

Malenka, R. C., J. A. Kauer, D. J. Perkel, and R. A. Nicoll (1989). The impact of postsynaptic calcium on synaptic transmission—its role in long-term potentiation. *Trends in Neuroscience* 12:444–450.

Malenka, R. C., D. V. Madison, and R. A. Nicoll (1986). Potentiation of synaptic transmission in the hippocampus by phorbol esters. *Nature* 321:695–697.

Malinow, R., D. V. Madison, and R. W. Tsien (1988). Persistent protein kinase activity underlying long-term potentiation. *Nature* 335:820–824.

Malinow, R., H. Schulman, and R. W. Tsien (1989). Inhibition of postsynaptic PKC or CaMKII blocks induction but not expression of LTP. *Science* 245:862–866.

McNaughton, B. L. (1982). Long-term synaptic enhancement and short-term potentiation in rat fascia dentata act through different mechanisms. *Journal of Physiology* 324:249–262.

Muller, D., P.-A. Buchs, Y. Dunant, and G. Lynch (1990). Protein kinase C activity is not responsible for the expression of long-term potentiation in hippocampus. *Proceedings of the National Academy of Sciences USA* 87:4073–4077.

Muller, D., M. Joly, and G. Lynch (1988a). Contributions of quisqualate and NMDA receptors in the induction and expression of LTP. *Science* 242:1694–1697.

Muller, D., and G. Lynch (1988b). Long-term potentiation differentially affects two components of synaptic responses in hippocampus. *Proceedings of the National Academy of Sciences USA* 85:9346–9350.

Muller, D., and G. Lynch (1989). Evidence that changes in presynaptic calcium currents are not responsible for long-term potentiation in hippocampus. *Brain Research* 479:290–299.

Muller, D., J. Turnbull, M. Baudry, and G. Lynch (1988). Phorbol ester–induced synaptic facilitation is different than long-term potentiation. *Proceedings of the National Academy of Sciences USA* 85:6997–7000.

Murakami, K., S. Y. Chan, and A. Routtenberg (1986). Protein kinase C activation by cis-fatty acid in the absence of Ca^{2+} and phospholipids. *Journal of Biology and Chemistry* 261:15,424–15,429.

Nishizuka, T. (1984). Turnover of inositol phospholipids and signal transduction. *Science* 225:1365–1370.

Otani, S., et al. (1989). Maintenance of long-term potentiation in rat dentate gyrus requires protein synthesis but not messenger RNA synthesis immediately post-tetanization. *Neuroscience* 28:519–526.

Reymann, K. G., R. Brodemann, H. Kase, and H. Matthies (1988). Inhibitors of calmodulin and protein kinase C block different phases of hippocampal long-term potentiation. *Brain Research* 461:388–392.

Reymann, K. G., et al. (1990). Activation of a K-252b–sensitive protein kinase is necessary for a postsynaptic phase of long-term potentiation in area CA1 of rat hippocampus. *European Journal of Neuroscience* 2:481–486.

Reymann, K. G., U. Frey, R. Jork, and H. Matthies (1988). Polymyxin B, an inhibitor of protein kinase C, prevents the maintenance of synaptic long-term potentiation in hippocampal CA1 neurons. *Brain Research* 440:305–314.

Routtenberg, A., et al. (1986). Phorbol ester promotes growth of synaptic plasticity. *Brain Research* 378:374–378.

Routtenberg, A., and D. M. Lovinger (1985). Selective increase in phosphorylation of a 47-kDa protein (F1) directly related to long-term potentiation. *Behavioral and Neural Biology* 44:186–200.

Skene, J. H. P. (1989). Axonal growth-associated proteins. *Annual Review of Neuroscience* 12:127–156.

Stanton, P. K., and J. M. Sarvey (1984). Blockade of long-term potentiation in rat hippocampal CA1 region by inhibitors of protein synthesis. *Journal of Neuroscience* 4:3080–3088.

11 Trans-synaptophobia Revisited

Aryeh Routtenberg

Last year I discovered an affliction that appeared to have a pernicious effect on those neurobiologists studying long-term potentiation. With tongue firmly in cheek I labeled it "trans-synaptophobia"—the fear of crossing to the other side of the synapse. Although there were signs that a vaccine for this disorder might be emerging soon, recurrent breakouts in various locations in the United States and United Kingdom necessitate a renewed appraisal of the disorder and a consideration of therapeutic treatments.

The main source of the problem is the apparent need to identify either the presynaptic or postsynaptic side of the synapse as the exclusive site for the maintenance of synaptic change. The reason for concern is that it may be important to incorporate proposals made as long as 40 years ago, which, I assert, are still eminently sensible today. Hebb (1949) implied and Schmitt, Dev, and Smith (1976) explicitly stated that alterations at synapses occur as a result of bidirectional communication at the synapse.

I would like to propose that this communication takes the form of a dialogue. It is useful to think of this dialogue as occurring between the transmitter-containing terminal and the postsynaptic density–containing target zone. Enhanced communication occurs when agreed to by both parties.

Most of the contributors to this book have at one time or another come down with this malady. In a seminal paper, Lynch and Baudry (1984) clearly put all their molecules (calpain, fodrin, glutamate receptors) on the postsynaptic side; no presynaptic terminal was in evidence in their proposed model. Other early presynaptic theories (Routtenberg, 1985) focused on the possibility that there was a physical growth of the synaptic terminal. A perfunctory bow to the postsynaptic mechanism was in evidence. Bliss and associates (1986) demonstrated that release of excitatory amino acid transmitters was correlated with long-term potentiation (LTP). This type of mechanism was found in the same ward with its phylogenetically disadvantaged cousin, the *Aplysia,* who also demonstrated a use-dependent enhanced presynaptic terminal release of transmitter (Kandel and Schwartz, 1982). In this latter model, no postsynaptic element was in evidence.

[I have noticed that people outside the field often view this disorder like an American football game with the teams lined up on each side of the junction and the latest report giving a thrust to the particular team, only to be thwarted by a subsequent report from the opposition. This makes for spirited grant proposals, but in my view, misplaced the focus of the scientific inquiry. My personal speculation here is that such an approach is indeed useful for U.S. grants in which harried reviewers and panel members have little time for complex configurations. I can recall, indeed, that in addition to the condemnatory phrases "handwaving" and "fishing expedition," the less-used but no less damning "talmudic" was sure to lower the priority score of a submitted application.]

At this point the informed reader might well think—yes, of course, this was true a few years ago, but now there is growing awareness of the potential for a retrograde message (e.g., Linden and Routtenberg, 1989; Lynch et al., 1989; Piomelli et al., 1987), and so the issue is essentially resolved.

But, dear reader, the illness has alas recurred, again in evidence in the two recent reports of Malinow and Tsien (1990) and Bekkers and Stevens (1990). Both indicated that the presynaptic site was indeed the site of persistent change. Their results are reviewed elsewhere in this book in chapters 6 and 8. Using recent advances in cellular recordings and techniques of quantal analysis, both laboratories concluded that after LTP there was a change in quantal content (presynaptic) but not quantal size (postsynaptic). The presynaptic team just pushed back to the postsynaptic and the shoot-out at the O\K corral may appear over.

More than acknowledgment by advocates of either stripe of the fact that "yes, to be sure, there are minor alterations occurring on the other side," one requires rather a description of the events over time on both sides as the enhanced communication at the synapse develops.

Here I propose that during the development of enhanced and persistent communication between presynaptic and postsynaptic sites a dialogue is occurring that deploys both orthograde and retrograde signals. As is discussed in later sections, this involves the essential activity of the same molecule, protein kinase C (PKC), which is present on both sides of the synapse. The approach taken here is to specify the precise time when PKC on each side of the synapse is critically important for maintaining the enhanced response.

PROTEIN KINASE C INVOLVEMENT IN BOTH PRESYNAPTIC AND POSTSYNAPTIC LTP

In the perspective of recent attempts to pinpoint LTP mechanisms to presynaptic or postsynaptic processes, it may be useful to return to earlier studies on PKC and LTP to determine if they provide any fresh insight into the current debate. Initial proposals (1984, 1985) and results (1983, 1985) from this laboratory indicated that a PKC substrate, protein F1 (GAP43; Benowitz and Routtenberg, 1987) was phosphorylated in direct relation to the extent of enhancement of LTP. We suspected then but know now that protein F1 is localized presynaptically, clearly suggesting involvement of the presynaptic mechanism in LTP (see Routtenberg, 1989; Colley, 1991 for review).

The increase in protein F1 phosphorylation, while demonstrating that the consequences of an in vivo treatment can be preserved ex vivo, leaves unanswered the question of the precise mechanism that is engaged in vivo. For example, the phosphorylation increase in vitro may not precisely reflect what is happening in vivo. Of concern is the possibility that a kinase that normally does not phosphorylate protein F1 would now do so, having access to it consequent to homogenization. That is, the presynaptic protein F1 could theoretically be phosphorylated by a PKC subtype (Nishizuka, 1988) that is localized postsynaptically. But because the compartmentalization would be partially disrupted, the postsynaptic PKC could then phosphorylate the presynaptic protein F1. Two points argue against this. First, kinases do not appear to be promiscuous with regard to what substrates they phosphorylate. In particular, gamma PKC, which is likely to be postsynaptic (Nishizuka, 1988), poorly phosphorylates protein F1 while beta PKC phosphorylates F1 quite readily (Sheu et al., 1990). Thus, kinases may wander, but they remain true to their substrate.

In this regard it is interesting that protein F1 is phosphorylated in vivo (Rodnight et al., 1985), and this in vivo phosphorylation can be increased by phorbol esters (De Graan et al., 1988). Whether F1 can be increased in phosphorylation in vivo after LTP remains unknown, although failures, particularly in the slice, would be suspect because the number of synapses activated would be small relative to the total. Nonetheless, it is clear that a presynaptic phosphorylation of protein F1 exists when synaptic morphology is intact, and this phosphorylation is increased by PKC activation.

A second issue concerns the mechanism for the increased in vitro phosphorylation after LTP. Is this an increase in vivo of PKC activity or an increase in the number of vacant sites available for phosphorylation, possibly caused by increased phosphatase activity? One approach to answering this question was taken by Dr. Shew Chan in my laboratory a few years ago (Chan et al., 1988). We compared the level of phosphorylation in tissue from LTP animals with the level of phosphorylation in the same tissue that had been subsequently dephosphorylated by alkaline phosphatase and then rephosphorylated. Reasoning that if there was an increase in phosphorylation in vivo after LTP, there would be a greater difference in phosphorylation between the conditions than if there was an increase in number of vacant sites (less sites to dephosphorylate by phosphatase). Their data were entirely consistent with the view that there was an in vivo increase in kinase activity.

This conclusion was strengthened by the recent observation that PKC inhibitors reduce LTP-induced increases in protein F1 phosphorylation (Colley et al., 1990). The reasoning behind this conclusion is as follows: if the assay we use measures PKC activity, then after application of inhibitor in vivo, we should observe a decrease in F1 phosphorylation in vitro. On the other hand, if the assay is measuring vacant sites, then after inhibitor there should be an increase in vacant sites in vivo and hence an increase in phosphorylation in vitro. What we found was that PKC inhibitors blocked the increased phosphorylation of F1 induced by the high-frequency stimulation that normally produces LTP. This finding then suggests that we are measuring kinase activation. To assess the issue of whether PKC inhibitors lingering in the test tube could then block kinase activity, we also injected the inhibitor immediately just before harvesting the animal so that the same amount of inhibitor was present in the test tube but had not any preceding physiological effect. In this case no reduction in F1 phosphorylation was observed.

In conclusion, converging lines of evidence suggest that after in vivo LTP the increase in phosphorylation of F1 observed in vitro is a consequence of increased kinase activity. One should recall in this regard that Akers and colleagues (1986) did observe that PKC activation occurs after LTP, so that the increased phosphorylation of F1 observed in vitro is likely to be caused by increased kinase activity. Because kinase activation in vivo could potentially reduce the number of sites in vivo, the reason that there is not a decrease in protein F1 phosphorylation in vitro is that the number of sites phosphorylated is small relative to the total available (estimated to be less than 1% in the case of pyruvate dehydrogenase). An abundance of sites are remaining to be phosphorylated by the activated PKC.

The reason why it is important to determine that the increased F1 phosphorylation does occur in vivo after LTP is that it points to a sequence of molecular events occurring on the presynaptic side during a particular time frame of LTP. This gives us an anchoring point to discover the time points at which other presynaptic and postsynaptic processes are recruited.

Another importance of this localization is that on the basis of studies with *N*-methyl-D-aspartate (NMDA) blockade (Linden et al., 1987) retrograde signaling is implied. We now turn to these considerations.

SYNAPTIC DIALOGUE REQUIRES A RETROGRADE SIGNAL

Years before retrograde signal ideas were fashionable (Piomelli et al., 1987; Lynch et al., 1989; Linden and Routtenberg, 1989), earlier reports and theories proposed such a mechanism. Indeed, it is almost perfunctory to say that such must exist, for without it there would be no mechanism for the postsynaptic cell to communicate with the presynaptic cell.

Hebb (1949) implied the necessity for a postsynaptic to presynaptic signal when he stated that activity in the postsynaptic cell was necessary for presynaptic terminal growth to occur. Because concurrent presynaptic and postsynaptic activity preceded axonal growth in Hebb's model, the idea of signaling back to the presynapse was certainly suggested.

Several model systems that clearly demonstrate the presence of a retrograde signal now exist. Perhaps the most well studied is the nerve growth factor (NGF) model, in which postsynaptic targets release growth factor, bind to a receptor, and are internalized and transported back to the cell body for action at the nuclear level (see Johnson et al., 1988). This type of terminal-target interaction was very much in the minds of Schmitt and associates (1976) when they described the "quiet revolution" in neurobiology back in 1976. They proposed, based on NGF data and other information such as reciprocal synapses in local circuits, that bidirectional communication was an inherent part of synaptic function. Our own ultrastructural studies of synapses within the hippocampus suggested that the synaptic spinule might well be a morphological substrate for retrograde signaling and bidirectional transport as was noted: " . . . the morphological observations of the synaptic spinule suggest the involvement in transport of material between the pre- and postsynaptic processes. The parallel apposed pre- and postsynaptic membranes would be ideal for such transport. The coated vesicles in particular may be important for the transfer of large molecules. . . . The presence of both active zones and extended apposition of membranes in the synaptic spinule could provide for the occurrence and compartmentalization of both electrophysiological and molecular events, respectively, at the same synaptic junction" (Tarrant and Routtenberg, 1977, p. 472).

The views of bidirectional communication appear not to have influenced the formulations of memory models of the early 1980s (Kandel and Schwartz, 1982; Lynch and Baudry, 1984), where only one side was the exclusive domain of change. With the evidence for an induction role for the NMDA receptor postsynaptically in LTP (Collingridge et al., 1983), two reports later suggested a role for retrograde signaling to the presynaptic terminal. These studies showed that presynaptic activation as evidenced by protein F1 phosphorylation (Linden et al., 1987) or by increased transmitter release (Errington, et al., 1987) was reduced or completely blocked by NMDA blockade, which prevented LTP expression. Both groups reasoned that, if the blockade were working postsynaptically, the retrograde signal was prevented in its presynaptic action by the initial postsynaptic blockade.

The only evidence claimed to directly support this idea is in a report of Williams and coworkers (1989), who suggest that arachidonic acid (AA) may be a retrograde signal. If so, it might work by activating PKC as demonstrated by Murakami and associates (1986) and be shown to influence LTP by Linden and coworkers (1986, 1987). But the results of the Bliss group do little to indicate the necessity for such a conclusion, particularly as it is not clear whether elevated AA is coming from presynaptic sites, postsynaptic sites, or both, and whether such fatty acids are then acting as signals. Moreover, their capacity to cross membranes is not unimpeded, as indicated by the comparison of their action extracellularly or through whole-cell patch pipettes (Linden and Routtenberg, 1989). Hence the amount of fatty acid that would be required and the time taken to cross the plasma membrane barrier might make this an unsuitable signal.

In contrast, we have proposed that the fatty acid elevation takes place within the presynaptic terminal and along with other signals, including a retrograde one, activates presynaptic PKC. In the review with Linden (1989), a postsynaptic to presynaptic signal was proposed but the nature of that signal remains unspecified. We do think that the cis-fatty acid activation of PKC is an important factor in the LTP process, but we favor the view that it is occurring within the cell, possibly within the plane of the presynaptic membrane on its cytoplasmic side.

WHERE IS WHAT KINASE ACTIVE WHEN? THE EVIDENCE FROM INTRACELLULAR INJECTION OF PKC INHIBITORS

To answer the question of the role of PKC in plasticity, we have studied the effects of PKC inhibitors on LTP (Lovinger et al., 1987). We discovered that inhibitors blocked the persistence of the response but had no effect on initiation. Colley, Sheu, and Routtenberg (1990) have shown that inhibitors are effective for up to 30 minutes after LTP and then are ineffective. Measurement of protein F1 phosphorylation after inhibitor treatment indicates that the inhibitor does have an effect on that process, suggesting a presynaptic action. Support for this view comes from the work of Malinow, Schulman, and Tsien (1989) and Malenka and colleagues (1989), using the intracellular application of PKC inhibitors. They showed that leakage of inhibitors blocked LTP of the recorded cell, but left extracellular LTP unchanged. If after LTP was established the cell was penetrated, leakage intracellularly was without effect. Because leakage was used, the time frame of PKC activity postsynaptically was not specified. Moreover, because injections after LTP were given to cells that were not monitored prior to and during LTP, it is not clear when PKC inhibitors are effective and when their effectiveness ceases. Malinow and colleagues (1989) observed that extracellular application of inhibitor did influence LTP 30 minutes after induction. They suggested that this effect of inhibitor was on the presynaptic side. In their study, however, the extracellular application was via bath application so the target site for the bath-applied inhibitor remains uncertain.

To deal with the problems of intracellular leakage and bath application just discussed, Y. Y. Huang in my laboratory has recently completed a study using hippocampal slice preparations in which application intracellularly is by iontophoretic means. A depolarizing pulse is sufficient to eject PKC inhibitor. Because it causes cells to fire on occasion, appropriate controls for depolarization are used as are leakage controls. Indeed, it is first established that leakage is minimal and not physiologically effective. To deal with the problem of bath application not specifying locus, we have used extracellular application by micropressure injection either onto the cell bodies or onto the region of the stratum radiatum. (The method and strategy are fully identical to that of Linden et al., 1987.)

Huang found that application of inhibitor 10 minutes before LTP blocked the long-term expression but left initiation for the first 10 minutes after LTP intact. If given 5 minutes after LTP there was no effect. Dr. T. Goldstick, a colleague in the Biomedical Engineering Department here at Northwestern and an expert in the field of active and passive diffusion, estimates the time of diffusion given a molecule of a molecular weight (mol. wt.) of 364 (polymyxin B) or 1385 (H-7), to a point 400 μm away in the stratum radiatum will take 26 to 99 seconds depending on molecular weight, and assuming the dendrite is a cylinder 900 μ. One assumption made is that 10% of material ejected reaches the postsynaptic PKC. This assumption may be reasonable, but another approach to this problem, which reduces the number of assumptions, involves the results of a modest dose-response study by Huang. Three durations of ejection were used: 15 seconds, 30 seconds, and 120 seconds. The results show a graded effect with a significant result even at 15 seconds. Calculations were made by Professor Goldstick, based on the formula of diffusion in a plane sheet, nonsteady state, in which a uniform concentration exists (as would be the case in the continuous application for up to 2 minutes). With a 2-minute ejection then, 20% of the amount in the cell body travels 400 μ in 2 minutes. Because there is an effect with a 15-second ejection, which is 12.5% of the 2 minutes, it is reasonable to assume that one-fifth or 20% of the amount is effective. We therefore concluded that it would take 2 minutes or less for the inhibitor to reach the cell body. It would seem likely that the time taken is no less than 10 seconds and no more than 2 minutes. That being the case, then the PKC inhibitor, when ejected 10 minutes before LTP, would be present at the postsynaptic membrane prior to the time of LTP. That also means that the inhibitor reaches the postsynaptic membrane no more than 7 minutes after LTP when intracellularly applied 5 minutes after LTP, 8 minutes before it is effective extracellularly when applied to that same region. These results suggest that there is a narrow time window of PKC activation postsynaptically where PKC is necessary for LTP. Presynaptically, this time window is longer: an approximate estimate is that PKC activation is critical postsynaptically for 0 to 5 minutes after LTP. If PKC is not active, LTP diminishes at 10 to 15 minutes. PKC is critical presynaptically for between 5 and 30 minutes after LTP; if PKC is not active presynaptically, then LTP diminishes to baseline within 60 to 120 minutes.

ARE DIFFERENT PKC SUBTYPES ACTIVE AT DIFFERENT SYNAPTIC LOCI AFTER LTP?

Given that PKC is active presynaptically and postsynaptically in two distinct time domains, the question arises as to whether the same PKC molecule is performing the function on both sides of the synapse. Recent evidence indicates that PKC is a family of enzymes with a particular distribution (Nishizuka, 1988). One approach to the problem is to determine whether a particular subtype phosphorylates the presynaptic PKC substrate protein F1. Sheu and coworkers (1990) have recently demonstrated that beta PKC preferentially phosphorylates protein F1 relative to gamma and alpha PKC. We therefore propose that postsynaptic PKC is of the gamma type, presynaptic of the beta.

FORGETTING MECHANISMS: MODELS AND THE REAL THING

One concern with the present focus on storage mechanisms is that the need for mechanisms of forgetting is ignored; otherwise, the system might suffer from information overload. Moreover, the fact of forgetting is real (Underwood and Ekstrand, 1966), and a physiological mechanism for it is necessary. Several reports of a phenomenon known as long-term depression (LTD) in the cerebellum (e.g., Crepel and Krupa, 1988) and similar phenomena in the hippocampus (Stanton and Sejnowski, 1989) and visual cortex (Artola et al., 1990) have suggested that LTD might represent a physiological model of forgetting. Although much controversy surrounds the existence of the phenomenon (Stevens, 1990), the attractiveness of having a mechanism that is the reverse image of LTP is compelling. It has been proposed that LTD depends on a discorrelation between presynaptic and postsynaptic activity, a partial depolarization within a narrow range, or both. Too much depolarization causes LTP, too little and the system is unaltered; the result of a middle range of depolarization is LTD.

These physiological models strike me as too demanding energetically. Although it has certain attractive features, the notion that forgetting requires maintained activation of a depressed state for long periods of time places a heavy load on the system. To be sure, the loss of this process could account for reminiscence (Alloway and Routtenberg, 1967) and would explain in a general way the recurrence of early memories in the aged as a loss of a memory inhibition mechanism.

Collier and associates (1982, 1987) and Collier and Routtenberg (1984) suggested a different type of forgetting mechanism that involves a specific hippocampal pathway. This mechanism contrasts with the LTD mechanism suggested for the hippocampus, visual cortex, and cerebellum where the process is engendered by the particular interplay of excitatory and inhibitory inputs: no specialized pathway is implicated in the forgetting process. In contrast, Collier et al. (1987) proposed that activation of the mossy fiber system acted to erase information. In our studies, animals were implanted with electrodes guided physiologically to the granule cells or the pyramidal cells. Animals were trained to go back to food located in one part of a radial arm maze. Delays up to 20 minutes were imposed, and the unstimulated animal had little difficulty finding the food. If, during this interval, stimulation of the granule cells was introduced (1 second at 5 μA), the animal behaved as if it had completely forgotten the food location. The animal was otherwise totally intact because once it did find the food it would remember where that location was if tested again. Moreover, the animal searched for food in a manner indicating intact "working memory."

Since naloxone blocked the effect of granule cell stimulation, and naloxone by itself actually facilitated performance, we concluded that the activity in the mossy fiber system in some manner negatively regulated memory formation.

The notion that there is a process that can prevent this storage of information is intriguing. Moreover, the possibility exists that this process could itself produce a form of LTD, though the evidence available does not seem to provide any clues how this might specifically occur (Miles, 1990; Bradler and Barrionuevo, 1990).

Finally, since pyramidal cell stimulation at the same intensity and duration as was used for granule cells was ineffective, the erasure effect is specific to a particular subpopulation of hippocampal cells, granule, not pyramidal. The fact that pyramidal cells express protein F1 mRNA, while the granule cells do not (Rosenthal et al., 1987; Meberg et al., 1990) has not escaped our attention!

REFERENCES

Akers, R., et al. (1986). Translocation of protein kinase C activity after long-term potentiation may mediate synaptic plasticity. *Science* 231:587–589.

Alloway, T. A., and A. Routtenberg (1967). "Reminiscence" in the cold flour beetle, *Tenebrio molitor. Science* 158:1066–1067.

Artola, A., S. Brocher, and W. Singer (1990). Different voltage-dependent thresholds for inducing long-term depression and long-term potentiation in slices of rat visual cortex. *Nature* 347:69–72.

Bekkers, J. M., and C. F. Stevens (1990). Presynaptic mechanism for long-term potentiation in the hippocampus. *Nature* 346:724–728.

Benowitz, L. I., and A. Routtenberg (1987). A membrane phosphoprotein associated with neural development, axonal regeneration, phospholipid metabolism, and synaptic plasticity. *Trends in Neuroscience* 10:527–532.

Bliss, T. V. P. (1990). Maintenance is presynaptic. *Nature* 346:698–699.

Bliss, T. V. P., R. M. Douglas, M. L. Errington, and M. A. Lynch (1986). Correlation between long-term potentiation and release of endogenous amino acids from dentate gyrus of anesthetized rats. *Journal of Physiology* (London) 377:391–408.

Bliss, T. V. P., and M. A. Lynch (1988). Long-term potentiation of synaptic transmission in the hippocampus; properties and mechanisms. In P. W. Landfield and S. A. Deadwyler (eds.), *Long-Term Potentiation: From Biophysics to Behavior,* New York: Allen R. Liss, pp. 3–72.

Bradler, J. E., and G. Barrionuevo (1990). Heterosynaptic correlates of long-term potentiation induction in hippocampal CA3 neurons. *Neuroscience* 35:265–271.

Chan, S., P. Colley, and A. Routtenberg (1988). LTP-induced protein F1 phosphorylation in vitro: does it represent an increase or decrease in phosphate incorporation in vivo? *Society for Neuroscience* 14:18.

Colley, P. A. (1991). Persistence of hippocampal long-term potentiation; regulation by protein kinase C. In T. W. Stone (ed.), *Aspects of Synaptic Transmission*, London: Taylor and Francis (in press).

Colley, P. A., F.-S. Sheu, and A. Routtenberg (1990). Inhibition of protein kinase C blocks two components of LTP persistence leaving initial potentiation intact. *Journal of Neuroscience* 10:3353–3360.

Collier, T. J., J. S. Miller, J. Travis, and A. Routtenberg (1982). Dentate gyrus granule cells and memory: electrical stimulation disrupts memory for places rewarded. *Behavioral and Neural Biology* 34:227–239.

Collier, T. J., G. S. Quirk, and A. Routtenberg (1987). Separable roles of hippocampal granule cells in forgetting and pyramidal cells in remembering spatial information. *Brain Research* 409:316–328.

Collier, T. J., and A. Routtenberg (1984). Electrical self-stimulation of dentate gyrus granule cells. *Behavioral and Neural Biology* 42:85–90.

Collingridge, G. L., and T. V. P. Bliss (1987). NMDA receptors—their role in long-term potentiation. *Trends in Neuroscience* 10:288–293.

Collingridge, G. L., S. J. Kehl, and H. McLennan (1983). Excitatory amino acids in synaptic transmission in the Schaffer collateral—commissural pathway of the rat hippocampus. *Journal of Physiology* (London) 334:33–46.

Crepel, F., and M. Krupa (1988). Activation of protein kinase C induces a long-term depression of glutamate sensitivity of cerebellar Purkinje cells. An in vitro study. *Brain Research* 458:397–401.

Davies, S. N., R. A. J. Lester, K. G. Reymann, and G. L. Collingridge (1989). Temporally distinct pre- and post-synaptic mechanisms maintain long-term potentiation. *Nature* 338:500–503.

De Graan, P. N. E., et al. (1988). Phorbol esters induce long- and short-term enhancement of B-50/GAP-43 phosphorylation in rat hippocampal slices. *Neuroscience Research Communications* 3:175–182.

Edwards, F. A., A. Konnerth, B. Sakmann, and T. Takahashi (1989). A thin slice preparation for patch clamp recordings from neurons of the mammalian central nervous system. *Pflügers Archives* 414:600–612.

Errington, M. L., M. A. Lynch, and T. V. P. Bliss (1987). Long-term potentiation in the dentate gyrus: induction and increased glutamate release are blocked by D-(-)aminophosphonovalerate. *Neuroscience* 20:279–284.

Hansson, A., et al. (1986). Activation of protein kinase C by lipoxin A and other eicosanoids. Intracellular action of oxygenation products of arachidonic acid. *Biochemical and Biophysical Research Communications* 134:1215–1222.

Hebb, D. O. (1949). Organization of behavior. New York: Wiley, p. 64.

Johnson, E. M., M. Taniuchi, and P. S. DiStefano (1988). Expression and possible function of nerve growth factor receptors on Schwann cells. *Trends in Neuroscience* 11(7):299–304.

Kandel, E. R., and J. H. Schwartz (1982). Molecular biology of learning: Modulation of transmitter release. *Science* 218:433–443.

Linden, D., K. Murakami, and A. Routtenberg (1986). A newly discovered protein kinase C activator (oleic acid) preserves synaptic plasticity and promotes the growth of long-term potentiation. *Brain Research* 379:358–363.

Linden, D. J., and A. Routtenberg (1989). Cis-fatty acids, which activate protein kinase C, attenuate voltage-dependent Na + current in mouse neuroblastoma cells. *Journal of Physiology* 419:95–119.

Linden, D., F.-S. Sheu, K. Murakami, and A. Routtenberg (1987). Cis fatty acid regulation of synaptic potentiation: relation to phospholipase A_2 and protein kinase C activation. *Journal of Neuroscience* 7:3783–3792.

Linden, D. J., K. L. Wong, F.-S. Sheu, and A. Routtenberg (1988). NMDA receptor blockade prevents the increase in protein kinase C substrate (protein F1) phosphorylation produced by long term potentiation. *Brain Research* 458:142–146.

Lovinger, D. M., K. L. Wong, K. Murakami, and A. Routtenberg (1987). Protein kinase C inhibitors eliminate hippocampal long-term potentiation. *Brain Research* 436:177–183.

Lynch, G., and M. Baudry (1984). The biochemistry of memory: a new hypothesis. *Science* 224:1057–1063.

Lynch, M. A., M. L. Errington, and T. V. P. Bliss (1989). Norihydroguaiaretic acid blocks the synaptic component of long-term potentiation and the associated increases in release of glutamate and arachidonate: in vivo study in the dentate gyrus of the rat. *Neuroscience* 30:693–701.

Malenka, R. C., et al. (1989). An essential role for postsynaptic calmodulin and protein kinase activity in long-term potentiation. *Nature* 340:554–557.

Malinow, R., H. Schulman, and R. W. Tsien (1989). Inhibition of postsynaptic PKC or CaMKII blocks induction but not expression of LTP. *Science* 245:862–866.

Malinow, R., and R. Tsien (1990). Presynaptic enhancement by whole-cell recordings of long-term potentiation in hippocampal slices. *Nature* 346:177–180.

Meberg, P., et al. (1990). Synaptic plasticity: molecular and cellular approaches to the study of protein kinase C (PKC) regulation of protein F1/GAP-43 phosphorylation. *Society for Neuroscience* 16:658.

Miles, R. (1990). Synaptic excitation of inhibitory cells by single CA3 hippocampal pyramidal cells of the guinea-pig in vitro. *Journal of Physiology* 428:61–77.

Miles, R., and R. K. S. Wong (1987). Latent synaptic pathways revealed after tetanic stimulation in the hippocampus. *Nature* 329:724–726.

Murakami, K., S. Y. Chan, and A. Routtenberg (1986). Protein kinase C activation by cis-fatty acid in the absence of Ca^{2+} and phospholipids. *Journal of Biology and Chemistry* 261:15,424–15,429.

Nicoll, R. A., J. A. Kauer, and R. C. Malenka (1988). The current excitement in long-term potentiation. *Neuron* 1:97–103.

Nishizuka, Y. (1988). The molecular heterogenicity of protein kinase C and its implications for cellular regulation. *Nature* 334:661–665.

Piomelli, D., et al. (1987). Lipoxygenase metabolites of arachidonic acid as second messengers for presynaptic inhibition of Aplysia sensory cells. *Nature* 328:38–43.

Rodnight, R., C. Perrett, and S. Soteriou (1985). Two-dimensional patterns of neural phosphoproteins from the rat labeled in vivo under anaesthesia, and in vitro in slices and synaptosomes. *Progress in Brain Research.* W. H. Gispen and A. Routtenberg (eds.), 69:373–381.

Rosenthal, A., et al. (1987). Primary structure and mRNA localization of protein F1, a growth-related protein kinase C substrate, associated with synaptic plasticity. *European Molecular Biology Organization* 6:3641–3646.

Routtenberg, A. (1985). The CA3 pyramidal cell in the hippocampus: site of intrinsic expression and extrinsic control of memory formation. In L. Squire and N. Butters (eds.), *Neuropsychology of Memory.* New York: The Guilford Press, pp. 536–546.

Routtenberg, A. (1989). Role of protein kinase C and protein F1 in presynaptic terminal growth leading to information storage. In H. Rahmann (ed.), "Fundamentals of memory formation," *Progress in Zoology,* Vol. 37. New York: Springer-Verlag, pp. 283–295.

Routtenberg, A., et al. (1983). Effects of long-term potentiation of perforant path synapses in the intact hippocampus on in vitro phosphorylation of a 47 kD protein (F-1). *Federation Proceedings* 42:755.

Routtenberg, A., D. M. Lovinger, and O. Steward (1985). Selective increase in phosphorylation state of a 47 kD protein (F1) directly related to long-term potentiation. *Behavioral and Neural Biology* 43:3–11.

Schmitt, F. O., P. Dev, and B. H. Smith (1976). Electronic processing of information by brain cells. *Science* 193:114–120.

Sheu, F.-S., et al. (1990). Neuron-specific protein F1/GAP-43 shows substrate specificity for the beta subtype of protein kinase C. *Biochemistry and Biophysics Research Communications* 171:1236–1243.

Sheu, F.-S., T. Kasamatsu, and A. Routtenberg (1990). Elevated protein kinase C activity and substrate (F1/GAP-43) phosphorylation in kitten visual cortex parallels critical period. *Brain Research* 524:144–148.

Stanton, P. K., and T. J. Sejnowski (1989). Associative long-term depression in the hippocampus induced by hebbian covariance. *Nature* 339:215–218.

Staubli, U., J. Larson, and G. Lynch (1990). Mossy fiber potentiation and long-term potentiation involve different expression mechanisms. *Synapse* 5:333–335.

Stevens, C. F. (1990). A depression long awaited. *Nature* 347:16.

Sugiyama, H., I. Ito, and C. Hirono (1987). A new type of glutamate receptor linked to inositol phospholipid metabolism. *Nature* 325:531–533.

Tarrant, S. B., and A. Routtenberg (1977). The synaptic spinule in the dendritic spine: electron microscopic study of the hippocampal dentate gyrus. *Tissue and Cell* 9(3):461–473.

Underwood, B. J., and B. R. Ekstrand (1966). An analysis of some shortcomings in the interference theory of forgetting. *Psychological Review* 73:540–549.

Williams, J. H., M. L. Errington, M. A. Lynch, and T. V. P. Bliss (1989). Arachidonic acid induces a long-term activity-dependent enhancement of synaptic transmission in the hippocampus. *Nature* 341:739–742.

Zalutsky, R. A., and R. A. Nicoll (1990). Comparison of two forms of long-term potentiation in single hippocampal neurons. *Science* 248:1619–1624.

12 An Integrated Biochemical Model for Long-Term Potentiation

Michel Baudry

One of the difficulties in studying the biochemical mechanisms involved in long-term potentiation (LTP) is that it is impossible to directly access the cellular compartments where LTP is taking place. Another difficulty arises from the current confusion in the literature because each laboratory involved in the search for the LTP mechanism is overemphasizing its own enzymatic or cellular processes (see Kuba and Kumamoto, 1990, for a recent review). One way to overcome these difficulties is to consider the possibility that LTP is a variant of a cell-cell interaction phenomenon and that it shares a number of basic mechanisms with cellular systems exhibiting rapid changes in function and structure as a result of brief exposures to some stimulus. Platelets or other types of blood cells (erythrocytes) have been widely used to study such mechanisms because they provide a homogeneous population of easily available cells that respond rapidly to a wide range of stimuli. Although the intimate details of the mechanisms underlying platelet aggregation are not fully known, the main steps have been identified and some models are available (see Siess, 1989, for a review). In particular, most models include an initial influx of calcium; activation of protein kinase C, phospholipase A_2 (PLA_2), and calpain; the degradation of phosphatidylinositol; and an increased availability of free arachidonic acid followed by the synthesis of oxygenated metabolites of this fatty acid. Some models also involve the interaction between phospholipids and the cell cytoskeleton (Williamson et al., 1982; Mohandas et al., 1985; Sune and Bienvenue, 1988) and the translocation of phosphatidylserine between the two leaflets of the lipid bilayer (Zwaal et al., 1989). It was originally proposed that the observed correlation between the extent of phosphatidylserine exposure to the outer leaflet of the membranes and the extent of spectrin degradation reflected a role for spectrin in maintaining phospholipid asymmetry in the lipid bilayer. More recently, it was shown that the asymmetry is in fact generated by an aminophospholipid translocase (Seigneuret et al., 1985) that translocates phosphatidylserine from the outside to the inside leaflet of the bilayer. Interestingly, the activation of calpain inhibits the translocase activity (Comfurius et al., 1990), indicating the existence of links between calpain and the distribution of phospholipids. A number of these events have been previously implicated in the postulated mechanisms underlying LTP (Kuba and Kumamoto, 1990), and the model we present in this chapter is an attempt to integrate several of these elements in a coherent framework. We think that this new and rather speculative model of LTP is not only simplifying but also useful as it makes more specific and testable predictions. The chapter first describes recent results that indicate a critical role for PLA_2 in LTP. We then discuss the arguments supporting our model.

LTP, GLUTAMATE RECEPTORS, AND PHOSPHOLIPASES

LTP is triggered by the activation of *N*-methyl-D-aspartate (NMDA) receptors and the resulting influx of calcium in postsynaptic structures and is expressed by an increase in synaptic responses generated by quisqualate receptors with little change in those produced by NMDA receptors (Muller et al., 1988; Kauer et al., 1988). We have therefore postulated that the process (or processes) underlying LTP have to be found among those that are calcium-dependent and that can produce a selective change in quisqualate receptors (Massicotte and Baudry, 1991). A number of membrane-associated phospholipases are calcium-dependent, and there is evidence linking glutamate receptor activation to phospholipases. Thus, the tetanic stimulation used to induce LTP and NMDA receptor agonists elicit the release of arachidonic acid, which suggests that NMDA receptor activation produces the in situ stimulation of PLA_2 (Dumuis et al., 1988; Lynch et al., 1989). Moreover, another subtype of glutamate receptor, the so-called quisqualate metabotropic receptor, is positively linked to the phosphatidylinositol pathway, indicating that glutamate is also able to stimulate phospholipase C (PLC; Sladeczek et al., 1988). Activation of phospholipases represents an important component of the effects of both neurotransmitters and hormones (Loh and Law, 1980). By cleaving membrane phospholipids, these enzymes perform a dual function: they modify the lipid microenvironment of cell membranes and they generate a number of metabolites that play a second messenger function inside or outside the cell (Berridge and Irvine, 1984). Treatment of membranes with exogenous phospholipases has been reported to alter the characteristics of the binding sites for various neurotransmitters or neuromodulators such as norepinephrine, γ-aminobutyric acid (GABA), and the opioid peptides (Limbird and Lefkowitz, 1976; Periyasamy and Somani, 1986; Toffano et al., 1981; Pasternak and Snyder, 1974). In a number of cases it was shown that the nonpolar or polar moieties of membrane phospholipids, as well as the lysophospholipids and fatty acids generated by phospholipase treatment, were responsible for the changes in receptor binding. In other cases it appears more likely that changes in the lipid microenvironment of the receptor produce alterations in the conformation of the receptor, leading to changes in receptor binding.

REGULATION OF GLUTAMATE RECEPTORS BY PHOSPHOLIPASES

Treatment of rat synaptic membranes with PLC produced a complex set of modifications of the different subtypes of glutamate receptors (Massicotte et al., 1990a). Whereas the kainate binding sites did not appear to be affected, the AMPA-quisqualate receptors exhibited an increased affinity for the ligand. The binding of ^{3}H-glutamate and ^{3}H-glycine to the NMDA receptor was not modified but there was a large decrease in the binding of the NMDA antagonist ^{3}H-CPP. Finally, there was a decreased affinity of ^{3}H-TCP for the open state of the channel associated with the NMDA receptor but also an increased accessibility of N-(1-[thyenyl]-cyclohexyl)piperidine (TCP) to the channel when it was closed. We interpreted these results as evidence that the lipid microenvironment of the NMDA receptor and the AMPA-quisqualate receptor has a marked influence on the conformation of these receptors.

Similarly, treatment of synaptic membranes with PLA_2 produced an increased affinity of the AMPA-quisqualate receptor for the ligand, while the binding of ^{3}H-kainate, ^{3}H-glycine, and ^{3}H-glutamate to the kainate and NMDA receptor complex respectively were not affected (Massicotte and Baudry, 1990). Here again the effect of PLA_2 on the AMPA-quisqualate receptor was likely due to a PLA_2-induced disturbance in the lipid environment of the receptors as the effect was not reversed by the addition of bovine serum albumin (BSA), a known scavenger of the metabolites generated by PLA_2. PLA_2 treatment also slightly decreased the maximal number of binding sites for ^{3}H-6-cyano-7-nitroquinoxaline-2,3-dione (CNQX), an antagonist of the receptor, but it clearly shifted to the left the concentration response curves for inhibition of ^{3}H-CNQX by the agonists AMPA and glutamate, further indicating that PLA_2 treatment increased the affinity of the receptors for agonists (Baudry et al., 1990). The effect of PLA_2 was blocked by several inhibitors including bromophenacyl bromide (BPB), a PLA_2 inhibitor, and nordihydroguaiaretic acid, a lipoxygenase-PLA_2 inhibitor.

EFFECT OF A PLA_2 INHIBITOR ON THE INDUCTION AND MAINTENANCE OF LTP

As discussed in previous section, several arguments suggested a role for PLA_2 in LTP induction. In particular, several reports have indicated that different compounds that inhibit PLA_2 activity interfered with LTP (Lynch et al., 1989; Okada et al., 1989; Williams and Bliss, 1989). We reinvestigated the effects of one of the PLA_2 inhibitors, BPB, on LTP induction and maintenance (Massicotte et al., 1990b). Pretreatment of hippocampal slices with BPB (50 μM) markedly reduced the amplitude of LTP in field CA1. The presence of BPB, however, did not modify the amount of paired-pulse facilitation nor the amount of short-term potentiation elicited by theta-burst stimulation. It also did not affect the burst responses evoked by the LTP-inducing stimulation, which reflect both the transient reduction of inhibitory postsynaptic potentials (IPSPs) and the activation of NMDA receptors. Finally, it did not affect the magnitude of pre-established LTP. This pattern of results suggests that this PLA_2 inhibitor interferes with the induction of LTP by disrupting a process (presumably the activation of endogenous PLA_2 or possibly another phospholipase, as this drug is not a totally selective inhibitor) that follows the activation of the ionic currents (NMDA receptor–elicited calcium currents) that serve as the initial trigger for LTP. Continuous activation of this process does not seem to be required for the maintenance of LTP.

IS PLA_2-INDUCED INCREASE IN ^{3}H-AMPA BINDING A NECESSARY STEP FOR LTP?

Several groups have reported that epileptiform activity in the limbic system disrupts the mechanisms that induce LTP (Hesse and Teyler, 1976; Racine et al., 1983; Anwyl et al., 1987). Similarly, neonatal rats do not express LTP as a result of high-frequency stimulation until postnatal day 10 (Baudry et al., 1981; Teyler et al., 1989), at least in the CA1 field of the hippocampus; there are reasons to believe that more generally, neonatal animals exhibit different forms of synaptic plasticity than those expressed in adult animals (Konishi and Nottebohm, 1969; Hubel and Wiesel, 1970; Rankin et al., 1987). We reasoned that such situations might provide unique opportunities to establish the roles of different calcium-dependent processes in LTP induction and especially that of calcium-dependent phospholipases. We thus examined the effects of kainate-induced epileptic seizures on the binding properties of hippocampal glutamate receptors, the modulation of AMPA-quisqualate receptors by PLA_2 and on the formation of LTP in hippocampal membranes and slices, respectively (Massicotte et al., 1991). Whereas the binding of various ligands to the NMDA receptor was not modified by kainate treatment, the maximal number of binding sites for ^{3}H-AMPA notably decreased. More importantly, the increase in ^{3}H-AMPA binding elicited by PLA_2 treatment of hippocampal, but not cerebellar membranes, was markedly decreased following kainate injection. LTP was also substantially reduced in CA1 after kainate treatment. The loss of LTP was not due to changes in postsynaptic responses elicited by the bursts that trigger the potentiation effect, which suggests that kainate treatment disrupts processes that follow NMDA receptor activation. Systemic administration of kainate was also associated with calpain activation because the amount of spectrin breakdown products was increased several fold in hippocampal but not cerebellar homogenates. Pretreatment of telencephalic membranes with calpain greatly reduced the PLA_2-induced increase in ^{3}H-AMPA binding. We therefore proposed that kainate-induced seizure activity produces a massive in situ calpain activation that results in a long-lasting disturbance in the phospholipid distribution in the membrane bilayer. Under these conditions, PLA_2 treatment of membranes no longer results in an increase in ^{3}H-AMPA binding.

We also measured the effect of PLA_2 on ^{3}H-AMPA binding in telencephalic membranes prepared from 5-day-old animals. Not only did we not observe any stimulation of ^{3}H-AMPA binding by PLA_2 treatment of the membranes, but we obtained a marked decrease in binding (Baudry et al., 1991a). This observation is quite interesting because preliminary experiments indicated that certain patterns of electrical stimulation in hippocampal slices prepared from neonatal rats induced a long-term depression (LTD) of synaptic transmission instead of LTP; this LTD was blocked by α-amino-5-phosphonopentanoate (AP5), indicating that it is also triggered by stimulation of NMDA receptors (and therefore possibly mediated through PLA_2 activation; Baudry et al., 1990, unpublished data). Moreover, hippocampal homogenates from neonatal animals also exhibited high levels of spectrin breakdown products compared with adult animals, suggesting that in situ calpain activity is much higher in neonatal rats than in adult rats.

Thus, in two very different situations, 16 hours after seizure activity and at postnatal day 5, the absence of LTP is associated with an absence of PLA_2-induced increase in affinity of the quisqualate-AMPA receptors. Considering the previous arguments supporting a role for PLA_2 in LTP, it is reasonable to assume that the PLA_2-induced modification of the AMPA-quisqualate receptor is a necessary step in LTP induction. Furthermore, these data also suggest that a specific order of activation of calcium-dependent processes might be important in producing changes in synaptic efficacy.

EFFECT OF PHOSPHOLIPIDS ON ^{3}H-AMPA BINDING

In view of the role of the lipid microenvironment in determining the binding properties of the AMPA-quisqualate receptors, we investigated the effects of exogenous phospholipids on the characteristics of ^{3}H-AMPA binding to rat telencephalic membranes. The preliminary results we obtained are quite interesting. Incorporating phosphatidylserine in membranes produced a large increase in the affinity of ^{3}H-AMPA for the AMPA-quisqualate receptor. Incorporating phosphatidylethanolamine, phosphatidylcholine, or cholesterol had no effect (Baudry et al., 1991b). This finding suggests that manipulation of the phospholipids by opposite means (i.e., PLA_2 and phosphatidylserine incorporation) produces the same effect on the AMPA-quisqualate receptor (an increase in affinity). To determine whether the effects of phosphatidylserine incorporation and PLA_2 treatment were additive, we first treated the membranes with phosphatidylserine before performing the PLA_2 treatment. Under these conditions, PLA_2 treatment produced a decrease in ^{3}H-AMPA binding to a level lower than in native membranes. These results are interesting in regard to the studies performed in blood platelets or erythrocytes mentioned previously (Williams et al., 1982; Mohandas et al., 1985; Sune and Bienvenue, 1988; Zwaal et al., 1989; Comfurius et al., 1990). In these cells at rest, most of the phosphatidylserine is localized in the inner leaflet of the lipid bilayer. After activation, a fraction of phosphatidylserine becomes exposed to the outside, and a phospholipid translocase has been shown to slowly translocate phosphatidylserine from outside to inside (figure 12.1). It is thus tempting to assume that a similar situation exists in synaptic membranes and that during LTP the activation of PLA_2 results in a redistribution of phospholipids and an exposure of phosphatidylserine to the outside leaflet. This in turn would produce an increased affinity of the quisqualate-AMPA receptor. The concomitant activation of calpain would inhibit the activity of the translocase, thus maintaining the asymmetrical distribution of phosphatidylserine, and the increase in affinity of the AMPA-quisqualate receptors, at least for a certain period of time.

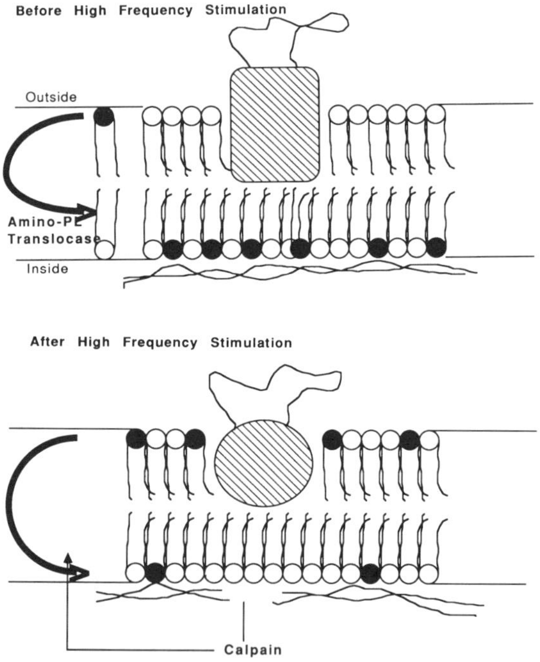

Figure 12.1 Schematic diagram of a postulated flip-flop mechanism. We propose that, as in platelets and erythrocytes, the majority of phosphatidylserine (filled polar heads) is located under resting conditions in the inner leaflet of the bilayer. An amino-phospholipid translocase is assumed to slowly translocate phosphatidylserine from the outside to the inside. Under these conditions, AMPA-quisqualate receptors are in a state of low affinity for agonists. After high-frequency stimulation and activation of NMDA receptors, the triggering of different Ca^{2+}-dependent processes produces a flip-flop of phosphatidylserine from the inside to the outside of the bilayer and the conversion of the AMPA-quisqualate receptors to a state of high affinity for agonists. In addition, the activation of calpain prevents the aminophospholipid translocase to reverse the distribution of phosphatidylserine.

CHANGES IN ^{3}H-AMPA BINDING WITH LEARNING AND LTP

In collaboration with the laboratory of Dr. R. Thompson at the University of Southern California, we have initiated studies aimed at evaluating the possibilities that changes in the properties of glutamate receptors take place in vivo as a result of the learning of specific tasks or as a result of manipulations producing changes in synaptic efficacy. In particular, we used quantitative autoradiography to study changes in the binding properties of AMPA-quisqualate and NMDA receptors in rabbit hippocampus as a result of the learning of a classical conditioned task. We used the conditioning of the eyelid nictitating membrane, a learning paradigm that has been shown to be accompanied by specific changes in the electrophysiological properties of hippocampal neurons (Berger and Thompson, 1978; Weisz et al., 1984). Our first study clearly showed that the learning of the pairing of a sound with an airpuff on the eye was associated with an increased binding of ^{3}H-AMPA to the AMPA-quisqualate receptor in hippocampus without modification of the binding of ^{3}H-TCP (a ligand for the NMDA receptor channel) to the NMDA receptor (Tocco et al., 1989). This result is important in that it is the first time that learning is shown to be associated with a change in a synaptic receptor in a mammalian species.

Experiments are also in progress to evaluate potential changes in the binding characteristics of the AMPA-quisqualate receptor after the induction of LTP in the rat dentate gyrus in vivo.

A REVISED MODEL FOR LTP

All the results just discussed form the basis of a new model that is an updated version of the one we previously proposed (Lynch and Baudry, 1984); it should be viewed as a working hypothesis rather than a final picture (figure 12.2).

The Induction Phase

Pattern stimulation at theta rhythm frequency produces a transient suppression of IPSPs and allows the temporal summation of excitatory postsynaptic potentials (EPSPs) and the activation of NMDA receptors. This activation results in an increase in calcium in postsynaptic structures.

The Development Phase

The development phase is probably relatively rapid (1–3 minutes) and is a period during which certain manipulations can prevent LTP formation (Arai et al., 1990; Gustafsson and Wigström, 1990). It represents the time during which a number of calcium-dependent processes are actively stimulated (proteases, lipases, kinases, etc.). Inhibition of any of these processes is likely to prevent the formation of LTP and leave intact some forms of short-term potentiation. Strong evidence exists for the involvement of proteases (calpain; Lynch and Baudry, 1984; Staubli et al., 1988; Oliver et al., 1989), phospholipases (PLA_2; Okada et al., 1989; Williams

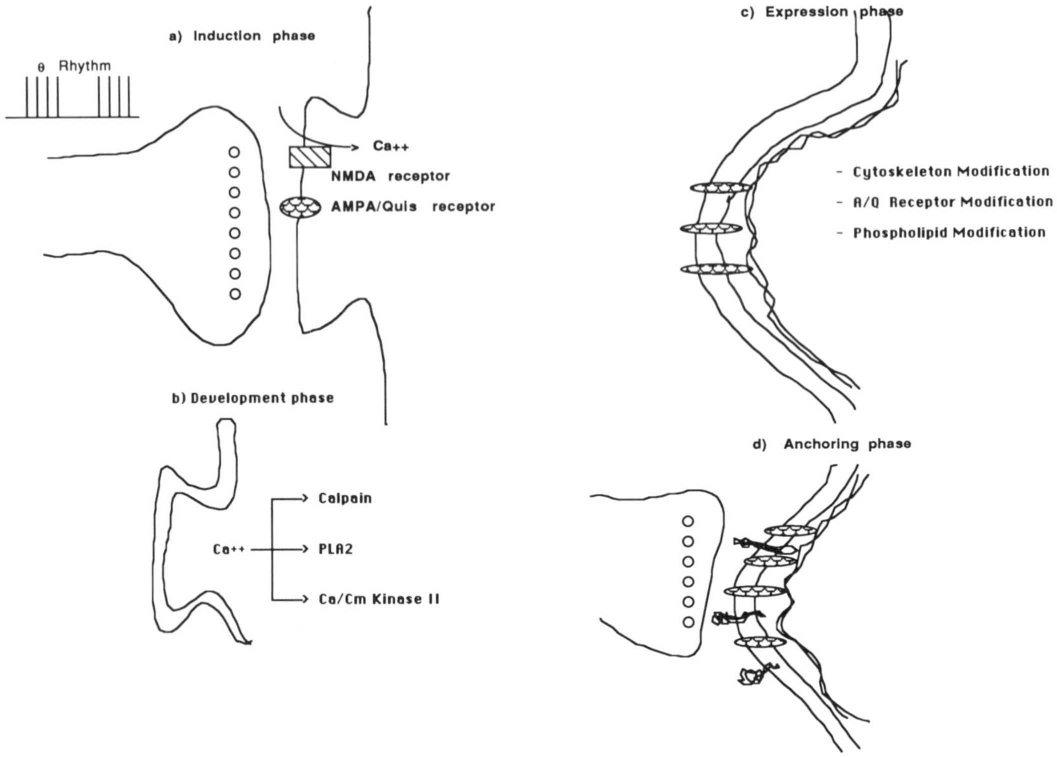

Figure 12.2 An integrated biochemical model of LTP. We propose that four phases are involved in the formation of LTP: (1) the induction phase, which leads to the activation of NMDA receptors and the influx of Ca^{2+} in the postsynaptic cell; (2) the development phase, which consists of the stimulation of a complex biochemical cascade involving proteases, lipases, and kinases; (3) the expression phase, which is associated with membrane modification, changes in configuration of the AMPA-quisqualate (A/Q) receptors, and changes in the shape of dendritic spines; and (4) the maintenance or anchoring phase, which represents the stabilization of the new configuration and involves cell-adhesion molecules and integrin proteins.

and Bliss, 1989), whereas only weak evidence is available for kinases (CaMKII; Malenka et al., 1989; Kennedy, 1989; Lisman and Goldring, 1988) or phosphatases. For PLA_2 there might well exist an autoamplifying process produced by the release of a "platelet-activating factor" (PAF) activating PAF receptors to further stimulate PLA_2 (del Cerro et al., 1990).

The Expression Phase

The combined activation of PLA_2 and calpain results in the degradation of cytoskeletal proteins and in a redistribution of phospholipids in the lipid bilayer with an increased exposure of phosphatidylserine to the outside of the membranes. This results in a change in configuration of the AMPA-quisqualate (synaptic) receptor, which is reflected by an increased affinity for the binding of agonists. At the functional level, it is not clear what such a change could produce.

In particular, it is conceivable that the AMPA-quisqualate receptors exist in two states: an active state, for which agonist binding produces channel opening, and an inactive state, for which agonist binding does not produce channel opening. A model of adaptive synapses based on such assumptions has been developed by Changeux and coworkers (Heidmann and Changeux, 1982).

Furthermore, the recent cloning of a family of AMPA receptors by two different groups (Keinanen et al., 1990; Boulter et al., 1990, Sommer et al., 1990) has indicated the existence of multiple genes (and thus gene products), and it has been suggested that the hippocampal receptors could be a heteromeric molecule. Moreover, the cloned receptors are encoded by four or more related genes, each of which exists in two closely similar versions generated by alternative splicing of the genes, and they have been defined as flip and flop. Expression of the genes in cell systems has shown that the flip elements provide larger currents than the flop. It is therefore conceivable that the modification of the configuration of the receptors we are proposing reflects a modification in the stoechiometry of the receptors, with for instance an increase in flip elements in the receptor molecules.

The Maintenance or Anchoring Phase

The maintenance, or anchoring, phase is postulated to stabilize the configuration generated in the earlier phases; it represents a combination of morphological changes (changes in the shape of dendritic spines; see chapter 14 for a review) and biochemical changes (stabilization of AMPA-quisqualate receptors in the new state), which could also involve extracellular matrix components and their corresponding membrane receptors (Staubli et al., 1990).

Recently, considerable excitement (Barinaga, 19900; Bliss, 1990) has been raised by results obtained from quantal analysis of the changes in parameters of synaptic transmission that gave the impression that the mechanism involved in LTP maintenance is presynaptic (Malinow and Tsien, 1990; Bekkers and Stevens, 1990; see also chapters 6 and 8). Another study (Foster and McNaughton, 1991; see also chapter 7), however, failed to reproduce the same results. A discussion of the different problems associated with these studies goes beyond the scope of this chapter, and we have addressed elsewhere some of the issues raised by these reports (Lynch and Baudry, 1991). Our conclusions are that the issue of the locus of the changes underlying LTP is far from being settled and that more work is needed.

CONCLUSION

The model we have discussed in this chapter potentially accounts for many features of LTP as well as many reports concerning the mechanisms involved in LTP. In particular it explains one puzzling aspect of LTP: that a wide range of inhibitors of a variety of calcium-dependent enzymes prevent LTP formation. This aspect would not be surprising if, as we propose, LTP results from the activation of a complex cascade of events involving cytoskeletal elements, integral membrane proteins, phospholipids, and enzymatic processes. The present model has also the advantage that, by strengthening the analogies between LTP and other cell biological mechanisms, it somewhat demystifies LTP and provides new ways of studying its mechanisms and functions. For instance, it is worth noting that there is a large amount of literature concerning the effects of phosphatidylserine on learning and memory (Corwin et al., 1985; Fagioli et al., 1989), and it is tempting to speculate that the effect of phosphatidylserine on the AMPA-quisqualate receptor we observed has something to do with its cognitive enhancer properties. Also keep in mind that even though we might understand the mechanisms of LTP by using "simpler" cells than neurons, we will still need to evaluate the functions of LTP in different neuronal networks to start understanding higher neuronal functions.

ACKNOWLEDGMENTS

This research was supported by Grant BNS 96284 from the National Science Foundation. The author wishes to thank Shelli Sedlak for her expert secretarial assistance.

REFERENCES

Anwyl, R., J. Walshe, and M. Rowan (1987). Electroconvulsive treatment reduces long-term potentiation in rat hippocampus. *Brain Research* 435:1–2.

Arai, A., J. Larson, and G. Lynch (1990). Anoxia reveals a vulnerable period in the development of long-term potentiation. *Brain Research* 511:353–357.

Barinaga, M. (1990). The tide of memory, turning. *Science* 248:1603–1605.

Baudry, M., D. Arst, M. Oliver, and G. Lynch (1981). Development of glutamate binding sites and their regulation by calcium in rat hippocampus. *Brain Research* 227:37–48.

Baudry, M., G. Massicotte, and S. Hauge (1991a). Opposite effects of phospholipase A2 on ^{3}H-AMPA binding in adult and neonatal membranes. *Brain Research* (in press).

Baudry, M., G. Massicotte, and S. Hauge (1991b). Phosphatidylserine increases the affinity of the AMPA/Quisqualate receptor in rat brain membranes. *Behavioral and Neural Biology* 55:137–140.

Bekkers, J. M., and C. F. Stevens (1990). Presynaptic mechanism for long-term potentiation in the hippocampus. *Nature* 346:724–729.

Berger, T. W., and R. F. Thompson (1978). Identification of the pyramidal cells as the critical elements in hippocampal neuronal plasticity during learning. *Proceedings of the National Academy of Sciences (USA)* 75:1572–1576.

Berridge, M. J., and R. F. Irvine (1984). Inositol triphosphate, a second messenger in cellular signal transduction. *Nature* 312:315–321.

Bliss, T. V. P. (1990). Maintenance is presynaptic. *Nature* 346:698–699.

Boulter, J., et al. (1990). Molecular cloning and functional expression of glutamate receptor subunit genes. *Science* 249:1033–1037.

Comfurius, P., et al. (1990). Loss of membrane phospholipid asymmetry in platelets and red cells may be associated with calcium-induced shedding of plasma membrane and inhibition of aminophospholipid translocase. *Biochimica Biophysica Acta* 1026:153–160.

Corwin, J., et al. (1985). Behavioral effects of phosphatidylserine in the aged Fischer 344 rat: amelioration of passive avoidance deficits without changes in psychomotor task performance. *Neurobiology of Aging* 6:11–15.

del Cerro, S., A. Arai, and G. Lynch (1990). Inhibition of long-term potentiation by an antagonist of platelet-activating factor receptors. *Behavioral and Neural Biology* 54:213–217.

Dumuis, A., et al. (1988). NMDA receptors activate the arachidonic acid cascade system in striatal neurons. *Nature* 336:69–70.

Fagioli, S., et al. (1989). Phosphatidylserine administration during postnatal development improves memory in adult mice. *Neuroscience Letters* 101:229–233.

Foster, T. C., and B. L. McNaughton (1991). Long-term synaptic enhancement in CA1 is due to increased quantal size, not quantal content. *Hippocampus* 1 (in press).

Gustafsson, B., and H. Wigström (1990). Long-term potentiation in the CA1 region: its induction and early temporal development. *Progress in Brain Research* 83:223–232.

Heidmann, T., and J. P. Changeux (1982). Un modele moleculaire de regulation d'efficacite d'une synapse chimique au niveau post-synaptique. *Comptes Rendus de l'Académie des Sciences (Paris)* 295:665–670.

Hesse, G. W., and T. J. Teyler (1976). Reversible loss of long-term potentiation following electroconvulsive seizures. *Nature* 264:562–564.

Hubel, D. H., and T. N. Wiesel (1970). The period of susceptibility to the physiological effects of unilateral eye closure in kittens. *Journal of Physiology* 206:419–436.

Kauer, J. A., R. C. Malenka, and R. A. Nicoll (1988). A persistent postsynaptic modification mediates long-term potentiation in the hippocampus. *Neuron* 1:911–917.

Keinanen, K., et al. (1990). A family of AMPA-selective glutamate receptors. *Science* 249:556–560.

Kennedy, M. B. (1989). Regulation of synaptic transmission in the central nervous system: long-term potentiation. *Cell* 59:777–787.

Konishi, M., and F. Nottebohm (1969). Experimental studies in the ontogeny of bird vocalizations. In R. A. Hind (ed.), *Bird Vocalizations*. Cambridge: Cambridge University Press.

Kuba, K., and E. Kumamoto (1990). Long-term potentiation in vertebrate synapses: a variety of cascades with common subprocesses. *Progress in Neurobiology* 34:197–269.

Limbird, L. E., and P. J. Lefkowitz (1976). Adenylate cyclase-coupled beta-adrenergic receptors: effect of membrane-perturbing agents on receptor binding and enzyme stimulation by catecholamines. *Molecular Pharmacology* 12:559–567.

Lisman, J. E., and M. A. Goldring (1988). Feasibility of long-term storage of graded information by the Ca^{++}/calmodulin dependent protein kinase molecules of the post-synaptic density. *Proceedings of the National Academy of Sciences (USA)* 83:5320–5324.

Loh, H. H., and P. Y. Law (1980). The role of membrane lipids in receptor mechanisms. *Annual Review of Pharmacology and Toxicology* 20:210–234.

Lynch, G., and M. Baudry (1984). The biochemical basis of learning and memory: a new and specific hypothesis. *Science* 224:1057–1063.

Lynch, G., and M. Baudry (1991). Re-evaluating the constraints on hypothesis regarding LTP expression. *Hippocampus* 1 (in press).

Lynch, M. A., M. L. Errington, and T. V. Bliss (1989). Nordihydroguaiaretic acid blocks the synaptic component of long-term potentiation and the associated increases in release of glutamate and arachidonate: an in vivo study in the dentate gyrus of the rat. *Neuroscience* 30:693–701.

Malenka, R. C., et al. (1989). An essential role for postsynaptic calmodulin and protein kinase activity in long-term potentiation. *Nature* 340:554–557.

Malinow, R., and R. W. Tsien (1990). Presynaptic enhancement shown by whole-cell recordings of long-term potentiation in hippocampal slices. *Nature* 346:177–180.

Massicotte, G., and M. Baudry (1990). Modulation of AMPA/Quisqualate receptors by phospholipase A_2 treatment. *Neuroscience Letters* 118:245–248.

Massicotte, G., and M. Baudry (1991). Triggers and substrates of hippocampal synaptic plasticity. *Neurological and Biobehavioral Review* (in press).

Massicotte, G., M. Kessler, G. Lynch, and M. Baudry (1990a). *N*-methyl-D-aspartate and quisqualate/AMPA receptors: differential regulation by phospholipase C treatment. *Molecular Pharmacology* 32:278–285.

Massicotte, G., M. W. Oliver, G. Lynch and M. Baudry (1990b). Effect of bromophenacylbromide, a phospholipase A_2 inhibitor, on the induction and maintenance of LTP in hippocampal slices. *Brain Research* 537:49–53.

Massicotte, G., P. Vanderklish, G. Lynch, and M. Baudry (1991). Modulation of AMPA/quisqualate receptors by phospholipase A_2: a necessary step in long-term potentiation. *Proceedings of the National Academy of Sciences (USA)* 88:1893–1897.

Mohandas, N., et al. (1985). The structural organization of skeletal proteins influences lipid translocation across erythrocyte membrane. *Journal of Biology and Chemistry* 260:14,264–14,268.

Muller, D., M. Joly, and G. Lynch (1988). Contributions of quisqualate and NMDA receptors to the induction and expression of LTP. *Science* 242:1694–1697.

Okada, D., S. Yamagishi, and H. Sugiyama (1989). Differential effects of phospholipase inhibitors in long-term potentiation in the rat hippocampal mossy fiber synapses and Schaffer commissural synapses. *Neuroscience Letters* 100:1–3.

Oliver, M. W., M. Baudry, and G. Lynch (1989). The protease inhibitor leupeptin interferes with the development of LTP in hippocampal slices. *Brain Research* 505:233–238.

Pasternak, G. W., and S. H. Snyder (1974). Opiate receptor binding: enzymatic treatments discriminate between agonist and antagonist interactions. *Molecular Pharmacology* 10:183–193.

Periyasamy, S., and P. Somani (1986). Effect of proteases and phospholipases on 3H-yohimbine binding to human platelet membranes. *Biochemical Pharmacology* 35:3131–3136.

Racine, R. J., N. W. Milgram, and S. Hafner (1983). Long-term potentiation phenomena in the rat limbic forebrain. *Brain Research* 260:217–231.

Rankin, C. H., M. Stopfer, E. A. Marcus, and T. J. Carew (1987). Development of learning and memory in Aplysa. I. Functional assembly of gill and siphon withdrawal. *Journal of Neuroscience* 7:120–132.

Seigneuret, M., E. Favre, G. Morrot, and P. F. Devaux (1985). Strong interactions between a spin-labeled cholesterol analog and erythrocyte proteins in the human erythrocyte membrane. *Biochimica Biophysica Acta* 813:174–182.

Siess, W. (1989). Molecular mechanisms of platelet activation. *Physiology Review* 69:58–178.

Sladeczek, F., M. Recasens, and J. Bockaert (1988). A new mechanism for glutamate receptor action: phosphoinositide hydrolysis. *Trends in Neuroscience* 11:545–549.

Sommer, B., et al. (1990). Flip and flop: a cell-specific functional switch in glutamate-operated channels of the CNS. *Science* 249:1580–1585.

Staubli, U., et al. (1988). Chronic administration of a thiol-proteinase inhibitor blocks long-term potentiation of synaptic responses. *Brain Research* 444:153–158.

Staubli, U., P. Vanderklish, and G. Lynch (1990). An inhibitor of integrin receptors blocks long-term potentiation. *Behavioral and Neural Biology* 53:1–5.

Sune, A., and A. Bienvenue (1988). Relationship between the transverse distribution of phospholipids in plasma membrane and shape change of human platelets. *Biochemistry* 27:6794–6800.

Teyler, T. J., A. T. Perkins, and K. M. Harris (1989). The development of long-term potentiation in hippocampus and neocortex. *Neuropsychologia* 27:31–39.

Tocco, G., et al. (1989). Quisqualate receptor binding in hippocampus following classical conditioning of the rabbit nictitating membrane. *Society for Neuroscience Abstracts* 15:463.

Toffano, G., et al. (1981). Regulation of GABA receptor binding to synaptic plasma membrane of rat cerebral cortex: the role of endogenous phospholipids. *Brain Research* 222:95–102.

Weisz, D. J., T. W. Clark, and R. F. Thompson (1984). Increased activity of dentate granule cells during nictitating membrane response conditioning in rabbits. *Behavioral Brain Research* 12:145–154.

Williams, J. H., and T. V. Bliss (1989). An in vitro study of the effect of lipoxygenase and cyclo-oxygenase inhibitors of arachidonic acid on the induction and maintenance of long-term potentiation in the hippocampus. *Neuroscience Letters* 107:1–3.

Williamson, P., et al. (1982). Involvement of spectrin in the maintenance of phase-state asymmetry in the erythrocyte membrane. *Cell* 30:725–733.

Zwaal, R. F., et al. (1989). Loss of membrane phospholipid asymmetry during activation of blood platelets and sickled red cells; mechanisms and physiological significance. *Molecular and Cellular Biochemistry* 91:23–31.

13 Protein Kinase C Substrate B-50 (F1, GAP-43) and Long-Term Potentiation

Pierre de Graan and
Willem Hendrik Gispen

Three mechanisms have been proposed for long-term potentiation (LTP) invoking the long-term activation of Ca^{2+}-sensitive enzymes. Two of these hypotheses propose that protein kinases are involved, and the third one concerns an increased sensitivity of postsynaptic glutamate receptors by the Ca^{2+}-activated enzymes (Lynch and Baudry, 1984; see chapter 12), a hypothesis that is strongly supported by recent findings showing that the expression of LTP is associated with an enhanced transmission mediated by kainate-quisqualate channels (see chapter 3). The kinases that have been implicated in the mechanism of LTP are the type II Ca^{2+}-calmodulin–dependent kinase (CaMKII; see chapter 10) and Ca^{2+}-phospholipid–dependent protein kinase C (PKC; see chapter 11). CaMKII is a major constituent of the postsynaptic density and is presumably activated by *N*-methyl-D-aspartate (NMDA) receptor–mediated Ca^{2+} influx. Long-term activation of protein kinases has been observed in vitro and may involve autophosphorylation of the enzyme (for a review see Soderling, 1990). Two laboratories (Malinow et al., 1989; Malenka et al., 1989) have independently provided strong evidence for the involvement of CaMKII in postsynaptic mechanisms underlying LTP by microinjecting synthetic peptides, which interfere with CaMKII activity in postsynaptic CA1 pyramidal cells. These studies do not address a possible presynaptic role for CaMKII in LTP.

PKC has been implicated in LTP for several reasons: (1) artificial activators of PKC, phorbol esters, evoke LTP-like phenomena (Malenka et al., 1986; Muller et al., 1988); (2) PKC inhibitors block LTP (Malinow et al., 1988, 1989; Malenka et al., 1989); (3) LTP is paralleled by a translocation of PKC activity (Akers et al., 1986); (4) PKC injection into hippocampal pyramidal cells elicits LTP-like phenomena (Hu et al., 1987); and (5) increased phosphorylation of PKC substrates has been reported after tetanization (Nelson et al., 1989). Although these studies provide strong evidence for a role of PKC in LTP, most of them either deal with postsynaptic mechanisms underlying LTP or do not distinguish between a presynaptic or postsynaptic involvement of PKC. Presynaptic PKC is thought to play an important role in the regulation of neurotransmitter release (for a review see Dekker et al., 1991). A sustained increase in glutamate release is thought to be part of the mechanisms underlying LTP (see chapters 1, 6, and 8).

One way to study presynaptic PKC activity is to monitor the degree of phosphorylation of a well-characterized presynaptic PKC substrate, the B-50 protein (also known as F1, GAP-43, and neuromodulin; for reviews see Skene, 1989, and chapter 11). B-50 is a nervous tissue–specific protein that is predominantly localized in the presynaptic membrane. The protein is associated with the inner face of the membrane, probably anchored by a thio-ester linkage to palmitate. B-50 is an endogenous substrate of PKC (Aloyo et al., 1983; De Graan et al., 1989). It has been suggested that B-50 plays a role in the regulation of polyphosphoinositide metabolism, G_0 activity (Strittmatter et al., 1990), and calmodulin binding. Furthermore, the protein has been implicated in neurite outgrowth, neurotransmitter release (Dekker et al., 1989), and LTP (for reviews see Benowitz and Routtenberg, 1987; Skene, 1989).

To investigate the role of B-50 phosphorylation in LTP Routtenberg (Benowitz and Routtenberg, 1987; see chapter 11) elicited LTP by in vivo tetanization and subsequently measured B-50 phosphorylation in the homogenate of the extirpated tetanized brain region using [γ-^{32}P] adenosine triphosphate (ATP). In these studies the tissue is homogenized before the phosphorylation assay. The results of such a "post hoc" assay are difficult to interpret: one reason is that the assay does not distinguish between presynaptic and postsynaptic or glial PKC. To tackle this problem we developed an in situ phosphorylation assay using ^{32}P-orthophosphate labeling combined with immunoprecipitation of B-50, which enables the measurement of B-50 phosphorylation in intact hippocampal slices (De Graan et al., 1989). With this method we could show that K^+ and phorbol esters induce a concentration-dependent increase in B-50 phosphorylation (De Graan et al., 1988).

A relatively short treatment of hippocampal slices with active phorbol esters elicits long-term synaptic enhancement, which resembles enhancement after tetanization (Malenka et al., 1986). Although some properties of phorbol-induced and tetanus-induced LTP may be different, they are thought to share at least some molecular mechanisms. In our hippocampal slice system we tested whether a 20-minute treatment with 10^{-6} M of phorbol 12,13-dibutyrate (PDB) produced long-lasting effects on the responsiveness of the Schaffer collateral/CA1 system and concomitantly on B-50 phosphorylation (figure 13.1). PDB induced a significant increase in the population spike (PS) amplitude and B-50 phosphorylation within 20 minutes. Despite removal of the PDB by extensive washing, PS amplitude and B-50 phosphorylation remained elevated for at least 60 minutes after removal of the phorbol. The nonactive phorbol ester 4α-phorbol 12,13-didecanoate (4αPDD) had no effect on either of the two parameters. Control experiments in which tracer amounts of ^{3}H-PDB were added showed that 30 minutes after removal of PDB, less than 1% of the PDB remained in the tissue.

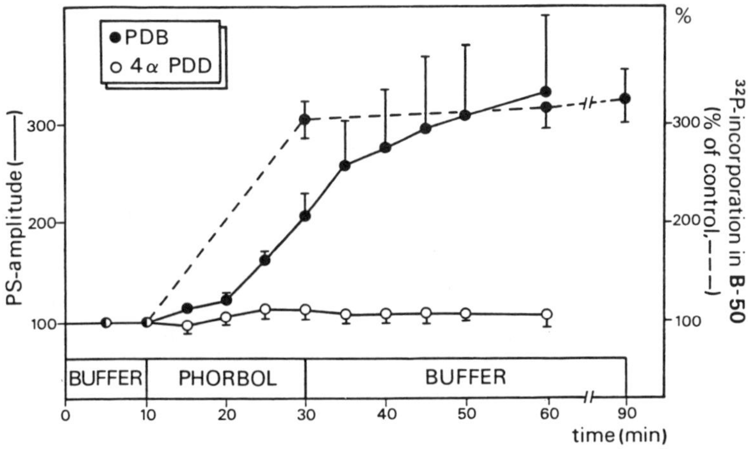

Figure 13.1 Long-lasting effects of a 20 minute treatment of hippocampal slices with 4β-phorbol 12,13-dibutyrate (PDB) on population spike (PS) amplitude and B-50 phosphorylation. After treatment with 10^{-6} M PDB (●) or 4α-PDB (○) slices were extensively washed or perfused with control buffer. Field potentials were recorded in the stratum pyramidale of CA1. The average PS amplitude (solid lines, mean ± SEM, n = 4) is expressed as % of the PS during the 10 min control period (prior to the phorbol treatment). In situ B-50 phosphorylation (broken lines, mean ± SEM, n = 4) was measured by quantitative immunoprecipitation from ^{32}P-orthophosphate prelabeled slices, and is expressed as % of the value obtained for untreated control slices at each time point.

The sustained increase in B-50 phosphorylation is most likely due to translocation of PKC from the cytosol to the membrane, a phenomenon that has also been reported after tetanization (Akers et al., 1986). Our data show that phorbol ester–induced LTP is paralleled by a sustained B-50 phosphorylation. Whether a similar increase in B-50 phosphorylation occurs after tetanus-induced LTP remains to be shown. As B-50 appears to be involved in the regulation of neurotransmitter release (Dekker et al., 1989), it is possible that B-50 is involved in the mechanisms underlying the long-term increase in glutamate release during LTP.

REFERENCES

Akers, R. F., et al. (1986). Translocation of protein kinase C activity may mediate hippocampal long-term potentiation. *Science* 231:587–589.

Aloyo, V. J., H. Zwiers, and W. H. Gispen (1983). Phosphorylation of B-50 by calcium-activated, phospholipid-dependent protein kinase and B-50 kinase. *Journal of Neurochemistry* 41:649–653.

Benowitz, L. I. and A. Routtenberg (1987). A membrane phosphoprotein associated with neural development, axonal regeneration, phospholipid metabolism and synaptic plasticity. *Trends in Neuroscience* 10:527–532.

De Graan, P. N. E., et al. (1988). Phorbol esters induce long- and short-term enhancement of B-50/GAP-43 phosphorylation in rat hippocampal slices. *Neuroscience Research Communication* 3:175–182.

De Graan, P. N. E., et al. (1989). Determination of changes in the phosphorylation state of the neuron-specific protein kinase C substrate B-50 (GAP-43) by quantitative immunoprecipitation. *Journal of Neurochemistry* 52:17–23.

Dekker, L. V., P. N. E. De Graan, and W. H. Gispen (1991). Transmitter release: target for regulation by PKC? *Progress in Brain Research* (in press).

Dekker, L. V., et al. (1989). Inhibition of noradrenaline release by antibodies to B-50 (GAP-43). *Nature* 342:74–76.

Hu, G.-Y., et al. (1987). Protein kinase C injection into hippocampal pyramidal cells elicits features of long term potentiation. *Nature* 328:426–429.

Lynch, M. A., and M. Baudry (1984). The biochemistry of memory: a new and specific hypothesis. *Science* 224:1057–1063.

Malenka, R. C., et al. (1989). An essential role for postsynaptic calmodulin and protein kinase activity in long-term potentiation. *Nature* 340:554–557.

Malenka, R. C., D. V. Madison, and R. A. Nicoll (1986). Potentiation of synaptic transmission in the hippocampus by phorbol esters. *Nature* 321:175–177.

Malinow, R., D. V. Madison, and R. W. Tsien (1988). Persistent protein kinase activity underlying long-term potentiation. *Nature* 335:820–824.

Malinow, R., H. Schulman, and R. W. Tsien (1989). Inhibition of postsynaptic PKC or CaMKII blocks induction but not expression of LTP. *Science* 245:862–866.

Muller, D., J. Turnbull, M. Baudry, and G. Lynch (1988). Phorbol ester-induced synaptic facilitation is different than long-term potentiation. *Proceedings of the National Academy of Sciences USA* 85:6997–7000.

Nelson, R. B., et al. (1989). The two major phosphoproteins in growth cones are probably identical to two protein kinase C substrates correlated with the persistence of long-term potentiation. *Journal of Neuroscience* 9:381–389.

Skene, J. H. P. (1989). Axonal growth-associated proteins. *Annual Review of Neuroscience* 12:127–156.

Söderling, T. R. (1990). Protein kinases: regulation by autoinhibitory domains. *Journal of Biological Chemistry* 265:1823–1826.

Strittmatter, S. M., D. Valenzuela, T. E. Kennedy, E. J. Neer, and M. C. Fishman (1990). G_0 is a major growth cone protein subject to regulation by GAP-43. *Nature* 344:836–841.

III Biophysical and Structural Changes in Long-Term Potentiation

14 Studies of Synaptic Structural Modifications after Long-Term Potentiation and Kindling: Context for a Molecular Morphology

Christopher S. Wallace, Nicholas Hawrylak, and William T. Greenough

The essential synaptic organization of the hippocampal formation has been known for more than half a century, and the devastating functional consequences of its absence have fascinated and illuminated several generations of neuroscientists. We have yet, however, to understand how plasticity in hippocampal synapses contributes to memory. This endeavor promises to be monumental. When one views fine hippocampal anatomy in Golgi stained sections, as Ramon y Cajal (1911) and Lorente de No (1934) originally did, one sees at once an order that is tantalizing and an intricacy that is daunting. Experimental access to the hippocampus requires that it be simplified, but authenticity can be compromised unless the accumulation of greater detail about a particular part of the system is balanced with a consistent effort to account for the roles of those cell types or synapses (both excitatory and inhibitory) excluded from the experimental preparation. Similarly, molecules extracted using biochemical methods must be placed in the context of synaptic function for their role in plasticity to be properly assessed.

As current issues in LTP research at the end of the twentieth century are considered, we are still contending with some of the questions raised by the pioneers of neuroscience at the end of the nineteenth century. For example, the question of whether long-term potentiation (LTP) leaves its print on the brain by forming new synapses, as Ramon y Cajal (1893) suggested, or by increasing the strength of existing synapses, as Tanzi (1893) proposed, remains an area of active debate today. In this chapter, we discuss morphological findings that bear on this question provided by studies of both LTP and kindling. We include the kindling work because, although it may be a pathological process, it shares many important features with LTP. Like LTP, kindling is a long-term modification of neuronal responsiveness that develops after patterned stimulation. Kindling has been observed at the same synapses as LTP and appears to arise via similar molecular mechanisms. It has yet to be resolved whether kindling and LTP are distinct entities with shared properties and mechanisms or whether they represent separate points on a continuum of plastic processes that enhance responses to patterned stimulation. (For a comprehensive comparison of the electrophysiological, biochemical, and pharmacological data reflecting possible commonalities in the mechanisms of LTP and kindling, see Cain [1989].)

Within the hippocampal formation, morphological changes have been reported after LTP and kindling that support the suggestion that changes in efficacy may result from modifications of existing synapses (Fifkova and Van Harreveld, 1977; Desmond and Levy, 1983; Geinisman et al., 1988, 1990a, 1990b), as well as from the addition of newly formed synapses (Lee et al., 1980, 1981; Chang and Greenough, 1984; Hawrylak et al., 1989; Chang et al., 1991a, 1991b, submitted). It is possible, however, that regions of the hippocampus may respond differently. As the following morphological studies indicate, synaptogenesis has tended to be observed in CA1 whereas dendritic spine shape change has been more frequently reported in the dentate gyrus.

Increasing electrophysiological and pharmacological evidence has suggested that LTP may not be a single phenomenon, but may instead be a family of analogous processes adapted to regional specialization (see Kuba and Kumamoto, 1990, and other chapters in this book). As the list of structures exhibiting LTP-like phenomena has grown past the boundaries of the trisynaptic circuit, the limbic forebrain, and the mammalian central nervous system (for a review of the distribution of LTP, see other chapters in this volume; Teyler and DiScenna, 1987; Bliss and Lynch, 1988; Kuba and Kumamoto, 1990), the catalogue of molecules implicated in potentiation in these systems has also burgeoned. At this point, as LTP is being pursued to its molecular essence in a vast array of systems, it is becoming even more important to discern the functional analogies among the molecular elements at work in different networks.

METHODOLOGICAL SCAFFOLDING FOR SYNAPTIC STRUCTURAL ANALYSIS

The hippocampus has provided a stable framework for pursuing the cellular and molecular mechanisms of plasticity because its properties have continued to resemble memory as studies have progressed across levels of organization from the cellular to the synaptic to the molecular. Nonetheless, as experiments focus on finer and finer details, we must remain aware of the ways in which we have simplified the system. Some examples are discussed in the following section.

Artificial Patterns and Levels of Stimulation

The demonstration of "behavioral LTP" (Sharp et al., 1985; Green and Greenough, 1986) was an important step in authenticating experimental LTP as it showed that LTP may parallel a natural information storage process, but it raises intriguing and yet unanswered questions about the properties of "natural LTP" and its induction by environmental stimulation (see chapter 7). The discovery of enhanced potentiation at the theta frequency in the Schaffer collateral–CA1 pathway (Larson et al., 1986;

Rose and Dunwiddie, 1986) has provided evidence that the simple high-frequency stimuli that demonstrated LTP initially may obscure the tuning of hippocampal pathways to patterned stimulation. This may mark the dawning of our understanding about how even more selective local activation might gate specific molecular cascades that lead to precise patterns of synaptic remodeling.

Overemphasis on Trisynaptic Circuit

The basic lamellar organization of intrahippocampal pathways is such that slices can be easily prepared that capture all the components of the trisynaptic circuit (Andersen et al., 1971). Although the regularity and accessibility of these excitatory pathways has provided a marvelous platform for the pursuit of mechanisms of excitatory potentiation, recent anatomical studies (Amaral and Witter, 1989; Yeckel and Berger, 1990) indicate that an emphasis on lamellar organization has obscured an appreciation of the longitudinal (and otherwise translamellar) organization of these projections originally described by Lorente de No (1934). While the hippocampus seems to be distinctive in its high ratio of principal neurons to inhibitory interneurons, it is nonetheless important to recognize that inhibitory neurons could play a substantial role in patterning the activation of excitatory pathways, and do themselves appear to exhibit LTP at their excitatory afferent sites in both CA1 (Buszaki and Eidelberg, 1982) and dentate gyrus (Kairiss et al., 1987). Plasticity in these cells could have an important role in adaptively filtering afferent input and modulating potentiation in excitatory circuits. Furthering our understanding of how the fine structure of hippocampus represents the integrative processes it performs requires that we consider these nonlamellar aspects of hippocampal circuitry.

Process of Imaging and Quantifying Ultrastructure May Introduce Aberrant Views

In morphological studies, images must be interpreted in the context of how they were gathered. Since the resolution of the electron microscope is required to distinguish synaptic structures, concerns arise about means of (1) fixation, (2) sampling, and (3) quantification. First, fixatives may interact differently with various cellular constituents. Most morphological studies of LTP have used aldehyde fixation, although a few have used rapid freezing and freeze substitution. These methods may generate different results in some cases. Second, sections suitable for viewing in the electron microscope provide limited two-dimensional views of the three-dimensional structures of interest. Serial section reconstruction can provide complete and accurate measurements of synaptic elements (e.g., Harris and Stevens, 1989; Harris et al., 1989), but is so labor intensive that it often becomes impractical for experimental comparison, although it has been used in a handful of LTP and kindling studies (Andersen et al., 1987; Geinisman et al., 1988; 1990a, 1990b; Harris et al., 1989). Direct measurements or counts of morphological entities, such as synapses, from single random sections are biased to the extent that their elements differ among treatment groups in size, shape, or orientation. A further caveat is that an *apparent* qualitative change in synapses could actually reflect a change in synapse numbers. That is, if new synapses form, all of which have a particular property (e.g., very large size or a particular shape), the fact that we infer processes from statistical averages could lead us to misinterpret the result (e.g., as an increase in size of pre-existing synapses or a transformation to a new shape). Proper detection of number change is thus as important to qualitative synapse measurements as to those actually directed at detecting numerical change. Correction of single section measurements based on simplifying geometrical assumptions similarly induces bias to the extent that the assumptions are not met. New stereological methods offer ways to achieve highly accurate, unbiased estimates economically (Gundersen et al., 1988; Geinisman et al., 1988, 1990a, 1990b). This added efficiency also permits more animals to be examined and thus further increases the accuracy of experimental comparisons.

SYNAPTIC STRUCTURAL CHANGES OBSERVED IN NON-LTP PARADIGMS

Behavioral Experience and Synaptic Number

There has been a dynamic interplay between the morphological studies of LTP induction and those manipulating behavioral experience ever since the LTP studies began in the mid-1970s. Here we review some exemplary behavioral studies separately as sources of both hypothesis generation and of comparison with the LTP studies. This section is restricted to effects on synapses; studies of glial cells are discussed separately. Throughout the chapter, all results discussed are statistically significant ones, unless specifically noted otherwise.

By far the most commonly reported consequence of differential experience on brain is the differential formation and/or loss of synapses. Such effects can arise in competing pathways within a sensory system, as in the case of monocular deprivation where deprived geniculostriate axons have fewer terminals than do those of the experienced eye (Tieman, 1984). In this case it is clear that the formation and loss of synapses generates an altered pattern of functional connections (LeVay et al., 1980), something that is presumably true in general when connections form or are lost. Differences in numbers of connections are also seen in a variety of comparisons between animals given laboratory-style housing with relatively low amounts of opportunity for novel physical and social stimulation and animals given complex-style housing with toys, several other animals, and otherwise more stimulating surroundings. Animals in the more stimulated groups have more highly branched dendrites and more synapses per neuron in visual cortex and other brain structures (Volkmar and Greenough, 1972; Beaulieu and Colonnier, 1985; Floeter and Greenough,

1979; Turner and Greenough, 1985). Synapse formation or loss, or compatible changes such as dendritic growth or shrinkage, have also been reported in association with learning various behaviors (Greenough et al., 1979; Greenough et al., 1985; Black et al., 1990). Comparable synaptic changes in association with habituation, sensitization, and associative conditioning have been reported in invertebrates (Bailey and Chen, 1986; Alkon et al., 1990). These changes would seem to occur quite rapidly, as the dendritic effects of a complex rearing environment on dendritic fields are detectable after as little as 4 days' experience (Kilman et al., 1988), and a considerable amount of change has to build up for it to be detectable in the average dendritic field parameters. Together these findings argue that, if the phenomena underlying LTP are the same phenomena that underlie memory and seemingly related effects of experience, then we should expect to see synaptogenesis in association with LTP.

Behavioral Experience and Qualitative Synapse Change

In addition to changes in synapse number, qualitative changes in preexisting synapses appear to occur after behavioral experiences similar to those just discussed. These changes could reflect synaptic efficacy alterations.

Examples of the changes in synapse properties that have been frequently reported and probably do reflect qualitative changes include the following:

Size Synapses have been reported to be larger in some parts of the cerebral cortex of animals reared in complex environments than in animals reared in standard laboratory housing (e.g., West and Greenough, 1972; Sirevaag and Greenough, 1987 [we excluded Mollgaard et al., 1971, here because it was retracted by Diamond et al.,1975]). Likewise, larger synapses are associated with the nondeprived eye in the monocular deprivation paradigm (Tieman, 1984). Size changes are often not reported in other paradigms seemingly fairly similar to these two, however, and there is substantial conflict in the literature as to the effects of manipulations such as binocular visual deprivation on synapse size (see Greenough and Chang, 1988, for review).

Vesicle Measurements Reports of differences in the number, density, and location of vesicles probably should be interpreted cautiously if they emanate from aldehyde-fixed preparations. As we have noted in somewhat more detail elsewhere (Greenough and Chang, 1985, 1988), aldehydes may cause neurotransmitter release and vesicle depletion at peripheral synapses (e.g., McKinlay and Usherwood, 1978; Smith and Reese, 1980). While we do not know of data that directly bear on this in the central nervous system (CNS), there are morphological indicants of aldehyde effects on vesicles. In unpublished work, we have observed differences in vesicle positioning between aldehyde-fixed boutons and those preserved by quick-freezing and substitution procedures, as noted in figure 14.1. In general, in the latter case, the vesicles exhibit a reduced tendency to clump toward the synaptic cleft and are more evenly distributed throughout the terminal. We also observed less clumping of vesicles toward the cleft in preparations that had been fixed in the presence of divalent cations (Mg^{2+}, Mn^{2+}, Co^{2+}; Birks, 1974) that would compete with Ca^{2+} to impede neurotransmitter release (Chang et al., 1979). A final problem that deserves mention is that the role of vesicles in neurotransmitter release at peripheral synapses remains controversial (see Oorschot and Jones, 1987), and we have no good evidence regarding the vesicle hypothesis in the CNS.

Nonetheless, reports of effects of LTP induction on vesicle distribution discussed in subsequent sections and several behavioral reports suggest that *something* may be going on even if the aldehyde effects may render the results hard to interpret. One particularly consistent behavioral effect is the tendency for subnormal amounts of sensory stimulation to reduce the average number of vesicles per terminal (e.g., Garey and Pettigrew, 1974; Gulley et al., 1978; Tieman, 1984, 1985). These effects may persist beyond the period of deprivation (e.g., Vrensen and DeGroot, 1974, 1975). Sirevaag and Greenough (1987) found larger vesicle aggregates in occipital cortical layer IV synapses of animals from complex rearing environments than in animals reared in individual laboratory cages. As an indicant shorter-term change, Bailey and Chen (1983) reported an increase in the number of vesicles near the active zone in sensitized synapses from Aplysia abdominal ganglia.

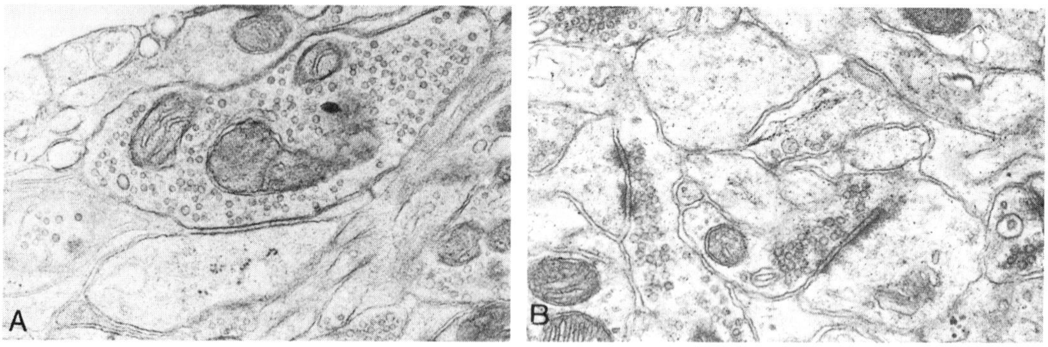

Figure 14.1 Comparison of synaptic structural views using freeze and chemical fixation. (A) View of a synapse from an upright dentate slice (Chang and Greenough, 1988) rapidly frozen with an inverted slam freezer (Wallace et al., 1988) and freeze-substituted in 3% osmium in acetone. Note the absence of a pronounced postsynaptic density (PSD) and the uniform distribution of vesicles. The tissue surface is visible at the upper left corner. (B) View of synapse from chemically fixed tissue (perfusion with 2% paraformaldehyde and 2.5% glutaraldehyde and post-fixed in 1% osmium). Magnification is 35,000× for both micrographs.

Shape A tantalizing series of light microscopic studies by Coss and coworkers has indicated that experience may modulate spine shape in some cases. In the first of these, Coss and Globus (1978) reported that spine density along dendrites was greater and spine necks were shorter on interneurons in the tectum of jewel fish that were socially housed in comparison with isolation housed fish. Likewise, spines on the Kenyon interneurons in the corpora pedunculata of honeybees became shorter as the bees progressed through the life cycle change from nurser to forager (Coss et al., 1980). Brandon and Coss (1982) reported that these changes occurred very rapidly, within the few minutes of the initial "orientation flight" with which the honeybee inaugurates her transition to forager. In contrast to these findings, Sirevaag and Greenough (1985) did not detect differences in the length, perimeter, area, or roundness of spines in visual cortex of rats reared in a complex environment compared with controls housed individually or in pairs. Since only spines connected to the dendrite by a neck were measured, the small sample of synapses (about 100 per group) may have precluded detection of a small length difference.

The shape of spines varies dramatically in many brain regions during development. Developmental studies suggest that spines often progress from a sessile form, as depicted in figure 14.2, in which there is no clearly discernable head and neck, to a mushroom-shaped mature form (Juraska and Fifkova, 1979; Miller and Peters, 1981). The functional consequences of this shift are unknown. The relation to LTP is surprising and is discussed in the section Spine Shape and LTP in Development and Recovery.

Conformation of the Apposition Zone Finally, the shape of the contact or apposition zone of synapses may vary with experience or the state of the synapse. Streit and associates (1972) described a more wrinkled or undulating presynaptic membrane, with the cleft and postsynaptic membrane invaginating the presynaptic terminal in waking, compared to

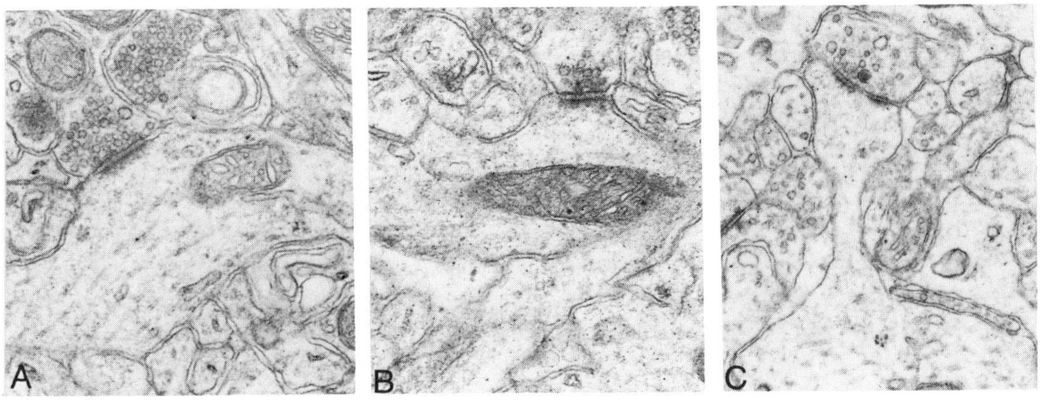

Figure 14.2 Synaptic types. (A) Shaft synapse. (B) Sessile synapse. (C) Synapse on a connected spine containing a perforated PSD.

anesthetized rats. Cooke and colleagues (1974) and Jones and Devon (1977) confirmed the greater curvature of the postsynaptic element into the presynaptic element in waking rats. Dyson and Jones (1980) found that the relative frequency of flatter synapses increased while that of presynaptically convex synapses decreased in molecular layer of rat occipital cortex as the animals approached adulthood. Tieman (1985) reported that geniculocortical synapses of monocularly deprived eyes in cats were more presynaptically convex than those associated with the open eye. Likewise, Wesa and associates (1982) reported that synapses were more presynaptically concave in visual cortex of rats from a complex environment than in individually housed rats. In each of these cases, the postsynaptic density (PSD) curvature was altered, such that the contact itself differed, as opposed to parts of the spine membrane outside of the PSD zone. The general rule is for the more experienced state to be shifted toward presynaptic concavity or away from postsynaptic concavity (toward flatness).

Perforated Postsynaptic Density Based on serial reconstruction, Peters and Kaiserman-Abramof (1969) first detailed the irregular perforations that are occasionally seen in the postsynaptic density. The frequency with which synapses exhibit these perforations in the visual cortex varies with a variety of experience manipulations including developmental age, social versus individual housing, rearing environment complexity (Greenough et al., 1978), and visual discrimination training (Vrensen and Cardozo, 1981). In hypothalamic regions governing lactation, pregnancy and nursing similarly increases the number of perforated synapses (Hatton and Ellisman, 1982). While no function of these perforations has been discerned, Geinisman and associates (1986) found a reduction in perforated synapses specific to a subpopulation of aged rats that exhibited a memory impairment, suggesting some sort of functional importance of this type of synapse (see Geinisman et al., 1988, 1990a, 1990b; and the following section on synaptic structural alterations after kindling for perforated synapse measurements in LTP and kindling).

Polyribosomal Aggregates One final qualitative change deserves brief mention. Greenough and coworkers (1985) reported increased numbers of synapses with spines containing polyribosomal aggregates in animals from a complex environment. This change appears to be related to synapse number changes, as polyribosomal aggregates characterize populations of synapses that are new or recently forming (Steward and Falk, 1985). In what could be a related phenomenon, Desmond and Levy (1990) reported a reduction in spines with polysomes at their bases (in the dendrite, not in the spine) after LTP in the dentate gyrus.

Conclusions from Experience Manipulation Studies

These studies indicate that both synapse formation and loss, and alterations in several different morphological characteristics of previously existing synapses, occur in response to behavioral manipulations. Whether the morphological alterations represent several independent changes or components of a coherent efficacy change mechanism remains uncertain, although there is no consistent association among them, or between them and synapse formation, across the studies reviewed in this chapter. If the morphological alterations represent a coherent process, it means that not all components are expressed at the same level across paradigms.

ALTERATIONS IN ULTRASTRUCTURE ASSOCIATED WITH SYNAPTIC MODIFICATION AFTER LTP AND KINDLING

We focus on three methodological aspects of these experiments that have attempted to correlate the activational history of a synapse with its structural condition: (1) the hippocampal region studied, (2) the stimulation parameters used, and (3) the latency between stimulation and fixation. These parameters reflect on the developing issues of regional specialization, selective cascade gating by stimulus pattern, and temporal spectrum of processes likely to be induced (e.g., both short-term [Racine and Milgram, 1983] and long-term [Racine et al., 1983] potentiation and depression phenomena), and stability of the synaptic modification. Additional considerations for interpretation also include in vitro and in vivo preparations, species differences, age effects, sex differences, and anesthetic effect on LTP threshold, as well as the aforementioned considerations of sampling bias and quantification. While anesthetic effects on LTP threshold have been reported (MacIver, et al., 1989; Engstrom et al., 1990), the confounding of anesthetic and region (see tables 14.1 and 14.2) makes it difficult to determine whether this has played any role in morphological studies. Gonadal steroid effects on hippocampal excitability (Teyler et al., 1980) and synaptic number (Gould et al., 1990; Wooley and McEwen, 1990), as well as stress and adrenal steroid effects on LTP induction (Shors et al., 1990), mandate more attention to both the sex of the subject and the conditions to which they are subjected before LTP induction. Available data, however, do not allow us to discern any effects of these endocrine variables on morphological studies. Other effects potentially attributable to these variables are discussed as they arise.

Our goal here is twofold: first, to provide a context for reported structural change as a complement to studies of LTP using electrophysiological, pharmacological, or biochemical approaches, and second, to identify the inconsistencies among previous studies to temper interpretation and highlight questions that still remain.

Reports of modifications in hippocampal synapses after potentiating stimulation continue to honor the predictions of both Ramon y Cajal

(1893) and Tanzi (1893). Bliss and Lømo (1973) focused on the latter perspective in their original description of LTP: "The potentiation of the synaptic wave can in our view be most simply accounted for in terms of facilitated synaptic transmission. . . . Facilitation could take the form of an increase in the number of terminals invaded by the constant test volley, an increase in the amount of transmitter released per synapse, an increase in the sensitivity of the post-synaptic junctional membrane, or a reduction of the resistance of the narrow stem by which spines are attached to the parent dendrite (Rall, 1970)." Neither synapse formation, nor the glial changes described in the following sections, were anticipated in that period of emphasis on the stability of neuronal and glial structure.

Changes in synapse number have been reported, as have changes in the structure of existing synapses, after LTP and kindling. Tables 14.1, 14.2, and 14.3 provide a summary of the methods used and results reported from these studies. For efficiency, we have been occasionally somewhat loose in the text in specifying the eliciting conditions and verification of LTP. The tables clarify these issues.

EVIDENCE FOR ALTERATIONS IN EXISTING SYNAPSES

Spine Area and Spine Dimension Changes in Dentate Gyrus

Freeze Substitution Studies Van Harreveld and Fifkova (1975) and Fifkova and Van Harreveld (1977) first reported structural change after LTP. This work proposed lowering of spine resistance by alterations in spine shape or neck dimensions. Rapid freezing and freeze-substitution were used to avoid inducing changes in tissue volume that might result during aldehyde fixation (Van Harreveld and Fifkova, 1975). Subsequently, some of these studies have been replicated using electrophysiological verification of LTP induction and aldehyde fixation (Fifkova, 1985), but no experiments appear to have used freeze substituted tissue in which LTP was verified.

These early experiments took advantage of the registry between regions of the entorhinal cortex and different laminae of the dentate molecular layer (DML) to which they project. Fibers in the perforant path arising from the medial entorhinal cortex form *en passant* synapses with granule cell dendrites in the middle third of the DML, whereas fibers from lateral entorhinal cortex project to the distal third of the DML (Hjorth-Simonsen and Jeune, 1972; Steward and Scoville, 1976). Van Harreveld and Fifkova (1975; Fifkova and Van Harreveld, 1977) stimulated the entorhinal cortex of mice, then exposed and froze the dentate molecular layer at time points ranging from 2 minutes to 23 hours poststimulation. Controls were either implanted, but unstimulated, or unoperated mice. In the earlier studies (Van Harreveld and Fifkova, 1975; Fifkova and Van Harreveld, 1977), the lateral entorhinal cortex was stimulated and the distal third of the DML, which receives its perforant path projection, was examined. Subsequently

(Fifkova and Anderson, 1981; Fifkova et al., 1982), both medial and lateral entorhinal cortex were stimulated and both middle and distal thirds were examined. In both cases, the proximal third of the DML served as a control as it receives no direct entorhinal projections. Because the freeze substitution procedure precluded concurrent electrophysiological recording, it must be presumed that sample regions were potentiated based on the anatomical projections and the stimulation parameters (Van Harreveld and Fifkova, 1975). The presence of LTP and the absence of seizures, however, was reported in a later study, using separate animals (Payne et al., 1982).

As figure 14.3 indicates, animals with lateral entorhinal cortex stimulation showed an increase in spine area in the distal third of the DML at each time point sampled (see also table 14.1). The proximal third of the molecular layer showed a transient decrease in spine area (22.6%) at 2 to 6 minutes. In addition, two transient presynaptic changes were observed in the distal molecular layer: (1) a decrease in axon terminal area at 2 to 6 minutes and (2) a decrease in vesicle density at 10 to 60 minutes.

When both lateral and medial entorhinal cortex were stimulated, an increase in spine area was observed in both regions of the DML receiving entorhinal projections. Both middle and distal DML had greater spine areas at both 4 minutes and 90 minutes after stimulation. In contrast to the results for lateral entorhinal stimulation alone, however, where the spine increases were restricted to the sublamina containing the activated afferents, joint medial and lateral entorhinal stimulation also increased spine area in the proximal third of the DML, which receives no direct entorhinal input. This effect suggests that associational and commissural projections to the proximal third of the DML were somehow transynaptically activated, although the pathway is unclear (Fifkova et al., 1982). These effects are intriguing, given that concurrent stimulation of the commissural pathway and the perforant path can block the formation of LTP at perforant-dentate granule synapses (Douglas et al., 1982) and under bicuculline blockade of γ-aminobutyric acid (GABA)-mediated inhibition, activation of the commissural pathway results in the formation of apparently *N*-methyl-D-aspartate (NMDA)-dependent LTP at commissural-dentate granule cell synapses in the proximal third of the DML (Steward et al., 1990). Discerning the functional relevance of the changes observed in the proximal third of DML by Fifkova and coworkers (1982) will require additional work, but these physiological results argue for consideration of both the inhibitory and excitatory contributions of this pathway in studies of LTP in the dentate gyrus, and underscore the dependence of LTP formation on the context of its induction. It should be noted that there were no spine area or perimeter increases in the proximal third of the DML in an experiment that used different stimulus parameters and aldehyde perfusion fixation and that verified LTP with electrophysiological recording (Fifkova, 1985).

In the lateral plus medial entorhinal stimulation study, detailed spine

Table 14.1 Summary of morphological studies of LTP in the dentate gyrus. DML = dentate molecular layer; IBI = interburst interval; ITI = intertrain (or interstimulus) interval; EPSP = excitatory postsynaptic potential; N_V = numerical density; N_A = areal density; S_V = surface area per unit volume; L_A = length per unit area; PSD = postsynaptic density; IO = input-output; CON = control. (See text for discussion.)

Preparation	Mouse in vivo (urethane anesthesia)	Mouse in vivo (urethane anesthesia)	Mouse in vivo (unspecified anesthesia)	Rat in vivo (urethane and chloralose)	Rat in vivo (urethane and chloralose anesthesia)	Adult male rats in vivo (unspecified anesthesia)	Young adult rat in vivo
Stimulated	Lateral entorhinal cortex	Lateral and medial entorhinal cortex	Lateral and medial entorhinal cortex	Angular bundle	Perforant path	Perforant path	Medial perforant path
Examined	Distal DML vs. proximal DML	Proximal (P), Middle (M), and distal (D) DML	Distal and middle DML	Middle one-third of DML	Middle one-fifth of DML	Middle and proximal DML	Middle DML
Potentiating stimulation	30 Hz for 30 sec; $n = 8$ (2 min); $n = 6$ (10–60 min); $n = 10$ (4–8 hr); $n = 7$ (23 hr)	30 Hz for 30 sec; $n = 10$ (4 min); $n = 10$ (90 min)	Fifteen 20 msec bursts at 400 HZ delivered at 0.2 Hz; $n = 8$	*Spaced:* 3–4 bouts; 8 trains of 8 pulses at 400 Hz, 0.1 sec IBI; 10 min ITI; $n = 6$ *Massed:* 24–8 pulse trains at 400 Hz, 1 burst each 1/5 sec; 5 sec ITI; $n = 6$ (2 min); $n = 6$ (10 min)	10 trains of 100 Hz for 1 sec with 30 sec ITI; $n = 3$	4 trains of 300 pulses made up of 20 pulses at 200 Hz, 5 sec between burst; 30 min ITI; $n = 4–5$	15 20 ms bursts at 400 Hz delivered at 0.2 Hz; delivered once-a-day for 4 days; $n = 7$
Control stimulation	Unoperated control; $n = 11$ Sham implant; $n = 5$ (15–18 hr)	Sham implant; $n = 10$ (4 min); $n = 10$ (90 min)	Sham implant; $n = 5$	(Contralateral hippocampus control) *Spaced:* Test stim every 15 sec *Massed:* 196 pulses at 1/15 sec	Unoperated rats; $n = 2$	Passive controls: only implanted $n = 4–5$ Active controls: 1200 pulses at 0.2 Hz; $n = 4–5$	Coulombic: control stimulation; $n = 7$ Unstimulated: implant only; $n = 7$
Verification of potentiation	None	None	35% increase over baseline of dentate evoked response	LTP = 50% increase in EPSP slope; no verification in massed 2 min group	30 min leftward shift in IO function	Separate animals show LTP lasting 2 min–7 days	Electrophysiological recording
Fixation	Rapid freezing and freeze substitution	Rapid freezing and freeze substitution	Aldehyde perfusion	Aldehyde perfusion	Aldehyde perfusion	Aldehyde perfusion	Aldehyde perfusion
Quantification	Direct measurements on single sections	Direct measurements on single sections	Direct measurements on single sections	Measurements from single sections	Measurements from serial sections	Direct measurements on single sections	Serial thin sections with

Stereology	No				No					No		Corrections: N_V from N_A; S_V from L_A	No	No		Disector
Time(s)	2–6 min	10–60 min	4–8 hr	23 hr	4 min M1/3	4 min D1/3	90 min P1/3	90 min M1/3	90 min D1/3	45–60 min M1/3	45–60 min D1/3	LTP vs. control (all LTP groups pooled)	30 min (?)	8 hr	48 hr	1 hr (after last stimulation)
Spine dimension																
Area	15.4%	38.6%	35.5%	24.1%	19.5%	32.0%	14.0%	28.2%	33.0%	27.2%	35.5%					
Perimeter	—	—	—	—	8.9%	13.7%	6.1%	11.4%	17.7%	18.3%	22.6%					
Head width	—	—	—	—	21.6%	23.2%	28.1%	33.6%	34.7%	—	—					
Neck length	—	—	—	—	—	−31.0%	—	—	−25.0%	—	—		15% LTP spines > longest CON			
Neck width	—	—	—	—	42.2%	61.7%	—	—	61.2%	20.0%	41.1%		Increased			
Spine Shape																
Concave synapse	—	—	—	—	—	—	—	—	—	—	—	44%				
Nonconcave	—	—	—	—	—	—	—	—	—	—	—	−16% (simple); −22% (ellipsoid)				
Spinule	—	—	—	—	—	—	—	—	—	—	—			37.6%	30.5%	
Apposition																
Contact length	—	—	—	—	—	—	—	—	—	11.8%	12.9%	Tot: concave: 33.4%; non-PSD: concave 32.5%				
PSD length	—	—	—	—	—	—	—	—	—	—	—	PSD: concave: 36.6% vs. nonconcave: −25.4%				↑ Perf/nonperf ratio: ~31%
Perforated syn	—	—	—	—	—	—	—	—	—	—	—					↓ Perf PSD dimensions
PSD length	—	—	—	—	—	—	—	—	—	—	—					
Axon Terminal																
Area	−15.6%	—	—	—	—	—	—	—	—	—	—					
Vesicles																
Number/density	—	−19.6%	—	—	—	—	—	—	—	—	—					
Distribution	—	—	—	—	—	—	—	—	—	—	—	↑ Frontline vesicles				
Ca+ contents	—	—	—	—	—	—	—	—	—	—	—					
Synapse Number																
Shaft synapse	—	—	—	—	—	—	—	—	—	—	—					
Sessile synapse	—	—	—	—	—	—	—	—	—	—	—					
Glia																
Surface area	—	—	—	—	—	—	—	—	—	—	—					
Reference	Van Harreveld and Fifkova, 1975; Fifkova and van Harreveld, 1977				Fifkova and Anderson, 1981; Fifkova et al., 1982					Fifkova, 1985		Desmond and Levy, 1986a; 1986b; 1986c; 1988a	Andersen et al., 1987	Schuster et al., 1990		Geinisman et al., 1990b; de Toledo-Morrell et al., 1990

Table 14.2 Summary of morphological studies of LTP in hippocampal subfield CA1. For explanations of abbreviations, see table 14.1. In addition, CV = coefficient of variation, TV = total vesicles; D = distant vesicles; LV = local vesicles; AV = attached vesicles; APV = 2-amino-5-phosphonovaleric acid. (See text for discussion.)

Preparation	Adult male rats in vivo (nembutal and chloral hydrate)	Young adult rats in vitro	Male and female rats in vitro	Young adult male rats in vivo (urethane anesthesia)	Female rat in vitro	Two-year-old male rats in vitro
Stimulated	Schaffer collateral–commissural fibers	Schaffer collateral–commissural fibers	Schaffer collateral–commissural fibers	Schaffer collateral–commissural fibers	Schaffer collateral–commissural fibers	Schaffer collateral–commissural fibers
Examined	Stratum radiatum	Stratum radiatum	Stratum radiatum	Stratum radiatum	Stratum radiatum	Stratum radiatum
Potentiating Stimulation	3 trains at 100 Hz for 1 sec; 10–15 min ITI; $n = 20$	3 high-frequency bursts (200 Hz for 0.5 sec); $n = 8$	6 trains at 100 Hz for 1 sec or 200 Hz for 0.5 sec; $n = 5$	1 sec burst at 100 Hz with 5 sec intervals between bursts, followed by 0.2 Hz test pulse, $n = 5$	1 second pulse at 100 Hz, followed by 0.2 Hz test pulses every 5 min; $n = 4$ (15 min); $n = 6$ (30 min); $n = 6$ (60 min)	6 trains at 100 Hz for 1 sec; $n = 5$
Control Stimulation	3 trains at 0.2 Hz for 3 min; 10–15 min ITI; $n = 11$	1 min train of low-frequency (1 Hz) pulses; $n = 7$	Low freqeuncy: 1 Hz for 600 sec; $n = 5$; Continuous stimulation: 40 Hz or 100 Hz for 10 min; $n = 4$	Implanted control, only 0.2 Hz test pulse; $n = 5$	No stimulation 100 pulses at 0.2 Hz 1 sec at 100 Hz in presence of 50 μM APV; $n = 6$ (pooled controls)	Activity control: 1 Hz for 600 sec; $n = 5$
Verification of Potentiation	Population spike nondecremental	Electrophysiological recordings	Population spike potentiation	Increase in population spike/population EPSP initial slope	Increased initial slope and amplitude of EPSP	Population spike potentiation
Fixation	Aldehyde perfusion	Aldehyde immersion	Aldehyde immersion	Aldehyde perfusion	Aldehyde immersion	Aldehyde immersion
Quantification	Direct measurements on single sections	Measurements on single sections	Direct measurements on single sections	Measurement on single sections	Direct measurements on single sections	Direct measures on single sections
Stereology	No	No	No	N_A corrected to yield N_V	No	No

Time(s)	10–15 min	10 min	10–15 min 2 hr 8 hr (Data below pooled LTP vs. CON)	20 min	15 min	30 min	60 min	30 min
Space Dimension								
Area	↓CV	↓CV; ↓median; ↓skew	↓CV	21%				
Perimeter	—	—	↓Length; ↓CV	11.4%				
Head width	—	—	—	—	—	—	—	—
Neck length	—	—	—	—	—	—	—	—
Neck width	↓CV; ↓skew	—	—	—	—	—	—	—
Spine Shape								
Concave Synapse	—	—	—	—	—	—	—	—
Non-Concave	—	—	—	—	—	—	—	—
Spinule	—	—	—	—	—	—	—	—
Apposition								
Contact Length	—	—	−10.6%	—	—	—	—	—
PSD Length	↓CV; ↓skew	↓Skew	—	—	—	—	—	—
Perforated Syn	—	—	—	—	—	—	—	—
PSD Length	—	—	—	—	—	—	—	—
Axon Terminal								
Area	—	—	—	—	—	—	—	—
Vesicles:								
Number/Density	—	—	—	↓TV; ↓DV; ↓LV; ↑AV	14%	15.4%	17.2%	—
Distribution				↑AV/LV; ↑LV/DV				
Ca++ Contents	—	—	—		−27.5%	−29.95%	−32.5%	
Synapse Number								
Shaft synapse	33%; Shaft-spine ratio: 40.0%	—	~100%	—	—	—	—	44%
Sessile Synapse	—	—	~175%	—	—	—	—	73%
Glia								
Surface Area	—	—	—	—	—	—	—	
Reference	Lee et al., 1980	Lee et al., 1981	Chang and Greenough, 1984	Applegate et al., 1987	Meshul and Hopkins, 1990			Chang et al., 1991a

Table 14.3 Summary of morphological studies of kindling in the dentate gyrus and in hippocampal subfield CA1. For explanations of abbreviations, see Table 14.1. In addition, ADs = afterdischarges. (See text for discussion.)

	Dentate gyrus kindling		CA1 kindling	
Preparation	Young adult rats in vivo; awake, freely moving	Rat in vivo; awake, freely moving	Adult male rat in vitro	Adult male rat in vivo; awake, freely moving
Stimulated	Medial perforant path	Angular bundle	Schaffer collateral–commissural fibers	Schaffer collateral–commissural fibers
Examined	Middle DML	DML	Stratum radiatum	Middle and distal stratum radiatum
Potentiating stimulation	1 msec pulses at 60 Hz for 2 sec at intensity that produced 10 sec ADs; twice daily until criterion below $n = 7$	1 sec trains of 62 Hz at 500–1100 μA intensity delivered twice daily; $n = 4$	1 sec train at 60 Hz, at 3 times the intensity required to produce population spike; $n = 6$	2 sec train at 60 Hz at 50–110 μA delivered twice daily until criterion; $n = 5$
Control stimulation	Stimulated: 120 pulses at 2 Hz; $n = 7$ Unstimulated controls: $n = 7$	62 pulse at 0.2 Hz pulses at 1.0 mA; $n = 6$	1 Hz for 1 min at an intensity that produced a half maximal population spike; $n = 6$	0.2 Hz for 10 min; $n = 5$
Verification of potentiation	Behavioral observation of 5 generalized seizures	Kindled animals: 3 generalized seizures Control: no ADs or seizures	Epileptiform ADs averaging 12 pop. spikes and lasting 154 msec	Experimental: 5 generalized seizures Control: No ADs, no seizures
Fixation	Aldehyde perfusion	Aldehyde perfusion	Aldehyde perfusion	Aldehyde perfusion
Quantification	Serial thin sections in conjunction with	Timm stain labeling (light microscopy)	Direct measures on single sections	Direct measurement of synapse N_A
Stereology	Disector	None		Correction for astrocytic process V_V
Time(s)	4 wk (after criterion)	18 hr (after last seizure)	15 min (after last train)	24–48 hr (after last seizure)
Spine Dimension				
Area	—	—	—	—
Perimeter	—	—	—	—

Table 14.3 (continued)

Preparation	Dentate gyrus kindling: Young adult rats in vivo; awake, freely moving	Dentate gyrus kindling: Rat in vivo; awake, freely moving	CA1 kindling: Adult male rat in vitro	CA1 kindling: Adult male rat in vivo; awake, freely moving
Head width	—	—	—	—
Neck length	—	—	—	—
Neck width	—	—	—	—
Spine Shape				
Concave	—	—	—	—
Synapse				
Non-Concave	—	—	—	—
Spinule	—	—	—	—
Apposition				
Contact Length	—	—	—	—
PSD Length	—	—	—	—
Perforated synapse PSD length	Ratio of perf to non-perf: 40% 12.1%; area: 18.2%	—	—	
Axon Terminal				
Area	—	—	—	—
Vesicles				
Number/ Density	—	—	—	—
Distribution	—	—	—	—
Ca + + Contents	—	—	—	—
Synapse Number	−18% (axo-spinous synapses)	Timm stain label for presynaptic terminals of mossy fiber projections suggested possible sprouting of an ectopic projection		
Shaft snapse	—		73%	25%
Sessile Synapse	—		103%	—
Glia				
Surface Area	—	—	—	V_V: 37% (middle); 33% (distal)
Reference	Geinisman et al., 1988; Geinisman et al., 1990	Sutula et al., 1988	Hawrylak et al., 1988; Chang et al., 1991b	Hawrylak et al., 1989

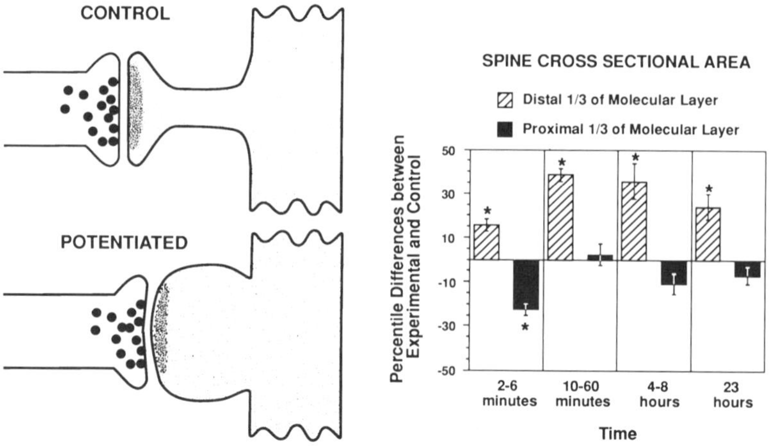

Figure 14.3 Evidence for spine swelling after LTP in the dentate gyrus. These studies used rapid freezing and freeze substitution (see text for details). (Drawn from data in Fifkova and Van Harreveld, 1977.)

measures were also made (Fifkova and Anderson, 1981). Spine head and neck width were both increased in both pathways at 4 minutes and in the lateral pathway at 90 minutes. Only head width was increased in the medial pathway at 90 minutes. However, concurrent electrophysiological characterization of the response would be necessary to properly interpret these effects and Fifkova (1985) did not repeat the dissociation using aldehyde fixatives (see the following section). Finally, spine neck length was reduced in the distal third of the molecular layer at both time points. This spine neck shortening contrasts with the spine neck lengthening reported in aldehyde fixed material (Andersen et al., 1987, and the following section). Figure 14.4 compares spine measurements on both freeze substituted and chemically fixed tissue.

Aldehyde Fixation Studies

While freeze substitution is well-suited to preserving cell volume, it is not easily combined with electrophysiology. The use of aldehyde perfusion fixation permitted electrophysiological assessment of the activational state of tissue examined morphologically. Fifkova (1985) stimulated both the medial and lateral entorhinal cortex. In this replication, however, a different stimulation pattern was used (see table 14.1) and only one time point was examined. Stimulated animals demonstrated a 35% enhancement of evoked response and had larger spine areas and perimeters, wider spine necks, and longer contact lengths in both middle and distal DML.

Another perfusion study of electrophysiologically monitored LTP reported similar spine widening (Andersen et al., 1987). Rats that received stimulation showed an enhancement in the input-output curve lasting at least 30 minutes. Compared with unoperated controls, spines in potentiated animals sampled from the middle fifth of the DML measured in serial

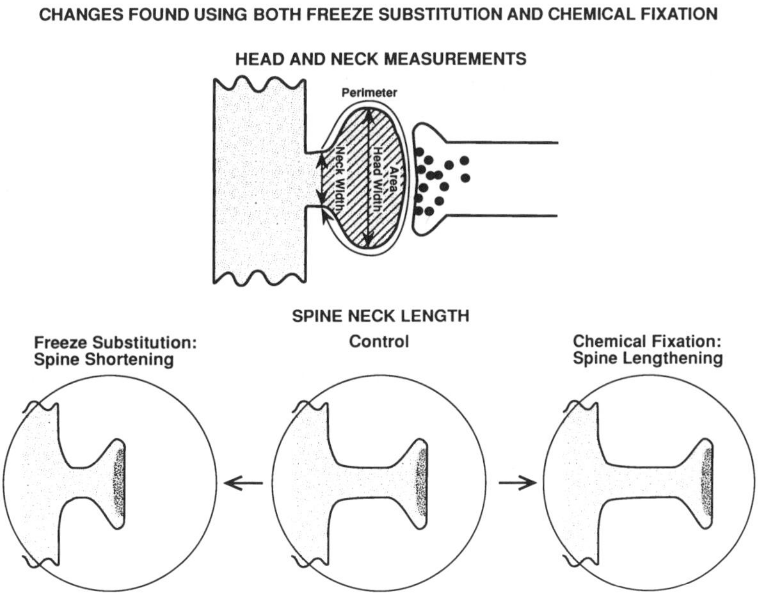

Figure 14.4 Summary of spine dimension changes after LTP in the dentate gyrus observed with chemical fixation and freeze substitution. Increases in spine area and spine width are consistent across studies using both methods, but measures of spine length differ, with a shortening reported in substituted tissue and a lengthening reported in chemically fixed tissue. (See text for details. Drawn from data in Fifkova and Van Harreveld, 1977; Fifkova and Anderson, 1981; Fifkova, 1985; Desmond and Levy, 1986a, 1988b; Andersen et al., 1987.)

sections had wider necks. Also, 15% of the LTP spines were longer than the longest control (this contrasts with the spine shortening observed in freeze substitution; Fifkova and Anderson, 1981). Spine neck widening is also compatible with the reports of spine shape interconversion discussed in the next section (Desmond and Levy, 1988b).

Spine Shape Interconversion

Another group has also examined the shapes of spines after LTP (Desmond and Levy, 1983, 1986a, 1986b, 1988a). Animals were bilaterally implanted with both stimulating (angular bundle) and recording electrodes, with one hippocampus serving as control. To determine which levels of the DML this stimulation would activate, one-dimensional current source density analysis was performed in animals not used for microscopy. This showed that the largest synaptic activation (i.e., greatest current sink) occurred in the middle one-third of the DML. Two patterns of unilateral conditioning stimulation have been used in these experiments, spaced and massed (detailed in table 14.1). The original report (Desmond and Levy, 1983) consisted only of animals that had received the spaced stimulation and were examined at 10 and 60 minutes after stimulation. Subsequent reports have included both these spaced animals (combined into a single group) and massed animals examined at 2 minutes and 10 minutes after stimulation (Desmond and Levy, 1986a, 1986b, 1988a,

1990; also considered in the following discussion). At least a 50% increase in the initial slope of the population excitatory postsynaptic potential (EPSP) over baseline was required for acceptance of an animal for morphological analysis. As a result of the short survival time of the 2 minute massed stimulation group, however, animals had to be sacrificed immediately after stimulation and the criterion could not be used. Synapses were first categorized on the basis of whether they appeared on dendritic shafts or dendritic spines. Dendritic spines were additionally classified by head shape as follows:

Simple: (1) if the ratio of its major axis (parallel to PSD) and minor axis (perpendicular) of the spine head was less than 1.5 : 1 and (2) if it did not have a concave contact shape.

Ellipsoid: (1) if the ratio of the major and minor axes was equal to or greater than 1.5 : 1 and (2) and the spines were convex in shape.

Concave: spines whose apposition had a U or W shape. The latter class includes the spinule (Tarrant and Routtenberg, 1977) and has been examined separately in another study (see the following discussion and Schuster et al., 1990).

The initial report (Desmond and Levy, 1983) did not use stereological corrections and is superseded by a subsequent report that used a stereological correction for size differences to estimate number per volume (N_V) from number per area (N_A) (Desmond and Levy, 1986a). Analysis of the spaced group N_V confirmed an increase for concave synapses, 48.4%, as a result of conditioning stimulation. Although not significant, both massed groups increased N_V of concave spines as well. Analysis of N_V of concave and nonconcave (i.e., simple and ellipsoid types) synapses in the activated region of DML as a function of stimulation (spaced and massed 2 minutes and 10 minutes combined) yielded an increase in concave and a decrease in nonconcave synapses. On the basis of these results, Desmond and Levy (1986a) proposed the "interconversion hypothesis," suggesting that these changes represent a remodeling of existing synapses to a more efficacious form, as shown in figure 14.5. Additional measurements from this same experimental tissue are discussed in several subsequent sections. Such separation of aspects of potentially synchronous and coordinated events could be artificial, but it is done with the view that distinctions in synaptic substructure could also imply separate regulatory mechanisms and functional impact.

A recent study has suggested that spinules might be selectively increased after LTP. Spinule synapses (Szentagothai and Hamori, 1969; Tarrant and Routtenberg, 1977) are characterized by an evagination of the postsynaptic element into the profile of the presynaptic element, bringing the postsynaptic and presynaptic membranes into especially close apposition or even contact. This protuberance of the postsynaptic element often penetrates the postsynaptic density, and consequently spinule syn-

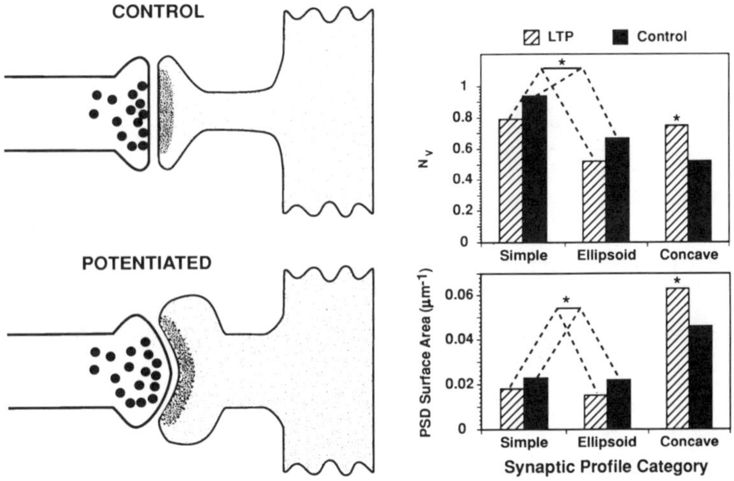

Figure 14.5 Evidence for spine shape interconversion after LTP in the dentate gyrus. According to Desmond and Levy (1988b), these results are consistent with spine swelling to the extent that concave synapses appear to have greater areas and wider necks, but concave synapses per se have not been observed in substituted dentate tissue (see text for details). (Redrawn with permission from Desmond and Levy, 1986a, and Desmond and Levy, 1986b.)

apses are frequently also perforated synapses (see "Perforated PSD" below). Spinule synapses are part of the category classed as "concave" by Desmond and Levy (1983) and have also been observed in freeze substituted tissue (Fifkova and Van Harreveld, 1977). Schuster and associates (1990) measured the N_A of synapses with a spinule after stimulation of the perforant pathway in vivo. These animals were compared with active controls and passive controls. LTP was not verified in the animals examined morphologically, but the same stimulation produced LTP lasting from 2 minutes to 7 days in separate animals. As shown in figure 14.6, animals examined 8 hours and 48 hours after potentiating stimulation showed a higher density of spinules in the middle third of the DML. At 8 hours (48 hours was not reported), spinule density in the proximal third of the DML after stimulation is similar to that seen in the middle and proximal DML of control animals. The intriguing increased association of presynaptic and postsynaptic elements observed in spinules, as well as the fact that these profiles occur in both aldehyde fixed and freeze-substituted material, encourage further examination of spinule density after LTP using stereological methods and expanding the small sample size. These same animals have been analyzed using other morphological measurements, such as vesicle distribution, density of shaft synapses, density of ribosomes in the cytoplasm, and frequency of invaginations of the presynaptic membrane, but to date, those results have not appeared in sufficient detail to permit adequate interpretation here (see Wenzel et al., 1986; Schuster et al., 1986).

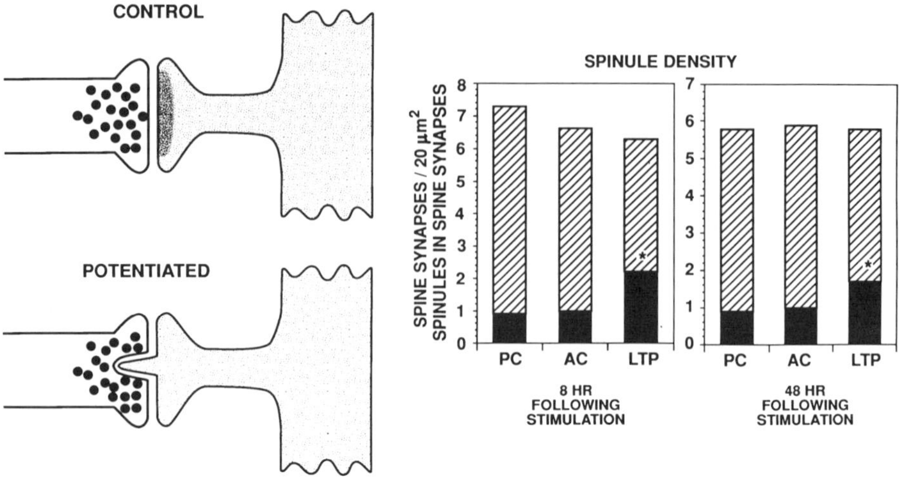

Figure 14.6 Evidence for an increase in the density of spinules after LTP in the dentate gyrus. This promising finding merits additional study with larger samples and stereological methods. (Redrawn with permission from Schuster, Krug, and Wenzel, 1990, Spinules in axospinous synapses of the rat dentate gyrus: changes in density following long-term potentiation. *Brain Research* 523:171–174.)

Spine Area and Spine Dimension Changes in Hippocampal Subfield CA1

In association with reports of an increase in synapse number after LTP (see the section "Evidence for Synaptic Number Changes After LTP"), two groups have also found evidence of shape changes in CA1. Using both in vivo and in vitro preparations, Lee and coworkers (1980, 1981) reported a reduction in the variance of spine dimension measures (see table 14.2) 10 to 15 minutes after LTP. The authors suggested that this effect might be produced by an overall rounding of spines. Lee and coworkers (1981) also noted that all spine area measures, but particularly neck width, are larger in slices than with in vivo perfusion, suggesting that a swelling process occurs in vitro that could obscure LTP-induced spine swelling. Chang and Greenough (1984), using an in vitro preparation, also found direct evidence for rounding of spine shape, such as decreases in perimeter length, a reduction in the perimeter-to-area ratio (a stereological index of roundness known as the "form factor"), and a decrease in apposition, but not PSD, length, as illustrated in figure 14.7, at 10 to 15 minutes. Such shape changes had declined at 2 hours and were no longer observed at 8 hours, however, which suggests that in CA1 this response is transient, whereas the synaptic number change is a more enduring alteration. In contrast to these reports, Applegate and associates (1987) found an increase in both spine perimeter and area 20 minutes after LTP.

These reports indicate that spine shape changes may occur in CA1, as in the dentate. In CA1, however, shape changes appear to be short-term modifications.

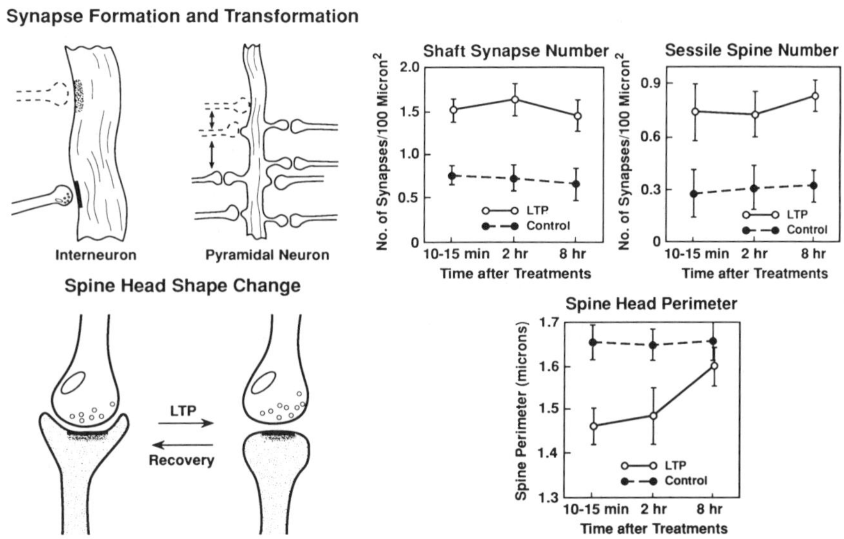

Figure 14.7 Evidence for transient shape changes and enduring synapse addition after LTP in CA1. This report replicates the findings of Lee and coworkers (1980, 1981) and extends the examination of changes to include later time points (see text). (Redrawn with permission from Chang and Greenough, 1984, Transient and enduring morphological correlates of synaptic activity and efficacy change in the rat hippocampal slice. *Brain Research* 309:35–46.)

Note on Comparisons of Freeze-substituted and Aldehyde-fixed Tissue

These two methods provide distinctly different styles of preservation, which requires consideration when interpreting morphological studies. Aldehyde fixation preserves an essentially unlimited sample area and is more readily combined with electrophysiological approaches. Compared with conventional chemical methods, rapid freezing has the advantages of permitting high temporal resolution because the tissue is frozen solidly within 2 milliseconds or less (Heuser et al., 1979), so that phases of rapidly occurring events can be captured for viewing, and maintaining more closely the natural distribution of soluble tissue elements and integrity of membrane compartments, to preserve tissue volume, extracellular space, certain elements of fine structure, and ionic distribution (Rash, 1983; Ornberg and Reese, 1980). Samples are limited to superficial regions of tissue, however, because rapid freezing rates sufficient to preserve ultrastructure without ice crystal damage occur only within the superficial 10 to 15 microns of tissue contacting the freezer surface (Rash, 1983). The absence of concave profiles in rapidly frozen freeze-substituted material (Desmond and Levy, 1988b), raises concerns about the influences of fixation on profile appearance. It is interesting, however, that spinules have been observed in both substituted and chemically fixed tissue (see Fifkova and Van Harreveld, 1977). In tissue substituted with osmium, a distinct PSD is not visible, in contrast to chemically fixed tissue (see figure 14.7). The destruction of actin filaments by osmium has been observed in vitro (Maupin-Szamier and Pollard, 1978) and may also occur during freeze substitution. No method is artifact free. Consequently, we are left with a cubistic view of synaptic structure: no single view is complete (see Landis et al., 1988), so one must combine several perspectives to approach a representation of the natural structure. The recent development of a rapid freezing instrument (Wallace, et al., 1988), in which a cooled copper surface descends upon an upright specimen, and the use of an appropriate hippocampal brain slice preparation that maintains an uncut pial surface (Chang and Greenough, 1988) promise to provide a complementary view to aldehyde studies by permitting the combination of freezing and electrophysiological recording.

Spine Shape and LTP in Development and Recovery

Studies correlating spine shape changes during development (Teyler et al., 1989) and recovery from deafferentation (Reeves and Steward, 1986) with the capability to support LTP appear to contrast with the LTP-induced spine neck dimensional changes in normal adults. Reeves and Steward (1986) used a unilateral entorhinal cortex lesion to induce reactive sprouting of the normally minor crossed entorhinal projection. The projections of the damaged entorhinal cortex degenerate and are replaced by sprouts from the contralateral entorhinal afferents. This crossed pathway expands to fill the vacated postsynaptic surface, and, about 8 days after the lesion, stimulation of the contralateral entorhinal cortex induces LTP in the ipsilateral dentate, a phenomenon not observed in the intact animal. Electron microscopic analysis showed that, in contrast to the intact DML, following sprouting synapses were predominately on "sessile" spines, whose width and length are roughly equal, rather than the "mushroom" shape characteristic of a mature spine (Reeves and Steward, 1986). A similar result has been reported in CA1 during development (Teyler et al., 1989), as depicted in figure 14.8. When about 15 days old, rats exhibit a distinct peak in the magnitude of LTP, during which the amplitude of LTP is markedly greater than in either younger animals or adult animals. Ultrastructural examination at this time reveals that a higher proportion of synapses are of the sessile type than in the adult (Teyler et al., 1989; Harris et al., 1989). Taken together, these results suggest that the ability to widen the spine head or neck is not necessary for LTP. One possibility is that these immature synapses are capable of a greater range of plastic response than more mature and, presumably functionally committed, synapses that possess less potential for additional modification (Teyler et al., 1989). Another consideration might be that at these early stages of LTP expression, the balance of inhibition and excitation is altered from that found in the mature or intact pathway, such that less efficacious synapses are capable of supporting potentiation in a context of lower inhibition. While these results undercut spine shape changes as the sole mechanism for LTP formation, the possibility remains

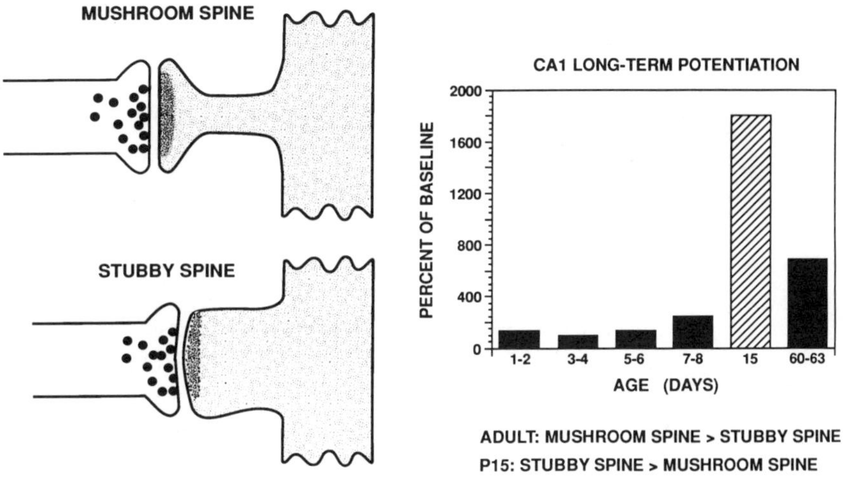

Figure 14.8 Association between spine shape and LTP peak amplitude during CA1 development. At about 15 days of age, rats exhibit a peak in the amplitude of LTP, which can be induced. At this age, the bulk of synapses are on neckless "stubby" or sessile spines. (Similar findings have been reported in dentate gyrus during reinnervation; see text.) (Reprinted with permission from Teyler, Perkins, and Harris, 1989, The development of long-term potentiation in hippocampus and neocortex. *Neuropsychologia* 27(1):31–40.)

that shape changes might be part of an orchestrated combination of efficacy changes in the adult dentate gyrus.

Alterations in the Synaptic Junctional Zone

Results from Postsynaptic Density Length Measurements Desmond and Levy (1986b) used the experimental tissue described under "Spine Shape Interconversion" to measure another synaptic structural element, the length of the PSD in concave and nonconcave synapses after potentiating and control stimulation. Direct measurements of length and tissue area were corrected to yield an estimate of the surface per volume of the DML (S_V). After potentiation, the combined stimulation groups showed an increase in PSD S_V. Conversely, the PSDs of nonconcave synapses were decreased. This pattern is reminiscent of the pattern seen in prior N_A and N_V measures and is consistent with the interconversion hypothesis proposed by Desmond and Levy (1986a; see the previous discussion). The exact functional relevance of increased PSD S_V in concave synapses is not clear, but in the frog neuromuscular junction, increases in the length of the active zone are correlated with increased efficacy (Herrera et al., 1985). Petukhov and Popov (1986) also found an increase in PSD length in CA3 giant synapses after potentiating stimulation of the mossy fibers.

Perforated PSDs Recently, there have been reports that the density of synapses containing a perforated postsynaptic density increase (Geinisman et al., 1990b) after LTP, as has been previously reported after kindling (Geinisman et al., 1988; 1990a; see the section on synaptic structural alterations after kindling). Geinisman and colleagues (1990b) used the unbiased stereological ''disector'' (Sterio, 1984) to estimate the number of synapses per neuron in the middle molecular layer. Animals in the LTP group received stimulation of the medial perforant path on each of 4 consecutive days. The formation of LTP was verified by a recording electrode placed in the dentate gyrus. These animals were perfused with aldehyde 1 hour after the stimulus train on the fourth day. Two control groups were used for comparison: Coulombic controls received equivalent stimulation at nonpotentiating frequencies, and implanted controls underwent the surgery and electrode implant but did not receive any stimulation. After LTP induction, there was no net increase in the number of shaft or spine synapses, but there was an increase in the proportion of perforated synapses in LTP animals relative to controls. Additional measures of PSD maximal profile length and PSD plate area were from serial sections in the same sample as previously mentioned (de Toledo-Morrell et al., 1990). Perforated synapses showed a shift toward smaller PSD dimensions after LTP. Against the backdrop of an increase in the number of perforated synapses as a consequence of LTP, the second result suggests that LTP might drive recruitment of smaller nonperforated synapses into the perforated class. This work is notable because it employed stereologically correct methods to generate unbiased estimates of the parameters examined. The finding of an increase in the proportion of perforated synapses after LTP is consonant with the increases in perforated synapses as a function of learning and experience just discussed. Additionally, the similarity of these results and those observed after kindling (Geinisman et al., 1990a; discussed in the following section) suggest that LTP and kindling may affect the same structure, although not necessarily in the same way.

Increased Apposition Length Two studies have reported an increase in synaptic contact length after LTP. Fifkova (1985) found that synaptic contact length was increased along with dendritic spine dimensions in the middle and distal DML 45 to 60 minutes after stimulation of medial and lateral entorhinal cortex (see ''Spine Area and Spine Dimension Changes in Dentrate Gyrus'' for details of the other measures). This measure is hard to interpret because it does not distinguish the PSD and non-PSD regions of the membrane. Desmond and Levy (1988a) measured the length of the synaptic apposition, which excluded the PSD to determine if non-PSD regions of apposition changed independently of the PSD (PSD length changes are reported separately, see Desmond and Levy, 1986b, and ''Results from Postsynaptic Density Length Measurements''), in the animals previously described. The contact length (minus the PSD) was corrected to estimate the amount of non-PSD surface per sample tissue volume S_V. In the stimulated middle third of DML, the S_V for the non-PSD apposition of concave synapses was increased in pooled LTP groups relative to controls. Interestingly, the massed 2-minute group does not show an increase, suggesting that at this earliest time point the change has not become manifest. The spaced group, which itself contains pooled 10-minute and 60-minute groups, displays the largest difference, as it did in the S_V value for the PSD. In contrast, in CA1 Chang and Greenough (1984) reported a decrease in apposition length, with no change in the PSD (see figure 14.7).

Presynaptic Changes in Existing Synapses

Measurements of vesicle position and number have been made in both CA1 and dentate gyrus and might provide insights into presynaptic mechanisms, but, as just noted, must be viewed with some qualification and caution. A constellation of facilitation processes may be triggered by tetanizing stimulation, such that early time samples could confound short-term changes with those associated with more enduring LTP (see Racine and Milgram, 1983; and Racine et al., 1983). Furthermore, vesicles may be affected by actions of aldehydes (McKinlay and Usherwood, 1978), as well as the stimulation itself (see Applegate and Landfield, 1988).

Findings from Dentate Studies Vesicle distribution and density have been described in two studies. Fifkova and Van Harreveld (1977) observed a transient 15.6% decrease in presynaptic vesicles in the distal DML frozen 2 to 6 minutes after stimulation. At the 10- to 60-minute sample points, stimulated tissue displayed a 19.6% decrease in vesicle density. Vesicle loss could reflect greater transmitter release. In the same tissue used for other measures, Desmond and Levy (1986c) examined vesicle number and position. Vesicles within one vesicle diameter of the presynaptic membrane were termed "front-line" and those between one and four vesicle diameters were called "distant." After LTP, the number of front-line vesicles in concave synapses increased 49% relative to controls, but overall number of vesicles did not increase.

Findings of CA1 Studies Applegate and colleagues (1987) also examined LTP effects on vesicles in CA1. Stimulation of the Schaffer collaterals was performed in vivo. Controls were implanted and stimulated with only the test pulses used to verify LTP in the stimulated animals. Animals were perfused 20 minutes after stimulation. The density of vesicles was counted in several locations in the presynaptic terminal: (1) total number of vesicles (TV) in a terminal; (2) local vesicles (LV—those within 150 nm of the active zone); (3) vesicles attached (AV) to the presynaptic membrane; and (4) distant vesicles (DV), calculated by subtracting LV from TV. As figure 14.9 indicates, the overall TV, DV, an LV decreased after LTP, but of the remaining vesicles, an increase was seen in the ratio of LV/DV and AV/LV, suggesting a redistribution of vesicles toward the presynaptic membrane.

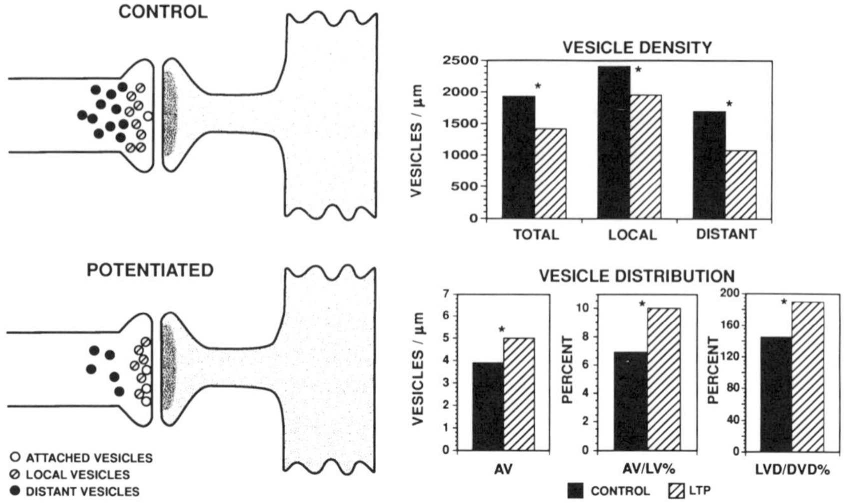

Figure 14.9 Reported decrease in vesicle number and redistribution of vesicles after LTP in CA1. AV = attached vesicles; LV = local vesicles; LVD = local vesicle density; DVD = distant vesicle density. Numerical changes make position changes difficult to interpret. (See figure 14.10 and text for further discussion.) (Redrawn with permission from Applegate, Kerr, and Landfield, 1987, Redistribution of synaptic vesicles during long-term potentiation in the hippocampus. *Brain Research* 401:401–406.)

Meshul and Hopkins (1990) examined Ca^{2+} in vesicles in the hippocampal slice. Calcium was detected using potassium oxalate precipitation in conjunction with chemical fixation. LTP was verified with electrophysiological recording. Potentiated animals were examined at 15, 30, and 60 minutes. Control animals were either unstimulated or given potentiating stimulation in the presence of the NMDA receptor agonist α-amino-5-phosphonovaleric acid (APV). Control groups did not differ and were pooled. (The APV blockade of the effect of stimulation is interesting as it may imply a retrograde signal of postsynaptic NMDA–receptor activation or presynaptic NMDA receptors.) In contrast to Applegate and coworkers (1987), Meshul and Hopkins (1990) found an increase in vesicles per presynaptic terminal in potentiated animals at each time point examined, as indicated in figure 14.10. The opposite results of these two groups could reflect different amounts of stimulation, in vitro versus in vivo responses, sex differences (because Applegate et al. used males and Meshul and Hopkins used females), or a combination of these. Finally, the number of vesicles that contained Ca^{2+} precipitates was decreased with LTP at each time point, as was the percentage of total vesicles containing Ca^{2+}. Although it is not clear what process this might reflect, calcium distribution has implications for a variety of processes from synaptic transmission to second messenger cascades.

Taken together, the vesicle results do not suggest any consistent pattern with regard to changes in vesicle number. Vesicle position effects occur

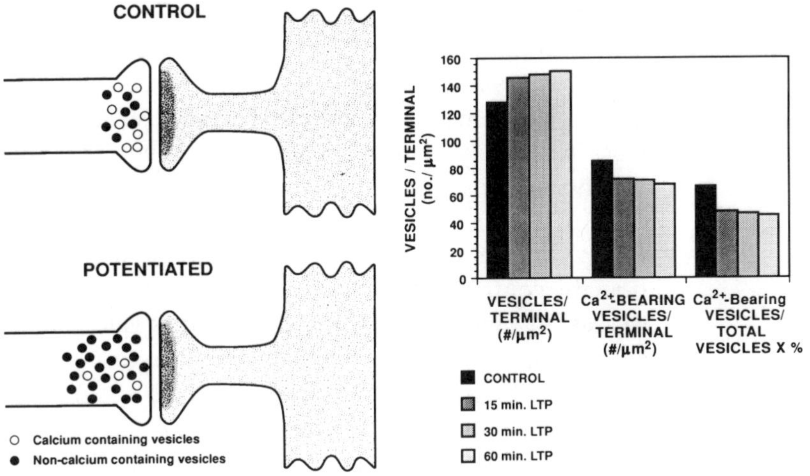

Figure 14.10 Reported increase in vesicle number and decrease in the proportion of Ca^{2+}-containing vesicles after LTP in CA1. (See figure 14.9 and text for discussion.) (Drawn from data in Moshal and Hopkins, 1990.)

against a background of changing vesicle number changes that also make them difficult to interpret. The most interesting result is the persisting vesicle depletion in the freeze-substituted tissue of Fifkova and Van Harreveld (1977), which occurs in the absence of aldehyde effects. This result could be compatible with reports of increased transmitter release after LTP induction (see, for example, chapter 1).

EVIDENCE FOR SYNAPTIC NUMBER CHANGES AFTER LTP

As discussed under "Synaptic Structural Changes Observed in Non-LTP Paradigms," change in the number of synapses through synaptogenesis and synapse loss is the most consistent form of plastic change evident in sensory development and behavioral studies. In hippocampal subfield CA1, synaptogenesis is also a consistent result of LTP induction. Two laboratories have examined CA1 stratum radiatum after potentiation of the Schaffer collateral–commissural pathway. Lee and coworkers (1980, 1981) examined synapses in stratum radiatum of CA1 after the induction of LTP using both in vivo and in vitro rat hippocampal preparations. Slices were immersion fixed 10 minutes after completing stimulation. Although the results for spine shape differed across the two studies, the number of synapses onto dendritic shafts increased in the stimulated groups in both studies. Chang and Greenough (1984) performed a similar slice experiment. Controls received the same number of stimuli at the same intensity over the same total time period but at 1 Hz. Immersion fixation was within 10 to 15 minutes after stimulation for one group and at 2 and 8 hours for two others. The results, which appear in figure 14.7, showed an immediate and complete (i.e., no further changes over the 8-hour period) increase in the density (NA) of two different types of synapses: shaft synapses, as indicated in the reports of Lee and associates (1980, 1981) and sessile spine synapses, similar to those shown in figure 14.2, which were separately counted when we believed that there was an unusual number of these early in the stages of examining our micrographs. The density of mushroom shaped spines did not increase in the stimulated group, but, as the number of mushroom spines was higher, not lower than the control, the results do not suggest a transformation of mushroom to sessile spines. Rather, the shaft and sessile spine results suggest that shaft and sessile spine synapses may be forms in transition to mature spines, as figure 14.7 illustrates. The aggregate increase in sessile spine and shaft synapses constituted only a 5% increase in the total number of synapses, although the relative number of both types was approximately doubled. Whether an increase of this size is sufficient to account for a 300% increase in the amplitude of the population spike (this had declined by 46% at 8 hours) is a question that we do not know how to answer.

It should be noted that an "overstimulation control" was also run in this study, which received continuous stimulation at either 40 or 100 Hz for 10 minutes and was similarly fixed after a 10- to 15-minute delay. This group showed no LTP and no increase in synapse number, although there was some mitochondrial swelling. Hence the synaptogenesis was tightly tied to the occurrence of LTP. We have also replicated the basic synaptogenesis findings in slices from 2-year-old rats (Chang et al., 1991a). This, combined with our results from the kindling paradigm following, constitutes strong evidence that synaptogenesis is a reliable consequence of events that induce plastic functional change in hippocampal subfield CA1.

One other feature of the results should be noted. We examined the dendritic diameter distribution where it could be measured for both the shaft and sessile spine synapses. The diameter distribution for the LTP group's shaft synapses had two peaks, one at 0.33 to 0.67 μm and one at about 2 μm and larger. These appeared to correspond to the average diameters for excitatory pyramidal cell dendrites and inhibitory dendrites (Lorente de No, 1934; Andersen et al., 1969; Harris and Stevens, 1989). Thus, it appears that both feed-forward excitatory and feed-forward inhibitory pathways exhibit a synapse number increase in this preparation.

Overall, the data from subfield CA1 make an overwhelming case for the association of synapse formation with the induction of plastic change. There are small indications of shape changes (previously discussed) in these areas, but these changes appear to be transient, outlasted by LTP (Chang and Greenough, 1984). Although it is possible that the shape changes represent a transient component of the increased responsiveness, it seems clear in subfield CA1 that the only morphological correlate of an enduring nature is the increased number of shaft and sessile spine synapses.

Synaptic Structural Alterations after Kindling

Findings from Dentate Gyrus Studies Recently, morphological investigations of synaptic plasticity after kindling stimulation have suggested possible shared mechanisms of LTP and kindling. Geinisman and associates (1988, 1990a) used the unbiased disector technique for estimating the number of synapses per neuron and PSD dimensions in the molecular layer of the hippocampal dentate gyrus after kindling of the medial perforant path. As figure 14.11 shows, the number of axospinous synapses per neuron was decreased in kindled animals. The loss was selective to nonperforated synaptic contacts while perforated synapses were retained. The ratio of perforated to nonperforated synapses was increased 45% in kindled rats. Furthermore, only the perforated synapses in kindled rats showed increases in the length and area of PSDs (compare this to the decrease in perforated PSD dimensions following LTP, de Toledo-Morrell et al., 1990). These results concern stable long-term kindling, because 4 weeks were allowed for the immediate effects of seizures to dissipate before sacrifice.

Sutula and coworkers (1988) also studied kindling stimulation in the dentate gyrus using the Timm stain to detect zinc, which is enriched in mossy fiber terminals. Timm granules, normally sparse in the inner molecular layer, were noticeably increased for as long as 5 months after kindling. Using electron microscopy, these particles were seen in pre-

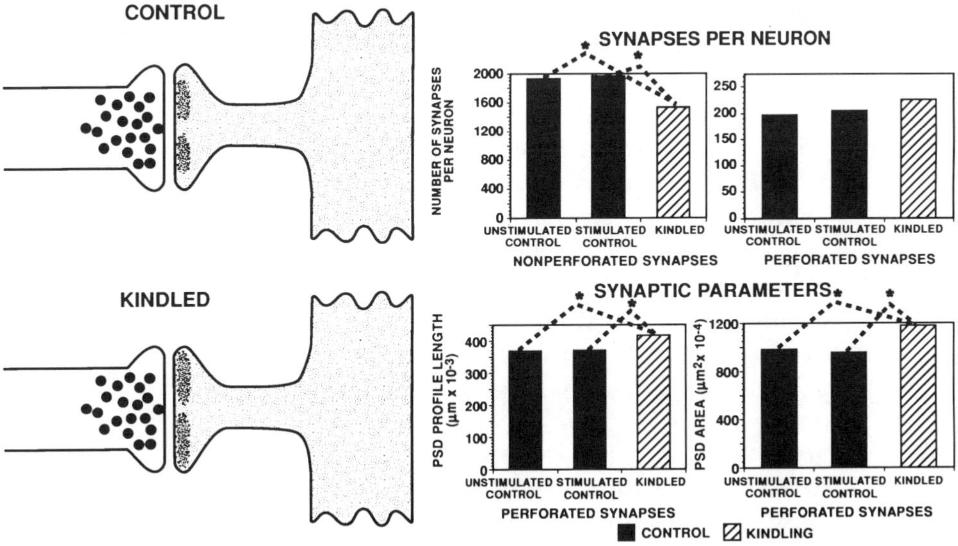

Figure 14.11 Evidence for selective changes of perforated and nonperforated synapses after kindling in the dentate gyrus. (See text for discussion of perforated synapses in LTP, experience, and learning.) (Drawn from data in Geinisman, Morrell and de Toledo-Morrell, 1988, 1990a.)

synaptic boutons in this zone. These data, however, must be interpreted cautiously until synapses are directly quantified using appropriate stereological methods, as changes in zinc concentrations in terminals might also account for the results. Sutula and colleagues (1988) used perforant path stimulation similar to that of Geinisman and associates (1988, 1990a), so it is possible that both remodeling of mossy fiber projections and selective retention of perforated synapses might occur concurrently in different regions of the DML. To date, no studies appear to have quantified synapses in both regions after kindling.

Findings from CA1 Studies An essential feature of the kindling model of epilepsy is that focal electrophysiological seizures known as afterdischarges (ADs) must be present for the development of kindling (for a review of kindling, see McNamara et al., 1985). To better understand the mechanisms contributing to synaptic plasticity and epileptogenesis, the in vitro hippocampal slice preparation has been used to examine the early morphological events associated with the initial expression of ADs in CA1. Kindling stimulation that produced as few as six ADs in hippocampal slices (aldehyde fixation 15 minutes after the last stimulation) resulted in increased density of shaft synapses by 73% and of sessile spine synapses by 103% (Hawrylak et al., 1988, Chang et al., 1991b submitted). The increases in the density of shaft and sessile spine synapses suggest that synapses form during kindling possibly through a sequence in which newly formed shaft synapses progress to sessile spine synapses and then to fully grown mature synapses, as proposed for LTP earlier in this chapter (see figure 14.7). An in vivo study may lend support to the transformation hypothesis, at least with regard to shaft synapses. Hawrylak and coworkers (submitted) kindled rats by inducing afterdischarges in CA1 twice daily until full tonic-clonic seizures occurred. Tissue was fixed 24 to 48 hours after the last stimulation. Although a shaft synapse increase was seen, there was no concomitant increase in sessile spines, suggesting that this change may have dissipated over either the long time-course of the study or the 24- to 48-hour prefixation period. These results suggest that LTP and kindling of CA1 involve a similar process of synaptogenesis. Alterations of the Timm staining pattern were observed by Sutula and colleagues (1988), with as few as five to ten ADs, also suggesting that new synapses may form early in the kindling process.

RECONCILING CHANGES IN SYNAPSE NUMBER VERSUS MODIFICATION OF EXISTING SYNAPSES AFTER LTP AND KINDLING

Substantial evidence for both synapse number change and synapse efficacy change is evident in the studies we have reviewed. There appear to be regional differences with a tendency for CA1 to increase numbers of shaft and sessile spine synapses and for dentate to exhibit remodeling of existing synapses. Measures of spine shape change are somewhat inconsistent, but there is reasonable consensus between the reports of Desmond and Levy (1983) and Fifkova and Van Harreveld (1977) that spines are bigger and spine necks are wider (Fifkova and Anderson, 1981; Desmond and Levy, 1988b) after LTP (also Andersen et al., 1987). Spine length measures remain inconsistent, reported as shorter in freeze substitution studies and longer in aldehyde studies (Fifkova and Anderson, 1981; Andersen et al., 1987). Interpretation that these changes might form a primary mechanism in LTP is constrained by the finding in developing and recovering systems that LTP capacity peaks at a time when neckless sessile spines are most abundant. Changes in the frequency of perforated synapses after LTP and kindling also seem rigorously documented in the dentate gyrus; in these studies, PSD length increased after kindling and decreased after LTP. These studies have used impeccable modern stereological procedures and present a standard that all others should emulate (Geinisman et al., 1988, 1990a, 1990b). Presynaptic changes (e.g., in vesicle location), though of interest, tend to be inconsistent and probably interact substantially with the effects of aldehydes. Much of the ambiguity in the results may arise from methodological inconsistencies. Future comparisons could be much more useful if:

1. Studies would employ physiologically plausible stimulation patterns to be compared with active (but nonpotentiating) controls.
2. Electrophysiological recording uniformly accompanied morphological analysis to both verify and characterize potentiation.
3. Time points be chosen to coincide with the phenomenology of LTP and samples taken throughout the life of potentiation to detect stages of structural modification, segments of biochemical cascades (i.e., time domain of Ca^{2+} protease vs. locally synthesized protein vs. immediate early gene product), or both.
4. Stereological methods be used to ensure that estimates are unbiased and accurate.
5. Investigators make "good faith" attempts to replicate representative measurements from prior studies accurately in addition to whatever new measurements they may add.

GLIAL CHANGES ACCOMPANYING SYNAPTIC PLASTICITY

Glial cells are no longer viewed only as buffers of extracellular K^+ and neurotransmitters, but also are regarded as a component of a dynamic system of cell-cell molecular interactions with neurons that serves diverse functions in the CNS that range from guiding migrating neurons during development (Rakic, 1971) to the exchange of molecules and nutrients with neurons (Hertz and Schousboe, 1986). Recent reports have demonstrated astrocytic responses to glutamate, suggesting that networks of astrocytes may provide an extraneuronal system for rapid long-distance signaling (Cornell-Bell et al., 1990; Marrero et al., 1989; and Usowicz et al., 1989). Whether the mechanisms of LTP use such a rapid signaling system, and whether they involve more enduring changes of glial function or structure is now an important question. Anatomical studies of astrocytes have indicated a possible role in LTP and kindling. A preliminary study by Isaacs (1989) employed stereological methods to quantify GFAP-positive cell processes in the dentate gyrus of the dorsal hippocampus after in vivo LTP. Twenty-four hours after LTP, the surface density of astrocytic processes was increased in sample regions from 100 to 400 μm distant from the recording electrode. The 400-μm sample area appeared to be free of gliotic response to the recording electrode. In experiments employing in vivo kindling, the ultrastructure of astrocytes was examined 24 to 48 hours after the last seizure in stratum radiatum of CA1 in the dorsal hippocampus using stereological methods (Hawrylak et al., 1991). After kindling, the volume fraction of astrocytic processes was increased 33% in the middle and 37% in the distal region of stratum radiatum of kindled rats. These two reports suggest that LTP and kindling stimulation induce astrocytic hypertrophy or hyperplasia that may contribute to increased neuronal excitability. In the short term, astrocytic hypertrophy is thought to occur mainly by decreasing the extracellular space (ECS). It could be hypothesized that the reduction of the ECS could increase neuronal excitability by exaggerating transient ionic changes or enhancing ephaptic excitation. Persisting astrocyte hypertrophy, if it plays a role in LTP or kindling, probably would not act through this transient mechanism.

We suggest that astrocytic hypertrophy represents a morphological plasticity associated with the role of astrocytes in either regulating the number of synaptic connections or in providing them with metabolic support. Modulation of synaptic contacts by morphological alteration involving glial cells has been described during the normal development of the spinal cord (Ronnevi, 1977). In this case, synapse elimination appeared to be mediated through the disconnection and subsequent phagocytosis of synapses by glial cells. Similar glial involvement in synapse elimination appears to occur when astrocytes are added to glial-free cerebellar cultures (Meshul and Seil, 1988). In contrast to synapse elimination, astrocytes have been implicated as a factor promoting synapse formation in the hypothalamo-neurohypophyseal system (Hatton et al., 1984). In this system, it has been hypothesized that glial retraction and associated synaptogenesis may be involved in synchronizing cellular activity that leads to pulsatile hormone release. With regard to glial retraction, it is of interest that glial processes tended also to become thicker in the LTP study just described (Isaacs et al., 1989). Recent studies suggest that environmental stimuli capable of inducing synaptogenesis also result in hypertrophy and increased numbers of astrocytes (Sirevaag and Greenough, 1990). In both that study and the present study of kindling, the astrocytic hypertrophy may reflect a glial plasticity involved in regulating synapse numbers, or it may reflect the increased metabolic demands of additional, or more active, synapses.

WORKING TOWARD A MOLECULAR MORPHOLOGY

In this chapter we discuss ways in which synaptic structure may change after LTP and kindling. We propose that these structural changes be adopted as a context for future studies of the mechanisms of these processes. Structural changes can serve as touchstones because they represent coherent functional adaptations that probably result from the coordination of multiple biochemical processes. Since molecules participating in the formation of a plastic response may have roles in a variety of cell types and functions, it is important to observe these elements in conjunction with the synaptic structure they are presumed to affect. While this work should ultimately involve the use of labels to image candidate molecules in conjunction with stereological measurements of synaptic parameters, a great deal can be gained by relating the structural changes already reported to the operational envelope for particular biochemical processes. One parameter ripe for such an analysis is the time point chosen for morphological examination. Among the studies reviewed in this chapter, time points examined range from 2 minutes to 48 hours. It is hard to imagine that all the changes observed across this time domain are the signatures of a unitary phenomenon or are driven by the same biochemical processes. Time points should be selected that would allow the stages of LTP formation to be defined with respect to mechanism as well as functional adaptation. For example, early time points constrain the tools for synaptic remodeling to interactions of pre-existing local enzymes and structural proteins; whereas at later time points, structure may be altered by the action of proteins whose local synthesis is affected by LTP and, ultimately, by proteins generated by an increase in nuclear expression and transported to the site of synaptic remodeling. By addressing morphological change in the temporal framework of induction, expression, and maintenance, the alteration of synaptic structural state can begin to be brought into register with molecular regulation and physiological manifestation of potentiation.

ACKNOWLEDGMENTS

Supported by the Office of Naval Research N00014-89-J-1556 and the Epilepsy Foundation of America.

REFERENCES

Alkon, D. L., et al. (1990). Contraction of neuronal branching volume: an anatomic correlate of Pavlovian conditioning. *Proceedings of the National Academy of Sciences USA* 87:1611–1614.

Amaral, D. G., and M. P. Witter (1989). The three-dimensional organization of the hippocampal formation: a review of anatomical data. *Neuroscience* 31(3):571–591.

Andersen, P., T. V. P. Bliss, and K. K. Skrede (1971). Lamellar organization of hippocampal excitatory pathways. *Experimental Brain Research* 13:222–238.

Andersen, P., et al. (1987). Dimensions of dendritic spines of rat dentate granule cells during long-term potentiation. *Proceedings of the Physiological Society,* p. 264P.

Andersen, P., G. N. Gross, T. Lømo, and O. Sveen (1969). Participation of inhibitory and excitatory interneurons in the control of hippocampal cortical output. In M. A. B. Brazier (ed.), *The Interneuron.* Los Angeles: University of California Press.

Applegate, M. D., D. S. Kerr, and P. W. Landfield (1987). Redistribution of synaptic vesicles during long-term potentiation in the hippocampus. *Brain Research* 401:401–406.

Applegate, M. D., and P. W. Landfield (1988). Synaptic vesicle redistribution during hippocampal frequency potentiation and depression in young and aged rats. *Journal of Neuroscience* 8(4):1096–1111.

Bailey, C. H., and M. Chen (1983). Morphological basis of long-term habituation and sensitization in Aplysia. *Science* 220:91–93.

Bailey, C. H., and M. Chen (1986). Long-term sensitization in Aplysia increases the total number of varicosities of single identified sensory neurons. *Society for Neuroscience Abstracts* 12:860.

Beaulieu, C., and M. Colonnier (1985). The effect of environmental complexity on the numerical density of neurons and on the size of their nuclei in the visual cortex of cat. *Society for Neuroscience Abstracts* 11:225.

Birks, R. I. (1974). The relationship of transmitter release and storage to fine structure in a sympathetic ganglion. *Journal of Neurocytology* 3:133–160.

Black, J. E., et al. (1990). Learning causes synaptogenesis, whereas motor activity causes angioenesis, in cerebellar cortex of adult rats. *Proceedings of the National Academy of Sciences USA* 87:5568–5572.

Bliss, T. V. P., and T. Lømo (1973). Long-lasting potentiation of synaptic transmission in the dentate area of the anaesthetized rabbit following stimulation of the perforant path. *Journal of Neurophysiology* 232:331–356.

Bliss, T. V. P., and M. A. Lynch (1988). Long-term potentiation of synaptic transmission in the hippocampus: properties and mechanisms. In P. W. Landfield and S. A. Deadwyler (eds.), *Neurology and Neurobiology, vol. 35, Long-Term Potentiation: From Biophysics to Behavior.* New York: Alan R. Liss, pp. 3–72.

Brandon, J. G., and R. G. Coss (1982). Rapid dendritic spine stem shortening during one-trial learning: the honeybee's first orientation flight. *Brain Research* 252:51–61.

Buszaki, G., and E. Eidelberg (1982). Direct afferent excitation and long-term potentiation of hippocampal interneurons. *Journal of Neurophysiology* 48:597–607.

Cain, D. P. (1989). LTP and kindling: how similar are the mechanisms? *Trends in Neuroscience* 12:(1)6–10.

Chang, F.-L., M. K. Floeter, and W. T. Greenough (1979). Application of high magnesium concentration perfusion-fixation to rat visual cortex. *Society for Neuroscience Abstracts* 5:426.

Chang, F.-L., W. T. Greenough (1984). Transient and enduring morphological correlates of synaptic activity and efficacy change in the rat hippocampal slice. *Brain Research* 309:35–46.

Chang, F.-L., and W. T. Greenough (1988). Long-term potentiation in upright tangential mouse dentate slices. *Society for Neuroscience Abstracts* 14:568.

Chang, F.-L., N. Hawrylak, and W. T. Greenough (1991b). Astrocytic and synaptic response to kindling in hippocampal subfield CA1. I. Synaptogenesis in response to kindling in vitro (submitted).

Chang, F.-L., K. R. Isaacs, and W. T. Greenough (1991a). Synapse formation occurs in association with the induction of long term potentiation in two-year old rat hippocampus in vitro (submitted).

Cooke, C. T., T. M. Nolan, S. E. Dyson, and D. G. Jones (1974). Pentobarbital-induced configurational changes at the synapse. *Brain Research* 76:330–335.

Cornell-Bell, A. H., S. M. Finkbeiner, M. S. Cooper, and S. J. Smith (1990). Glutamate induces calcium waves in cultured astrocytes: long-range glial signaling. *Science* 247:470–473.

Coss, R. G., J. G. Brandon, and A. Globus (1980). Changes in the morphology of dendritic spines on honeybee calycal interneurons associated with cumulative nursing and foraging experiences. *Brain Research* 192:49–59.

Coss, R. G., and A. Globus (1978). Spine stems on tectal interneurons in jewel fish are shortened by social stimulation. *Science* 200:787–790.

Desmond, N. L., and W. B. Levy (1983). Synaptic correlates of associative potentiation/depression: an ultrastructural study in the hippocampus. *Brain Research* 265:21–30.

Desmond, N. L., and W. B. Levy (1986a). Changes in the numerical density of synaptic contacts with long-term potentiation in the hippocampal dentate gyrus. *Journal of Comparative Neurology* 253:466–475.

Desmond, N. L., and W. B. Levy (1986b). Changes in the postsynaptic density with long-term potentiation in the dentate gyrus. *Journal of Comparative Neurology* 253:476–482.

Desmond, N. L., and W. B. Levy (1986c). More front-line synaptic vesicles with long-term synaptic potentiation in the hippocampal dentate gyrus. *Society for Neuroscience Abstracts* 12:504.

Desmond, N. L., and W. B. Levy (1988a). Synaptic interface surface area increases with long-term potentiation in the hippocampal dentate gyrus. *Brain Research* 453:308–314.

Desmond, N. L., and W. B. Levy (1988b). Anatomy of associative long-term synaptic modification. In P. W. Landfield and S. A. Deadwyler (eds.), *Neurology and Neurobiology, vol. 35, Long-Term Potentiation: From Biophysics to Behavior.* New York: Alan R. Liss, pp. 265–305.

Desmond, N. L., and W. B. Levy (1990). Morphological correlates of long-term potentiation imply the modification of existing synapses, not synaptogenesis, in the hippocampal dentate gyrus. *Synapse* 5:139–143.

de Toledo-Morrell, L., Y. Geinisman, and F. Morrell (1990). Selective reduction in the average size of perforated postsynaptic densities in long-term potentiation (LTP). *Society for Neuroscience Abstracts* 407:2.

Diamond, M. C., et al. (1975). Differences in occipital cortical synapses from environmentally enriched, impoverished, and standard colony rats. *Journal of Neuroscience Research* 1:109–119.

Douglas, R. M., G. V. Goddard, and M. Riives (1982). Inhibitory modulation of LTP: evidence for a postsynaptic locus of control. *Brain Research* 240:259–272.

Dyson, S. E., and D. G. Jones (1980). Quantitation of terminal parameters and their interrelationships in maturing central synapses: a perspective for experimental studies. *Brain Research* 183:43–59.

Engstrom, D., et al. (1990). Modulation of hippocampal primed burst potentiation by anesthesia. *Brain Research* 521:148–152.

Fifkova, E. (1985). Synaptic hypertrophy of the dentate fascia of the hippocampus. In Eccles and Dimitrijevic (eds.), *Recent Achievements in Restorative Neurology 1: Upper Motor Neuron Functions and Dysfunctions.* Basel: S. Karger, pp. 263–271.

Fifkova, E., and C. L. Anderson (1981). Stimulation-induced changes in dimensions of stalks of dendritic spines in the dentate molecular layer. *Experimental Neurology* 74:621–627.

Fifkova, E., C. L. Anderson, S. J. Young, and A. Van Harreveld (1982). Effect of anisomycin on stimulation-induced changes in dendritic spines of the dentate granule cells. *Journal of Neurocytology* 11:183–210.

Fifkova, E., and A. Van Harreveld (1977). Long-lasting morphological changes in dendritic spines of dentate granular cells following stimulation of the entorhinal area. *Journal of Neurocytology* 6:211–230.

Floeter, M. K., and W. T. Greenough (1979). Cerebellar plasticity: modification of Purkinje cell structure by differential rearing in monkeys. *Science* 206:227–229.

Garey, L. J., and J. D. Pettigrew (1974). Ultrastructural changes in kitten visual cortex after environmental modification. *Brain Research* 66:165–172.

Geinisman, Y., L. de Toledo-Morrell, and F. Morrell (1986). Loss of perforated synapses in the dentate gyrus: morphological substrate of memory deficit in aged rats. *Proceedings of the National Academy of Sciences USA* 83:3027–3031.

Geinisman, Y., F. N. Morrell, and L. de Toledo-Morrell (1988). Remodelling of synaptic architecture during hippocampal "kindling." *Proceedings of the National Academy of Sciences USA* 85:3260–3264.

Geinisman, Y., L. de Toledo-Morrell, and F. Morrell (1990a). The brain's record of experience: kindling-induced enlargement of the active zone in hippocampal perforated synapses. *Brain Research* 513:175–179.

Geinisman, Y., L. de Toledo-Morrell, and F. Morrell (1990b). Increase in the proportion of perforated axospinous synapses induced by long term potentiation (LTP). *Society for Neuroscience Abstracts* 16:407–411.

Gould, E., C. S. Wooley, M. Frankfurt, and B. S. McEwen (1990). Gonadal steroids regulate dendritic spine density in hippocampal pyramidal cells in adulthood. *Journal of Neuroscience* 10(4):1286–1291.

Green, E. J., and W. T. Greenough (1986). Altered synaptic transmission in dentate gyrus of rats reared in complex environments: evidence from hippocampal slices maintained in vitro. *Journal of Neurophysiology* 55:(4)739–749.

Greenough, W. T., and F.-L. Chang (1985). Synaptic structural correlates of information storage in mammalian nervous systems. In C. W. Cotman (ed.), *Synaptic Plasticity.* New York: Guilford Press, pp. 335–372.

Greenough, W. T., and F.-L. Chang (1988). Plasticity of synapse structure and pattern in the cerebral cortex. In A. Peters and E. G. Jones (eds.), *Cerebral Cortex.* New York, Plenum Press, 7:391–440.

Greenough, W. T., J. M. Juraska, and F. R. Volkmar (1979). Maze training effects on dendritic branching in occipital cortex of adult rats. *Behavioral and Neural Biology* 26:287–297.

Greenough, W. T., J. Larson, and G. Withers (1985). Effects of unilateral and bilateral training in a teaching task on dendritic branching of neurons in the rat motor-sensory forelimb cortex. *Behavioral and Neural Biology* 44:301–314.

Greenough, W. T., R. W. West, and T. J. DeVoogd (1978). Subsynaptic plate perforations: changes with age and experience in the rat. *Science* 202:1096–1098.

Gulley, R. L., R. J. Wenthold, G. R. Neises (1978). Changes in the synapses of spiral ganglion cells in the rostral anteroventral cochlear nucleus of the waltzing guinea pig following hair cell loss. *Brain Research* 158:279–294.

Gundersen, H. J. G., et al. (1988). Some new, simple and efficient stereological methods and their use in pathological research and diagnosis. *Acta Pathologica Microbiologica et Immunologica Scandinavia* 96:379–394.

Harris, K. M., F. E. Jensen, and B. H. Tsao (1989). Ultrastructure, development, and plasticity of dendritic spine synapses in area CA1 of the rat hippocampus: extending our vision with serial electron microscopy and three dimensional analyses. In *The Hippocampus—New Vistas.* New York: Alan R. Liss, pp. 33–52.

Harris, K. M., and J. K. Stevens (1989). Dendritic spines of CA1 pyramidal cells in the rat hippocampus: serial electron microscopy with reference to their biophysical characteristics. *Journal of Neuroscience* 9(8):2982–2997.

Hatton, J. D., and M. H. Ellisman (1982). A restructuring of hypothalamic synapses is associated with motherhood. *Journal of Neuroscience* 2:704–707.

Hatton, G. I., L. S. Perlmutter, A. K. Salm, and C. D. Tweedle (1984). Dynamic neuron-glial interactions in the hypothalamus and pituitary: implications for hormone synthesis and release. *Peptides 5(Suppl.)*1:121–138.

Hawrylak, N., F.-L. Chang, and W. T. Greenough (1989). Astrocytic response to in vivo kindling of the hippocampus. *Society for Neuroscience Abstracts* 15:779.

Hawrylak, N., F.-L. Chang, and W. T. Greenough (1991). Astrocytic and synaptic response to kindling in hippocampal subfield CA1. II: Synaptogenesis and astrocytic process increases to in vivo kindling (submitted).

Hawrylak, N., et al. (1988). Synaptogenesis in kindling. *Society for Neuroscience Abstracts* 14:881.

Herrera, A., A. Grinnell, B. Wolowske (1985). Ultrastructural correlates of experimentally altered transmitter release efficacy in frog motor nerve terminals. *Neuroscience* 16:491–500.

Hertz, L., and A. Schousboe (1986). Role of astrocytes in compartmentation of amino acid and energy metabolism. In S. Fedoroff and A. Vernadakis (eds.), *Astrocytes* (Vol. 2). Orlando, Florida: Academic Press, pp. 179–208.

Heuser, J. E., et al. (1979). Synaptic vesicle exocytosis captured by quick freezing and correlated with quantal release. *Journal of Cell Biology* 81:275–300.

Hjorth-Simonsen, A., and B. Jeune (1972). Origin and termination of the hippocampal perforant path in the rat studied by silver impregnation. *Journal of Comparative Neurology* 144:215–232.

Isaacs, K. R., et al. (1989). Long-term potentiation alters glial processes in the dentate gyrus. *Society for Neuroscience Abstracts* 15:610.

Jones, D. G., and R. M. Devon (1977). The influence of pentobarbitone on the distribution of membrane in cortical synapses. *Neuroscience Letters* 6:177–182.

Juraska, J. M., and E. Fifkova (1979). An electron microscope study of the early postnatal development of the visual cortex of the hooded rat. *Journal of Comparative Neurology* 183:833–883.

Kairiss, E. W., W. C. Abraham, D. K. Bilkey, and G. V. Goddard (1987). Field potential evidence for long-term potentiation of feed-forward inhibition in the rat dentate gyrus. *Brain Research* 401:87–94.

Kilman, V. L., C. S. Wallace, G. S. Withers, and W. T. Greenough (1988). 4 days of differential housing alters dendritic morphology of weanling rats. *Society for Neuroscience Abstracts* 14:1135.

Kuba, K., and E. Kumamoto (1990). Long-term potentiation in vertebrate synapses: a variety of cascades with common subprocesses. *Progress in Neurobiology* 34:197–269.

Landis, D. M. D., A. K. Hall, L. A. Weinstein, and T. S. Reese (1988). The organization of cytoplasm at the presynaptic zone of a central nervous system synapse. *Neuron* 1:201–209.

Larson, J., D. Wong, and G. Lynch (1986). Patterned stimulation at the theta frequency is optimal for the induction of hippocampal LTP. *Brain Research* 368:347–350.

Lee, K., M. Oliver, F. Schottler, and G. Lynch (1981). Electron microscopic studies of brain slices: the effects of high-frequency stimulation on dendritic ultrastructure. In G. A. Kerkut and H. V. Wheal (eds.), *Electrophysiology of Isolated Mammalian CNS Preparations*. New York: Academic, pp. 189–211.

Lee, K. S., F. Schottler, M. Oliver, and G. Lynch (1980). Brief bursts of high-frequency stimulation produce two types of structural change in rat hippocampus. *Journal of Neurophysiology* 44(2):247–258.

LeVay, S., T. N. Wiesel, and D. H. Hubel (1980). The development of ocular dominance columns in normal and visually deprived monkeys. *Journal of Comparative Neurology* 191:1–51.

Lorente de No, R. (1934). Studies on the structure of the cerebral cortex. II. Continuation of the study of the ammonic system. *Journal Für Psychologie und Neurologie* 46:113–177.

MacIver, M. B., D. L. Tauck, and J. J. Kendig (1989). General anaesthetic modification of synaptic facilitation and long-term potentiation in hippocampus. *British Journal of Anaesthesia* 62:301–310.

Marrero, H., M. L. Astion, J. A. Coles, and R. K. Orkand (1989). Facilitation of voltage-gated ion channels in frog neuroglia by nerve impulses. *Nature* 339:378–380.

Maupin-Szamier, P., and T. D. Pollard (1978). Actin filament destruction by osmium tetroxide. *Journal of Cell Biology* 77:837–852.

McKinlay, R., and P. Usherwood (1978). The effects of magnesium ions on the fine structure of the insect neuromuscular junction. *Journal of Ultrastructural Research* 62:83–93.

McNamara, J., et al. (1985). Kindling model of epilepsy: a critical review. *Critical Review of Clinical Neurobiology CRC Press* 1:341–391.

Meshul, C. K., W. F. Hopkins (1990). Presynaptic ultrastructural correlates of long-term potentiation in the CA1 subfield of the hippocampus. *Brain Research* 514:310–319.

Meshul, C., F. Seil (1988). Transplanted astrocytes reduce synaptic density in the neuropil of cerebellar cultures. *Brain Research* 441:23–32.

Miller, M., A. Peters (1981). Maturation of rat visual cortex. II. A combined Golgi-electron microscope study of pyramidal neurons. *Journal of Comparative Neurology* 203:555–573.

Mollgaard, K., et al. (1971). Qualitative synaptic changes with different experience in rat brain. *International Journal of Neuroscience* 2:113–128.

Oorschot, K. E., and D. G. Jones (1987). The vesicle hypothesis and its alternatives: a critical assessment. In D. G. Jones (ed.), *Current Topics in Research on Synapses.* New York: Alan R. Liss, pp. 85–153.

Ornberg, R. L., and T. Reese (1980). A freeze substitution method for localizing divalent cations: examples from secretory systems. *Federation Proceedings* 39:2802–2808.

Payne, K., et al. (1982). Evoked potentials and long-term potentiation in the mouse dentate gyrus after stimulation of the entorhinal cortex. *Experimental Neurology* 75:134–148.

Peters, A., and I. R. Kaiserman-Abramof (1969). The small pyramidal neuron of the rat cerebral cortex: the synapses upon dendritic spines. *Zeitshrift Zellforsh Mikroskopic Anatomie* 100:487–506.

Pertukhov, V. V., and V. J. Popov (1986). Quantitative analysis of ultrastructural changes in synapses of the rat hippocampal field CA3 in vitro in different functional states. *Neuroscience* 18(4):823–835.

Racine, R. J., and N. W. Milgram (1983). Long-term potentiation phenomena in the rat limbic forebrain. *Brain Research* 260:217–231.

Racine, R. J., and N. W. Milgram (1983). Short-term potentiation phenomena in the rat limbic forebrain. *Brain Research* 260:201–216.

Rakic, P. (1971). Neuronal-glial relationships during granule cell migration in the developing cerebellar cortex. A Golgi and electron microscopic study in the Macacus rhesus. *Journal of Comparative Neurology* 141:282–312.

Rall, W. (1970). Cable properties of dendrites and effects of synaptic location. In P. Andersen and J. K. S. Jansen (eds.), *Excitatory Synaptic Mechanisms.* Oslo: Universitetsforlaget, pp. 175–187.

Ramon y Cajal, S. (1893). New findings about the histological structure of the central nervous system. *Archiv fur Anatomie und Physiologie (Anatomie)* 1893:319–428.

Ramon y Cajal, S. (1911). Histologie du systeme nerveux de l'homme et des vertebres. Paris: A. Maloine.

Rash, J. E. (1983). The rapid freeze technique in neurobiology. *Trends In Neuroscience* 6:208–212.

Reeves, T. M., and O. Steward (1986). Emergence of the capacity for LTP during reinnervation of the dentate gyrus: evidence that abnormally shaped spines can mediate LTP. *Experimental Brain Research* 65:167–175.

Ronnevi, L.-O. (1977). Spontaneous phagocytosis of boutons on spinal motoneurons during early postnatal development. An electron microscopical study in the cat. *Journal of Neurocytology* 6:487–504.

Rose, G. M., and T. V. Dunwiddie (1986). Induction of hippocampal LTP using physiologically patterned stimulation. *Neuroscience Letters* 69:244–248.

Schuster, T., et al. (1986). Ultrastructural changes of hippocampal neurons and synapses following LTP—a morphometric study. *Advances in the Biosciences* 59:115–118.

Schuster, T., M. Krug, and J. Wenzel (1990). Spinules in axospinous synapses of the rat dentate gyrus: changes in density following long-term potentiation. *Brain Research* 523:171–174.

Sharp, P., B. McNaughton, and C. Barnes (1985). Enhancement of hippocampal field potentials in rats exposed to a novel, complex environment. *Brain Research* 339:361–365.

Shors, T. J., M. R. Foy, S. Levine, and R. F. Thompson (1990). Unpredictable and uncontrollable stress impairs neuronal plasticity in the rat hippocampus. *Brain Research* 24:663–667.

Sirevaag, A. M., and W. T. Greenough (1985). Differential rearing effects on rat visual cortex synapses. II. Synaptic morphometry. *Developmental Brain Research* 19:215–226.

Sirevaag, A. M., and W. T. Greenough (1987). Differential rearing effects on rat visual cortex synapses. III. Neuronal and glial nuclei, boutons, dendrites, and capillaries. *Brain Research* 424:320–332.

Sirevaag, A. M., and W. T. Greenough (1991). Plasticity of GFAP-immunoreactive astrocyte size and number in visual cortex of rats reared in complex environments. *Brain Research* 540:273–278.

Smith, J., and T. S. Reese (1980). Use of aldehyde fixatives to determine rate of synaptic transmitter release. *Journal of Experimental Biology* 89:19–29.

Staubli, U., J. Larson, and G. Lynch (1990). Mossy fiber potentiation and long-term potentiation involve different expression mechanisms. *Synapse* 5:333–335.

Sterio, D. C. (1984). The unbiased estimation of number and sizes of arbitrary particles using the dissector. *Journal of Microscopy* 134:127–136.

Steward, O., and P. M. Falk (1985). Polyribosomes under developing spine synapses: growth specializations of dendrites at sites of synaptogenesis. *Journal of Neuroscience Research* 13:75–88.

Steward, O., and S. A. Scoville (1976). Cells of origin of entorhinal cortical afferents to the hippocampus and fascia dentata of the rat. *Journal of Comparative Neurology* 169:347–370.

Steward, O., R. Tomasulo, and W. Levy (1990). Blockade of inhibition in a pathway with dual excitatory and inhibitory action unmasks a capability for LTP that is otherwise not expressed. *Brain Research* 516:292–300.

Streit, P., et al. (1972). Dynamic ultrastructure of presynaptic membranes at nerve terminals in the spinal cord of rats: anesthetized and unanesthetized preparations compared. *Brain Research* 48:11–26.

Sutula, T., X. X. He, J. Cavazos, and S. Grayson (1988). Synaptic reorganization in the hippocampus induced by abnormal functional activity. *Science* 239:1147–1150.

Szentagothai, J., and J. Hamori (1969). Growth and differentiation of synaptic structures under circumstances of deprivation of function and of distant connections. In G. E. W. Wolstenholme and M. O'Conner (eds.), *Cellular Dynamics of the Neuron*. New York: Academic Press, pp. 301–320.

Tanzi, E. (1893). Facts and inductions in current histology of the nervous system. *Rivista Sperimentale di Freniatriae Medicina Legale Delle Mentali Alienazioni* 19:419–472.

Tarrant, S. B., and A. Routtenberg (1977). The synaptic spinule in the dendritic spine: Electron microscopic study of the hippocampal dentate gyrus. *Tissue & Cell* 9:461–473.

Teyler, T. J., and P. DiScenna (1987). Long-term potentiation. *Annual Review of Neuroscience* 10:131–161.

Teyler, T. J., A. T. Perkins, and K. M. Harris (1989). The development of long-term potentiation in hippocampus and neocortex. *Neuropsychologia* 27(1):31–40.

Teyler, T. J., D. L. Vardaris, D. L. Lewis, and A. B. Rawitch (1980). Gonadal steroids: effects on excitability of hippocampal pyramidal cells. *Science* 209:1017–1019.

Tieman, S. B. (1984). Effects of monocular deprivation on geniculocortical synapses in the cat. *Journal of Comparative Neurology* 222:166–176.

Tieman, S. B. (1985). The anatomy of geniculocortical connections in monocularly deprived cats. *Cellular and Molecular Neurobiology* 5:35–45.

Turner, A. M., and W. T. Greenough (1985). Differential rearing effects on rat visual cortex synapses. I. Synaptic and neuronal density and synapses per neuron. *Brain Research* 309:373–376.

Usowicz, M. M., V. Gallo and S. G. Cull-Candy (1989). Multiple conductance channels in type-2 cerebellar astrocytes activated by excitatory amino acids. *Nature* 339:380–383.

Van Harreveld, A., and E. Fifkova (1975). Swelling of dendritic spines in the fascia dentata after stimulation of the perforant fibers as a mechanism of post-tetanic potentiation. *Experimental Neurology* 49:736–749.

Volkmar, F. R., and W. T. Greenough (1972). Rearing complexity affects branching of dendrites in the visual cortex of the rat. *Science* 176:1445–1447.

Vresen, G., and J. N. Cardozo (1981). Changes in size and shape of synaptic connections after visual training: an ultrastructural approach of synaptic plasticity. *Brain Research* 218:79–97.

Vrensen, G., and D. DeGroot (1974). The effect of dark-rearing and its recovery on synaptic terminals in the visual cortex of rabbits: a quantitative electron microscope study. *Brain Research* 78:263–278.

Vrensen, G., and D. DeGroot (1975). The effect of monocular deprivation on synaptic terminals in the visual cortex of rabbits: a quantitative electron microscope study. *Brain Research* 93:15–24.

Wallace, C. S., F.-L. Chang, and W. T. Greenough (1988). Applications of a freezing system designed to capture CNS dynamic morphology. *Society for Neuroscience Abstracts* 14:568.

Wenzel, J., M. Krug, T. Ott, and T. Schuster (1986). Ultrastructural changes in neurons and the synapses of the dentate area accompanying LTP induced by perforant path stimulation. *Advances in Biosciences* 59:109–114.

Wesa, J. M., F.-L.F. Chang, W. T. Greenough, and R. W. West (1982). Synaptic contact curvature: effects of differential rearing on rat occipital cortex. *Developmental Brain Research* 4:253–257.

West, R. W., and W. T. Greenough (1972). Effect of environmental complexity on cortical synapses of rats: preliminary results. *Behavioral Biology* 7:279–284.

Woolley, C. S., and B. S. McEwen (1990). Estradiol regulates synapse density in the CA1 region of the hippocampus in the adult female rat. *Society for Neuroscience Abstracts* 16:328.

Yeckel, M. F., and T. W. Berger (1990). Feedforward excitation of the hippocampus by afferents from the entorhinal cortex: redefinition of the role of the trisynaptic pathway. *Proceedings of the National Academy of Sciences USA* 87:5832–5836.

15 Long-Lasting Maintenance of Long-Term Potentiation and Macromolecular Synthesis

Hansjuergen Matthies

In the course of our investigations on molecular and cellular correlates of long-term memory formation, we became interested in posttetanic long-term potentiation (LTP) because the remarkably long persistence of this synaptic change suggested its role as a mechanism of memory. Probably because LTP was first investigated by electrophysiological methods and also because only a single mechanism was assumed to effect this long-lasting potentiation, attention was mainly focused on induction and early maintenance.

Because of our data from learning experiments and the resulting concept assuming the existence of subsequent stages of memory formation with different underlying mechanisms, we directed our attention to more than the relatively early course of LTP. We assumed that if LTP actually represents a mechanism of lasting memory, it should also reveal different phases similar to those observed in memory formation. Additionally, it should consequently require protein synthesis for the formation of longer-lasting LTP maintenance. This approach differed somewhat from the original electrophysiological view that mainly considered synaptic events and disregarded the longer duration of anabolic processes as well as their control by the entire neuron. Even the second messenger systems and the phosphorylation of preexisting presynaptic or postsynaptic proteins as cellular mechanisms of LTP, which entered the foreground of LTP research, did not sufficiently explain the final realization of a semi-persistent synaptic enhancement. In my mind, a permanently activated state of protein kinases contradicts their general role in the control of cellular metabolism, even if a long-lasting and nearly irreversible switching can be obtained under relatively unphysiological conditions. To better explain our approach, we present a few key results obtained in our learning experiments that lead to our multistage concept and to our assuming that macromolecular synthesis is involved in LTP maintenance.

The existence of different kinds of memory and the time-dependent formation of a permanent memory trace was already suggested by numerous psychological and behavioral studies when we started our investigations on biochemical correlates of long-term memory formation. We therefore looked first for a learning model in rats, which enabled us to prove short and transient retention of learned behavior and to separate by suitable experimental conditions these early stages from a more or less permanent trace. We also wanted our model to account for more intense biochemical changes in ample neuronal structures than were expected to occur in the widely used one-trial passive-avoidance learning or in similar learning tasks. Our methodological preparatory work finally resulted in our choosing a footshock-motivated brightness discrimination task, which teaches the animals to escape into a bright alley against their innate behavior to flee into the dark. We also regarded this task as a conditioned active darkness avoidance. It enabled us to produce long-lasting retention of the learned behavior using 40 to 60 trials during a single training session of at most 60 minutes; we were thus still able to investigate the relatively slow biochemical processes during consolidation of long-term memory. The data obtained with this learning model further supported the suggestions that the retention of a learned behavior after completion of training is maintained by subsequent different processes and not by a single cellular mechanism (Ott and Matthies, 1978; figures 15.1, 15.2, 15.3):

The time-course of retention fluctuated with two significant minima 1 hour and 4 to 5 hours after training, respectively.

The application of an electroconvulsive shock (ECS) after training did not suppress the retention during the following 2 to 3 hours, but completely extinguished the trace 5 hours after acquisition.

The ECS-gradient of long-term retention tested 1 or 2 days after acquisition indicated that the formation of long-term memory showed a decreas-

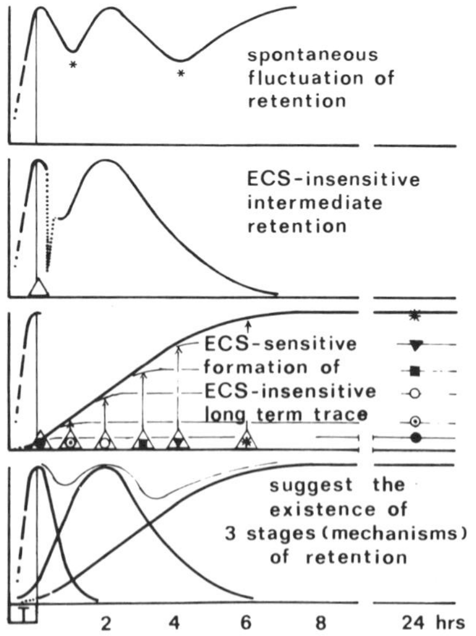

Figure 15.1 Retention of brightness discrimination in rats. ECS = electroconvulsive shock. T = training period.

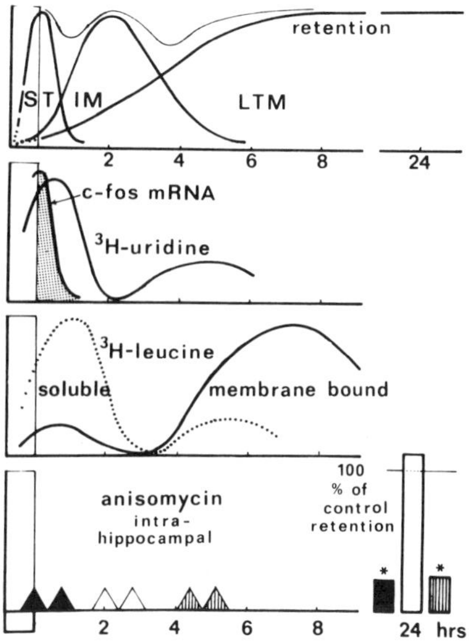

Figure 15.2 Macromolecular changes during and after rats acquired brightness discrimination. (Top) Time-course of the assumed memory stages (see figure 15.1). (Top middle) Incorporation of ^{3}H-uridine into hippocampal neurons indicating increased RNA-synthesis and induction of c-fos mRNA in the hippocampus. (Bottom middle) Time-course of increased incorporation of ^{3}H-leucine into hippocampal proteins. (Bottom) Effects of inhibition of protein synthesis by anisomycin at three different times after learning: during and immediately after learning, which results in severe amnesia; 2–3 hrs after learning, which does not influence long-term memory; and 4–5 hr after learning, which produces amnesia. ST = short-term memory; IM = intermediate memory; LTM = long-term memory.

ing ECS-sensitivity during the 5 to 6 hours after learning; thereafter, memory was ECS-insensitive.

The inhibition of brain protein synthesis by anisomycin during learning did not influence the acquisition of the new behavior, but it did prevent the formation of long-term memory.

These results suggested that the retention of the learned darkness avoidance used in our studies is maintained by at least three subsequent and probably overlapping processes that differed in their time-course of origin and decay as well as in their sensitivity to experimental interventions. In addition, a slowly developing long-term memory obviously requires newly synthesized proteins already produced during and after learning. The following biochemical investigations on the macromolecular changes related to the formation of a semi-permanent memory trace have provided these main results:

c-fos mRNA became expressed in the hippocampus immediately after training (Tischmeyer et al., 1990).

Labeled RNA precursors and amino acids were increasingly incorporated into RNA of hippocampal neurons and of some neocortical structures during and after training (Pohle and Matthies, 1971, 1974).

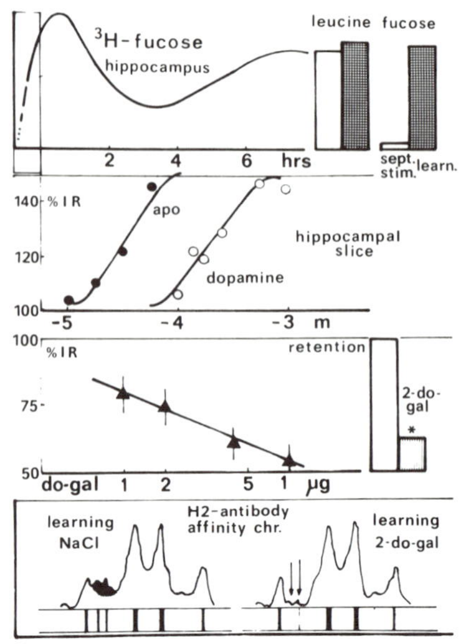

Figure 15.3 Formation of glycoproteins after rats acquired brightness discrimination. (Top) Time-course of increased incorporation of ^{3}H-fucose into hippocampal proteins. (Top middle) Influence of dopaminergic agonists on the incorporation of ^{3}H-fucose into proteins of hippocampal slices. (Bottom middle) Inhibition of fucose incorporation by pretreatment of rats with 2-deoxy-galactose and the amnesic action of 2-deoxy-galactose. (Bottom) Separation of hippocampal fucosyl-glycoproteins with H2-antibody-affinity chromatography (chr.). An increase of two bands in the 37 kDa range occurs in trained animals (left), they are considerably suppressed after pretreatment of trained rats with amnesic doses of 2-deoxy-galactose (right).

The learning-related increase of protein synthesis showed two maxima: one during and immediately after training, which mainly represented soluble proteins, and, after a silent phase, a second peak 4 to 8 hours after learning, which was mainly attributed to membrane proteins (Popov et al., 1975, 1976).

The incorporation of labeled fucose increased during and after learning in hippocampal neurons (Popov et al., 1980).

Whereas the increase of protein synthesis in hippocampal structures also occurred after septal stimulation, an increased fucose incorporation was only obtained after learning (Jork et al., 1978).

An increase of fucose incorporation was induced in hippocampal slices by dopaminergic agonists, as well as in vivo by intrahippocampal application. This increase induced an improvement of the retention of the learned behavior (Jork et al., 1979).

2-Deoxy-galactose treatment produced a severe suppression of long-term memory without influencing its acquisition. This amnesia was accompanied by a marked decrease of fucose incorporation into two hippocampal glycoprotein bands, which are increasingly labeled in untreated trained animals (Jork et al., 1986).

Disposing of these data and the resulting conclusions, and assuming LTP as a mechanism of memory, we tried to show whether similar stages and corresponding time-courses as well as macromolecular changes occur after induction of a posttetanic synaptic potentiation. For this end, suitable conditions for long-term experiments on hippocampal slices were elaborated (Reymann et al., 1985) to investigate maintenance of LTP at least 7 to 8 hours after tetanization, considering that the consolidation of a long-term memory trace requires at least 6 to 8 hours.

First we tried to prove an involvement of protein synthesis in LTP, using anisomycin as an inhibitor. We showed that the intraventricular application of 400 μg of anisomycin before and after tetanization of the perforant path in vivo did not prevent the induction and early maintenance of LTP, but completely suppressed the late maintenance 5 hours after tetanization (Krug et al., 1984). Furthermore, Frey and colleagues (1988) demonstrated that the presence of anisomycin during tetanization did not influence the induction of LTP in the CA1 region of hippocampal slices; anisomycin also prevented its maintenance after 5 to 6 hours (figure 15.4). To obviate

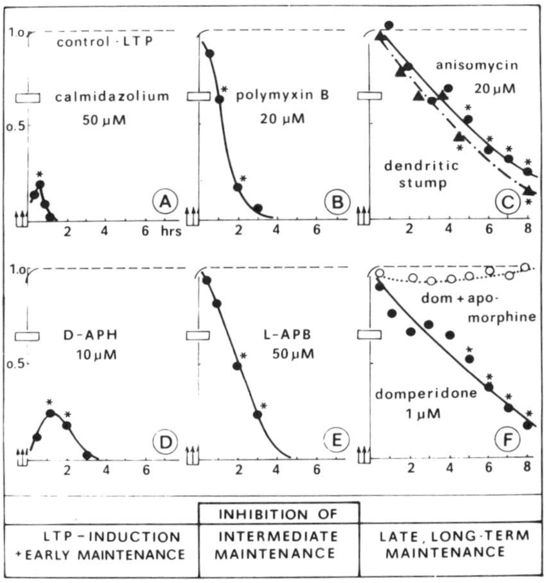

Figure 15.4 Effects of the presence of different inhibitors during tetanization of Schaffer collaterals on the timecourse of long-term potentiation in the rat hippocampal CA1 region in vitro. Values as fraction of potentiation in control slices. (A) Effect of 50 μM calmidazolium, an inhibitor of calmodulin. (B) Effect of 20 μM polymyxin B, an inhibitor of proteinkinase C. (C) Effect of 20 μM anisomycin, an inhibitor of protein synthesis (filled circles) and timecourse of potentiation in dendrites separated from their cell bodies as the main site of neuronal protein synthesis. (D) Effect of 10 μM D-2-amino-5-phosphonoheptanoate (D-APH), an antagonist of the NMDA-subtype of glutamate receptors. (E) Effect of 50 μM L-2-amino-5-phosphonobutyrate (L-APB), an antagonist of a glutamate receptor subtype probably coupled to the phosphoinositol-system. (F) Effect of 1 μM domperidone (dom), a blocker of dopamine receptors (filled circles) and of the simultaneous action of 1 μM dom and 1 μM apomorphine, a potent dopamine agonist (open circles).

objections considering possible side effects of anisomycin not related to an inhibition of protein synthesis, we investigated the time-course of posttetanic excitatory postsynaptic potential (EPSP) in dendrites separated from the CA1 cell bodies as the main source of neuronal protein synthesis (Frey et al., 1989). In this preparation, LTP can be induced as in uncut control slices; the synaptic enhancement, however, reveals the same decay as that after tetanization in the presence of anisomycin (see figure 15.4). Finally, we showed that the induction of LTP by tetanization of the perforant path in vivo is followed by a notably increased incorporation of labeled leucine into the proteins of the rat dentate area (Lössner et al., 1990; figure 15.5). These findings clearly show that newly synthesized proteins are necessary for a long-lasting maintenance of LTP, but not for its induction and early maintenance; the existence of different LTP stages was therefore proved. These results and conclusions were recently confirmed by Otani and associates (1989), who also demonstrated the postsynaptic site of this macromolecular synthesis. Stanton and Sarvey (1984) also investigated the effects of inhibitors of protein synthesis on LTP in the hippocampal CA1 region in vitro; their experimental conditions and results, however, differed in some ways. According to their data, anisomycin did not

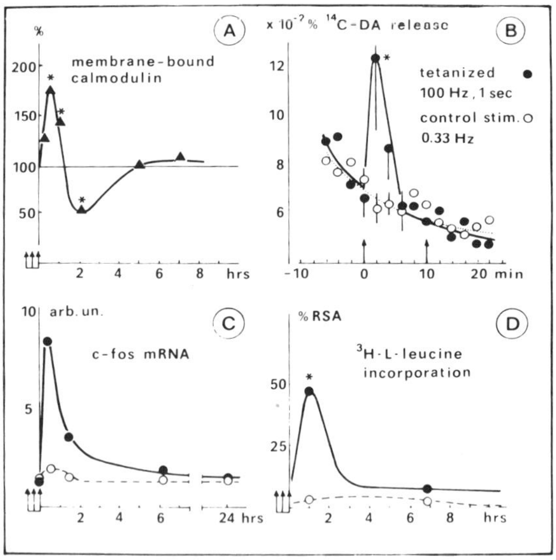

Figure 15.5 (A) Translocation of calmodulin in rat hippocampal slices after tetanization of Schaffer collaterals. Membrane-bound calmodulin determined by an immunochemical method. Values in % of control slices. (B) Release of ^{14}C-dopamine (^{14}C-DA) in hippocampal slices after control stimulation (0.33 Hz) and after tetanization (100 Hz) of Schaffer collaterals. The slices were preloaded with ^{14}C-DA. Values as % of total radioactivity. (C) Induction of c-fos mRNA by LTP-producing tetanization (100 Hz) of the perforant path of freely moving animals. Open circles control stimulation (0.33 Hz), arb.un. arbitrary units. (D) Increase of incorporation of ^{3}H-leucine into proteins of the dentate gyrus after LTP-producing tetanization of the perforant path of freely moving rats. RSA relative specific activity.

influence the occurrence of LTP, but only slightly decreased the population spike amplitude 30 minutes after tetanization. They concluded that anisomycin is not able to block LTP. Their observation time of 30 minutes, however, was too short for an evaluation of the effects on the late maintenance of LTP. On the other hand, they did not produce such a late stage because the tetanization used in their study was insufficient. Their low frequency of 20 Hz only induced a transient potentiation that decayed over 4 to 5 hours. This time-course, however, interestingly corresponded to the anisomycin-resistant intermediate stage of LTP, which is blocked by inhibitors of protein kinase C (Reymann et al., 1988). Therefore, the immediate prevention of LTP by emetine, puromycin, and cycloheximide observed by Stanton and Sarvey (1984) may be rather due to side effects of these drugs and not be related to their inhibition of protein synthesis. Similar objections also apply to a later study of Deadwyler and coworkers (1987). They also observed an immediate effect of cycloheximide, but they only used a 15-Hz tetanization and a 15-minute observation time; they therefore did not clearly produce and record effects on late maintenance. Controversial results and conclusions were also obtained with regard to the posttetanic induction of proto-oncogenes, particularly of c-fos proto-oncogene, which was proposed to play a role by its gene product in the control of expression of specific neuronal proteins. Bliss and colleagues (1988) and Douglas and coworkers (1988) did not obtain an induction of c-fos–like protein in granule cells after LTP-producing tetanization of the perforant path, but they used anesthetized animals in their experiments. After repeated tetanization of the perforant path (sufficient to produce LTP longer than 24 hours), we obtained a significant expression of c-fos mRNA in the hippocampus in freely moving rats. Additionally, Dragunow and colleagues (1989) observed an induction of both c-fos mRNA and protein in the dentate gyrus after LTP-producing tetanization. This occurrence, however, was not clearly related to the size of LTP. They therefore suggested that the induction of c-fos possibly plays a role in the induction of LTP maintenance. This proposal exactly corresponds to our assumption, considering that the late maintenance of LTP obviously depends on newly synthesized proteins. They may be expressed under control of a set of early genes induced by an adequate tetanization, because we induced not only c-fos mRNA after tetanization of the perforant path, but also a transient increase of raf protein kinase–like immunoreactivity in the dentate gyrus (Mihaly et al., 1990).

Moreover, like long-term memory in learning experiments, the induction of a late stage of LTP maintenance seems to involve not only the expression of early genes and the synthesis of new proteins but also their further processing by fucosylation. Pretreating rats with amnesic doses of 2-deoxy-galactose was found to block the fucose–1-2 galactose linkage of the glycan moiety of hippocampal glycoproteins (Jork et al., 1986). Such a pretreatment did not influence the induction of LTP in the dentate gyrus after tetanization of the perforant path in vivo or in the CA1 region of the hippocampal slices prepared from these animals; in addition, it completely prevented the expression of the late maintenance 4 to 6 hours after induction of LTP (figure 15.6). Considering the dopaminergic control of fucosylation in hippocampal slices (Jork et al., 1979), we also investigated the effect of dopaminergic agonists on the time-course of LTP in the CA1 region of hippocampal slices. It was shown that the presence of 1 μM of domperidone, sulpiride, and flupenthixol, respectively, did not influence induction of posttetanic potentiation, but prevented late maintenance and thus revealed a similar time-course of LTP as that observed after inhibition of protein synthesis by anisomycin (Frey et al., 1990). This effect of the dopaminolytic drugs can be prevented by the simultaneous presence of 1 μM apomorphine (see figure 15.4), indicating that the effects of the neuroleptics on LTP maintenance are actually mediated by dopamine receptors and not caused by other mechanisms such as calmodulin inhibition. To prove that dopamine was involved in the induction of a long-lasting maintenance of LTP in the CA1 region, we measured the release of the transmitter by LTP-producing tetanization of the Schaffer collaterals in hippocampal slices after preloading the cells with labeled dopamine (Frey et al., 1990; see also figure 15.5). It was shown that a high-frequency stimulation of 100 Hz (but not low-frequency stimulation of 0.33 Hz) resulted in a markedly increased release of (14C)-dopamine, supporting the assumption that a dopaminergic signal contributes to the induction of the late LTP maintenance at least in the CA1 region. With regard to corresponding mechanisms in the dentate area, the studies of Stanton and Sarvey (1985) should be mentioned, in which they suppressed the norepinephrine-induced long-lasting potentiation in the dentate gyrus by inhibition of protein synthesis. Considering these results, it can be speculated that norepinephrine improves the neuronal connectivity in the dentate area by mediating attention or arousal, similar to the way in which dopamine acts in the CA1 region by mediating emotional influences. The molecular mechanism underlying the norepinephrine action, however, has still to be elucidated. According to our studies, it does not enhance the fucosylation of neuronal glycoproteins.

Summarizing these experimental data and considering our studies on

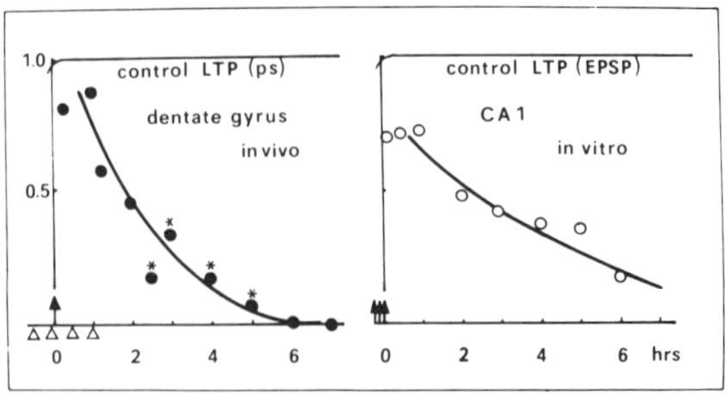

Figure 15.6 Time-course of LTP after pretreatment of rats with 2-deoxy-galactose. (Left) LTP in the dentate gyrus in vivo. (Right) LTP in the CA1 region in slices.

the mechanisms of LTP induction and early maintenance (Matthies, 1990), we suggest that there are at least three subsequent and overlapping stages of LTP in the CA1 region of the rat hippocampus accomplished by different mechanisms of transmitter-receptor interaction, signal transduction, and effectuation (figure 15.7):

A glutamatergic NMDA–receptor mediated, calmodulin-dependent, anisomycin-insensitive postsynaptic induction of LTP.

A protein kinase C–dependent, anisomycin-insensitive intermediate stage, probably related to activation of glutamatergic non-NMDA receptors, transiently maintaining LTP by increased release of glutamate possibly induced or supported by a sustained postsynaptic release of a retrograde chemical signal.

A long-lasting maintenance, involving a postsynaptic synthesis and fucosylation of proteins and their insertion into postsynaptic membranes.

This late maintenance is controlled by at least two convergent inputs to the postsynaptic neuron: at first, a glutamatergic signal possibly mediated by a metabotropic glutamate receptor and a resulting activation of protein kinase C. This transduction induces the expression of a set of early genes and the subsequent synthesis of target proteins and is sensitive to inhibitors of protein kinase C and anisomycin. The second input, a dopaminergic signal, controls the fucosylation of the pre-existent or newly synthesized target proteins and is sensitive to dopaminolytic drugs and premedication with 2-deoxy-galactose, which block the fucosylation at the fucose–1-2 galactose linkage and thus prevent the final processing of a

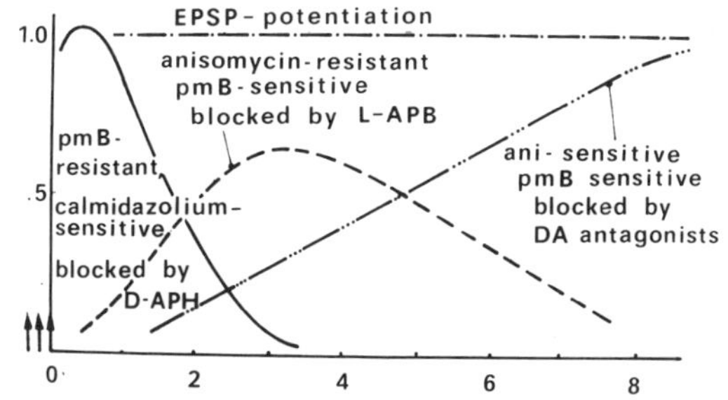

Figure 15.7 Assumed stages of LTP in the Ca 1 region of the rat hippocampus. The first stage induction of LTP and early maintenance—is sensitive to a blockade of NMDA-receptors by D-2-amino-5-phosphonoheptanoate (D-APH), and to an inhibition of calmodulin by calmidazolium, but is resistant to an inhibition of protein kinase C by polymyxin B (pmB). The second stage—intermediate maintenance—is sensitive to L-2-amino-5 phosphonobutyrate (L-APB), an antagonist of a glutamate receptor subtype probably coupled to a phosphoinositol-system, to Polymyxin B (pmB), an inhibitor of protein kinase C, but is resistant to anisomycin, an inhibitor of protein synthesis. The third stage—long lasting maintenance—is prevented by a blockade of dopamine receptors, and sensitive to an inhibition of protein kinase C by polymyxin B (pmB), to an inhibition of protein synthesis by anisomycin, as well as to a prevention of a specific fucosylation by pretreatment with 2-deoxy-galactose (do-gal).

functional membrane protein. Considering such a two-step control of induction of late maintenance by different transmitters, which may be released at somewhat differing stimulus intensities or frequencies, the importance of the parameters of tetanization with regard to the duration of LTP becomes more comprehensible. It seems that the induction and intermediate stage of LTP, which lasts only a few hours, can already be obtained by lower frequencies of tetanization, whereas the release of dopamine mediating the completion of target proteins necessary for the late maintenance possibly requires a high-frequency tetanization of at least 100 Hz. Even if some steps and conditions of these mechanisms involved in the induction and effectuation of long-lasting LTP have to be more precisely elucidated, the present data obviously suggest the necessary role of protein for synthesis for the late maintenance of LTP.

REFERENCES

Bliss, T. V. P., M. L. Errington, G. Evan, and S. P. Hunt (1988). Induction of c-fos-like protein in rat hippocampus following electrical stimulation. *Journal of Physiology* 398:96.

Deadwyler, S. A., T. Dunwiddie, and G. Lynch (1987). A critical level of protein synthesis is required for long-term potentiation. *Synapse* 1:90–95.

Dragunow, M., et al. (1989). Long-term potentiation and the induction of c-fos mRNA and proteins in the dentate gyrus of unanaesthetized rats. *Neuroscience Letters* 101:274–280.

Frey, U., et al. (1989). Long-term potentiation induced in dendrites separated from their CA1 pyramidal somata does not establish a late phase. *Neuroscience Letters* 97:135–139.

Frey, U., M. Krug, K. Reymann, and H. Matthies (1988). Anisomycin, an inhibitor of protein synthesis, blocks late phases of LTP-phenomena in the hippocampal CA-region in vitro. *Brain Research* 452:57–65.

Frey, U., H. Schroeder, and H. Matthies (1990). Dopaminergic antagonists prevent long-term maintenance of posttetanic LTP in the CA1 region of rat hippocampal slices. *Brain Research* 522:69–75.

Jork, R., B. Lössner, and H. Matthies (1978). Hippocampal activation and incorporation of macromolecule precursors. *Pharmacology Biochemistry and Behavior* 9:709–712.

Jork, R., B. Lössner, and H. Matthies (1979). Dopamine and macromolecule synthesis in rat hippocampus. *Pharmacology Biochemistry and Behavior* 11:247–249.

Jork, R., G. Grecksch, and H. Matthies (1986). Impairment of glycoprotein fucosylation in rat hippocampus and the consequences on memory formation. *Pharmacology Biochemistry and Behavior* 25:1137–1144.

Krug, M., B. Lössner, and T. Ott (1984). Anisomycin blocks the late phase of long-term potentiation in the dentate gyrus of freely moving rats. *Brain Research Bulletin* 13:39–42.

Lössner, B., C. Schweigert, M. Krug, and H. K. Matthies (1990). Posttetanic long-term potentiation in the dentate gyrus of freely moving rats is accompanied by an increase in protein synthesis. *Biomedica Biochimica Acta* 49:385–392.

Matthies, H. (1989). In search of cellular mechanisms of memory. *Progress in Neurobiology* 32:277–349.

Mihaly, A., et al. (1990). Transient increase of rat protein kinase-like immunoreactivity in the rat dentate gyrus during long-term potentiation. *Neuroscience Letters* 116:45–50.

Otani, S., C. J. Marshall, W. P. Tate, and G. V. Goddard (1989). Maintenance of long-term potentiation in rat dentate gyrus requires protein synthesis but not messenger RNA synthesis immediately postetanization. *Neuroscience* 28:519–526.

Ott, T., and H. Matthies (1978). Lernen und Gedächtnis. In R. A. Stamm und H. Zeier (eds.), *Die Psychologie des 20. Jahrhunderts. Bd. VI, Lorenz und die Folgen.* Zürich: Kindler Verlag AG, pp. 988–1018.

Pohle, W., and H. Matthies (1971). The incorporation of (3H)-uridine monophosphate into the rat brain during a training period. A microautoradiographic study. *Brain Research* 29:123–127.

Pohle, W., and H. Matthies (1974). Incorporation of 3H-leucine into brain cells after learning. *Pharmacology Biochemistry and Behavior* 2:573–577.

Popov, N., et al. (1976). Increased fucose incorporation into rat hippocampus during learning. A biochemical and microautoradiographic study. *Brain Research* 101:295–304.

Popov, N., S. Schulzeck, S. Schmidt, and H. Matthies (1975). Changes in labeling of soluble and insoluble rat brain proteins using (3H)-tyrosine as precursor during a learning experiment. *Acta Biologica Medica Germanica* 34:1863–1867.

Reymann, K. G., et al. (1985). The duration of long-term potentiation in the CA1 region of the hippocampal slice preparation. *Brain Research Bulletin* 15:249–255.

Reymann, K. G., U. Frey, R. Jork, and H. Matthies (1988). Polymyxin B, an inhibitor of protein kinase C, prevents the maintenance of synaptic long-term potentiation in hippocampal CA1 neurons. *Brain Research* 440:305–314.

Stanton, P. K., and J. M. Sarvey (1984). Blockade of long-term potentiation in rat hippocampus CA1 region by inhibitors of protein synthesis. *Journal of Neuroscience* 4:3080–3088.

Stanton, P. K., and J. M. Sarvey (1985). Blockade of norepinephrine induced long-lasting potentiation in the hippocampal dentate gyrus by an inhibitor of protein synthesis. *Brain Research* 361:276–283.

Tischmeyer, W., et al. (1990). Accumulation of c-fos mRNA in rat hippocampus during acquisition of a brightness discrimination. *Behavioral and Neural Biology* 54:165–171.

IV Relationship Between Long-Term Potentiation and Learning and Memory

16 Behaviorally Induced Synaptic Enhancement: Memory or Modulation?

Carol A. Barnes, Bruce L. McNaughton, and Cynthia A. Erickson

LTE AS AN INFORMATION STORAGE MECHANISM

For the past two decades, our knowledge of the ways in which the mammalian central nervous system can be modified through electrically induced synaptic activity has increased remarkably. For example, as in the peripheral nervous system, synaptic efficacy in the hippocampal formation can be increased for relatively short periods ranging from milliseconds (facilitation; Landau et al., 1973; McNaughton, 1980), seconds (augmentation; Magleby and Zengel, 1976; McNaughton, 1982), to minutes (potentiation; Birks, 1977; Magleby, 1973; Magleby and Zengel, 1975; McNaughton, 1982). In addition to these short-lasting processes of synaptic modification, the brain also possesses a more durable form of synaptic change originally described by Bliss, Lømo, and Gardner-Medwin (Lømo, 1966; Bliss and Lømo, 1973; Bliss and Gardner-Medwin, 1973) that can last anywhere from several hours to several weeks, depending on stimulus conditions and other variables. This phenomenon has been called long-lasting potentiation (Bliss and Lømo, 1973), long-term potentiation (LTP; Douglas and Goddard, 1975), or long-term enhancement (LTE; McNaughton et al., 1978). Primarily to distinguish the long-lasting synaptic change observed after high-frequency stimulation from shorter-lasting synaptic changes (e.g., potentiation; see McNaughton, 1982), we refer to the phenomenon as LTE in this chapter.

Although LTE has been studied primarily in the hippocampal formation, it is not exclusively found there (Artola and Singer, 1987; Bindman et al., 1988; Lee, 1982; Racine et al., 1983; Voronin, 1985; Wilhite et al., 1986; Wilson, 1984). The emphasis on the hippocampus probably reflects the ease with which recordings can be made from this structure and the ability to make relatively straightforward interpretations of the extracellular field potentials elicited there. It is also of some importance that the hippocampus, a structure strongly implicated in mnemonic function (Kesner and Dimattia, 1987; Mishkin et al., 1984; O'Keefe and Nadel, 1978; Olton et al., 1979; Scoville and Milner, 1957; Squire et al., 1984; Sutherland and Rudy, 1989; Teyler and Discenna, 1986) also shows forms of stimulation-induced plasticity that are quite durable (Barnes, 1979; Barnes and McNaughton, 1980, 1985; Bliss and Gardner-Medwin, 1973; de Toledo-

Morrell and Morrell, 1985; Douglas and Goddard, 1975; Racine et al., 1983; Staubli and Lynch, 1987). These observations have engendered questions concerning whether this form of synaptic alteration actually underlies behaviorally relevant information storage when elicited by natural patterned neural activity. This is a technically difficult question to address, although modest inroads to this problem are being achieved using freely behaving animals (as we discuss in this chapter).

Because obtaining direct proof that LTE is involved in learning is difficult, the basic approach taken by most researchers has been to design experiments in such a way that, if unambiguous results were obtained, it would be possible to disprove, or to cast into serious doubt, the hypothesis that associative memory is based on LTE-like synaptic changes. The results obtained from experiments using this approach have, to this date, been positive rather than negative. Examples of such data include the findings of correlations between the persistence of LTE and memory (e.g., Barnes, 1979), and the disruption of memory and new learning by bilateral saturation of the LTE process (McNaughton et al., 1986; Castro et al., 1989) or by blocking the NMDA receptors that are necessary for the induction of LTE (Morris et al., 1986; Morris, 1989). Another approach to this question attempts to relate artificially induced LTE to a process of synaptic strengthening that is behaviorally induced and may share common mechanisms with LTE. It is this behaviorally induced synaptic change that is the primary topic of this chapter.

Extracellular field potential recording methods have been used in the search for experience-dependent LTE-like synaptic modification because, at present, this is the only way in which this problem can be studied in freely behaving animals. Detecting changes resulting from a learning event in a large population of synaptic responses, such as that represented by the field potential may, at first consideration, seem to be unrealistic. It would be particularly difficult to detect learning-related changes in systems that have a large, long-term information storage capacity and presumably must therefore use only a small proportion of their modifiable synapses for any given memory (or alternatively, a small proportion of their total modifiability). Because the synaptic modification found at the perforant path–granule cell synapse in the hippocampus does not appear to be permanent (e.g., Barnes, 1979; Castro et al., 1989), the original idea was that it may, therefore, be possible to detect learning-related changes in this system. In the case of a system that stores information only temporarily, more of the modifiable synapses might conceivably be used for any given event (e.g., see Marr, 1971).

SHORT-TERM EXPLORATORY MODULATION (STEM)

In fact, the first indication that a behaviorally induced synaptic change might be detectable from field potential records in the hippocampus came from the observation that if one recorded a series of 10 responses sequentially immediately after the rat had been connected to the recording apparatus, and then again 5 minutes later, the averaged synaptic response recorded on the second series was always larger than the one elicited soon after being transported to the recording room (Barnes, 1979). The reasons for this reliable synaptic increase were unknown at that time. Sharp and her colleagues (1989), however, clarified the conditions under which such increases in perforant path–granule cell synaptic responses can be obtained: specifically, the magnitude of the synaptic change appears to be related to the occurrence of exploratory behaviors that rats exhibit when they are placed into relatively novel environments. For this reason we have referred to this phenomenon as short-term exploratory modulation (STEM).

A clear demonstration of this effect was provided in an experiment in which a rat was simply removed from its home cage where it had been sitting quietly and placed into a relatively novel recording chamber. This simple manipulation induced the rat to explore freely without any particular reward. The exploration of the new recording chamber was accompanied by a gradual increase in the synaptic response over the period of exploration. The synaptic growth was of a magnitude that is at least equal to the changes seen after electrically induced LTE. In fact, the change in synaptic strength is rather well described by the time integral of exploratory behavior less a decay ("forgetting") term. Using the behavioral scores as input, Sharp and coworkers (1989) computed the numerical integral of the equation:

$$d(\mathrm{EPSP})/dt = -k_1(\mathrm{EPSP} - 1) + k_2(B)$$

where EPSP (excitatory postsynaptic potential) is the amplitude of the EPSP normalized to a baseline value of 1.0, and B is the behavioral score (1 for exploration, 0 otherwise) at the time of the evoked potential. The only two free empirical parameters, k_1 and k_2, are constants that regulate the decay of the enhanced component of the EPSP and the fractional growth per unit of exploration respectively. As can be seen in figure 16.1, this simple mathematical description of the data can account quite closely for the empirical responses obtained. The importance of this simple relationship is that it reinforces the observation that the STEM phenomenon is not at all related to the *moment-to-moment* behavior of the animal, but rather to the *recent history* of exploratory behavior. Because these synaptic alterations outlast changes in the behavior that produced them, they are distinguishable from the behavioral state "gating" effect described by Winson and Abzug (1977, 1978). It appears, therefore, that the fascia dentata may exhibit a form of temporary memory for recent exploration activity.

In addition to STEM's not being caused by momentary behavioral state changes, a number of other possible nonspecific factors have been ruled out. These include the fact that STEM has been dissociated from the effects of the electrical stimulation used to measure it and the manipula-

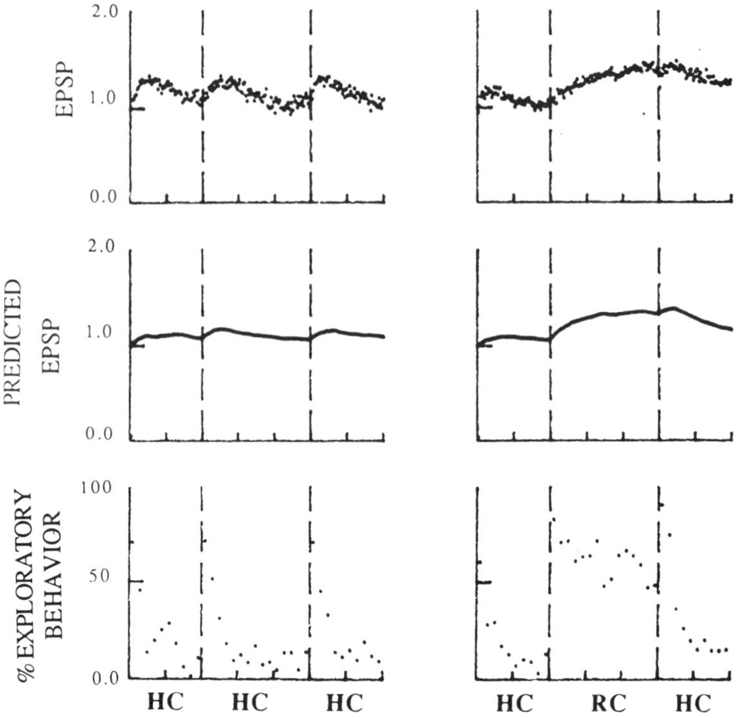

Figure 16.1 Averaged normalized values from 6 rats of the field EPSP (top row), group means of percentage of observations during which exploratory behavior occurred during these sessions (averaged over 1-minute bins, bottom row), and predicted EPSP values obtained from the application of the equation described in the text (middle row). Use of this temporal-integration model provided a much better fit to the overall data pattern than could be obtained by taking into account only the instantaneous behavioral state. The vertical dashed lines indicate the time at which the rats were picked up, handled briefly, and then either replaced into the home (HC) or placed into the recording chamber (RC). (Data from Sharp et al., 1989; figure 3.)

tions involved in the handling and transport of the rat to a new environment do not, alone, produce the STEM effect (Sharp et al., 1989). Furthermore, changes in presynaptic excitability are not involved. This was demonstrated by showing that the amplitude of the presynaptic fiber potential remains constant during the synaptic growth (Green et al., 1990a). Also, there is no change in the threshold level of the EPSP at which the population spike begins, thus indicating that the state of polarization of the granule cells does not change during STEM (Green et al., 1990a). As with electrically induced LTE, STEM is not due to posttetanic potentiation (PTP). That is, there is no apparent change in the probability of transmitter release during STEM as assessed indirectly by the paired-pulse method (McNaughton, 1982; Green et al., 1990a). In addition, the EPSP change during STEM is of equal magnitude whether the response is recorded at the current source in the granule cell layer or at the current sink in the stratum moleculare (Green et al., 1990a). This observation is important, as it implies that the effect does not involve a redistribution of current sources and sinks in the granule cell dendrites and that the effect is localized to the fascia dentata and not volume conducted from elsewhere.

Because of the close relationship between exploratory behavior and the synaptic response increases observed during STEM it was possible that the growth was related to motor activity or to the hippocampal EEG theta rhythm, both of which accompany such behavior. To test for the contribution of motor behavior to the synaptic changes generated during STEM, rats were forced to locomote in a motorized treadmill. In this situation the sensory input to the animal does not change as a result of movement, but there is robust locomotor behavior and hippocampal theta rhythm. The synaptic response recorded in the treadmill, however, does not increase as it does during exploration-related movement. This tends to argue against the idea that STEM is a result of the locomotor activity per se that normally accompanies exploration. These data also suggest that the theta rhythm may not be critically involved in the STEM effect because theta is even more robust under treadmill conditions than under normal exploratory activity. This conclusion was verified in two additional ways: by inactivating the medial septal projection and fibers of passage to the hippocampus temporarily, with microapplication of a local anesthetic (Green et al., 1990a), or permanently with electrolytic lesions of the medial septum (Green et al., 1990b). When tetracaine is injected into the medial septum (a treatment that temporarily abolishes hippocampal theta; Mizumori et al., 1989), the perforant path–granule cell evoked field synaptic response still exhibits normal growth when the animal explores its environment. In addition, septal lesions have no effect on the behaviorally induced EPSP growth at that synapse (Green et al., 1990b). Thus, neither the septum nor the fibers coursing through that area contribute to the STEM phenomenon.

It appears, therefore, to be the exploration rather than the accompanying movement or EEG theta rhythm that is the necessary condition for the EPSP growth during STEM. Whether this behaviorally induced change in the synaptic response elicited in the fascia dentata involves any of the same mechanisms as electrically induced LTE remains to be determined.

One aspect of STEM that clearly distinguishes it from LTE is that the population spike amplitude actually becomes smaller during exploratory behavior, whereas the population spike amplitude is larger after LTE (see figure 16.2). Paradoxically, however, the population spike onset latency and peak shift to the left both in STEM and in LTE. This shift suggests that the granule cells are in fact being depolarized during STEM, but that some additional process is influencing the spike amplitude. Our working model of how these apparently discrepant changes in the perforant path–granule synapse may arise is that exploration in a given environment results in the strengthening and firing of a small, specific set of perforant path afferents. These afferents are presumably driven by the particular sensory

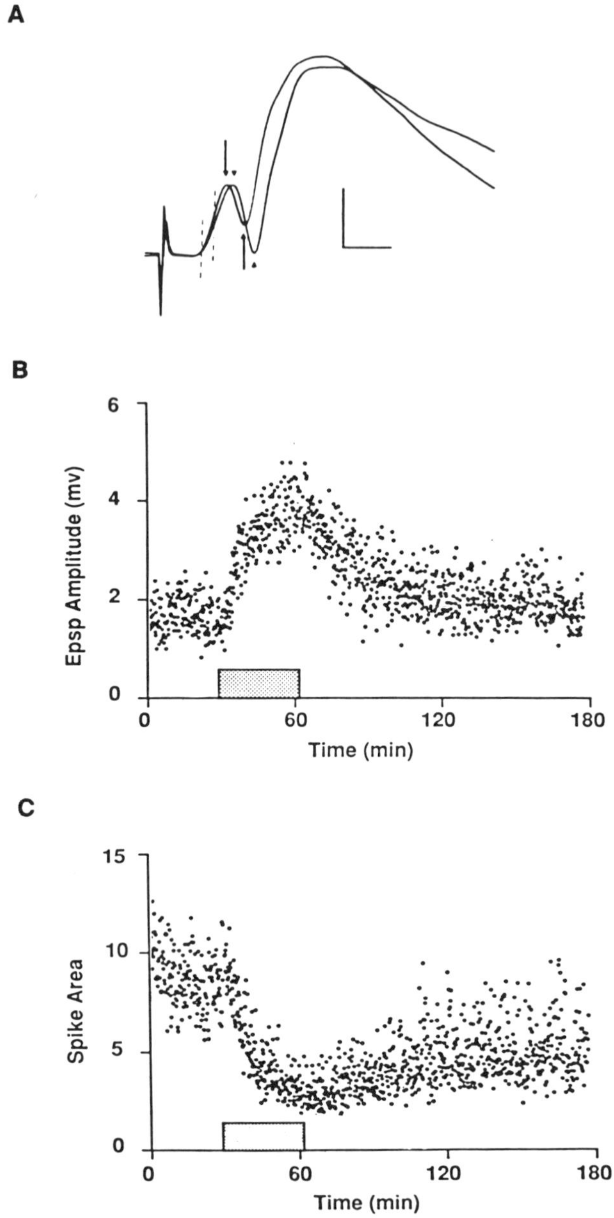

Figure 16.2 (A) Representative evoked responses elicited at the perforant path–granule cell synapse before exploration and 16 minutes after transferring a rat from its home environment. The dashed lines show the approximate points of measurement of the EPSP, the falling arrows depict the onset of the population spike, and the rising arrows indicate the peak of the population spike. Note that although the population spike amplitude gets smaller during exploration the onset and peak latency shift to the left. (B, C) Example of the STEM effect, characterized by increases in the synaptic response (B) and a decline in population spike amplitude (C). The shaded bar indicates the time period during which the rat was actively exploring on an open platform. During the time period before and after the bar the rat was relatively inactive in its home cage. Note that these two components of the synaptic response behave independently of one another, although they are both influenced by the onset of exploratory behavior. (Data after Green et al., 1990a.)

features present in a given environment. This strengthening of a subset of afferents would be enough to explain the overall increase observed in the EPSP. The persistent decline in population spike amplitude while the latency of the spike shifts to the left might be explained by a combination of two factors. First, perforant path fibers also make contact onto inhibitory interneurons, and it is possible that, during exploration, the strength of excitatory connections onto the inhibitory interneurons also increases. This increase could at least partly account for the reduced spike amplitude. There may also be some contribution to the general decline in spike amplitude from changes in the excitability of inhibitory interneurons as a result of some secondary, possibly subcortical source. This source is not the medial septum, as has just been discussed, but perhaps, for example, the locus coeruleus or median raphe. Whatever the exact mechanism, the overall pattern of change suggests the possibility that exploration may result in a substantial increase in the specificity of granule cell output. One function of such a change might be the formation of an efficient representation of the local environment involving relatively few granule cells.

DO STEM AND LTE SHARE COMMON MECHANISMS?

One way to begin to test the ideas about STEM's potential relation to LTE is to determine whether this behaviorally induced synaptic change involves the same pharmacological receptors as electrically induced LTE. To address this question we examine the effects of the noncompetitive NMDA receptor antagonist MK-801 on the STEM phenomenon at the perforant path–granule cell synapse.

For this experiment rats were prepared for chronic recording of granule cell evoked field potentials elicited by stimulation of the perforant path (essentially as described in Barnes, 1979). Responses were recorded over a baseline period of 90 minutes while the rats were alert but not moving in their home cages, and then for 20 minutes while they were encouraged to explore on an open platform in the same room. Recording continued for an additional 90 minutes after the rats had been returned to their home cages. One hour before the exploratory period, saline or doses of 0.30 mg/kg or 0.08 mg/kg of the NMDA receptor blocker MK-801 were administered intraperitoneally. These treatments were counterbalanced across animals. (For preliminary reports see also Erickson et al., 1990, and Barnes et al., 1990.)

In control (saline) sessions, exploratory activity produced a gradual but robust growth in the field EPSP that persisted long after the rat was returned to its home cage (figure 16.3). This EPSP growth was significantly reduced ($F\ [2, 6] = 15.98$; $p < .001$) in a dose-dependent fashion during MK-801 sessions (see figure 16.3). The population spike, however, was unaffected by this treatment.

The fact that NMDA receptors are involved in producing the synaptic

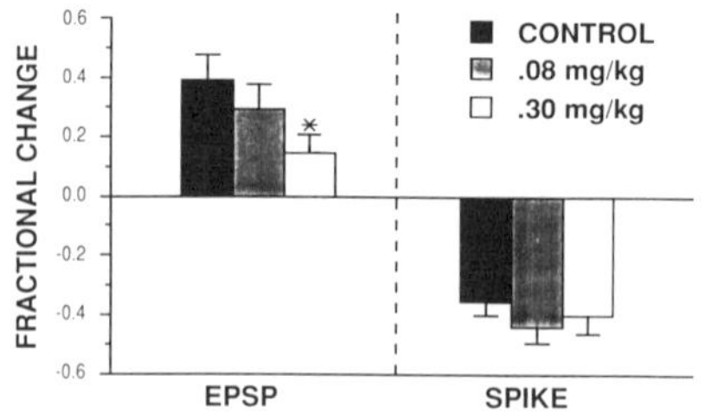

Figure 16.3 Averaged data from rats given either saline, 0.08 or 0.30 mg/kg of MK-801 in a counterbalanced fashion 1 hr before they were encouraged to explore on an open platform. The fractional change is measured between baseline (quiet in home cage) compared with responses obtained after 15 min of exploration. Notice that the synaptic response increase normally seen during exploration was blocked in a dose-dependent fashion after the MK-801 treatment (see text), while the decline of population spike amplitude was unaffected by this treatment.

increases seen during STEM, much as they are involved in the induction of stimulation-induced LTE (Abraham and Mason, 1988) suggests that these processes may use certain common mechanisms. The lack of effect on the population spike by an NMDA antagonist also supports the general notion that these components of modification of the field potential can be clearly dissociated. On the other hand, it remains possible that MK-801 disrupts the neural activity patterns that are necessary for the induction of the exploration effect, rather than acting directly on the synapses recorded. To examine this issue directly, experiments must be designed that apply NMDA antagonists in a restricted fashion to the synapses in question. Furthermore, it will be of interest to determine how artificially induced LTE and STEM interact in the same animal. With these questions answered, a clearer assessment of the relationship, if any, between LTE and STEM will be possible. Even if it develops that this exploration-induced synaptic change uses different mechanisms than those invoked in LTE, exploring whether STEM reflects nonspecific modulatory processes with little information content or whether it reflects memory or information storage of specific environments will still be important. The possibility should not be overlooked that a naturally occurring plastic process such as STEM may, in fact, reflect actual information storage mechanisms, and that LTE may be the epiphenomenon.

ACKNOWLEDGMENTS

This work was supported by grants AG03376 and MH00897 and the National Science Foundation.

REFERENCES

Abraham, W. C., and S. E. Mason (1988). Effects of the NMDA receptor/channel antagonists CPP and MK-801 on hippocampal field potentials and long-term potentiation in anesthetized rats. *Brain Research* 462:40–46.

Artola, A., and W. Singer (1987). Long-term potentiation and NMDA receptors in rat visual cortex. *Nature* 330:649–652.

Barnes, C. A. (1979). Memory deficits associated with senescence: a neurophysiological and behavioral study in the rat. *Journal of Comparative and Physiological Psychology* 93:74–104.

Barnes, C. A., C. A. Erickson, and B. L. McNaughton (1990). Links between synaptic plasticity and behavior. *Clinical Neuropharmacology* (in press).

Barnes, C. A., and B. L. McNaughton (1980). Spatial memory and hippocampal synaptic plasticity in senescent and middle-aged rats. In D. Stein (ed.), *Psychobiology of Aging: Problems and Perspectives*. Amsterdam: Elsevier, pp. 253–272.

Barnes, C. A., and B. L. McNaughton (1985). An age comparison of the rates of acquisition and forgetting of spatial information in relation to long-term enhancement of hippocampal synapses. *Behavioral Neuroscience* 99:1040–1048.

Bindman, L. J., K. P. S. J. Murphy, and S. Pockett (1988). Postsynaptic control of the induction of long-term changes in efficacy of transmission at neocortical synapses in slices of rat brain. *Journal of Neurophysiology* 60:1053–1065.

Birks, R. I. (1977). A long-lasting potentiation of transmitter release related to an increase in transmitter stores in a sympathetic ganglion. *Journal of Physiology (London)* 232:331–356.

Bliss, T. V. P., and A. R. Gardner-Medwin (1973). Long-lasting potentiation of synaptic transmission in the dentate area of the unanaesthetised rabbit following stimulation of the perforant path. *Journal of Physiology (London)* 232:357–374.

Bliss, T. V. P., and T. Lømo (1973). Long-lasting potentiation of synaptic transmission in the dentate area of the anaesthetized rabbit following stimulation of the perforant path. *Journal of Physiology (London)* 232:331–356.

Castro, C. A., L. H. Silbert, B. L. McNaughton, and C. A. Barnes (1989). Recovery of spatial learning deficits following decay of electrically induced synaptic enhancement in the hippocampus. *Nature* 342:545–548.

de Toledo-Morrell, L., and F. Morrell (1985). Electrophysiological markers of aging and memory loss in rats. *Annals of the New York Academy of Science* 444:296–311.

Douglas, R. M., and G. V. Goddard (1975). Long-term potentiation of the perforant path-granule cell synapse in the rat hippocampus. *Brain Research* 86:205–215.

Erickson, C. A., B. L. McNaughton, and C. A. Barnes (1990). Exploration-dependent enhancement of synaptic responses in rat fascia dentata is blocked by MK-801. *Society for Neuroscience Abstracts* 16:442.

Green, E. J., B. L. McNaughton, and C. A. Barnes (1990a). Exploration-dependent modulation of evoked responses in fascia dentata: dissociation of motor, EEG and sensory factors, and evidence for a synaptic efficacy change. *Journal of Neuroscience* 10:1455–1471.

Green, E. J., B. L. McNaughton, and C. A. Barnes (1990b). Role of the medial septum and hippocampal theta rhythm in exploration-related synaptic efficacy changes in rat fascia dentata. *Brain Research* 529:102–108.

Kesner, R. P., and B. V. Dimattia (1987). Neurobiology of an attribute model of memory. *Progress in Psychobiology and Physiological Psychology* 12:207–277.

Landau, E. M., A. Smolinsky, and Y. Lass (1973). Post-tetanic potentiation and facilitation do not share a common calcium-dependent mechanism. *Nature* 244:155–157.

Lee, K. S. (1982). Sustained enhancement of evoked potentials following brief, high-frequency stimulation of the cerebral cortex in vitro. *Brain Research* 239:617–623.

Lømo, T. (1966). Frequency potentiation of excitatory synaptic activity in the dentate area of the hippocampal formation. *Acta Physiologica Scandinavia (Supplement)* 68:128.

Magleby, K. L. (1973). The effect of tetanic and post-tetanic potentiation on facilitation of transmitter release at the frog neuromuscular junction. *Journal of Physiology (London)* 234:353–371.

Magleby, K. L., and J. E. Zengel (1975). A quantitative description of tetanic and post-tetanic potentiation of transmitter release at the frog neuromuscular junction. *Journal of Physiology (London)* 245:183–208.

Magleby, K. L., and J. E. Zengel (1976). Augmentation: a process that acts to increase transmitter release at the frog neuromuscular junction. *Journal of Physiology (London)* 257:449–470.

Marr, D. (1971). Simple memory: a theory for archicortex. *Philosophical Translations of the Royal Society (London)* B262:23–81.

McNaughton, B. L. (1980). Evidence for two physiologically distinct perforant pathways to the fascia dentata in rat. *Brain Research* 199:1–19.

McNaughton, B. L. (1982). Long-term enhancement and short-term potentiation in rat fascia dentata act through different mechanisms. *Journal of Physiology (London)* 324:249–262.

McNaughton, B. L., R. M. Douglas, and G. V. Goddard (1978). Synaptic enhancement in fascia dentata: cooperativity among coactive afferents. *Brain Research* 157:277–293.

McNaughton, B. L., et al. (1986). Long-term enhancement of hippocampal synaptic transmission and the acquisition of spatial information. *Journal of Neuroscience* 6:563–571.

Mishkin, M., B. J. Malamut, and J. Bachevalier (1984). Memories and habits: two neural systems. In G. S. Lynch, J. L. McGaugh, and N. M. Weinberger (eds.), *Neurobiology of Learning and Memory*. New York: Guilford Press, pp. 65–88.

Mizumori, S. J. Y., B. L. McNaughton, C. A. Barnes, and K. B. Fox (1989). Preserved spatial coding in hippocampal CA1 pyramidal cells during reversible suppression of CA3c output: evidence for pattern completion in hippocampus. *Journal of Neuroscience* 9:3915–3928.

Morris, R. G. M. (1989). Synaptic plasticity and learning: selective impairment of learning in rats and blockade of long-term potentiation in vivo by the *N*-methyl-D-aspartate receptor antagonist AP5. *Journal of Neuroscience* 9:3040–3057.

Morris, R. G. M., E. Anderson, G. S. Lynch, and M. Baudry (1986). Selective impairment of learning and blockade of long-term potentiation by an *N*-methyl-D-aspartate receptor antagonist, AP5. *Nature* 319:774–776.

O'Keefe, J., and L. Nadel (1978). *The Hippocampus as a Cognitive Map*. Oxford: Clarendon Press.

Olton, D. S., J. T. Becker, and G. E. Handelmann (1979). Hippocampus, space, and memory. *Behavioral and Brain Sciences* 2:313–365.

Racine, R. J., N. W. Milgram, and S. Hafner (1983). Long-term potentiation phenomena in the rat limbic forebrain. *Brain Research* 260:217–231.

Scoville, W. B., and B. Milner (1957). Loss of recent memory after bilateral hippocampal lesions. *Journal of Neurology, Neurosurgery, and Psychiatry* 20:11–21.

Sharp, P. E., B. L. McNaughton, and C. A. Barnes (1989). Exploration-dependent modulation of evoked responses in fascia dentata: fundamental observations and time course. *Psychobiology* 17:257–269.

Squire, L. R., N. J. Cohen, and L. Nadel (1984). The medial temporal region and memory consolidation: a new hypothesis. In G. Weingartner and E. Parker (eds.), *Memory Consolidation*. Hillsdale, N.J.: Erlbaum, pp. 185–210.

Staubli, U., and G. Lynch (1987). Stable hippocampal long-term potentiation elicited by "theta" pattern stimulation. *Brain Research* 435:227–234.

Sutherland, R. J., and J. W. Rudy (1989). Configural association theory: the role of the hippocampal formation in learning, memory, and amnesia. *Psychobiology* 17:129–144.

Teyler, T. J., and P. Discenna (1986). The hippocampal memory indexing theory. *Behavioral Neuroscience* 100:147–154.

Voronin, L. L. (1985). Synaptic plasticity at archicortical and neocortical levels. *Neurofiziologiya* 16:651–665.

Wilhite, B. L., T. J. Teyler, and C. Hendricks (1986). Functional relations of the rodent claustral-entorhinal-hippocampal system. *Brain Research* 365:54–60.

Wilson, D. A. (1984). Comparison of the postnatal development of postactivation potentiation in the neocortex and dentate gyrus of the rat. *Developmental Brain Research* 16:61–68.

Winson, J., and C. Abzug (1978). Neuronal transmission through hippocampal pathways dependent on behavior. *Journal of Neurophysiology* 41:716–732.

Winson, J., and C. Abzug (1978). Neuronal transmission through hippocampal pathways dependent on behavior. *Journal of Neurophysiology* 41:716–732.

17 Memory Facilitation Induced by *N*-methyl-D-aspartate Blockade

Cesare Mondadori
and Lawrence Weiskrantz

The discovery of *N*-methyl-D-aspartate (NMDA) blockers as pharmacological tools has raised hopes that they may help clarify some of the fundamentals of the physiology of memory. One of the central questions is whether, as suggested by Teyler and Discenna (1987) and Collingridge and Bliss (1987), learning and memory are basically mediated by a process analogous to long-term potentiation (LTP; i.e., the sustained enhancement of synaptic efficacy that can be induced experimentally by short bursts of high-frequency stimulation).

Induction of LTP has been shown to be prevented by blockade of the NMDA receptors (Collingridge et al., 1983; Harris et al., 1984; Wigström et al., 1986; Coan et al., 1987), which are present in high density in the hippocampus (Monaghan and Cotman, 1985). If the fundamental mechanisms of LTP and learning are the same, it was argued, acute blockade of the NMDA receptors should affect learning in the same way as a lesion of the hippocampus: for example, spatial learning should be impaired (see e.g., Olton et al., 1979; Aggleton et al., 1986; Barnes, 1988). In line with these expectations, Morris and associates (1986) found that intracerebroventricular administration of 2-amino-5-phosphopentanoate (AP5), a competitive NMDA antagonist, disturbs the acquisition performance of rats in a water maze but not in a visual discrimination task.

At first sight, these data present a coherent picture, but many questions remain. Of particular importance within the context of this theory is whether the disparate effects of NMDA blockade in the two tasks were really the result of one task's involving spatial learning and the other task's involving nonspatial learning. In the pharmacology of learning and memory, task-dependency is such a common phenomenon (see e.g., Mondadori, 1981; Mondadori, 1987) that it seemed necessary to examine this aspect more closely. In an extensive series of experiments using a variety of learning tasks, Mondadori and coworkers (1989) showed that the disruptive effects of acute NMDA blockade on memory were strongly dependent on the nature of the learning tasks and not obviously related to their spatial learning components. The most important finding was that disruptive effects on memory were only observed when the antagonist was administered *before* the learning task. Under such conditions, however, there is always a possibility that a disturbance of performance can occur indirectly (e.g., through interference with perception during the learning trial). Under experimental conditions in which such indirect interference effects were excluded by administering the drug immediately after the learning trial, and, again, depending on the task, NMDA blockade had either *positive* effects or no effects at all on the animals' retention performance. The absence of negative effects after post-trial administration has also been reported by other investigators (Venable and Kelly, 1990; Danysz et al., 1988). The observation that in our experiments MK-801, a noncompetitive NMDA antagonist, and AP7, a competitive antagonist, both displayed the same activity profile supports the view that these effects are in fact attributable to an interaction with NMDA mechanisms.

As this memory-facilitating action of NMDA blockers apparently contradicts a general NMDA-blocker-LTP hypothesis of memory, the present experiments were conducted to ascertain whether the facilitatory effect is a general phenomenon (i.e., whether it is also induced by the new, orally active competitive NMDA blocker CGP 37849; Fagg et al., 1990).

The experimental conditions, methods, and procedures and the experimental animals were the same as in our previous studies (Mondadori et al., 1989). Groups of 25 male white mice (Tif:MAGf [SPF]; 20–22 gm) were used in the experiments. They were housed in plastic cages in a room lighted between 6 AM and 6 PM and had free access to food and water throughout the study. The step-down passive-avoidance apparatus consisted of an electrifiable grid enclosed by gray PVC walls 50 cm high. In the middle of the grid was a wooden platform 10 mm high and 67 mm in diameter, surrounded by a removable gray PVC tube. The mice were placed one by one on the platform inside the tube, which was removed after 10 seconds. With a few exceptions, they stepped down from the platform within 20 seconds to explore. As soon as the animals had all four feet on the grid, they received a footshock (1 mA for 1 second) and were then immediately removed from the apparatus. Twenty-four hours after training, each animal was placed on the platform and the step-down latency recorded (retest latency) up to a cutoff time of 150 seconds. Under these conditions, our animals showed low levels of learning: the retest latencies remained low, so that the paradigm was sensitive to facilitation of retention. The retests were carried out blind: the experimenter was unaware of the kind of treatment the animals were receiving.

MK-801 and CGP 37849 were dissolved in methylcellulose (Methocel) and administered intraperitoneally either 30 minutes (MK-801) or 60 minutes (CGP 37849) before the learning trial, or immediately after its completion (post-trial). MK-801 was given in doses ranging from 0.001 to 10 mg/kg and CGP 37849 in doses of 0.001 to 30 mg/kg.

The following results were noted: When administered pretrial, both substances induced a clear-cut, dose-related facilitation of retention performance. As in the initial study (Mondadori et al., 1989), facilitation was only seen in response to low doses (0.003–1 mg/kg MK-801 and 0.01–3 mg/kg CGP 37849); higher doses had no facilitatory effect (figures 17.1 and 17.2). It is interesting that the initial step-down latencies were shortened in a dose-related fashion by MK-801, but not by CGP 37849. The results of post-trial administration differed: whereas MK-801 improved retention performance at all doses tested (in confirmation of our earlier experiments), the effect of CGP 37849 was dose-related: as in the "pre-trial" experiments, low doses led to an improvement, but the higher doses were ineffective. These results are shown in figures 17.3 and 17.4.

These observations clearly confirm our earlier findings and demonstrate that the improvement of memory evoked by low doses of NMDA blockers is a robust and reproducible phenomenon. The similarity between the results obtained with competitive and noncompetitive NMDA blockers indicates that the observed effects were most probably due to blockade of the NMDA receptors. The similarity between the results of

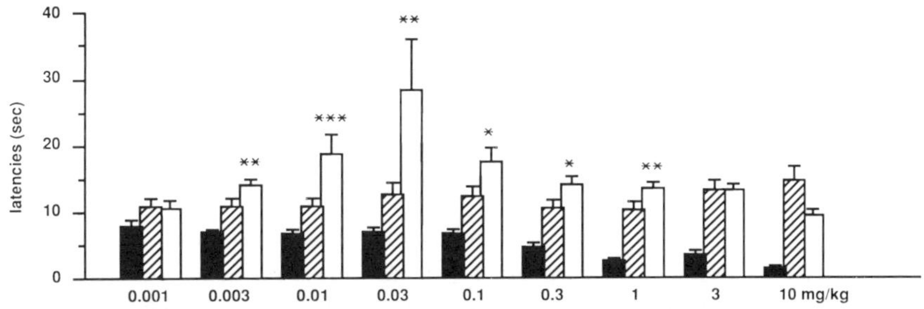

Figure 17.1 Step-down passive avoidance. Effects of MK-801 on retention performance of mice. The compound or vehicle (methylcellulose) was administered intraperitoneally 30 min before the learning trial. Retest was performed after 24 hr. Solid columns: baseline latencies (± SEM). Hatched columns: retest latencies of the vehicle-treated controls. Blank columns: retest latencies of the MK-801–treated animals. All groups, $N = 25$. Prolonged retest latencies (in comparison to vehicle-treated controls) are indicative of (drug-induced) better learning. * = $p < .05$; ** = $p < .01$; *** = $p < .001$ (Mann-Whitney U-test, two-tailed).

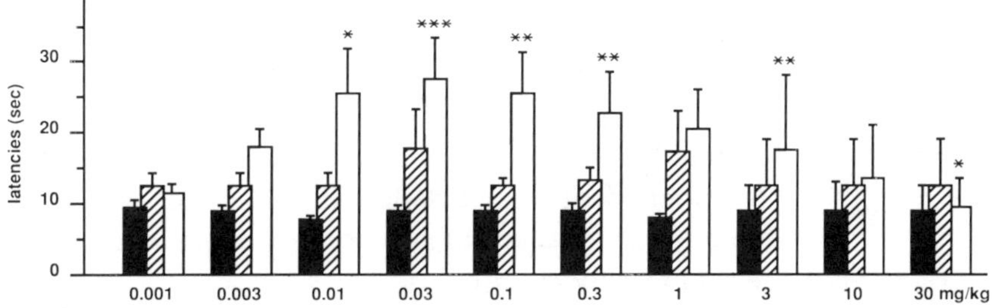

Figure 17.2 Step-down passive avoidance. Effects of CGP 37849 on retention performance of mice. The compound or vehicle (methylcellulose) was administered intraperitoneally 60 min before the learning trial. Retest was performed after 24 hr. Blank columns: retest latencies of the CGP 37849–treated animals. For further explanation see legend to figure 17.1.

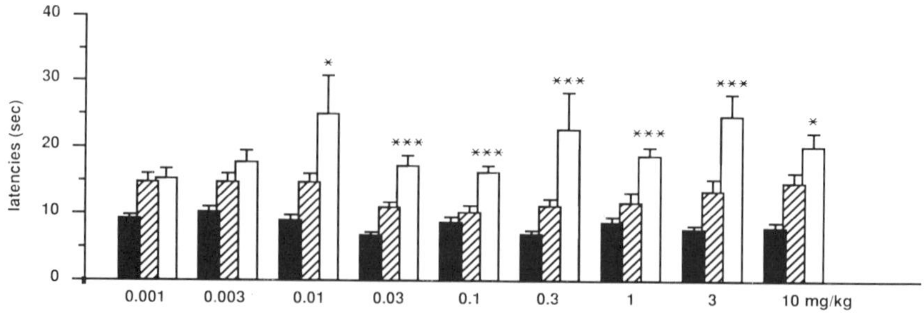

Figure 17.3 Step-down passive avoidance. Effects of MK-801 on retention performance of mice. The compound or vehicle (methylcellulose) was administered intraperitoneally immediately after the learning trial. Retest was performed after 24 hr. For further explanation see legend to figure 17.1.

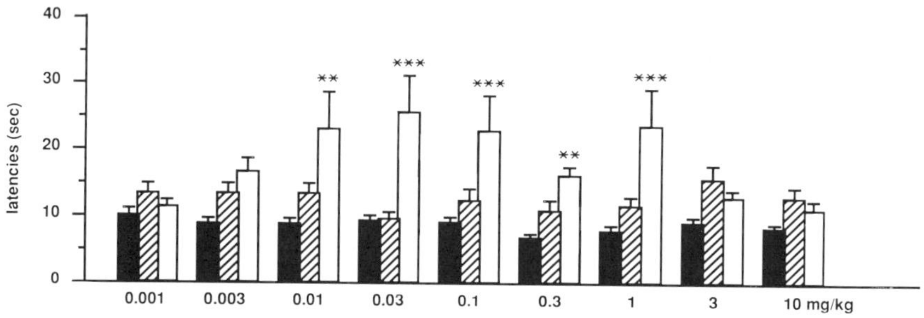

Figure 17.4 Step-down passive avoidance. Effects of CGP 37849 on retention performance of mice. The compound or vehicle (methylcellulose) was administered intraperitoneally immediately after the learning trial. Retest was performed after 24 hr. Blank columns: retest latencies of the CGP 37849–treated animals. For further explanation see legend to figure 17.1.

the experiments performed pretrial and post-trial indicates that the positive effects are likely due to an influence on memory processes, and are not mediated by indirect effects resulting from alterations of perception, emotion, motivation, and so on. The differences between the results produced by MK-801 and CGP 37849 on post-trial administration show that competitive NMDA blockers (the same effects were induced by CGP 39551; unpublished results) only elicit the observed effects on memory within a certain range of doses, whereas MK-801 is active over the entire dose range tested, even at doses causing severe side-effects. The suspicion that MK-801 already provokes side-effects in the dose-range used is strengthened by the curtailment of the step-down (baseline) latencies seen after pretrial administration (compare figure 17.1).

All modulations of retention performance after post-trial administration of drugs are ascribed to direct effects on still unconcluded memory processes (compare, e.g., McGaugh and Herz, 1972). Up to now, the length of time after a learning trial during which modulations were still possible has been assumed to range from some minutes to about 1 hour (McGaugh and Herz, 1972); Inhibitors of protein synthesis are the sole exceptions being active after even longer intervals (Gibbs and Ng, 1977). Recent experiments with memory-enhancing substances (nootropics) now disclose interesting new aspects: piracetam and oxiracetam can still improve the retention performance of laboratory animals when given 8 hours, but not as long as 16 hours, after the learning trial (Mondadori et al., 1991). In a series of experiments, it was demonstrated that the sensitivity period depends on the substance administered: strychnine was still active if given 1, but not 2, hours after the learning trial; physostigmine after 2, but not 4 hours (Mondadori et al., 1991). It therefore seemed important to determine the duration of the sensitivity of memory to the effects of NMDA blockers.

To examine this aspect experimentally, we administered MK-801 and CGP 37849 at different times (0, 1, 2, 4, 8, and 16 hours) after the learning situation and tested retention performance 3 days later. The long retention interval was chosen to exclude any possibility that the substances might still be active at the time of the retention trial. The results were unequivocal: both MK-801 and CGP 37849 improved the animals' retention performance when given 1, 2, 4, or 8 hours after the learning trial, but not 16 hours after. The results are shown in figures 17.5 and 17.6. Concurrent control experiments without footshock gave no indication of drug-induced changes in the retest latencies. These control experiments and the time-dependency of the effect (no effect at an interval of 16 hours) rule

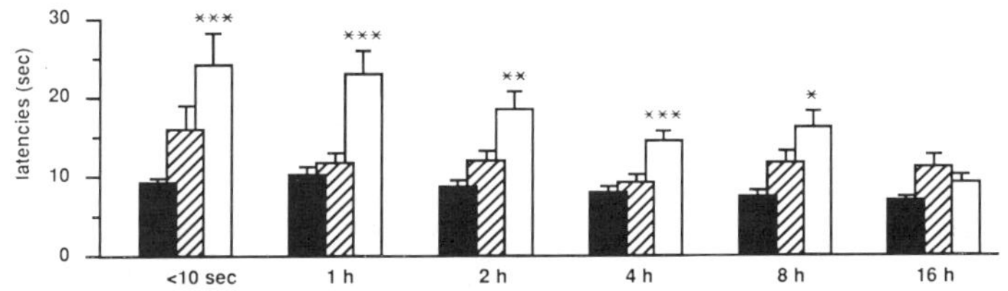

Figure 17.5 Step-down passive avoidance. Effects of MK-801 on retention performance of mice. The compound or vehicle (methylcellulose) was administered intraperitoneally at various intervals (10 sec, 1 hr, 2 hr, 4 hr, 8 hr, and 16 hr) after the learning trial. Retest was performed after 3 days. For further explanation see legend to figure 17.1.

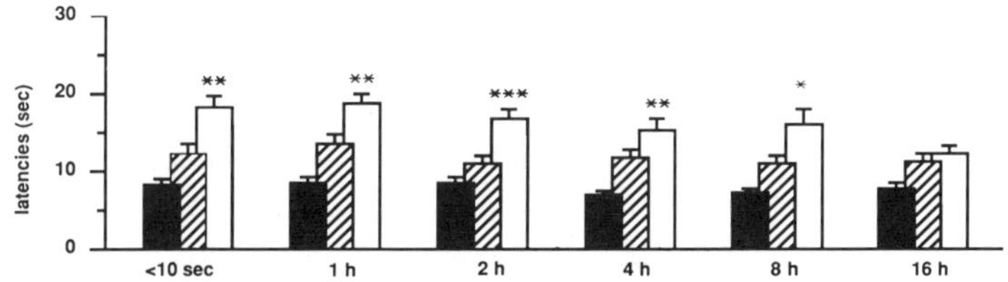

Figure 17.6 Step-down passive avoidance. Effects of CGP 37849 on retention performance of mice. The compound or vehicle (methylcellulose) was administered intraperitoneally at various intervals (10 sec, 1 hr, 2 hr, 4 hr, 8 hr, and 16 hr) after the learning trial. Retest was performed after 3 days. Blank columns: retest latencies of the CGP 37849–treated animals. For further explanation see legend to figure 17.1.

out any inference that the prolongation of the retest latencies might be due to merely a drug-induced inhibition of behavior.

The standard interpretation of such findings is, as already mentioned, that the substances exert an influence on still unconcluded memory processes. If the effects of MK-801 and CGP 37849 are in fact attributable to blockade of the NMDA receptors, it follows that some phase of memory processing lasting at least 8 hours must include NMDA-receptor activity, or can still be modulated by influences acting via NMDA receptors. It must be stressed once again that effects observed after post-trial administration could not be ascribed to modulations of recall: the animals were under the influence of the drug neither during the learning trial, nor during retest (3 days later).

In attempting to arrive at an overall evaluation of our findings, it is first of all helpful to suspend judgment based on what is known about the biochemical effects of the test substances and consider these general propositions. There are conditions under which the retention performance of experimental animals can be facilitated by NMDA blockade. NMDA blockers thus belong, without any particular distinction, to the large category of preparations that under clearly defined experimental conditions can have positive effects on memory but under other conditions have no effects or negative effects (compare Mondadori 1981, 1987). NMDA blockers' ability to improve subsequent retention performance even if administered after the learning trial could be attributed to a specific action on memory processes that outlast the learning situation. Negative effects (i.e., impairments of retention performance) have thus far only been demonstrated under conditions in which the drugs were administered before the learning trial, and hence indirect effects via modulation of perception, emotion, and motivation could not be excluded. The improvement of retention performance brought about by NMDA blockade is still demonstrable after a retention interval of 3 days: it involves a long-lasting modulation, or in other words, long-term memory.

Considering the known biochemical properties of the substances and supposing that LTP is indeed the basis of some form of memory and NMDA blockade does in fact inhibit LTP in vivo, the question arises whether our results are open to any interpretation consistent with such assumptions. The obvious recourse would be to postulate that low doses of NMDA blockers do not block LTP. The memory-facilitating effect could therefore be based either on facilitation or prolongation of LTP, or on still unknown neural functions of NMDA receptors. The first possibility calls for experiments to clarify the question of how NMDA receptor blockade influences neuronal networks already modulated by LTP. Alternatively, it could be postulated that passive avoidance is not one of the forms of memory that depend on LTP. Another argument often adduced is that LTP is only involved in the initial short-lasting phase of memory processing, which is not susceptible to modulation by post-trial administration because of the lapse of time preceding the onset of the drug effect. This argument is hardly compatible with the data presented here: in view of the similarity of the results produced by pretrial and post-trial administration of CGP 37849, it can be assumed that the physiological site of action of the substance is exactly the same under both conditions.

All in all, our results may challenge any LTP hypothesis of learning. If the observed memory facilitation is independent of LTP, our results might indicate the existence of new and still undiscovered functions of the NMDA receptors.

ACKNOWLEDGMENTS

Special thanks are due to T. Ducret, J. Borkowski, R. Mayer, and H. Buerki for performing the experiments and preparing the art.

REFERENCES

Aggleton, J. P., P. R. Hunt, and J. N. P. Rawlins (1986). The effects of hippocampal lesions upon spatial and non-spatial tests of working memory. *Behavioural Brain Research* 19:133–146.

Barnes, C. A. (1988). Spatial learning and memory processes: the search for their neurobiological mechanisms in the rat. *Trends in Neurosciences* 11:163–169.

Coan, B. J., W. Saywood, and G. L. Collingridge (1987). MK 801 blocks NMDA receptor–mediated synaptic transmission and long-term potentiation in rat hippocampal slices. *Neuroscience Letters* 80:11–114.

Collingridge, G. L., and T. V. P. Bliss (1987). NMDA receptors—their role in long term potentiation. *Trends in Neurosciences* 10:288–293.

Collingridge, G. L., S. J. Kehl, and H. McLennan (1983). Excitatory amino acids in synaptic transmission in the Schaffer collateral–commissural pathways of the rat hippocampus. *Journal of Physiology* 334:33–46.

Danysz, W., J. T. Wroblewski, and E. Costa (1988). Learning impairment in rats by *N*-methyl-D-aspartate receptor antagonists. *Neuropharmacology* 27:653–656.

Fagg, G. E., et al. (1990). CGP 37849 and CGP 39551: novel and potent competitive *N*-methyl-D-aspartate receptor antagonists with oral activity. *British Journal of Pharmacology* 99:791–797.

Gibbs, M. E., and K. T. Ng (1977). Psychobiology of memory: towards a model for memory formation. *Biobehavioral Reviews* 1:113–136.

Harris, E. W., A. H. Ganong, and C. W. Cotman (1984). Long-term potentiation in the hippocampus involves activation of *N*-methyl-D-aspartate receptors. *Brain Research* 323:132–137.

McGaugh, J. L., and M. J. Herz (1972). *Memory Consolidation*. San Francisco: Albion Publishing Company.

Monaghan, D. T., and C. W. Cotman (1985). Distribution of NMDA-sensitive 1-H-glutamate binding sites in the rat brain as determined by quantitative autoradiography. *Journal of Neuroscience* 5:2909–2919.

Mondadori, C. (1981). Pharmacological modulation of memory: trends and problems. *Acta Neurologica Scandinavica* 64:(Suppl.) 89:129–140.

Mondadori, C. (1987). Pharmacology of memory: science or art? In E. Mutschler and E. Winterfeld (eds.), *Trends in Medicinal Chemistry.* Proceedings of the Ninth International Symposium on Medicinal Chemistry, Berlin 1986. New York: Weinheim, pp. 263–279.

Mondadori, C., T. Ducret, and J. Borkowski (1991). How long does consolidation take? New compounds can facilitate memory storage, even if administered up to 24 hours after the learning experience. *Brain Research* (in press).

Mondadori, C., et al. (1989). NMDA receptor antagonists can enhance or impair learning performance in animals. *Experimental Brain Research* 75:449–456.

Morris, R. G. M., E. Anderson, G. S. Lynch, and M. Baudry (1986). Selective impairment of learning and blockade of long-term potentiation by an *N*-methyl-D-aspartate receptor antagonist AP5. *Nature* 319:774–776.

Olton, D. S., J. T. Becker, and G. E. Handelman (1979). Hippocampus, space and memory. *Behavioral and Brain Sciences* 2:316–365.

Teyler, T. J., and P. Discenna (1987). Long-term potentiation. *Annual Review of Neuroscience* 10:131–161.

Venable, N., and P. H. Kelly (1990). Effects of NMDA receptor antagonists on passive avoidance learning and retrieval in rats and mice. *Psychopharmacology* 100:215–221.

Wigström, H., B. Gustafsson, and Y. Y. Huang (1986). Mode of action of excitatory amino acid receptor antagonists on hippocampal long lasting potentiation. *Neuroscience* 17:1105–1115.

18 Hippocampal Synaptic Plasticity and *N*-methyl-D-aspartate Receptors: A Role in Information Storage?

Richard G. M. Morris, Sabrina Davis, and Steven P. Butcher

The hypothesis that the physical basis of information storage in the mammalian brain resides in alterations of synaptic efficacy has long been proposed (Cajal, 1911; Konorski, 1948; Hebb, 1949), is central to several neurobiological models of memory (see, for example, Marr, 1971), and is widely accepted by many neuroscientists. However, whereas synaptic plasticity is a neurobiological concept referring to the capacity of synapses to alter as a function of injury, development, or patterns of activation, learning and memory are psychological concepts inferred from alterations of behavior in response to experience. It follows that valid tests of the hypothesis that certain types of synaptic plasticity play a role in information storage require experimental studies to map between two different levels of analysis. Such work should evaluate whether identified neural mechanisms underlying a particular form of synaptic plasticity are in practice activated during certain kinds of learning, and whether they are necessary for information storage to occur. Theoretical work is also essential to evaluate the computational and neurobiological adequacy of formal models that make use of synaptic plasticity to store information (see, for example, Willshaw and Buckingham, 1990).

This chapter describes experimental work conducted within the spirit of such an inquiry but that falls far short of the ideal. It focuses on only one type of learning (namely spatial navigation) and on only one type of synaptic plasticity (hippocampal long-term potentiation [LTP]). However, we defend this limited starting point on the grounds that the physiological properties of LTP are now reasonably well understood; that its induction can be experimentally controlled by drugs that may be used in controlling the behavior of animals; and that the type of learning we are investigating, although poorly understood psychologically, is nevertheless known to depend on the integrity of the hippocampal formation. Thus, there are grounds for believing that the role of synaptic plasticity in learning can be evaluated rigorously and the learning paradigm we are using is, neuropsychologically, a reasonable behavioral assay. More spe-

---

This chapter first appeared in *Philosophical Transactions* 329:187–204, and is reprinted with permission from the Royal Society, London.

cifically, the experiments are intended to test the hypothesis that the underlying neural mechanisms of one form of hippocampal LTP are involved in the storage of information by examining whether the pharmacological blockade of LTP causes a behaviorally specific learning impairment that can be dissociated from sensorimotor side-effects, impairments in retrieval, or both.

HIPPOCAMPAL SYNAPTIC PLASTICITY

Different Forms of Synaptic Plasticity

Synaptic plasticity is a very general concept referring to structural and functional alterations of neural efficiency including reactions to injury (e.g., lesion-induced synaptogenesis; Liu and Chambers, 1958), developmental changes (e.g., synapse elimination; Brown et al., 1976) and alterations induced by specific patterns of neural activity. This latter type of plasticity is our primary concern.

High-frequency activation of presynaptic afferents within hippocampal circuitry results in both short- and long-lasting changes of synaptic efficacy. Facilitation and augmentation refer to changes that are exclusively presynaptic and have a time-course of less than a few seconds (Magelby and Zengel, 1976; McNaughton, 1983). Posttetanic potentiation is, as its name implies, also induced by high-frequency stimulation and has a decay time-course of a few minutes. However, the discovery of a long-lasting or long-term potentiation (Bliss and Lømo, 1973) with a decay time-course that, in chronic preparations, can be as long as days, weeks, or even months has, understandably, attracted considerable attention as a phenomenon whose underlying mechanisms could be involved in long-term memory. LTP is not the only long-lasting change in neural function known to occur in hippocampus. Others include kindling, an epileptiform discharge induced by repetitive subthreshold stimulation (Goddard et al., 1969); long-lasting decreases in after-hyperpolarizing currents, first identified as correlates of learning in *Hermissenda* (see Alkon, 1987), but also found in hippocampus after classical conditioning (Disterhoft et al., 1986); and long-term depression including both heterosynaptic depression (Lynch et al., 1977) and, more controversially, associative homosynaptic depression (Stanton and Sejnowski, 1989). The remainder of this chapter focuses on LTP because several of its physiological properties are suggestive of a memory mechanism.

Long-Term Potentiation

LTP was discovered in the late 1960s and first reported in detail by Bliss and Lømo (1973). The original experiments, conducted by using anesthetized rabbits, involved the bilateral placement of stimulating electrodes in the perforant path entering the hippocampus and recording electrodes in the molecular layer and hilus of the dentate gyrus. One three-phase experiment began with repetitive low-frequency electrical stimulation (one per 30 seconds) to evoke field potentials consisting of a mixture of fiber potentials, excitatory postsynaptic potentials (EPSPs), inhibitory postsynaptic potentials (IPSPs), and population spikes. These remained stable throughout the preliminary "baseline" phase. However, when a brief tetanic burst of stimulation (100 Hz for 2 seconds) was given unilaterally (phase 2) followed by a return to low-frequency stimulation (phase 3), the field potentials recorded on the side of the brain that had received the high-frequency burst were found to be substantially enhanced relative to their pretetanic baseline. Bliss and Lømo (1973) showed that this increased responsiveness consisted of both a synaptic component (LTP) and a reduced threshold for cell firing for a given size of EPSP (E-S potentiation). Both components of the response are long-lasting (Bliss and Gardner-Medwin, 1973). Subsequent work in many laboratories has confirmed and expanded on these original observations by using both in vivo and in vitro preparations (see Brown et al., 1988; Nicoll et al., 1988; Deadwyler and Landfield, 1988, for recent reviews).

Physiological Properties of LTP

Research on LTP has revealed several other physiological properties relevant to a possible role in learning (table 18.1): (1) it was discovered and occurs prominently in the hippocampus, which has long been implicated in learning and memory (see, for example, Scoville and Milner; 1957; (2) it can be induced by extremely brief patterns of afferent stimulation, including both single stimuli paired with postsynaptic depolarization and rhythmic bursts of presynaptic activation that mimic naturally occurring patterns of neural activity (Wigström et al., 1986; Larson and Lynch, 1986; Pavlides et al., 1988); (3) it is induced rapidly, reaching a peak within 30–60 seconds (McNaughton, 1973; Gustaffson et al., 1989) but, according to one report, giving rise to postsynaptic changes over a longer time period (Davies et al., 1989); (4) its induction can be associative in the sense that activity at one point on the dendritic tree can influence whether synaptic change will occur at another point (McNaughton et al., 1978; Levy and Steward, 1979; Barrionuevo and Brown, 1983), a property relevant to a possible role in associative learning; (5) it is synapse-specific (Andersen et

Table 18.1 Properties of LTP Relevant to Its Putative Role in Learning

Occurs in hippocampus	Also occurs in other brain areas, and other brain areas are involved in learning
Induced by brief patterns of stimulation	Large field-potential changes are not observed naturally after learning
Rapid induction	Always decays over time
Associative	Temporal parameters of associative induction more specific than those of conditioning
Synapse-specific change	
Saturates	

al., 1977), thereby permitting massive information storage capacity and a parallel distributed processing "style" of computation; and (6) it saturates on repeated activation (McNaughton, 1983).

However, suggestive as these properties may seem, there are further properties of LTP that complicate hypotheses about its functional significance (see table 18.1): (1) it occurs outside the hippocampus (notably in cortex; Lee, 1983; Artola and Singer, 1987), and other brain regions are clearly involved in learning. Thus a preoccupation with hippocampal LTP may be misleading. (2) Although induced by patterns of stimulation that might occur naturally, there is controversy about whether LTP actually occurs as a correlate of learning. Increases in the population spike in the dentate hilus of rabbits that have undergone nictitating membrane conditioning (Thompson, 1990), although consistent with an LTP mechanism, may also be caused by changes in excitability induced by some other mechanism. In comparison, only modest changes in the slope function of field potentials are seen in animals that have been given considerable opportunity to explore a complex environment (Sharp et al., 1985). Part of the problem is whether one would really expect to see gross changes in a physiologically activated field potential as a consequence of the subtle spatially distributed subset of synaptic changes that might accompany a single learning experience (see Morris, 1989b, for discussion). (3) The time-window within which the presynaptic and postsynaptic events for inducing associative LTP must occur ($\approx$100 milliseconds) maps onto the temporal parameters of associative learning (e.g., classical conditioning) poorly. (4) Once induced, LTP seems to involve a heterogeneous family of synaptic changes with dissociable time-courses lasting a few hours, or several days (referred to as LTP1 and LTP2, respectively; Racine et al., 1983), time-courses that have no obvious parallel in extant behavioral findings. (5) The mechanisms of LTP might not be involved in long-term memory because nondecremental LTP has never been observed.

Our own view of these problems is that although they must be addressed, none are fatal for the hypothesis. To take one example, the phenomenon of associative long-term depression (LTD; Stanton and Sejnowski, 1989, throws new light on the time-course problems (4) and (5) above). Nondecremental LTP is not seen in freely moving animals; this may be because the conditions for producing LTD are inadvertently but necessarily produced by naturally occurring patterns of activity. Bearing in mind that LTP is an "artificial" phenomenon demonstrated by stimulating large numbers of afferent fibers synchronously, its decline over time may be due to a naturally occurring but activity-dependent LTD on small subsets of these fibers rather than a strictly time-dependent decay. Interestingly, Pavlides and coworkers (1988) have recently shown that short tetanic bursts on the trough of the naturally occurring theta wave can cause a depression of synaptic efficacy.

Thus LTP displays several suggestive properties that, although not without problems, are at least suggestive of an underlying memory mechanism. Several research groups have sought to exploit these properties in studies of its functional significance. Barnes (1979) has found correlations between behavioral learning and the decay time-course of LTP, whereas both McNaughton and coworkers (1986) and Castro and associates (1989) have shown that saturation of LTP is associated with an anterograde spatial amnesia. New avenues for exploring the functional significance of LTP have also opened up following the discovery that activation of a subtype of excitatory amino receptor is necessary for the induction of LTP.

Role of NMDA Receptor Activation in Induction of LTP

The last few years have seen striking advances in our understanding of excitatory neurotransmission in the central nervous system (CNS) made possible through the development of several selective agonists and antagonists of excitatory amino acid (EAA) receptors. Studies making use of techniques such as ligand binding, intracellular recording and patch-clamping have led to our current understanding of there being at least three main classes of receptor. The most widely characterized receptors are called kainate-, quisqualate- and *N*-methyl-D-aspartate (NMDA)-preferring receptors, so named after the preferential agonist at each site (Watkins and Evans, 1981; Foster and Fagg, 1984; Mayer and Westbrook, 1987; Watkins and Collingridge, 1989). Certain antagonists (e.g., 6-cyano-7-nitroquinoxaline [CNQX] and 6,7-dinitroquinoxaline-2,3-dione [DNQX]) interact preferentially at kainate and quisqualate receptors, whereas others (e.g., 2-amino-5-phosphonopentanoate [AP5]) bind to the NMDA receptor. Neurophysiological studies reveal that in the hippocampus, activation of kainate-quisqualate (KQ) receptors mediates fast synaptic transmission whereas NMDA receptors are not involved in this component of the synaptic response. This may not be the case in other brain areas (Thomson et al., 1985; Salt, 1986; Fox et al., 1989; Sillito et al., 1990). The NMDA-associated iontophore does, however, have the unusual property of responding to postsynaptic depolarization (Nowak et al., 1984; Mayer et al., 1984). At the resting potential (≈ -80 mV), the NMDA ion channel is blocked by the divalent cation magnesium such that binding of an endogenous transmitter to NMDA receptors is unable to open the channel. However, if the neuron is partially depolarized (e.g., to -35 mV), the magnesium block is released and subsequent activation of NMDA receptors can then open these channels. NMDA receptor ion channels are thus dually regulated, being both ligand- and voltage-gated (figure 18.1). Furthermore, it is now also known that fast synaptic transmission depends on the passage of Na^+ ions through the KQ receptor ion-channel, whereas the opening of the NMDA-receptor channel allows the preferential passage of Ca^{2+} ions into postsynaptic dendritic spines (McDermott et al., 1986).

A particularly important discovery has been that the selective NMDA antagonist AP5, although having no effect upon normal fast synaptic transmission in hippocampus, blocks the induction of LTP (Collingridge

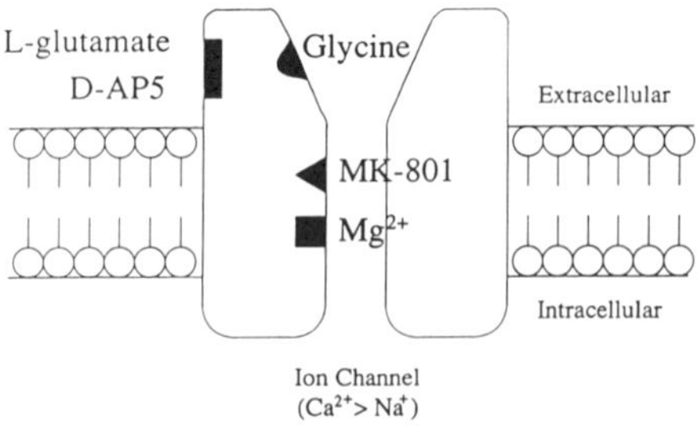

Figure 18.1 Simplified cartoon of NMDA receptor complex. The receptor protein is associated with an ion-channel, which, when open, is preferentially permeable to Ca^{2+} rather than Na^+. Ordinarily, the channel is blocked by Mg^2. D-AP5 binds competitively to the receptor recognition site for the endogenous transmitter (e.g., L-glutamate). Channel-opening is modulated by glycine and may be blocked by noncompetitive antagonists such as MK-801.

et al., 1983). Harris and associates (1984) extended this finding by showing that AP5's blockade of LTP was stereospecific; the D-isomer blocked LTP (at an ED_{50} of $\approx 8\ \mu M$) whereas the L-isomer was essentially without effect. The importance of this discovery is that, together with the work on receptor pharmacology, it has led to an understanding of the likely sequence of events occurring during the induction of LTP that, in turn, explains several of its properties outlined in the section Physiological Properties of LTP. Specifically, a high-frequency tetanus results in a sufficiently large and sustained depolarization such that the voltage-dependent block of the NMDA receptor ion channel is released. Ca^{2+} ions, rather than just Na^+, then enter the postsynaptic spine where they can act on one or several biochemical processes that may eventually result in the alteration of synaptic efficacy. AP5 blocks LTP by binding competitively to the NMDA receptor recognition site such that, even when the voltage-dependent block of the ion channel is released during a tetanus, the endogenous transmitter (e.g., L-glutamate) cannot gain access to its receptor to open the channel. AP5 is without effect on the expression of LTP because, once induced, LTP involves an alteration of fast synaptic transmission, i.e., the mediation of EPSPs via KQ receptors.

This brief account of the events occurring during the induction of LTP helps explain several of its physiological properties. Thus, LTP is induced by brief patterns of stimulation because Ca^{2+} can enter postsynaptic dendritic spines during either a short-lasting tetanus or when single pulses of afferent stimulation occur in instantaneous conjunction with postsynaptic depolarization. LTP is synapse-specific because the NMDA-associated ion channel is ligand-gated and so, under normal physiological conditions, requires the binding of transmitter released from specific presynaptic terminals. And LTP is associative because induction also requires postsynaptic depolarization caused by neural activation that, under normal conditions, will have been induced elsewhere on the dendrite other than at the site of presynaptic activity. Thus, NMDA receptors are "conjunction devices" endowing neurons with the biophysical capacity to detect the co-occurrence of presynaptic activity with postsynaptic depolarization, i.e. with the capacity to function as "Hebb-like" synapses (Kelso et al., 1986; Wigström et al., 1986).

Selective amino acid antagonists, such as DNQX and AP5, are marvelous tools with which to dissect various aspects of excitatory neurotransmission. Newer compounds are also becoming available that act as NMDA-receptor channel blockers (e.g., MK-801; Wong et al., 1986), or on the glycine regulatory site (Johnson and Ascher, 1987), which forms part of the NMDA-receptor complex (Kemp et al., 1988). One recent example of their use has been in a study concerned with whether the expression of LTP involves an increase in transmitter release, as proposed by Bliss and Lynch (1988), or a selective alteration in the number of postsynaptic receptors (Lynch and Baudry, 1984). Muller and coworkers (1988) examined the effects of DNQX and AP5 on LTP, and also, for purposes of calibration, a phenomenon called "paired-pulse potentiation" that is known to involve increased transmitter release. By using a stimulation paradigm in which the voltage-dependent block of the NMDA-receptor ion channel was partially released, they found that LTP is associated with an increase in the component of the EPSPs seen in the presence of AP5 (i.e., those caused by activation of KQ receptors) without any change in the smaller EPSPs induced in the presence of DNQX. This was not because of a lack of sensitivity for detecting changes in the current flowing through NMDA receptors because increases in both the DNQX- and AP5-sensitive components of the EPSP were seen in paired-pulse potentiation. A related finding has been reported by Kauer and colleagues (1988). The implication is that the expression of LTP is more likely to be associated with a selective postsynaptic change (e.g., in the number of KQ receptors, or the number of ions flowing through the KQ iontophore with each channel opening) than with a sustained increase in transmitter release. However, somewhat different results have been found by Collingridge (personal communication) and Tsien (1990) who both find that a small component of the increase in the EPSP remains in the presence of low concentrations of CNQX and that this is sensitive to AP5. One complication in analyzing the expression of LTP is the finding of Davies and coworkers (1989) that the altered sensitivity to iontophoretic application of the quisqualate agonist α-amino-3-hydroxy-5-methyl-4-isoxazole propionic acid (AMPA) develops only gradually over a period of 2 hours (see also Horn (1990).

ROLE OF NMDA RECEPTOR ACTIVATION IN LEARNING AND MEMORY

Design Requirements

In addition to being useful tools for exploring excitatory neurotransmission, selective excitatory amino acids (EAA) antagonists can also be used in behaving animals to investigate learning. One straightforward prediction of the hypothesis that the neural mechanisms underlying LTP are involved in information storage is that blockade of NMDA receptor action in vivo should cause impairments of learning. However, because NMDA receptors are widely distributed in the CNS, generalized NMDA receptor blockade is likely to have functional consequences over and beyond effects on learning. It follows that, if an NMDA antagonist such as AP5 is used to investigate the role of LTP in learning, it is essential that experiments incorporate the following:

1. Neurophysiological observations to check that the drug is actually impairing or blocking LTP in vivo.
2. Control procedures to dissociate primary and secondary effects of the drug.

The first of these requirements is straightforward, although it is remarkable how few behaviorial studies of NMDA antagonists have included neurophysiological measures. The disquiet is more than academic because noncompetitive NMDA antagonists, such as MK-801, may not block LTP in vivo if the attempt to induce it is made within the same short interval after drug administration as typically used in behaviorial studies between drug injection and behavioral testing (e.g., 30 minutes). Halliwell and Morris (1987) found no change in either the magnitude or decay time-course of LTP when tetanic stimulation was given 20 minutes after a 1 mg/kg^{-1} intraperitoneal injection of MK-801 in urethane anesthetized rats. A more detailed study by Abraham and Mason (1988), but also in anesthetized animals, did find blockade of LTP but only when stimulation was given 150 minutes after intraperitoneal injections at the equally high dose of 1 mg/kg^{-1}. In vitro observations by Coan and coworkers (1987) confirmed that use dependency, characteristic of MK-801's action as an NMDA-receptor channel blocker (Wong et al., 1986), may take up to 2 hours to develop fully in hippocampal slices. Until this channel block is fully developed, there is no reason why sufficient Ca^{2+} should not pass through the channel during brief periods of presynaptic activation coupled with postsynaptic depolarization. Interestingly, there is evidence suggestive of use-dependency in learning paradigms (Clineschmidt et al., 1982), but its occurrence is complicated by the fact that agonist activation will surely vary across brain regions. Thus, MK-801 may induce a rapid channel block in, for example, globus pallidus (where baseline cell firing rates are high) but have much slower effects in the CA1 region of the hippocampus (where they are low). The spirit if not the detail of this idea may help us understand why MK-801 causes its pronounced behavioral syndrome (ataxia, head-bobbing) within 15 minutes but fails to block LTP until 2 hours have elapsed since drug-injection. In our view, the convenience of noncompetitive antagonists in crossing the blood-brain barrier is offset by this ambiguity concerning their capacity to block hippocampal LTP in vivo. Not withstanding their use by several behavioral-research groups (Robinson et al., 1989; Mondadori et al., 1989; Whishaw and Auer,

1989), there clearly are obstacles to basing firm conclusions about the role of LTP in learning on experiments that use noncompetitive antagonists.

The second design requirement—the need for control procedures—divides into two logically separate issues. First, it is essential to investigate whether "side-effects" caused by drug action outside the hippocampus could be responsible for the apparent impairment of hippocampally mediated learning. Secondly, there may be effects of neurophysiological function within hippocampus in addition to the impairment of LTP. Both of these points follow from a crucial logical point (which we have stressed repeatedly in previous papers: Morris et al., 1986a; McNaughton and Morris, 1987; Morris, 1989a, b; Morris et al 1989b): namely, the drug-induced blockade of LTP and its impairment of learning are each dependent consequences of a single independent treatment. It is logically fallacious to presume, in the absence of further evidence, that one dependent consequence (e.g., a blockade of LTP) is necessarily the cause of the other (e.g., an impairment of learning).

Effects Outside Hippocampus It is known that AP5 can cause sensorimotor effects outside the hippocampus on sensory transduction (Cahusac et al., 1985; Salt, 1986) motor control and motor patterning (Dale and Roberts, 1984; Klockgether et al., 1986; Dale, 1989), muscle flaccidity (Turski et al., 1985), and suprasegmental reflexes (Davies and Watkins, 1983), any or all of which could give rise to a behavioral profile of impairment deceptively like that caused by hippocampal lesions. Exactly how these sensorimotor disturbances would mimic hippocampal disruption is unclear because hippocampectomized rats can see and move around properly, and they have both normal muscle tone and normal spinal reflexes. However, the mere possibility that a complex profile of extra-hippocampal disturbance might mimic the effects of a lesion should always be borne in mind.

Effects Within Hippocampus AP5 can also cause effects within the hippocampus other than on LTP induction, including a decrease in hippocampal theta activity (Leung and Desborough, 1988), reductions in hippocampal excitability (Errington et al., 1987; Abraham and Mason, 1988), and truncation of normal complex-spike firing (Abraham and Kairiss, 1988). Even more than the sensorimotor side-effects listed above, these drug-induced alterations of normal hippocampal function might be expected to cause behavioral disturbances similar to those produced by partial or complete hippocampal lesions. It should be noted, however, that in Leung and Desborough's 1988 study, the reduction in hippocampal theta was only apparent at their highest dose when 100 nmol of AP5 was infused intracerebroventricularly over 3 minutes, a rate of infusion 60 times faster than our 20 nmol h^{-1} chronic infusion protocol. Furthermore, they reported that at this dose, their animals "became ataxic and assumed an unsteady gait with the abdomen held near the floor during walking."

Such behavior is never seen in our animals chronically treated with AP5 at doses up to those sufficient to block LTP completely.

The pharmacological method of investigating the role of LTP in learning is, therefore, fraught with several interpretative difficulties. In the experiments described below, we have endeavored to address some of these problems, some directly, others indirectly. The cardinal features of our strategy have been as follows.

1. The use of a variety of neuropsychologically dissociable tasks, to search for behavioral specificity.

2. The conduct of both neurophysiological and behavioral measures whenever possible, sometimes in the same animal.

3. The precise measurement of drug levels in the CNS by using both whole-tissue and extracellular sampling techniques together with high-performance liquid chromatography (HPLC) fluorometric methods, to afford comparison with in vitro studies of NMDA receptors and a sound basis for comparing successive behavioral studies.

Behavioral and Anatomical Specificity

Morris and coworkers (1986a) showed that chronic intraventricular infusion of 40 mM D,L-AP5, a dose shown to be sufficient to block LTP in vivo, caused an impairment of spatial learning in the water-maze while leaving visual discrimination learning (tested in the same apparatus) intact (figure 18.2). This profile of impairment is similar to, although less severe than, that caused by hippocampal lesions (O'Keefe and Nadel, 1978; Morris et al. 1986b). The behavioral specificity was also borne out in Tonkiss and coworkers' (1988) discovery that AP5 impairs DRL performance (a non-spatial operant schedule involving differential reinforcement of low rates of an operant response for food reward) in a qualitatively similar way to that caused by hippocampal lesions, whereas the anatomical specificity is supported by observations that local, intrahippocampal infusions of nanomolar quantities of AP5 cause a dose-dependent impairment of both LTP in vivo and place-navigation (Morris et al., 1989b; two doses tested only). It is tempting to interpret these results as supporting the general hypothesis that activation of the neural mechanisms responsible for hippocampal LTP is necessary for those types of learning that require the integrity of hippocampal function but unnecessary for other types of learning. However, although consistent with this general hypothesis, it would be premature to draw so bold a conclusion on this evidence alone for the reasons outlined in the section Design Requirements.

First, as pointed out by Goddard (1986), the behavioral specificity seen after intracerebroventricular infusions might arise from differential drug diffusion in the brain. Given that intracerebral drug concentrations have been reported to decline with distance from the infusion cannula (Urquhart et al., 1984; Kleinschmidt et al., 1987), the latter's proximity to hippocampus but greater distance from, for example, visual cortex, may

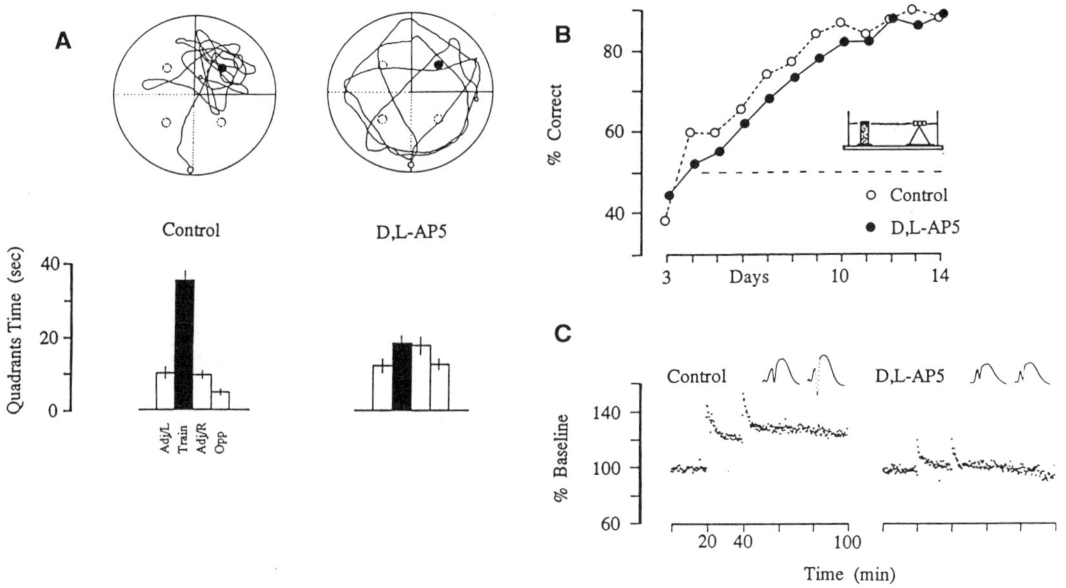

Figure 18.2. Intraventricular infusion of AP5 impairs spatial learning. Rats were implanted with an intracerebroventricular cannula connected to osmotic minipumps chronically delivering 40 mM D,L-AP5 at 0.5 μl h^{-1} over a period of up to 14 days. (A) Spatial learning. Paths taken during a 60 sec transfer test (platform absent) after 15 trials of training over 5 days. The former position of the platform is shown as (●). (B) Visual discrimination. Choice performance on a two-platform visual-discrimination task (inset) over 12 days of training (10 trials per day. ○ = control; ● = D,L-AP5. (C) LTP. Mean normalized early-rising slope values of field-potentials evoked in the hilus of the dentate gyrus after perforant path stimulation. Brief tetanic stimulation was given at the 20- and 40-min points.

have resulted in higher and more effective drug concentrations in hippocampus. We have addressed this problem by directly measuring whole-tissue levels of AP5 in various brain regions, and by conducting a second visual discrimination experiment in which the drug was infused bilaterally (20 mM D,L-AP5, 0.5 μl h^{-1} from each of two minipumps) into a cortical area just anterior to the visual cortex (Occ2; Zilles, 1985; we did not infuse into the visual cortex itself because of the 500 μm gliosis that can develop around an indwelling cannula). The results showed a remarkably uniform distribution of AP5 throughout the rodent forebrain after intracerebroventricular infusions whereas, with intracortical infusions, concentration only showed an appreciable decline at distances greater than approximately 8 mm (Butcher et al., 1991). Furthermore, the rate of visual-discrimination learning was unaffected by intracortical infusion of AP5 despite a measured whole-tissue concentration in visual cortex comparable to that which, in hippocampus, is associated with impairments of place learning. The issue raised by Goddard (1986) was an important and legitimate one but we believe that these results render it less tenable as an explanation of behavioral specificity.

Secondly, the apparent behavioral specificity reflects only a "single dissociation." No "double dissociation," such as an impairment of visual discrimination but not spatial learning following some other drug or lesion treatment, has been either sought or found (see Weiskrantz, 1968; Shallice, 1989). The most immediate worry that this fosters is that the dissociation may reflect nothing more than task difficulty. However, the visual discrimination task is learned more slowly by normal rats than either the standard place-navigation task (ca. 120 trials vs. 20 trials, respectively) or a two-platform spatial discrimination task whose motivational, reinforcement, and sensorimotor demands are equated to those of the visual discrimination task (120 against 50 trials; Morris et al., 1986b). Thus AP5 impairs the easier rather than the operationally more difficult task (cf. Mondadori et al., 1989).

However, there are deeper issues at stake. The failure to find any effects of a potent competitive NMDA antagonist on cortically mediated visual-discrimination learning is in contrast to the marked impairment of ocular dominance reversal following reverse suture after monocular rearing in kittens (Kleinschmidt et al., 1987). Bear (1987) and Singer (1990) have interpreted this and other related findings as evidence that activation of cortical NMDA receptors is essential for self-organization in the developing nervous system. But what of their role in the adult animal? If our visual discrimination findings are reliable, they imply that mechanisms other than NMDA-receptor mediated plasticity must be responsible for storing information about the association of a visual cue with reward or nonreward. A second implication is that, at doses sufficient to block LTP and impair spatial learning (but not necessarily at higher doses), chronic AP5 infusion cannot be causing a gross sensory impairment. In the watermaze, AP5-treated rats can see well enough to head toward a visible target, and they can discriminate a gray platform from one painted with black-and-white stripes of roughly equivalent luminosity. In contrast, studies of the effects of iontophoretic application of NMDA antagonists to lateral geniculate nucleus (LGN) and visual-cortex neurons point to participation of NMDA receptors in the normal throughput of information on the geniculo-striate pathway and in contrast sensitivity (Sillito et al., 1990; Fox et al., 1989; Daw et al., 1990). The inconsistency between these and our own behavioral findings may be partly due to dose dependency. Rats who, at sacrifice, are found to have substantially higher whole-tissue drug concentrations than those sufficient to block LTP do show abnormalities of behavior consistent with a partial loss of vision (we have not attempted any formal testing). However, the inconsistency may also be due to our use of a relatively unsophisticated visual discrimination task. A more subtle task, such as one involving discrimination between stripes of differing spatial frequency, or of lower contrast discriminability, may show performance (as against learning) impairments at cerebral concentrations equivalent to those that impair spatial learning. The question would then arise of whether the apparent spatial-learning impairment might actually be due to the AP5-treated animals having difficulty seeing distal cues (but see the section "Storage or Retrieval?" later in this chapter).

Sensorimotor Side-Effects

Rats given chronic intracerebroventricular infusion of AP5 at rates of up to 15 nmol h^{-1} (30 mM D-AP5, 0.5 μl h^{-1}) show remarkably normal behavior. They are certainly not ataxic, appear to show normal exploratory movements, can swim normally (with appropriate forelimb inhibition) and, in the water-maze, use the hidden platform as a refuge in much the same way as untreated rats. However, it is also true that their range of movements is not entirely normal. Some rats show a slight muscle flaccidity, a slower righting reflex, or have difficulty in holding onto the top of a wire cage when it is tilted from horizontal to vertical. In the first of our water-maze experiments (Morris et al., 1986a), a few rats fell off the hidden platform after a "wet-dog" shake early in training. This abnormality diminished over days and, we now know, is only inevitable in animals whose hippocampal-tissue AP5 concentration is very high.

Clearly these disturbances could be contributing to the AP5-induced impairment of some hippocampally mediated tasks (spatial learning, DRL performance) although for others, such as odor-potentiated taste aversion (Crooks et al., 1989), the proposal strains credibility. For example, rats that fall off the escape platform in the water-maze (and normal rats do this, too) might come to find the platform aversive. As escape is the only source of reinforcement in the task, learning might then proceed more slowly, not because of a direct participation of NMDA receptors in spatial learning but secondarily, because the incentive to learn was diminished. This possibility has been ruled out following the accidental observation during some pilot work that the behavior of falling-off the platform is greatly diminished by pretraining before administering the drug. Morris (1989a, expt 3) examined this formally by looking at the effects of non-spatial pretraining upon the AP5-induced impairment of place-navigation. Rats were first trained (as normals) to use an escape platform as a refuge, under conditions that prevented spatial learning: by successively hiding the platform in different locations over trials within a water-maze surrounded by black curtains that occluded sight of distal cues. Escape performance remained random during this pretraining but the rats did learn to climb onto the platform whenever they bumped into it. Following surgery to implant minipumps containing AP5 or artificial cerebrospinal fluid (aCSF) in these and other naive rats, spatial training was instituted by withdrawing the curtains and putting the platform in a fixed location (i.e., a protocol identical to that of the original 1986 study). Pre-training caused a striking reduction in the number of occasions rats fell off the platform but the drug-induced place-navigation impairment remained (figure 18.3). The analysis of variance showed no statistical

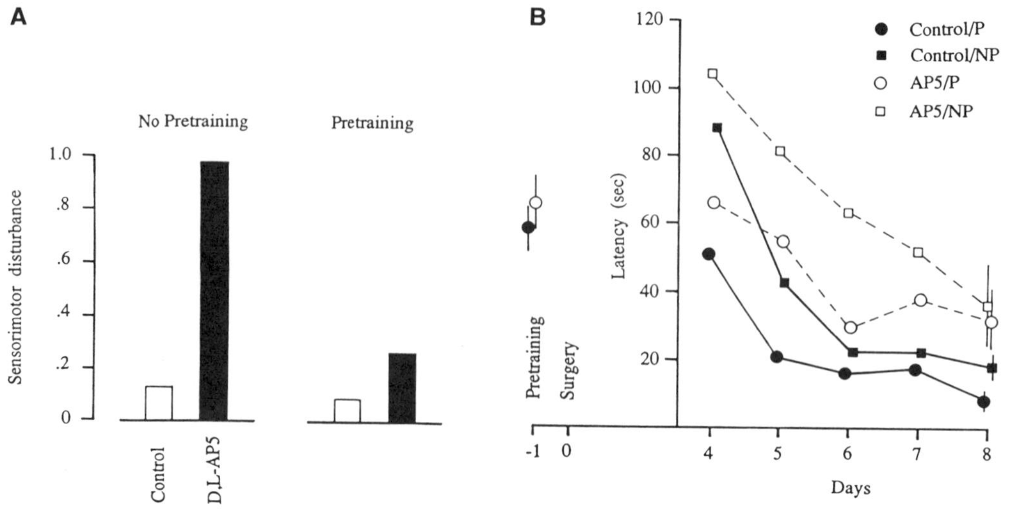

Figure 18.3 The spatial learning impairment can be partly dissociated from a gross sensorimotor disturbance. (A) Nonspatial pretraining caused a reduction in falls off the platform during the drug phase. (B) The extent of the AP5-induced learning impairment was unaffected by nonspatial pretraining. Escape latencies were lower at the outset of the drug phase in pretrained rats but the AP5/aCSF difference was maintained. ● = control/P; ■ = control/NP; ○ = AP5/P; □ = AP5/NP.

interaction between the drug-induced learning impairment and pretraining (the F-ratio was less than 1). The reason for this somewhat unexpected result is that rats have to learn that the hidden platform is a refuge and that AP5 interferes with this learning process as well as that of learning where the platform is located. Thus delaying the administration of AP5 until after the rats have learned to use the escape platform diminishes the sensorimotor disturbance. The irony is that the "sensorimotor disturbance" turns out to be a secondary consequence of a failure to learn rather than a viable explanation of the apparent learning impairment. Nonspatial pretraining is now used routinely in all our AP5 experiments and the procedure works well except in animals receiving very high drug doses (in whom the sensorimotor disturbances become so pronounced that the rats are virtually untestable).

The dose dependency of the sensorimotor disturbances induced by both competitive and noncompetitive antagonists is a fitting reminder that great care must be exercised in using these drugs to investigate learning. We had hoped to do some work with MK-801 (the minipump surgery necessary for AP5 infusions being both expensive and time consuming) but our experience of this drug's pronounced sensorimotor abnormalities (ataxia, head-bobbing) at doses near to the ED_{50} values for its anticonvulsant effectiveness (ca. 0.3 mg/kg^{-1}; Tricklebank et al., 1989) led to our abandoning this approach. It is still not clear whether the disturbances induced by competitive antagonists, such as AP5, AP7, and DL-3-(2-carboxypiperazin-4-yl) propyl-1-phosphonic acid (CPP), are qualitatively dissimilar but we do know that they are minimal at doses useful for investigating hippocampal-dependent learning.

Dose-Response Analysis

Over the past 2 years, we have conducted a detailed dose-response analysis of the effects of AP5 on spatial learning and LTP in vivo. Although preliminary reports of this experiment have appeared elsewhere (see, for example, Morris et al., 1989b), the description below is the first comprehensive summary of the results.

There were two main reasons for conducting a dose-response analysis. First, the hypothesis that activation of the neural mechanisms responsible for LTP is required for normal hippocampal-dependent learning would be disproved if conditions were found in which LTP was completely blocked but learning proceeded normally.* Conversely, finding parallel, overlapping dose-response functions would put the original observations of an AP5-induced impairment of spatial learning on a firmer footing. Secondly, measurements of both whole-tissue and extracellular AP5 in the CNS of animals subject to both behavioral and physiological procedures would provide an excellent opportunity to assess the specificity of AP5's mode of action in vivo in comparison with its now well understood action in vitro. Our reason for taking both measures of AP5 concentration was because we already suspected that the whole-tissue level was substantially higher than the effective extracellular concentration.

The general plan of the experiment is shown in figure 18.4. The behavioral protocol began with 3 days of nonspatial pretraining. The rats were then given surgery for implanting minipumps containing either aCSF or various concentrations of D-AP5, or given a sham operation (i.e., no minipump). Beginning 3 days later, all rats were given 5 days of spatial training followed, on the last day, by a transfer test. On the next day, or any of the succeeding 3 days, an attempt was made to induce hippocampal LTP in vivo (under urethane anesthesia). Following this, and while still under anesthesia, the extracellular fluid in hippocampus was sampled for 2 hours by using microdialysis probes. Finally, each animal was killed, their brains removed, and various brain regions dissected for whole-tissue measurements of AP5 and endogenous excitatory amino acids by using HPLC.

It did not always prove possible to collect the complete set of data from all animals. However, out of a total of more than 100 rats that began nonspatial pretraining, 56 rats completed all phases. All correlational analyses were conducted by using individual animal scores but it proved convenient to subdivide the rats into groups on the basis of either their

*Note that there is an asymmetry about this prediction. The hypothesis is silent about the opposite finding: a behavioral impairment in the absence of any blockade of LTP. The neural mechanisms underlying LTP are no more the be-all and end-all of learning among advocates of the hypothesis than they are among its critics.

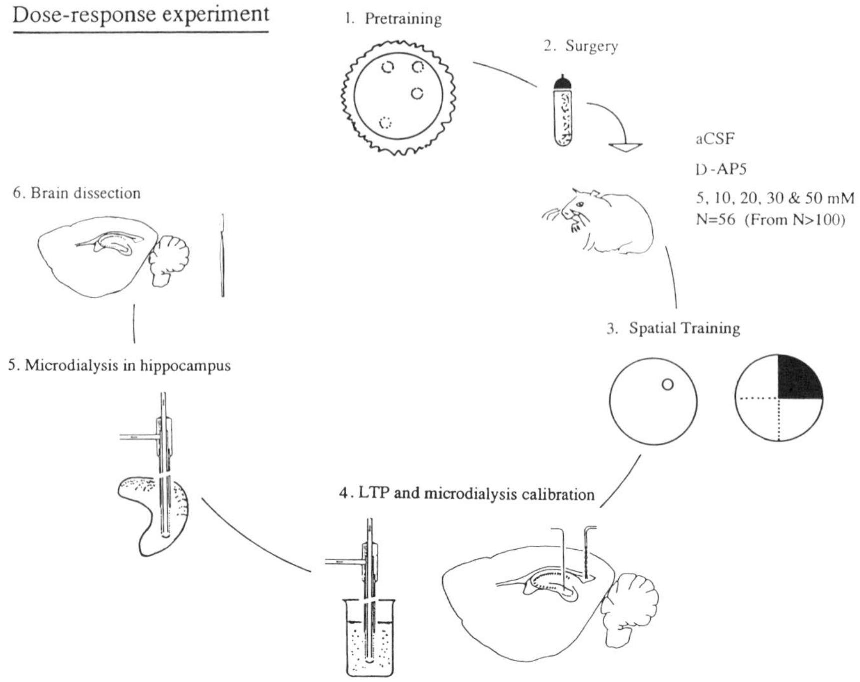

Figure 18.4 Plan of dose-response experiment: nonspatial pretraining, 12 trials, curtains around the pool, platform moved between trials. Surgery: minipumps containing aCSF or D-AP5 (5, 13, 20, 30, 40, and 50 mM), chronic pumping rate 0.5 μl h^{-1}. Spatial training: 30 trials, curtains open, platform in a fixed counterbalanced location for individual animals and removed for the 60 sec transfer test, all paths tracked by using an automatic image-analyzing system. Attempted LTP induction: rats given urethane anaesthesia 1.5 gm/kg^{-1}, bipolar-stimulating electrode in angular bundle and recording electrode in dentate hilus, field potentials amplified and monitored on-line by using an 11/23 computer with the early-rising slope calculated by linear regression, low-frequency stimulation = 0.1 Hz, tetanus = 3 trains of 33 pulses at 400 Hz given at least 45 min after assumption of stable low-frequency baseline, potentials monitored for a further 60 min, input/output functions (0–9 V) taken before and after the main series. The microdialysis probes were calibrated by using 5 μM D-AP5 during this electrophysiology phase. Microdialysis: the probe was positioned in hippocampus, aCSF perfused at 1.5 μl min^{-1}, six samples at 20 min per sample. Dissection: samples taken from left and right hippocampus; HPLC was used to analyse AP5 content from both extracellular and whole-tissue samples, AP5 being separated from other amino acids and detected as a fluorescent derivative following precolumn derivitization with o-pthaldialdehyde (the separation procedure involved a gradient elution between two buffers: buffer A, 50 mM sodium dihydrogen phosphate, pH 5.14, + 2.5% tetrahydrofuran; buffer B, methanol + 1.25% tetrahydrofuran) and a 5 μm C-18 Nucleosil column (250 mm × 4.6 mm), calibration by injection of 50 pmole D-AP5, data handling by computerized integration system.

whole-tissue or extracellular AP5 concentration. Thus groups were created whose whole-tissue AP5 concentration in hippocampus was 0 (i.e., aCSF and control rats), between 0.01 and 0.10, 0.11 to 0.20, 0.21 to 0.30, and, finally, above 0.31 nmol mg^{-1} wet mass. This sorting process immediately enabled us to identify the nine animals with very high AP5 concentrations as including all of the eight animals who showed persistent sensorimotor abnormalities of the kind discussed above. All data from these nine "very-high-dose" animals were disregarded in subsequent data analyses.

Analyses of the remaining 47 animals showed a dose-related impairment of both spatial learning and LTP (figure 18.5). Mean escape latency (averaged across the 30 spatial trials) increased as a function of whole-tissue content whereas the amount of LTP that could be evoked declined. The relationships between AP5 content and both percentage LTP and mean escape latency were highly significant correlations (figure 18.6).

The correlations did, however, indicate that the whole-tissue AP5 content was very high, disturbingly high if these values are any reflection of the effective AP5 concentration at NMDA receptors. The first clue that this was not the case lay in the electrophysiological data. This revealed the surprising finding that LTP could still be induced in vivo at a hippocampal tissue concentration that causes a complete blockade in vitro by using bath-applied AP5 at the same concentration (Harris et al., 1984). For

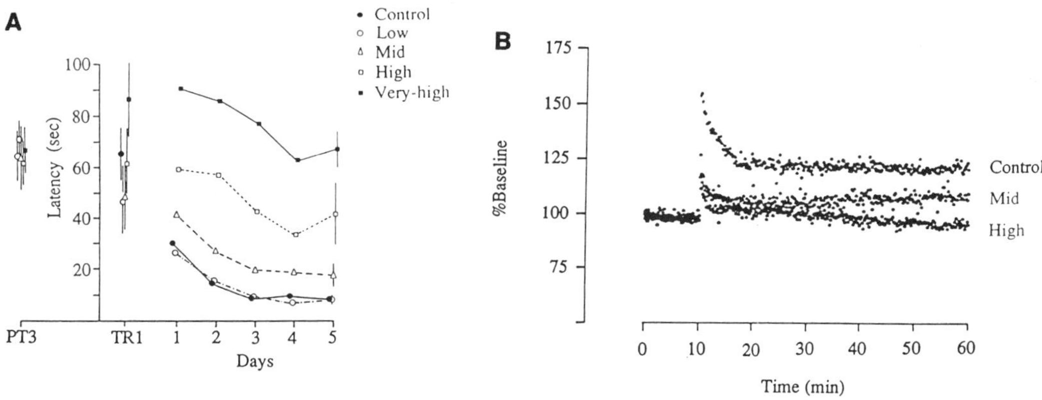

Figure 18.5 (A) Escape latency (s) on the last day of nonspatial pretraining (PT3), the first trial of spatial training (TR1) and throughout the 5 days of the spatial learning phase. Rats were divided into groups on the basis of whole-tissue AP5 content (control, aCSF rats (●); low 0.01–0.10 (○); mid, 0.11–0.20 (Δ); high, 0.21–0.30 (□); very high, >0.31 (■), all in nanomoles per milligram wet mass). A dose-response relation is apparent, with the "very high group" performing worse than at the end of pretraining; only these rats showed any signs of a sensorimotor impairment. (B) LTP as a percentage of the base line early-rising slope of the field-potential. Only three groups are shown for the sake of clarity. The "low group" was indistinguishable from "controls," whereas the "very high group" was like the "high group" in showing no LTP.

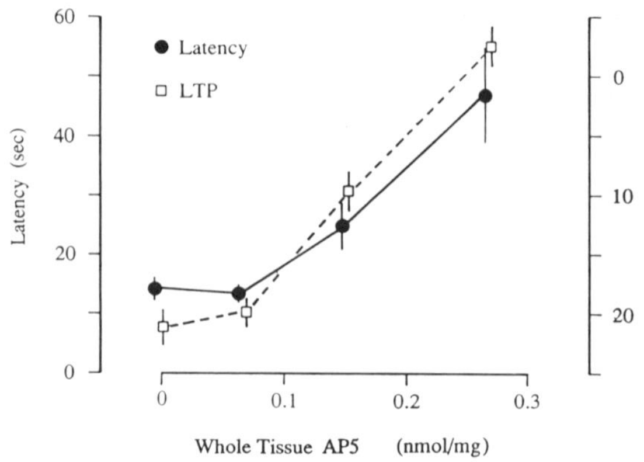

Figure 18.6. A plot of mean escape latency across the spatial learning trials and of mean percentage LTP 40 min after the tetanus against hippocampal whole-issue AP5 in brain (at sacrifice). Note inversion of LTP *y*-axis. ● = latency; □ = LTP.

example, the mid-level whole-tissue concentration, 0.11–0.20 nmol/mg^{-1} wet mass (mean = 0.15; i.e., ≈150 μM) was associated with 10% LTP (see figure 18.6). Might it be that the action of AP5 in vivo is radically different from its action in vitro? Such a possibility seemed unlikely, but the mere possibility brings us to the reasons why we examined both whole-tissue AP5 and the effective extracellular concentration by using dialysis.

Whole-tissue AP5 provides a measure of the total amount of AP5 remaining in hippocampus at sacrifice. However, it does not indicate in which of several "compartments" the drug is located: in plasma, cells or the interstitial space. To meet the second of our aims for this experiment, the comparison with in vitro studies of NMDA receptors, we needed to know the effective extracellular concentration. The analysis proceeded in a series of steps. First, we calibrated the percentage recovery of AP5 from our microdialysis probes by using a solution of known concentration (a value of 6.1% was obtained). Secondly, we checked that the dialysis perfusate was at steady-state (figure 18.7A) by using values obtained from later time points in the collection period (i.e., the 40-minute period beginning 60 minutes after starting perfusion). Thirdly, we conducted a regression analysis of dialysis perfusate against whole-tissue values of AP5 (figure 18.7B). The slope of this line, when percentage recovery is taken into consideration, indicates that the effective extracellular concentration is approximately 30 times lower than the whole-tissue concentration across a wide dose range. We therefore repeated the correlation analyses using extracellular concentration rather than whole-tissue content and found, for example, that the correlation with mean escape latency rose to a value of $r = 0.84$ that, in addition to being highly significant (d.f. 55, $p < .001$), implies that extracellular concentration accounts for 71% of the variability in escape latency. Furthermore, having obtained a measure of extracellular concentration, we were finally in a position to

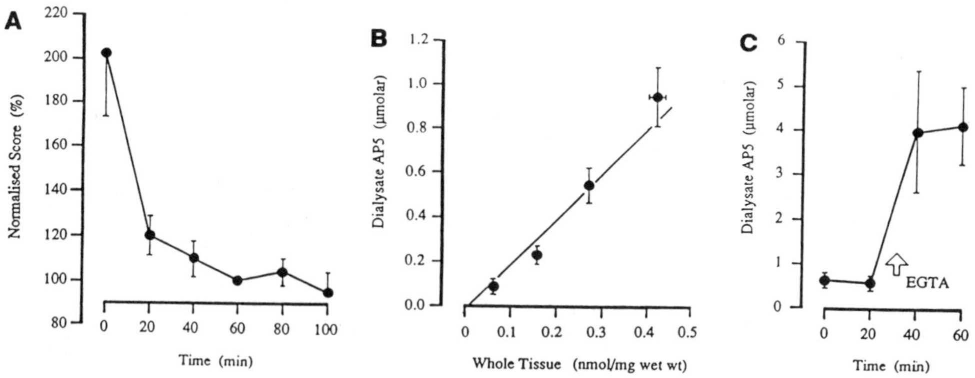

Figure 18.7 (A) Recovery time-course for microdialysis perfusate from 0–120 in 20-min samples. The high initial value probably reflects tissue damage. The mean values for the 60- and 80-min time periods were used in all subsequent calculations. (B) Relation between dialysate AP5 concentration and whole-tissue concentration. The calculated recovery rate from the microdialysis cannulae was 6.1% and thus the ratio of whole-tissue to effective extracellular concentration is ca. 30:1. (C) perfusion of 20 mM of EGTA in Ca^{2+}-free aCSF caused massive release of AP5 indicating that at least part of the difference between the whole-tissue and extracellular concentrations can be accounted for in terms of a Ca^{2+}-dependent "trapping" mechanism.

compare our results with those of certain in vitro studies.* Figure 18.8 shows a comparison with two pertinent experiments: Monaghan and colleagues' (1988) data on the displacement of D-[^{3}H]AP5 by D-AP5 in a ligand binding assay, and Harris and coworkers' (1984) data on AP5-induced impairment of LTP in the in vitro hippocampal slice. Our learning data has been normalized by comparing, across a range of AP5 extracellular concentrations, the savings in spatial escape latency relative to that of controls. The LTP in vivo data have also been normalized. Plotting the results in this way points to a remarkable parallel: the impairment in spatial learning occurs across exactly the same dose range as the AP5-induced blockade of both LTP in vivo and LTP in vitro and each of these three functions is, as anticipated, slightly to the right of the ligand binding results (these having been collected in the absence of L- glutamate).

But the story does not end there. The 30-fold discrepancy between the whole-tissue and extracellular concentrations implies that there must be some "trapping" of AP5 rendering it inaccessible to the microdialysis probes and, presumably, also to NMDA receptors. As this discrepancy between these two AP5 concentrations began to emerge through the series of replications, we naturally wondered about the fate of the AP5 remaining in brain that was unavailable to receptors. Biochemical experi-

*We appreciate that the method used to convert dialysate into extracellular concentration (in vitro bath recovery) does not precisely reflect in vivo recovery (Benveniste, 1989). However, the calibration procedure provides the closest approximation to in vivo conditions available without resorting to intricate mathematical modeling.

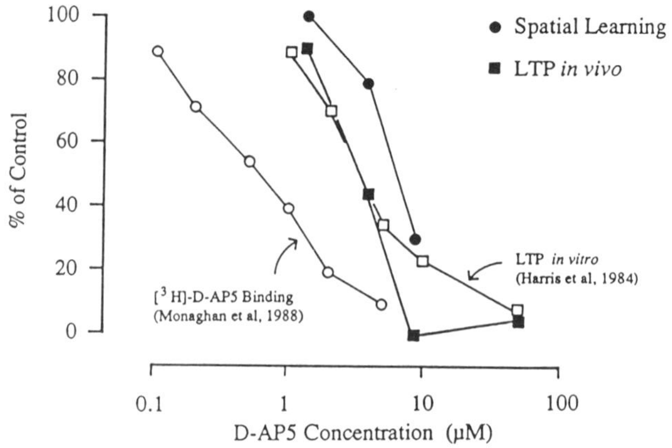

Figure 18.8 Comparison of spatial learning and LTP in vivo with in vitro binding and LTP data from published studies. Spatial learning was calculated as the normalized savings between the overall mean escape latency during the 30 spatial training trials and the latency on the last day of pretraining (PT3 in figure 18.5). LTP in vivo was calculated as the percentage of that shown by the control group. ● = spatial learning; ■ = LTP in vivo; □ = LTP in vitro (Harris et al., 1984); ○ = [^{3}H] D-AP5 binding (Monaghan et al., 1988).

ments conducted in collaboration with M. Kessler and R. Griffiths established that D-AP5 does not inhibit the uptake of L-[^{3}H]-glutamate on the high-affinity glutamate uptake carrier, nor is D-[^{3}H]AP5 itself taken up. However, following a suggestion of J. C. Watkins, we added 20 mM of ethylene-bis(oxyethylenenitrate)tetra-acetic acid (EGTA) to the infusion medium of the microdialysis probes and found a dramatic, eightfold increase in AP5 concentration in the perfusate lasting at least 40 minutes (see figure 18.7c). This finding suggests that a significant proportion of the whole-tissue AP5 is "trapped" in extracellular space by a Ca^{2+}-dependent mechanism.

In summary, parallel dose-response functions were obtained for both spatial learning and LTP. Importantly, we could find no intracerebral concentration of AP5 capable of blocking LTP completely that was without effect on learning. At sacrifice, most of the infused AP5 had escaped the brain but, of that left, over 96% was "trapped" and inaccessible to NMDA receptors. Nevertheless, direct measurement of the residual extracellular concentration of AP5 indicated that the concentration sufficient to block LTP in vivo and severely impair learning corresponded to data obtained from in vitro studies of NMDA receptor function. These findings provide striking support for the hypothesis that learning dependent on normal hippocampal function involves activation of hippocampal NMDA receptors.

Storage or Retrieval?

If blocking NMDA receptors impairs spatial learning, is this due to an encoding deficit, faster forgetting, impaired retrieval, or to interruption of some other psychological process involved in memory? We have begun the task of dissecting which subset of memory processes is impaired with an experiment specifically comparing storage with retrieval.

A clue to the nature of the impairment is provided by the neuropharmacological studies summarized in the section Role of NMDA Receptor Activation in Induction of LTP, indicating that activation of NMDA receptors is required for the induction of LTP but not its expression or maintenance, and that the increase in the EPSP may consist exclusively of a component sensitive to the non-NMDA antagonists CNQX and DNQX (Collingridge et al., 1983; Kauer et al., 1988; Muller et al., 1988; cf. Tsien, 1990). In a behavioral parallel to these findings, the following experiment indicates that AP5 has no effect on the retrieval of previously learned information at a dose that, in the same animals, impairs new learning.

The effect of a drug on retrieval is usually investigated by training animals in its absence but later testing them in its presence. This design suffers from the weakness that the lack of an effect on retrieval is revealed solely as a null result. Accordingly, we extended the usual design by including other groups required, at the time we introduced the drug, to learn a reversal of the task trained initially. This extended design permits a more rigorous examination of dissociable subprocesses of memory by providing both a second index of retrieval and confirmation that the drug is behaviorally effective in impairing learning.

Rats were given *initial training* in the water-maze as normal animals with the hidden platform in either the NE (half the animals) or SW quadrant of the water-maze (26 trials, last 4 days at 1 trial per day). The good performance shown over the final four trials indicated that information about the platform's location was well represented and easily retrieved from long-term memory. The animals were then divided into four groups for surgery (implantation of minipumps). Two groups received aCSF, whereas two others received D-AP5 at a minipump concentration of 30 mM, this being the concentration calculated, from the previous study, as just sufficient to block LTP completely. Beginning 3 days later, retraining in the presence of the drug was conducted at one trial per day. Two groups (AP5-same and aCSF-same) were retrained with the platform in the same place it had occupied during initial training; groups AP5-different and aCSF-different had the platform moved to the opposite location (i.e., SW instead of NE and vice versa). At the end of behavioral training, the rats were sacrificed, their brains removed, and samples from various brain regions dissected for subsequent analysis of AP5 whole tissue content using HPLC.

During initial training, all rats learned to approach the escape platform with short escape latencies and relatively direct paths. On the crucial first trial following surgery (i.e., before any effects of retraining), rats in groups different swam persistently in the former location of the platform (figure 18.9). Consequently, their mean escape latency was very high (82 ± 10 seconds) with some animals not finding the platform in its new location within the maximum permitted swim time of 120 seconds. Importantly,

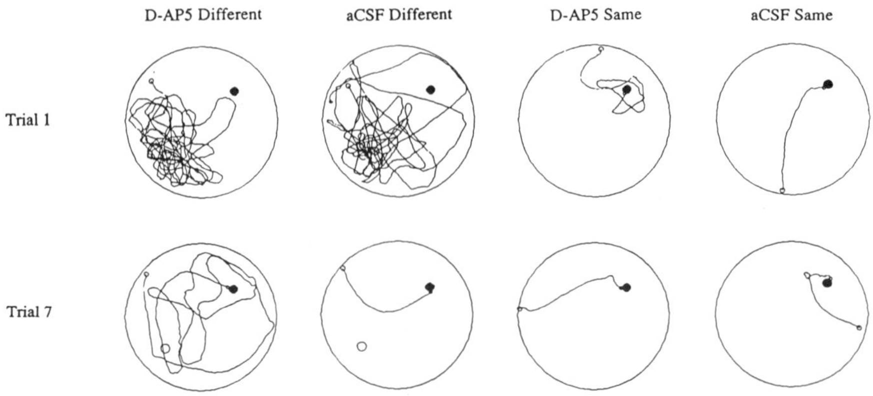

Figure 18.9 Storage against retrieval study. Paths taken by representative animals on the first and seventh trials of the drug-phase. The two "different groups" rats were originally trained to find the hidden platform in SW. Both show good memory of this former location on trial 1 but only the "aCSF-different" rat learns to approach the new platform location accurately over the course of reversal training. The two rats of the "same groups" both approach the originally learned platform location without difficulty.

on this first trial, the AP5-different and aCSF-different rats did not differ. The AP5-same and aCSF-same groups did not differ on this trial either, these rats swimming directly to the platform's original training location. However, they escaped relatively rapidly (latency = 15 ± 5 seconds) because the platform was still in the same place. To obtain a measure of performance that would be independent of escape latency, an "index of spatial bias" was calculated on the basis of time spent in two areas of the pool. This index measures the tendency of animals to revisit the old training quadrant versus their tendency to visit the opposite one (i.e., the new quadrant for groups different) and was calculated according to the formula:

$$\text{index of spatial bias} = \frac{\text{old} - \text{opposite}}{\text{old} + \text{opposite}}$$

This index can vary from +1.0 (all time spent in training quadrant) to −1.0 (all time in opposite quadrant) and should be relatively insensitive to escape latency. Figure 18.10 shows the results of this analysis. Note that the two aCSF groups showed an index of +0.55 on trial 1, irrespective of their widely differing escape latencies. The AP5 groups also showed an equivalent spatial bias. It follows that AP5 cannot be impairing retrieval.

Retraining continued over eight trials and, by the end of this phase, groups AP5-same, aCSF-same, and aCSF-different were all escaping via relatively direct paths with short escape latencies (see figure 18.9). However, rats in group AP5-different failed to learn the new platform location well and continued to take circuitous routes. Their poor performance was also reflected in a significantly slower decline and reversal of the index of spatial bias than that of group aCSF-different.

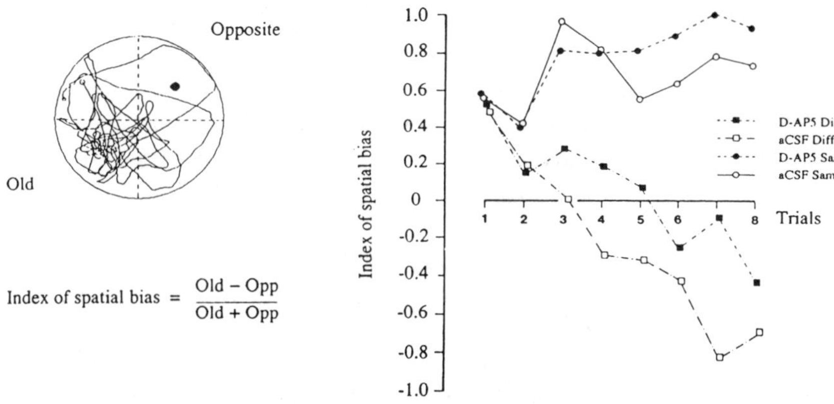

Figure 18.10 Index of spatial bias. All groups begin with an equivalent bias to the originally trained platform location. The index moves gradually negative for "groups different" as reversal proceeds with "group aCSF-different" learning significantly faster. ■ = D-AP5 different; □ = aCSF different; ● = D-AP5 same; ○ = aCSF same.

The analysis of hippocampal AP5 content revealed an overall mean whole tissue content of 0.28 nmol/mg^{-1} wet mass, which did not differ between the two AP5 groups. Although we did not examine LTP in vivo, the drug infusion protocol was identical to that used in the dose-response study described above. Accordingly, we can extrapolate from the regression function relating whole-tissue content and LTP (see figure 18.6) to ascertain that, at this concentration, LTP in vivo would have been just completely blocked. The intracerebral AP5 concentration was not so high as to cause gross sensorimotor disturbances and, as it happens, none were observed.

Taken together, these data imply that at an intracerebral concentration sufficient to block LTP in vivo, AP5 impairs storage but not retrieval. Quite apart from the parallel to the neuropharmacological findings referred to above, this result has implications for one of the alternative accounts of this series of experiments: the possibility of a drug-induced disturbance of sensorimotor control. We have earlier ruled out the possibility that AP5 causes a gross sensory disturbance on the basis of the successful learning of visual discrimination tasks by drug-treated rats, but we noted that this finding left open the possibility of a more subtle disturbance affecting sight of distal cues. However, the present findings (that AP5-treated rats were equally spatially biased as aCSF rats on the first trial) suggest that distal cues can be seen equally well by AP5-treated rats.

CONCLUSIONS

The discovery of the NMDA receptor and its role in one type of activity-dependent synaptic plasticity is one of the most important recent developments in neuroscience. Its property of being both ligand- and voltage-gated explains several of the physiological properties of hippocampal LTP, notably the associativity requirement of induction and that its expression is synapse-specific. Both properties are clearly relevant to the possible role of NMDA receptors in learning. The central finding of the experiments described above is that blocking this receptor pharmacologically also causes an anterograde learning impairment for at least one of the several types of learning known to depend on the integrity of the hippocampus. It is worth emphasizing that this result was in no way a foregone conclusion; part of its force is that NMDA antagonists might have had no effect on hippocampal-dependent learning despite causing a complete blockade of LTP.

This main finding has several theoretical and clinical implications. However, before turning to these, a word of caution is appropriate. The history of research on the physical basis of memory is littered with false leads (e.g., work on RNA-synthesis and "memory molecules"; see Byrne, et al., 1966) and, in the particular case of systemic pharmacological work, inappropriate inferences drawn from poorly controlled experiments (e.g., work on the "cholinergic hypothesis" of memory; see Collerton, 1986; Hagan and Morris, 1988). Conscious of this background, we make no apology for our emphasis on the theoretically uninteresting but experimentally crucial need for control experiments at every step of the analysis. These include explicit attempts to dissociate primary and secondary effects of drug action, checking that AP5 does actually block LTP in vivo in the same animals as those subject to behavioral training, and precise measurement of interstitial drug levels in vivo. Such strictures offer no guarantee of avoiding inappropriate inferences, but we hope they have helped us from being led astray. More specifically, the present paper refers to experiments whose results indicate that (1) one of the sensorimotor side-effects of AP5 can be statistically dissociated from the drug-induced impairment of spatial learning; (2) AP5-treated rats can see proximal and distal cues sufficiently well to learn a visual discrimination task at normal rate and to retrieve spatial information as well as untreated rats; and (3) the drug-induced impairment of spatial learning occurs across an equivalent range of interstitial drug concentrations in hippocampus as that responsible for blocking hippocampal LTP in vitro. However, many more control experiments are required, particularly studies exploring the other effects of NMDA antagonists within hippocampus in addition to their blockade of LTP.

Leaving these problems aside, what are the theoretical implications of the present results? First, they raise the possibility that at least some of the neural mechanisms of LTP are activated during certain kinds of learning and play a causal role in information processing or storage or both. If this is true, under what circumstances does NMDA-receptor activation normally occur? Secondly, why does the hippocampus possess at least two different kinds of long-lasting synaptic plasticity and how do these interact? Thirdly, can these findings contribute information useful for the development of formal "neural-network" models of hippocampal function?

With respect to the first issue, it is important to appreciate that NMDA receptors are not "learning receptors." Their function cannot be adequately described in psychological terms, the appropriate level of discourse being pharmacological. NMDA receptors are a molecular device for detecting the conjunction of presynaptic activity and postsynaptic depolarization, and for signaling this detection by means of a different ionic signal (namely Ca^{2+}) to that used ordinarily to mediate fast EPSPs (Na^{+}). Although this pharmacological property is potentially relevant to the psychological processes of associative learning, such as the detection of contiguity, it is important to appreciate that "detection" is not the same as "representation." Thus although activation of NMDA receptors may help us understand aspects of associative learning (e.g., how the nervous system detects that one stimulus occurs in association with another), a fuller understanding will depend critically on how stimulus information is represented neurally and into what circuitry these receptors are embedded (see McNaughton, 1989). In other circuits, or at different stages of development, NMDA receptors perform a myriad of different functional roles through this same pharmacological property. Thus activation of NMDA receptors during development seems to play a role in experience-dependent self-organization (Kleinschmidt et al., 1987; Cline et al., 1987; Bear et al., 1987; Singer, 1990; Horn, 1990), whereas, in the adult spinal cord, their activation is involved in the integration of suprasegmental reflexes (Davies and Watkins, 1983). In *Xenopus* embryos, activation of NMDA receptors provides a convenient way of turning on a Ca^{2+}-dependent K^{+} current, which repolarizes neurons and thus stabilizes the rhythmic activation characteristic of swimming (see Dale, 1989).

With respect to studies of learning, blockade of NMDA receptors seems to cause a behaviorally selective impairment. In addition to effects on spatial learning, competitive NMDA antagonists cause impairments of DRL schedules and odor-potentiated taste-aversion (Tonkis et al., 1988; Crooks et al., 1989; chronic infusion), passive avoidance and delayed conditional discrimination (Danysz and Wroblewski, 1989; Tan et al., 1989; intraperitoneal injection) and fear-potentiated startle (Miserindino et al., 1990; intra-amygdala infusion). They cause no significant impairment of visual or olfactory discrimination learning at short ITIs (although there may be an impairment at long ITIs; Staubli et al., 1989; chronic infusion), nor, when injected intracerebrally post-trial, do they significantly impair step-through avoidance learning (Mondadori et al., 1989). In one case, analysis of the impairment reveals that it may be secondary to a deficit in stimulus discriminability (Tan et al., 1989), whereas in another case, relevant control experiments show no change in the processing of conditional or unconditional stimuli (Miserindino et al., 1989). There are also reports of correlations between the number of NMDA receptors and certain types of learning (McCabe and Horn, 1988; Wenk et al., 1989). In our view, it is still too early to draw any clear theoretical picture concerning the role of NMDA receptor activation in information processing or storage (or both) from the profile of results obtained so far.

However, if hippocampal NMDA receptors are activated during a subset of hippocampal-dependent types of learning, their activation may, at least partially, be modulated by hippocampal rhythmic slow activity (RSA or "theta"). The hippocampal theta rhythm is a prominent pattern of 7 to 10 Hz electroencephalographic activity that, in rodents and other species, accompanies stimulus processing and certain types of movement (Robinson, 1980). Many previous efforts to understand its psychological function have been of limited success but the discovery of the voltage dependence of the NMDA receptor iontophore suggests a new hypothesis. Specifically, we propose that the rhythmical fluctuations of voltage characteristic of hippocampal theta play a role in regulating the probability that afferent input to the hippocampus from layers II and III of entorhinal cortex (Witter et al., 1989) can trigger NMDA receptor channel opening. Neural activity arriving on the crest of the theta rhythm would have a higher probability of activating the channel than input timed to arrive on the trough of the theta wave. Pavlides and coworkers (1988) have recently reported results confirming this prediction, and also indicating that activity on the trough of the theta wave may cause a depression of synaptic efficacy (see Stanton and Sejnowski, 1989). Larson and Lynch's (1986) earlier work on "primed-burst" potentiation showed that very short bursts of activity at the theta frequency can induce LTP, whereas Abraham and Kairiss (1988) have found that NMDA antagonists "truncate" the complex-spike (burst) firing characteristic of certain hippocampal neurons. Further, our proposal implies that, in rodents, information is presented to the hippocampal matrix no faster than at intervals of $\approx$150 milliseconds. This timing would be commensurate with the need to allow sufficient time (1) for separate neural inputs to disparate parts of a cell's dendritic tree to be "associated" via the relatively slow NMDA-dependent Ca^{2+} current and (2) for subsequent cellular repolarization.

With respect to the important third and fourth issues, we can do little more than stress the need for neuropharmacological and behavioral experiments addressing the mechanisms and functional significance of the nonassociative, AP5-independent form of hippocampal LTP shown at mossy fiber terminals onto CA3 pyramidal cell dendrites (Harris and Cotman, 1986; Nicoll et al., 1988). Lesion studies indicate that the retention of reference- and working-memory in the radial maze survives neurotoxin induced damage to CA3 neurons (Jarrard, 1986). However, this leaves open the possibility that CA3 plays an important role in acquisition. Further, with respect to relatively short-term memory, Frederickson and colleagues (1991) have shown that chelation of mossy fiber bouton zinc by diethyldithiocarbamic acid (DEDTC) does impair a delayed matching-to-place (working-memory) procedure in the water-maze (the zinc content of mossy fibers is the highest in the rodent forebrain and there is evidence that it is coreleased with the endogenous transmitter at these synapses). A critical theoretical issue is why the hippocampal network possesses two distinct forms of synaptic plasticity, with apparently different synaptic learning rules, and why these occur at the terminals of afferents having radically different connection probabilities onto a common set of principal neurons. Rolls' (1989) proposal that such an arrangement would be useful for constructing "episodic" memories deserves to be followed up with formal analysis. However, until more is known about the psychological function of area CA3, indeed of the hippocampus as a whole, the task of building "realistic" neural-network models is probably overambitious. Some progress can, however, be made by examining "simplifying models" (Willshaw and Buckingham, 1990).

Finally, there is great interest in the clinical potential of NMDA antagonists as anticonvulsants and for their capacity to limit brain damage in stroke (Meldrum, 1985; Iversen et al., 1989). That these drugs might also cause memory impairments in humans need not limit their usefulness when administered acutely (e.g., as soon as possible after a stroke), but may be more problematic if they had to be taken regularly (e.g., as anticonvulsants). At the very least, such a possibility points to the need for neuropsychological testing of cognitive function to accompany trials of these compounds' clinical effectiveness.

ACKNOWLEDGMENTS

This work was supported by an MRC Programme Grant held by R.G.M.M. and D. J. Willshaw and by Project Grants from the MRC and the Wellcome Trust. S. P. B. is a Royal Society University Research Fellow. We are grateful to Leslie Chapman for assistance in preparing the manuscript.

REFERENCES

Abraham, W. C., and E. W. Kairiss (1988). Spontaneous complex spikes of hippocampal pyramidal cells are truncated by APV in urethane anaesthetised rats. *Neurosci. Lett.* 89:36–42.

Abraham, W. C., and S. E. Mason (1988). Effects of the NMDA receptor/channel antagonists CPP and MK801 on hippocampal field potentials and long-term potentiation in anaesthetized rats. *Brain Res.* 462:40–46.

Alkon, D. L. (1987). *Memory Traces in the Brain.* Cambridge University Press.

Andersen P., S. H. Sundberg, O. Sveen, and H. Wigström (1977). Specific long-lasting potentiation of synaptic transmission in hippocampal slices. *Nature* 226:736–737.

Artola, A., and W. Singer (1987). Long-term potentiation and NMDA receptors in rat visual cortex. *Nature* 330:649–652.

Barnes, C. A. (1979). Memory deficits associated with senescence: a neurophysiological and behavioral study in the rat. *J. Comp. Physiol. Psychol.* 93:74–104.

Barrionuevo, G., and T. H. Brown (1983). Associative long-term potentiation in hippocampal slices. *Proc. Natn. Acad. Sci. U.S.A.* 80:7347–7251.

Bear, M. F., L. N. Cooper, and F. F. Ebner, (1987). A physiological basis for a theory of synapse modification. *Science* 237:42–48.

Benveniste, H. (1989). Brain microdialysis. *J. Neurochem* 52:1667–1679.

Bliss, T. V. P., and A. R. Gardner-Medwin (1973). Long-lasting potentiation of synaptic transmission in the dentate area of the unanaesthetised rabbit following stimulation of the perforant path. *Physiol. (Lond.)* 232:357–374.

Bliss, T. V. P., and T. Lømo (1973). Long-lasting potentiation of synaptic transmission in the dentate area of the anaesthetised rabbit following stimulation of the perforant path. *J. Physiol. (Lond.)* 232:331–356.

Bliss, T. V. P., and M. A. Lynch (1988). Long-term potentiation of synaptic transmission in the hippocampus: properties and mechanisms. In S. A. Deadwyler and P. Landfield (eds.), *Long-Term Potentiation: From Biophysics to Behavior.* New York: Alan R. Liss, pp. 3–72.

Brown, T. H., P. F., Chapman, E. W. Kairiss, and C. L. Keenan (1988). Long-term synaptic potentiation. *Science* 242:724–728.

Brown, M. C., J. K. S. Jansen, and D. Van Essen (1976). Polyneuronal innervation of skeletal muscle in new born rats and its elimination during maturation. *J. Physiol. (London)* 261:387–422.

Butcher, S. P., A. Hamberger, and R. G. M. Morris (1990). Intracerebral distribution of D, L-2-amino-phosphono-pentanoic acid (AP5) and the dissociation of different types of learning (in press).

Byrne, W. L., et al. (1966). Memory transfer. *Science (Wash.)* 153:658–659.

Cahusac, P. M. B., et al. (1985). The behavioural effects of an *N*-methylasparate receptor antagonist following application to the lumbar spinal cord. *Neuropharmacology* 23:719–724.

Cajal, S. Ramon y (1911) *Histologie du systeme nerveux de l'homme et des vertebres,* Vol. II. Paris: Maluine.

Castro, C. A., L. H. Silbert, B. L. McNaughton, and C. A. Barnes (1989). Recovery of spatial learning following decay of experimental saturation of LTE at perforant path synapses. *Nature* 342:545–548.

Cline, H. T., E. A. Debski, and M. Constantine-Paton (1987). *N*-methyl-D-aspartate receptor antagonist desegregates eye-specific stripes. *Proc. Natn. Acad. Sci. U.S.A.* 84:4342–4345.

Clineschmidt, B. V., et al. (1982). Restoration of shock-suppressed behaviour by treatment with (+)-5-methyl-10,11,-dihydro-5H-dibenzo[a,d]cyclohepten-5,10-imine (MK-801), a substance with potent anticonvulsant, central sympathomimetic and apparent anxiolytic properties. *Drug Dev. Res.* 2:147–163.

Coan, E. J., W. Saywood, and G. L. Collingridge (1987). MK-801 blocks NMDA receptor-mediated synaptic transmission and long-term potentiation in rat hippocampal slices. *Neurosci. Lett* 80:111–114.

Collerton, D. (1986). Cholinergic function and intellectual decline in Alzheimer's Disease. *Neuroscience* 19:1–28.

Collingridge, G. L., S. J. Kehl, and H. McLennan (1983). Excitatory amino acids in synaptic transmission in the Schaffer collateral-commissural pathway of the rat hippocampus. *J. Physiol. (Lond.)* 334:33–46.

Crooks, E. B., et al. (1989). Intraventricular administration of the NMDA antagonist APV disrupts learning of an odor aversion that is potentiated by taste. *Soc. Neurosci. Abstr.* 15:464.

Dale, N. (1989). The role of NMDA receptors in synaptic integration and the organisation of complex neural patterns. In J. C. Watkins and G. L. Collingridge (eds.), *The NMDA Receptor.* Oxford: IRL Press, pp. 93–108.

Dale, N. and A. Roberts (1984). Excitatory amino acid receptors in *Xenopus* embryo spinal cord and their role in the activation of swimming. *J. Physiol. (Lond.)* 348:527–543.

Danysz, W., and J. T. Wroblewski (1989). Amnesic properties of glutamate receptor antagonists. *Neurosci. Res. Commun.* 5:9–18.

Davies, S. N., R. A. Lester, K. G. Reymann, and G. L. Collingridge, (1989). Temporally distinct pre- and post-synaptic mechanisms maintain long-term potentiation. *Nature* 338:500–503.

Davies, J., and J. C. Watkins (1983). Role of excitatory amino acid receptors in mono- and polysynaptic excitation in the spinal cord. *Expl. Brain Res.* 49:293–318.

Daw, N., K. Fox, and H. Sato (1990). The effect of varying stimulus intensity on NMDA-receptor activity in cat visual cortex. *J. Physiol. (Lond.)* 420:46P.

Deadwyler, S. A. and P. Landfield (1988). *Long-Term Potentiation: From Biophysics to Behavior.* New York: Alan R. Liss.

Disterhoft, J. F., D. A. Coulter, and D. L. Alkon (1986). Conditioning-specific changes of rabbit hippocampal neurons measured in vitro. *Proc. Natn. Acad. Sci. U.S.A.* 83:2733–2737.

Errington, M. L., M. A. Lynch, and T. V. P. Bliss (1987). Long-term potentiation in the dentate gyrus: induction and increased glutamate release are blocked by D(−)amino phosphonovalerate. *Neuroscience* 20:279–284.

Frederickson, R. E., C. J. Frederickson, and G. Danscher (1991). *In situ* binding of bouton zinc reversibly disrupts hippocampal function. *Behavl. Brain Res.* (in press).

Foster, A. C., and G. E. Fagg (1984). Acidic amino-acid binding sites in mammalian neuronal membranes: their characteristics and relationship to synaptic receptors. *Brain Res. Rev.* 7:103–164.

Fox, K., H. Sato, and N. W. Daw (1989). The location and function of NMDA receptors in cat and kitten visual cortex. *J. Neurosci.* 9:2443–2454.

Gilbert, M. E., and C. M. Mack (1990). The NMDA antagonist MK-801 suppresses long-term potentiation, kindling, and kindling-induced potentiation in the perforant path of the unanaesthestised rat. *Brain Res.* (in press).

Goddard, G. V. (1986). A step nearer a neural substrate. *Nature* 319:721–722.

Goddard, G. V., D. C. McIntyre, and C. K. Leech (1969). A permanent change in brain function resulting from daily electrical stimulation. *Expl. Neurol.* 25:295–330.

Gustafsson, B., F. Asztely, E. Hanse, and H. Wigström (1989). Onset characteristics of long-term potentiation in the guinea-pig-hippocampal CA1 region *in vitro*. *Eur. J. Neurosci.* 1:382–394.

Hagan, J. J., and R. G. M. Morris (1988). The cholinergic hypothesis of memory: a review of animal experiments. In L. L. Iversen, S. D. Iversen, and S. H. Snyder (eds.), *Handbook of Psychopharmacology.* New York: Plenum Press, vol.20, pp. 237–323.

Halliwell, R. F., and R. G. M. Morris (1987). Anticonvulsant doses of MK-801 fail to block long-term potentiation *in vivo*, or impair spatial memory in the rat. *Neurosci. Lett. Suppl.* 29:599.

Harris, E. W., and C. W. Cotman (1986). Long-term potentiation of guinea pig mossy fibre responses is not blocked by *N*-methyl-D-asparatate antagonists. *Neurosci. Lett.* 70:132–137.

Harris, E. W., A. H. Ganong, and C. W. Cotman (1984). Long-term potentiation in the hippocampus involves activation of *N*-methyl-D-aspartate receptors. *Brain Res.* 323:132–137.

Hebb, D. O. (1949). *The Organization of Behavior.* New York: John Wiley.

Horn, G. (1990). Neural bases of recognition memory investigated through an analysis of imprinting. *Phil. Trans. Roy. Soc. B,* 329:133–142.

Iversen, L. L., et al. (1989). Noncompetitive NMDA antagonists as drugs. In J. C. Watkins and G. L. Colingridge (eds.), *The NMDA Receptor.* Oxford: IRL Press, pp. 217–226.

Jarrard, L. F., (1986). Selective hippocampal lesions and behavior: implications for current research and theorising. In R. L. Isaacson and K. H. Pribram (eds.), *The Hippocampus.* New York: Plenum Press, vol. 4, pp. 93–126.

Johnson, J. W., and P. Ascher (1987). Glycine potentiates the NMDA response in cultured mouse brain neurones. *Nature* 325:529–531.

Kauer, J. A., R. C. Malenka, and R. A. Nicoll (1988). A persistent postsynaptic modification mediates long-term potentiation in the hippocampus. *Neuron* 1:911–917.

Kelso, S. R., A. H. Ganong, and T. H. Brown (1986). Hebbian synapses in hippocampus. *Proc. Natn. Acad. Sci. U.S.A.* 83:5326–5330.

Kemp, J. A., et al. (1988). 7-Chlorokynurenic acid is a selective antagonist at the glycine modulatory site of the *N*-methyl-D-aspartate receptor complex. *Proc. Natn. Acad. Sci. U.S.A.* 85:6547–6550.

Kleinschmidt, A., M. F. Bear, and W. Singer (1987). Blockade of 'NMDA' receptors disrupts experience dependent plasticity of kitten striate cortex. *Science* 238:355–358.

Klockgether, T., M. Schwarz, L. Turski, and K-H. Sontag (1986). The rat ventromedial thalamic nucleus and motor control: role of *N*-methyl-D-aspartate-mediated excitation, gaba-ergic inhibition and muscarinic transmission. *J. Neurosci.* 6:1702–1711.

Konorski, J. (1948). *Conditioned Reflexes and Neuron Organisation.* Cambridge University Press.

Larson, J. and G. S. Lynch (1986). Induction of synaptic potentiation in hippocampus by patterned stimulation involves two events. *Science* 232:985–990.

Lee, K. (1983). Sustained modification of neuronal activity in the hippocampus and neocortex. In W. Siefert (ed.), *Neurobiology of the Hippocampus.* London: Academic Press, pp. 265–272.

Leung, L-W. S, and K. A. Desborough (1988). APV, and *N*-methyl-D-aspartate receptor antagonist, blocks the hippocampal theta rhythm in behaving rats. *Brain Res.* 463:148–152.

Levy, W. B. Jr, and O. Steward (1979). Synapses as associative memory elements in the hippocampal formation. *Brain Res.* 175:233–245.

Liu, C-N., and W. W. Chambers (1958). Intraspinal sprouting of dorsal root axons. *Arch. Neurol. Psych.* 79:46–61.

Lynch, G., and M. Baudry (1984). The biochemistry of memory: a new and specific hypothesis. *Science* 224:1057–1063.

Lynch, G. S., T. Dunwiddie, and V. Gribkoff (1977). Heterosynaptic depression: a post synaptic correlate of long-term potentiation. *Nature* 266:737–739.

McCabe, B. J., and G. Horn (1988). Learning and memory: regional changes in *N*-methyl-D-aspartate receptors in the chick brain after imprinting. *Proc. Natn. Acad. Sci. U.S.A.* 85:2849–2853.

MacDermott, A. B., et al. (1986). NMDA receptor activation increases cytoplasmic calcium concentration in cultured spinal cord neurons. *Nature* 321:519–522.

McNaughton, B. L. (1983). Activity-dependent modulation of hippocampal efficacy: some implications for memory processes. In W. Siefert (ed.), *Neurobiology of the Hippocampus.* London: Academic Press, pp. 233–252.

McNaughton, B. L. (1989). Neuronal mechanisms for spatial computation and information storage. In L. Nadel, L. A. Cooper, P. Culicover, and R. M. Harnish (eds.), *Neural Connections, Mental Computations.* Cambridge, Massachusetts: Bradford, MIT Press, pp. 285–350.

McNaughton, B. L., et al. (1986). Long-term enhancement of hippocampal synaptic transmission and the acquisition of spatial information. *J. Neurosci.* 6:563–571.

McNaughton, B. L., R. M. Douglas, and G. V. Goddard (1978). Synaptic enhancement in fascia dentata: cooperativity among coactive afferents. *Brain Res.* 157:277–293.

McNaughton, B. L., and R. G. M. Morris (1987). Hippocampal synaptic enhancement and information storage within a distributed memory system. *Trends Neurosci.* 10:408–415.

Magelby, K. L., and J. E. Zengel, (1976). Augmentation: a process that acts to increase transmitter release at the frog neuromuscular junction. *J. Physiol. (Lond.)* 257:449–470.

Marr, D. (1971). Simple memory. A theory for archicortex. *Phil. Trans. R. Soc.* B 262:23–81.

Mayer, M. L., and G. L. Westbrook (1987). The physiology of excitatory amino acids in the vertebrate central nervous system. *Prog. Neurobiol.* 28:197–276.

Mayer, M. L., G. L. Westbrook, and P. B. Guthrie (1984). Voltage-dependent block by Mg^{2+} of NMDA response in spinal cord neurons. *Nature* 309:261–263.

Meldrum, B. S. (1985). Possible therapeutic applications of antagonists of excitatory amino acid neurotransmitters. *Clin. Sci.* 68:113–122.

Miserindino, M. J. D., C. B. Sananes, K. R. Melia, and M. Davis (1989). Blockade of fear-potentiated startle by *N*-methyl-D-aspartate antagonists infused into the amygdala. *Soc. Neurosci. Abstr.* 15:167.

Monaghan, D. T., and C. W. Cotman (1985). Distribution of *N*-methyl-D-aspartate-sensitive L-[^{3}H]-glutamate-building sites in rat brain. *J. Neurosci.* 5:2909–2919.

Monaghan, D. T., et al. (1988). Two classes of *N*-methyl-D-aspartate recognition sites: differential distribution and differential regulation by glycine. *Proc. Natn. Acad. Sci U.S.A.* 85:9836–9840.

Mondadori, C., et al. (1989). NMDA receptor antagonists can enhance or impair learning performance in animals. *Expl. Brain Res.* 75:449–456.

Morris, R. G. M. (1989a). Synaptic plasticity and learning: selective impairment of learning in rats and blockade of long term potentiation in vivo by the *N*-methyl-D-aspartate receptor antagonist AP5. *J. Neurosci.* 9:3040–3057.

Morris, R. G. M. (1989b). Does synaptic plasticity play a role in learning in the vertebrate brain? In R. G. M. Morris (ed.), *Parallel Distributed Processing: Implications for Psychology and Neurobiology.* Oxford: Clarendon Press, pp. 248–285.

Morris, R. G. M., E. Anderson, G. S. Lynch, and M. Baudry (1986a). Selective impairment of learning and blockade of long term potentiation by a *N*-methyl-D-aspartate receptor antagonist, AP5. *Nature* 319:774–776.

Morris, R. G. M., J. J. Hagan and J. N. P. Rawlins, (1986b). Allocentric spatial learning by hippocampectomised rats: a further test of the 'spatial mapping' and 'working memory' theories and hippocampal function. *Q. J. Expl. Psychol.* 38B:365–395.

Morris, R. G. M., S. Davis, and S. P. Butcher (1989a). The role of NMDA receptors in learning and memory. In J. C. Watkins and G. L. Collingridge (ed.), *The NMDA Receptor.* Oxford: IRL Press, pp. 137–152.

Morris, R. G. M., R. F. Halliwell, and N. Bowery, (1989b). Synaptic plasticity and learning II: do different kinds of plasticity underly different kinds of learning? *Neuropsychologia* 27:41–59.

Muller, D., M. Joly, and G. Lynch, (1988). Contributions of quisqualate and NMDA receptors to the induction and expression of LTP. *Science* 242:1694–1697.

Nicoll, R. A., J. A. Kauer, and R. C. Malenka (1988). The current excitement in long-term potentiation. *Neuron* 1, 97–103.

Nowak, L., et al. (1984). Magnesium gates glutamate-activated channels in mouse central neurones. *Nature* 307:462–465.

O'Keefe, J., and L. Nadel, (1978). *The Hippocampus as a Cognitive Map.* Oxford University Press.

Pavlides, C., Y. J. Greenstein, M. Grudman, and J. Winson (1988). Long-term potentiation in the dentate gyrus is induced preferentially in the positive phase of theta rhythm. *Brain Res.* 439:383–387.

Racine, R. J., N. W. Milgram, and S. Hafner (1983). Long-term potentiation phenomena in the rat limbic forebrain. *Brain Res.* 260:217–231.

Robinson, T. E. (1980). Hippocampal rhythmical slow activity (RSA-theta): a critical analysis of selected studies and discussion of possible species differences. *Brain Res. Rev.* 2:69–101.

Robinson, G. S. Jr., G. B. Crooks, Jr., P. G. Shinkman, and M. Gallagher (1989). Behavioral effects of MK-801 mimic deficits associated with hippocampal damage. *Psychobiology* 17:156–164.

Rolls, E. T. (1989). Parallel distributed processing in the brain: implications of the functional architecture of neuronal networks in the hippocampus. In R. G. M. Morris (ed.), *Parallel Distributed Processing: Implications for Psychology and Neurobiology.* Oxford: Clarendon Press, pp. 286–307.

Salt, T. E. (1986). Mediation of thalamic sensory input by both NMDA receptors and non NMDA-receptors. *Nature* 322:263–265.

Scoville, W. B., and B. Milner (1957). Loss of recent memory after bi-lateral hippocampal lesions. *J. Neurol. Neurosurg. Psychiatry* 20:11–21.

Shallice, T. (1989). *From Neuropsychology to Mental Structure.* Cambridge University Press.

Sharp, P. E., B. L. McNaughton, and C. A. Barnes (1985). Enhancement of hippocampal field potentials in rats exposed to a novel complex environment. *Brain Res.* 339:361–365.

Sillito, A., P. C. Murphy, T. E. Salt, and C. I. Moody (1990). The dependence of retinogeniculate transmission in the cat on NMDA receptors. *J. Neurophysiol.* 63:347–355.

Singer, W. (1990). Otogenetic self-organisation and learning. In J. L. McGaugh, N. M. Weinberger, and G. Lynch (eds.),. *Brain Organisation and Memory: Cells, Systems and Circuits.* New York: Oxford University Press.

Stanton, P., and T. J. Sejnowski (1989). Associative long-term depression in the hippocampus induced by hebbian covariance. *Nature* 339:215–218.

Staubli, U., O. Thibault, M. DiLorenzo, and G. Lynch (1989). Antagonism of NMDA receptors impairs acquisition but not retention of olfactory memory. *Behav. Neurosci.* 103:54–60.

Tan, S., R. C. Kirk, W. C. Abraham, and N. McNaughton (1989). Effects of the NMDA antagonists CPP and MK-801 on delayed conditional discrimination. *Psychopharmacology* 98:556–560.

Thomson, R. F. (1990). Neural mechanisms of classical conditioning in mammals. *Phil. Trans. Roy. Soc. B,* 329:161–170.

Thomson, A. M., D. C. West, and D. Lodge (1985). An *N*-methyl-D-aspartate receptor-mediated synapse in rat cerebral cortex: a site of action of ketamine? *Nature* 313:479–481.

Tonkiss, J., R. G. M. Morris, and J. N. P. Rawlins (1988). Intraventricular infusion of the NMDA antagonist AP5 impairs DRL performance in the rat. *Expl. Brain Res.* 73:181–188.

Tricklebank, M. D., et al. (1989). The behavioural effects of MK-801: a comparison with antagonists acting non-competitively and competitively at the NMDA receptor. *Eur. J. Pharmacol.* 167:127–135.

Tsien, R. W. (1990). Calcium delivery and synaptic function in peripheral and central neurones. Hoescht Lecture to the Brain Research Association. *Neurosci. Lett.* 38 (Suppl.):57.

Turski, L., et al. (1985). Muscle relaxant actions of excitatory amino acid antagonists. *Neurosci. Lett.* 53:321–326.

Urquhart, J., J. W. Fara, and K. L. Willis (1984). Rate-controlled delivery systems in drug and hormone research. *Ann. Rev. Pharmacol. Toxicol.* 24:199–236.

Watkins, J. C., and G. L. Collingridge (1989). *The NMDA Receptor.* Oxford: IRL Press.

Watkins, J. C., and R. H. Evans (1981). Excitatory amino acid neurotransmitters. *Ann. Rev. Pharmacol. Toxicol.* 21:165–204.

Weiskrantz. L. (1968). Some traps and pontifications. In L. Weiskrantz (ed.), *Analysis of Behavioral Change.* New York: Harper & Row.

Weiskrantz, L. (1982). Comparative aspects of studies of amnesia. *Phil. Trans. R. Soc. Lond. B.* 298:97–109.

Wenk, G. L., et al. (1989). Retention of maze performance inversely correlates with *N*-methyl-D-aspartate receptor number in hippocampus and frontal neocortex in the rat. *Behav. Neurosci.* 103:688–690.

Whishaw, I. Q. and R. N. Auer (1989). Immediate and long-lasting effects of MK-801 on motor activity, spatial navigation in a swimming pool, and EEG in the rat. *Psychopharmacology* 98:500–507.

Wigström. H., B. Gustafsson, Y-Y. Huang, and W. C. Abraham (1986). Hippocampal long-lasting potentiation is induced by pairing single afferent volleys with intracellularly injected depolarising current pulses. *Acta Physiol. Scand.* 126:317–319.

Willshaw, D. J., and J. T. Buckingham (1990). An assessment of Marr's theory of the hippocampus as a temporary memory store. *Phil. Trans. Roy. Soc. B,* 329:205–215.

Witter, M. P., H. T. Groenewegen, F. H. Lopes da Silva, and A. H. M. Lohman (1989). Functional organisation of the extrinsic and intrinsic circuitry of the parahippocampal region. *Prog. Neurobiol.* 33:161–253.

Wong, E. H. F., et al. (1986). The anti-convulsant MK801 is a potent *N*-methyl-D-aspartate antagonist. *Proc. Natn. Acad. Sci. U.S.A.* 83:7104–7108.

Zilles, K. (1985). *The Cortex of the Rat.* Berlin: Springer-Verlag.

19 What Role for Long-Term Potentiation in Learning and the Maintenance of Memories?

Serge Laroche, Valérie Doyère, and Catherine Rédini Del Négro

INTRODUCTION: LTP AND LEARNING AND MEMORY

Long-term potentiation (LTP) is a paradigm example of activity-dependent strengthening of pre-existing synaptic connections of the kind that have long been invoked as a potential substrate for information storage, even long before the phenomenon itself was discovered (Fessard and Szabo, 1961). "There exists at least one group of synapses in the hippocampus whose efficiency is influenced by activity which may have occurred several hours previously—a time scale long enough to be potentially useful for information storage," wrote Bliss and Lømo in 1973 in their first report of LTP in the mammalian brain.

After 18 years, what is the state of our understanding of the link between LTP and learning and memory? Notwithstanding Bliss and Lømo's cautious statement, the question of whether LTP *is* a model of memory is frequently encountered. The semantic shift (trap) is obvious. From a psychological standpoint, the question, as it is phrased, is not likely to be meaningful because a restricted mechanistic ability is implicitly converted into a global description. It is pointless therefore to engage in an argument about how LTP and memory are related until the term *memory* is clarified. Memory is a psychological construct. It refers to an organized collection of representations of events and relationships between events, and therefore the concept of central representation is a key concept in both psychological and physiological models of memory. How are memories stored in the brain? The details are unknown, and we must depend on working models. The cognitive approach emphasizes that the emergence, organization, and evolution of central representations are dynamic processes, and it is largely believed that sensory and memory representations are emergent properties of patterns of neural activities in complex circuits. The building up of these patterns reflects the capacity of the brain to fracture reality and to simulate it within a neural frame, not as a passive projection onto a mental screen, but as a self-organizational construction that creates information. What must be deciphered therefore is both the syntax and semantics of neural representations: understanding how information in the brain is created, organized, retrieved, and used is a major challenge. At the physiological level, one seeks the nature of internal representations and the elementary operations that control their building-up/combination/storage/utilization. If we seek to define the neural mechanisms by which the brain makes learning and memory possible, then the following questions about the link between LTP and learning and memory can at best be posed: is LTP *one* of the necessary, or at least useful, elementary mechanisms involved? If so, what is the process (or processes) of the global function implemented by this mode of local interaction?

Ideally, whenever the potential importance of neural machinery like LTP is questioned, cross-examination of at least four research axes, if separated only for operational purposes, is desired. Let us put on the first axes the level or organization, or unit of complexity, of the system. One can easily recognize different levels of organization such as molecules, neurons, local circuits, and more diffuse assemblies, and each level is outlined by its appropriate methodology. This is an obvious distinction from a neurobiological point of view, but one that may or may not overlap with a hierarchical chain of explanations for memory. Internal representations are obviously not to be found at the single neuron level but require a number of processing elements constituting a widespread, distributed network, even if particular parts of the brain are highly modality specific and if some cells appear to possess specific extractor functions. A given property of a single neuron merely informs us about the property of the circuit to which it is a component. Looking at a diversity of indices is the only way of questioning the rules of interactions and translation between levels within the system.

The second axes describe topology. The distributed and redundant nature of the memory trace is a dominant position. A serious problem with topological analysis of candidate elementary mechanisms is that so far no delineation of the wiring diagram of any memory network exists. Parallel studies of learning and LTP often foster a search for a change at a focused locus, most frequently the perforant path synapses in the dentate gyrus in electrophysiological studies in behaving animals. Yet forms of LTP have now been described in a number of nonhippocampal areas including cortical sensory and association areas (Racine et al., 1983; Artola and Singer, 1987; Bindman et al., 1988; Iriki et al., 1989; Laroche et al., 1990a). Whether LTP-like weighting rules at different locations are properties that account for properties of learning and memory is still a matter of conjecture.

The third and fourth axes concern the forms or kinds of memories and time-related processes. Memory is a general term for many embedded systems, separated, at least for heuristic purposes, on the basis of empirical analyses. Because memory is not an observable entity but a multifaceted function whose properties—multidimensionality, time-dependent lability, and variable access, to cite but a few—and even existence are inferred through behavioral analyses, a variety of well-defined, rigorously controlled procedures are needed to gain access to the nature of stored information and to time-dependent processes such as encoding, consolidation, evolution, accessibility, and retrieval.

After two decades, it is fair to say that tremendous advances have been made in the description of properties and mechanisms of induction, maintenance, and expression of LTP at certain pathways within the hippocampus. Uncertainties and controversies still exist, but from current research, it may be advocated that none of the data available so far contradict the predictions that can be formulated if LTP is to be viewed as a neural model of synaptic changes in learning. This is not surprising, because knowledge of intimate mechanistic details, although certainly enlarging the horizons of behavioral analyses of the role of LTP processes in learning and memory, will not considerably affect the broad problem of learning and memory. What memory theorists first want to know in this line is whether synaptic efficiency changes do occur during learning and whether learning and memorizing is possible because of these changes. Second, if so, where and when these changes occur, and what exact function do they serve?

A critical appraisal of the various approaches and main experimental data on the behavioral importance of LTP has been the subject of several recent publications (Teyler and DiScenna, 1987; Bliss and Lynch, 1988; Buzsáki, 1989; Matthies, 1989), and our views are presented in a companion article (Laroche et al., 1991). In this chapter, we summarize results that we have obtained in testing the LTP hypothesis in the context of associative learning and memory. We also present a set of experiments designed to ask whether the magnitude of synaptic changes induced through LTP procedures is directly predictive of the strength of associative learning, and whether the maintenance of these synaptic efficacy changes has any importance for long-term retention and forgetting.

CLASSICAL CONDITIONING: THE HIPPOCAMPAL COMPONENT OF AN ASSOCIATIVE TRACE

In these experiments, we studied associative learning—the way in which an animal acquires knowledge about the relationships or associations between events in its environment. In rats, we used classical conditioning to a tone-shock association, the acquisition and retention of which is measured by the suppression of lever-pressing for a food reward during the tone (standard conditioned suppression). We chose this method because a large literature based on well-defined behavioral procedures allows analysis of the learning processes underlying response change under a well-defined conceptual framework (e.g., Dickinson, 1980).

We studied the firing rate of hippocampal cells during acquisition of this task. Basically, the results conform to what is seen in other associative learning tasks (Olds et al., 1972; Berger et al., 1976; Wiener et al., 1989). During conditioning, neurons in both the dentate gyrus and hippocampus, but not in the entorhinal cortex, exhibit bursts of discharges linked to behaviorally significant events of the task. This associative cell response develops within a few learning trials, parallels behavioral conditioning, can be maintained for periods of several months, and exhibits extinction under an appropriate paradigm (see Laroche et al., 1991, for review). One characteristic of the hippocampal associative response is that it correlates with the association being learned between environmental events, whatever the actual behavior or response tendency exhibited as a direct consequence of this knowledge (Laroche et al., 1987b). Hippocampal associative responses can therefore be viewed as a reflection of an active state of a central representation of the learned association. The functional role of hippocampal circuits in the emergence and organization of associative representations is not known. Presumably, the cell response is a consequence of activity organized into dynamic patterns in neuronal networks, hippocampal pathways being a part or a branch of a more widespread network engaged in processing and possibly storage of the associative link.

LEARNING MODIFIES HIPPOCAMPAL SYNAPTIC PHYSIOLOGY AND CHEMISTRY

Do synaptic changes in the hippocampal formation occur during acquisition of this task? Are these changes common to both learning and LTP? We have approached these questions in different ways. In one recent series of experiments in collaboration with Bliss and his colleagues we asked whether biochemical changes associated with LTP are also associated with learning. That the expression of LTP in certain hippocampal pathways is at least in part due to persistent presynaptic increases in neurotransmitter release has been largely discussed on the basis of both biochemical and, more recently, quantal analyses. At the origin of the proposed presynaptic mechanism is the demonstration that induction of LTP at the perforant path–granule cell synapses is correlated with a sustained increase in the release of glutamate, the putative transmitter for this pathway (Bliss et al., 1986; Bliss and Lynch, 1988; Lynch et al., 1989; see also the rest of this book for full presentation of current data).

Figure 19.1 summarizes results that we obtained in three different studies of glutamate release in the dentate gyrus after associative learning. We have used the so-called ex vivo technique, successfully applied to investigation of neurotransmitter release in LTP (Feasey et al., 1986), in which the dentate gyrus is removed after training to examine in slices or synaptosomes the release of radiolabeled glutamate. Release is stimulated by depolarization in high potassium in the presence and absence of calcium. The calcium-dependent component of potassium-stimulated release is taken as a measure of the ability of terminals to release glutamate from the vesicular pool of transmitter (Collins et al., 1981). In all these experiments, rats are first trained to press a lever for a food reward at

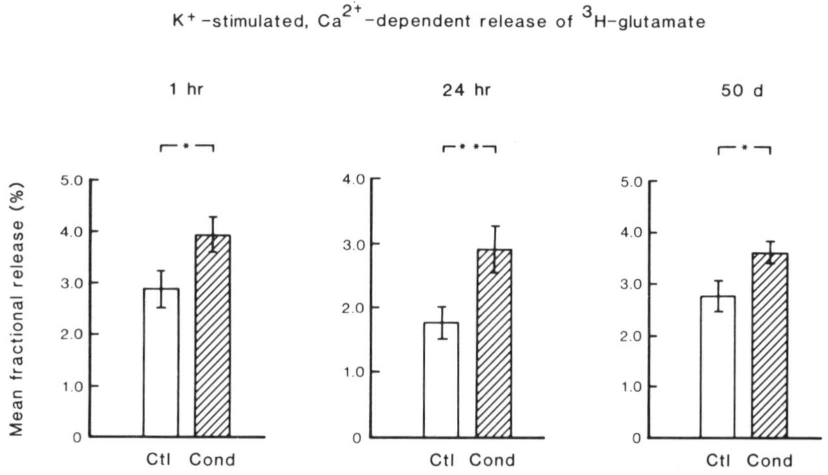

Figure 19.1 In vitro analysis of potassium-stimulated, calcium-dependent release of radiolabeled glutamate in the dentate gyrus after associative learning. Values are mean fractional release ± SEM obtained from dentate tissue prepared from pseudoconditioned controls (Ctl, open bars) and conditioned (Cond, hatched bars) animals. Significant increases in potassium-stimulated, calcium-dependent release of glutamate are seen in slices of dentate tissue taken 1 hr (left panel), or in synaptosomes obtained 24 hr (middle panel), after conditioning relative to control dentate taken at the same time intervals after pseudoconditioning. A significant increase in release is also obtained in slices taken 50 days (right panel) after a single conditioning session.

variable intervals of reinforcement until they reach a stable rate of lever pressing. During associative learning, a tone (the conditioned stimulus, or CS) is repeatedly paired with a footshock (the unconditioned stimulus, or US). This procedure results in a robust suppression of lever pressing for food during the period of the CS: the behavioral measure of associative learning.

In the first experiment (Laroche et al., 1987a), the dentate gyrus was removed 1 hour after the last of a series of four training sessions. Slices were then prepared for in vitro analysis of glutamate release. Measurements were also made on slices obtained from pseudoconditioned animals that were given explicitly unpaired presentations of the CS and US. As can be seen in figure 19.1 (left panel), the release of glutamate was significantly greater in the conditioned group than in the pseudoconditioned group. A similar increase in glutamate release in conditioned animals was obtained in a second experiment (Laroche et al., 1990b) in which synaptosomes (consisting predominantly of resealed synaptic terminals) were prepared from the dentate gyrus taken 24 hours after associative learning (see figure 19.1, middle panel). From these results we can conclude that associative learning is correlated with an increase in the ability of glutamatergic terminals in the dentate gyrus to release transmitter.

That this change can last for periods of time compatible with what is expected for the long-term maintenance of memories is suggested by the results of a third experiment. Rats were given only five conditioning trials in a single session and left for 50 days with no further practice, except that of lever-pressing for a food reward. Submitted to a test of long-term memory consisting of the CS alone, they showed no memory loss after the 50-day interval. In vitro analysis of glutamate release was examined on slices prepared from the dentate gyrus taken 1 hour after the test session. As shown on the right panel of figure 19.1, the increased capacity of terminals in the dentate gyrus to release glutamate in conditioned compared to pseudoconditioned rats is still present.

We also examined phosphoinositide turnover to determine its possible relationship to learning-induced increases in transmitter release (Laroche et al., 1990b). An increase in phosphoinositide turnover is one potential mechanism that can contribute to increased transmitter release in LTP (Bär et al., 1984; Lynch et al., 1988; Clements et al., 1990). Receptor-mediated hydrolysis of phosphatidylinositol-4,5-bisphosphate by phospholipase C leads to the production of inositol-1,4,5-trisphosphate (IP_3) and 1,2-diacylglycerol (1,2-DG), which both play second messenger roles (see Berridge and Irvine, 1989). IP_3 releases calcium from intracellular stores, and 1,2-DG is an endogenous activator of protein kinase C, the implication of which for LTP maintenance is well documented (Routtenberg et al., 1985; see chapter 10). To measure phosphoinositide turnover after associative learning, synaptosomes were prepared from the dentate gyrus taken 24 hours after training, incubated in radiolabeled inositol or radiolabeled arachidonic acid (see Lynch et al., 1988, for a full description of these methods). As illustrated in figure 19.2, significant increases in incorporation of both labeled inositol into inositol phosphates and labeled arachidonic acid into 1,2-diacylglycerol were observed in conditioned relative to pseudoconditioned animals. The increased incorporation of labeled inositol into phosphoinositides also observed here (figure 19.2, left panel) suggests that increase in inositol phosphates labeling in associative learning may occur through an increase in substrate availability rather than in the rate of hydrolysis of phosphoinositides by phospholipase C. In any event, the increased labeling of both inositol phosphates and 1,2-diacylglycerol suggests that the increase in glutamate release after conditioning may at least in part be explained by an increase in second messenger activity.

Two general conclusions can be drawn from these studies of transmitter release and second messenger activation in the dentate gyrus after learning: (1) learning is associated with a rapid and persistent synaptic change in the dentate gyrus, and (2) this change, at least to the extent that the presynaptic side is concerned, is highly similar to that occurring in LTP.

Similar conclusions can be drawn from the results obtained in electrophysiological experiments in which it was demonstrated that learning and the correlated development of hippocampal associative cell responses are accompanied by a robust and persistent (48 hours) increase in the capacity of perforant path synapses to display LTP, a learning-dependent, LTP-

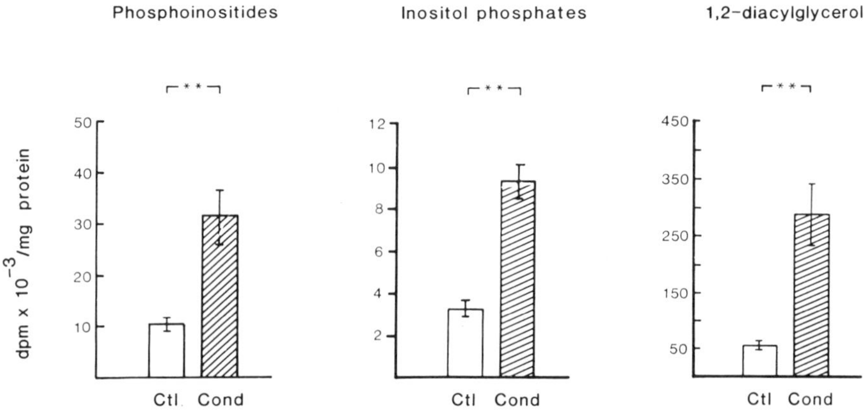

Figure 19.2 In vitro analysis of total labeling of phosphoinositides (left panel) and inositol phosphates (middle panel) by ^{3}H-inositol, and of 1,2-diacylglycerol by ^{14}C-arachidonic acid (right panel), in synaptosomes prepared from the dentate gyrus 24 hr after classical conditioning. Values are expressed as dpm $\times$ 10^{-3}/mg protein $\pm$ SEM. Significant increases in the incorporation of labeled inositol into both phosphoinositides and inositol phosphates, and of labeled arachidonic acid into 1,2-diacylglycerol, are obtained in synaptosomes from dentate tissue prepared from conditioned (Cond, hatched bars) relative to pseudoconditioned (Ctl, open bars) animals.

strengthening effect that appears to be dependent on the amount of learning (Bergis et al., 1990).

ARE LTP-LIKE SYNAPTIC CHANGES A NECESSARY, OR AT LEAST USEFUL, ELEMENTARY MECHANISM FOR LEARNING AND MEMORY?

One of the most compelling arguments in favor of a positive answer to this question comes from the observation by Morris and colleagues that chronic infusion of 2-amino-5-phosphonopentanoic acid (AP5), a selective antagonist of the *N*-methyl-D-aspartate subtype of glutamate receptor that is known to prevent the induction of LTP in certain (although not all) hippocampal pathways, into the lateral ventricle produces severe deficits in learning a spatial problem in a water maze (Morris et al., 1986). Although the glutamate antagonist may exert other effects than LTP blockade and may act at many synaptic relays both within the hippocampus and in nonhippocampal structures, a closer link between spatial learning impairment and LTP blockade in the hippocampus has been provided by later analyses (see chapter 18); as well as in other experiments in which saturation of LTP in the dentate gyrus, a maneuver assumed to impede the development of further synaptic modification, also produced spatial learning deficits (McNaughton et al., 1986). In classical conditioning, chronic infusion of AP5 into the dentate gyrus prevents both LTP and acquisition of associative memory in a task in which a perforant path stimulation is used as a CS (Laroche et al., 1989; see also figure 19.4), a technique that is described in detail later in this chapter.

ON THE ROLE OF LTP IN LEARNING AND MEMORY: A HYPOTHESIS

At this point, let us speculate and ask what function could such synaptic changes serve. During memory registration and processing, neurodynamic engrams are conceived of as a pattern of activation in a network with branching characteristics standing for the multidimensional nature of memory. In this state, the network is settled into a particular dynamic configuration of activity along the connectivity diagram. This is the active state of memory representing the actual support of information. The model asserts that memory traces cannot be left in this active state for the time memory lives, and that in the absence of excitation from a sufficient subset of relevant input signal, engrams are in a latent, or dormant state (inactive memory). Retrieval therefore is based on the capacity for a specific spatiotemporal distribution of activity to be restored during the read out, or reconstruction, of internal representations (see Bloch and Laroche, 1984, for full details).

Learning-dependent synaptic potentiation is thought to selectively strengthen the synapses initially activated during memory registration and processing and hence to participate in active-to-inactive memory shifting, a process that allows dormant engrams to be created. Such a mechanism is called *synaptic marking*. Presumably, it is initiated as consolidation proceeds and could serve two functions: selective stabilization of the network and reliability of its response to afferent activation.

PREDICTIONS

If LTP mechanisms are involved for the purpose of synapse strengthening and network stabilization during the consolidation or information-processing phase, then these mechanisms should be modulated by treatments known to affect learning when applied during a short period that follows acquisition. This possibility has been examined in experiments in which the effects of an electrical stimulation of the mesencephalic reticular formation, a memory-enhancing treatment, was studied on LTP in the dentate gyrus. Activation of the reticular formation was found to enhance both the amplitude and duration of LTP, provided that reticular stimulation was applied within 1 minute after LTP induction (Bloch and Laroche, 1985). The deleterious effect of protein synthesis inhibitors on both LTP and memory formation is another example of such a parallel (see Otani et al., 1989).

Central to several physiological and theoretical models of memory are two other predictions that relate quantitative aspects of synaptic changes to both the strength and the maintenance, or forgetting, of memories.

More specifically, a first, strong prediction is that the amount of learning should be directly dependent on the magnitude of synaptic changes (amplitude of LTP?) within the activated network. A second prediction is that the capacity for remembering might be related to the maintenance of synaptic changes (duration of LTP?) induced by learning. The latter prediction is less obvious than the former, however, because LTP can be viewed just as an intermediate mechanism leading to other changes in the properties of the network accounting for long-term memory.

BEHAVIORAL TEST OF THE HYPOTHESIS: LTP AMPLITUDE AND LEARNING STRENGTH

One difficulty that arises when attempting to test these predictions is that the multidimensional nature of memory makes the detection of a correlation between performance—the end result of many different processes—and LTP at a single locus in the brain unlikely. For example, memory of an event is not limited to the target memory built up under the control of the experimenter but is composed of a collection of attributes or features of the training episode (Underwood, 1969; Spear, 1978). Access to memory is therefore highly variable and can occur after the presentation of a partial and apparently secondary element of the initial situation, including contextual information. At the physiological level, this is accounted for by the distributed nature of memory networks.

To short-circuit the problem of multidimensionality of memory and of the weak localization of the engram, we have used a task in which direct activation of the pathway being investigated—the perforant path—is used as a cue signal. In this task, a unilateral high-frequency stimulation of the perforant path is given an informational content by conditioning, and projection cells form a functional module whose activation is both *imposed* by the training procedure and *necessary* for learning. The task here consists of learning the association between a stimulation of the perforant path as the CS and a footshock as US. As in preceding experiments, the amount the animals learn and remember about the CS-US relationship is quantified by measuring conditioned suppression of lever-pressing for food reward. We have shown previously that if parameters of perforant path stimulation are selected so that reliable LTP is induced, rats can learn this task and reach near asymptotic levels of performance within 10 to 15 trials (Laroche et al., 1989). In subsequent experiments, it was found that some rats learned the task in significantly more trials than others. Figure 19.3 summarizes behavioral and electrophysiological data obtained in three different experiments. As can be seen in the figure, rats with fast acquisition and near maximum levels of performance displayed significantly larger LTP of both the population excitatory postsynaptic potentials (EPSP) and population spike than rats who learned the task to a lesser extent. No significant differences were observed between the two groups in either the intensity at which the perforant path stimulus was given or in

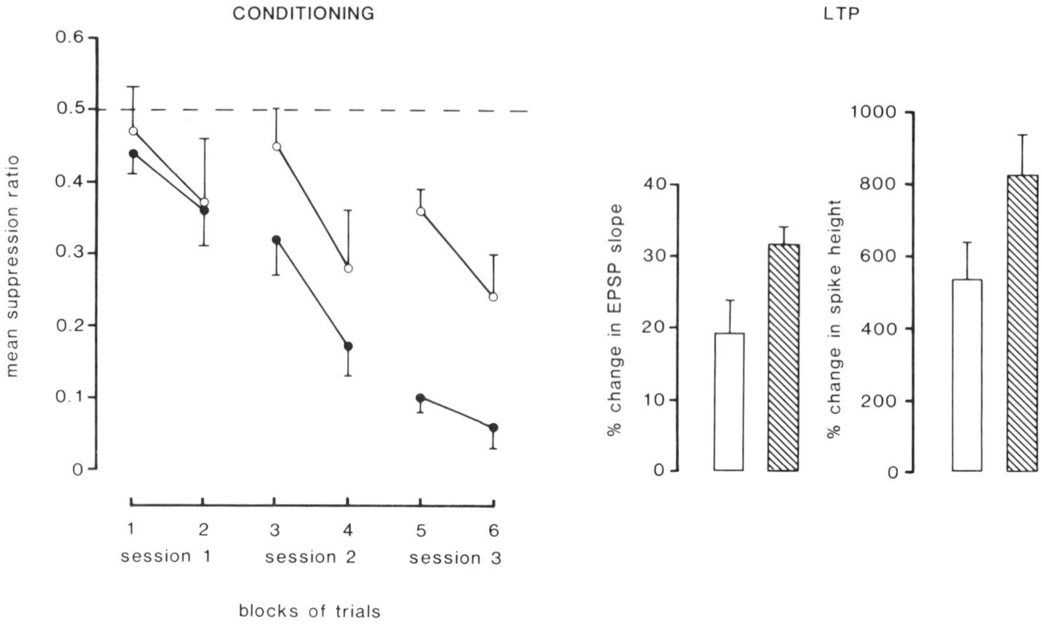

Figure 19.3 Associative learning and magnitude of LTP in the dentate gyrus when high-frequency stimulation of the perforant path is used as a conditioned stimulus. (Left panel) Associative learning is measured by conditioned suppression of lever-pressing for food and expressed as the mean suppression ratio ± SEM. A score of 0.5 (dashed line) indicates no learning, a score of 0.0 indicates maximum learning. Acquisition curves are from two subgroups separated on the basis of performance at the end of conditioning. (Right panel) Saturation level of LTP expressed as a percentage change from preconditioning baseline for both the population excitatory postsynaptic potential (EPSP) and population spike. LTP amplitude is significantly greater (hatched bars) in rats with near maximum performance (filled circles in acquisition curves) than in the second subgroup of rats (open bars) who learned the association to a lesser extent (open circles in acquisition curves).

the absolute amplitude of the dentate response obtained after conditioning. These results are indicative of a correlation between the magnitude of LTP and the amount of learning.

To examine this relationship more closely, we used three different strategies to block LTP, or reduce its magnitude, during conditioning (see Laroche et al., 1989). Figure 19.4 compares performance at the end of the three conditioning sessions with the magnitude of LTP of both the population EPSP and population spike in different groups. When the perforant path cue stimulus is given at an intensity above threshold for eliciting LTP (LTP group), animals learned the association and displayed LTP to a level comparable to controls. Chronic infusion of AP5 into the dentate gyrus on the stimulated side blocked the induction of LTP and completely prevented associative learning. Reduction of the perforant path stimulation intensity below LTP threshold resulted in no LTP and learning failure (PTP group). Finally, inhibitory modulation of LTP by near concomitant activation of commissural inputs resulted in a learning deficit propor-

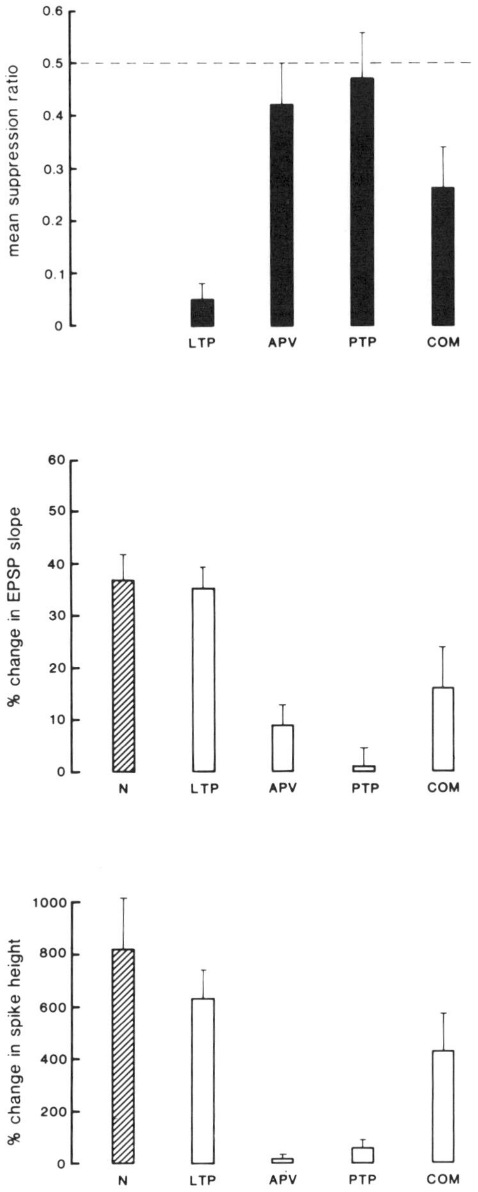

Figure 19.4 Effect of LTP reduction or blockade on acquisition of associative learning. (Top) Learning scores at the end of acquisition. (Middle) Amplitude of LTP of the population EPSP. (Bottom) Amplitude of LTP of the population spike. LTP group: rats for which stimulus trains to the perforant path as CS were given at an intensity for which a spike of approximately 1 mV was observed before conditioning. APV group: animals conditioned in the same way under chronic infusion of APV into the dentate gyrus. PTP group: animals for which the intensity of perforant path stimulus trains was reduced to a value below spike threshold. COM group: animals who received near concomitant stimulus trains to commissural and perforant path fibers. N-naive controls. Other details provided in legend to figure 19.3.

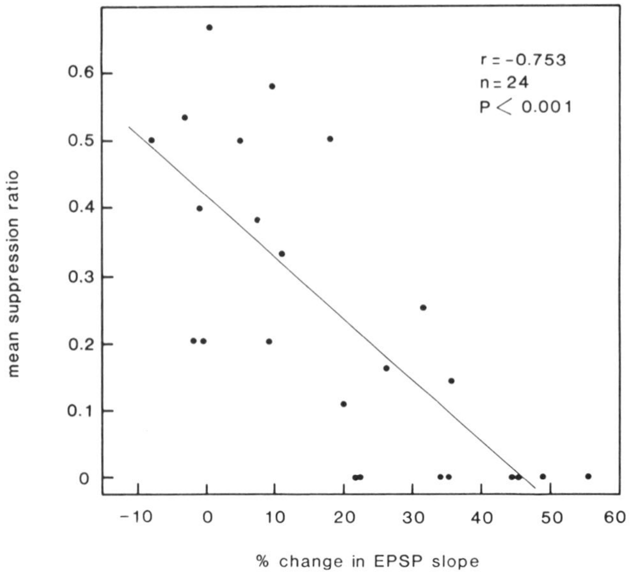

Figure 19.5 Linear relationship between the magnitude of LTP in the dentate gyrus and acquisition of associative learning. Ordinates-learning scores (see legend to figure 19.3); abscissae-amplitude of LTP of the EPSP.

tional to the reduction in LTP amplitude (COM group). Analyzing individual data from this study, a highly significant correlation was found between the magnitude of synaptic potentiation and the amount the animals learned about the CS-US associative link (figure 19.5). This linear relationship provides strong support to the hypothesis that the more synaptic potentiation that is produced in the activated network, the more the animals learn.

BEHAVIORAL TEST OF THE HYPOTHESIS: LTP DECAY AND FORGETTING

The second prediction was examined in a further experiment in which rats were trained in a manner similar to the previous LTP group. In this experiment, animals achieved equivalent levels of performance and LTP magnitude by the end of training. The decay function of LTP was examined during the following 31-day period, after which a long-term memory test was presented. Rats for which LTP had a slow decaying function and for which LTP was therefore preserved a month after learning displayed good retention of the CS-US association, while forgetting was observed when LTP had decayed to a negligible level. As can be seen in figure 19.6, a significant correlation was obtained between the magnitude of LTP just prior to the retention test and performance at this retention test. In this experiment, the retention test consisted of the presentation of the CS alone with the direct consequence of this procedure to trigger LTP back to

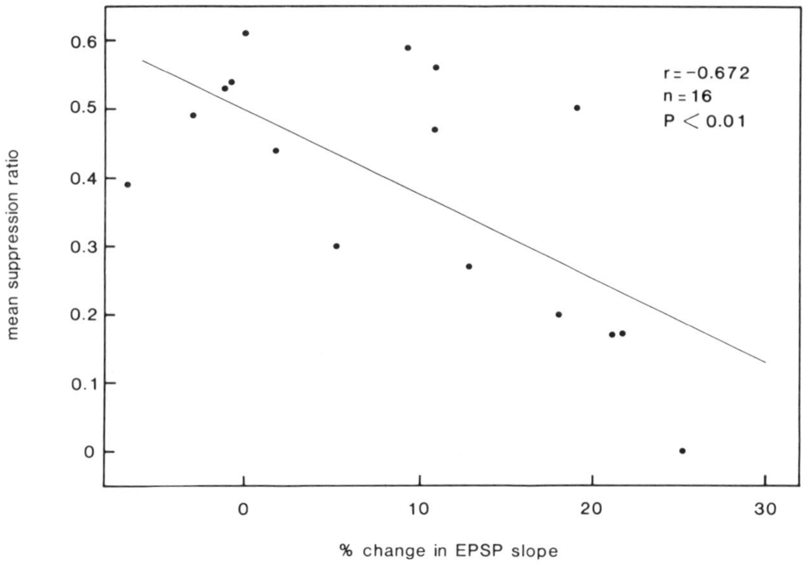

Figure 19.6 Linear relationship between the amplitude of LTP preserved 31 days after associative learning and retention of the CS-US association. Ordinates-retention scores at the test of long-term memory (see legend to figure 19.3); abscissae-amplitude of LTP of the EPSP observed just prior to the test of long-term memory.

its maximum level. This effect, however, had no detectable consequence on performance to subsequent test trials, a result that suggests that the amplitude of LTP, induced during learning and therefore supposedly linked to the association being learned, is the critical factor for remembering rather than the absolute amplitude of the dentate response per se. From these results, it can be suggested that long-term associative memory depends at least in part on the maintenance of synaptic changes induced in the pathway activated during learning.

These experiments are indicative of a role for LTP not only in acquisition, but also in long-term memory and forgetting: the strength of the memory trace, both during acquisition and a long time after, seems to depend on the magnitude of synaptic changes within the relevant network.

CONCLUDING REMARKS

Summarizing the results presented here, four conclusions can be drawn. First, associative learning in the rat appears to be correlated with changes in synapse properties in the dentate gyrus. Second, these synaptic changes have at least some features of LTP as induced by tetanization of the perforant path. Third, there is fairly good indication that these changes are useful, if not necessary, for the building up of the hippocampal component of an associative memory trace. Finally, the magnitude of synaptic changes seems to affect the strength of acquisition, and the decay of these changes with time affects the maintenance of memory.

It remains to be seen how this simple rule could apply to widespread distributed networks at a higher-order organizational level. Presumably, although not proven, the strength and maintenance of the memory trace should rely on a function of all synaptic weight values allocated along the network, each of its points having a particular past of consolidation, decay, and possibly refreshment.

To come again to the four research axes defined earlier, it is clear that generalization of the results should await many empty cells along the four scales to be filled. How far we are from the lesser unequivocal explanatory level where the two orders of events—LTP on the one hand, memory function on the other—can be integrated within a coherent picture? No one knows: revolutions still await us. Perhaps what we are missing most is a sufficiently powerful (predictive) scientific theory to guide us toward the right kind of observations.

REFERENCES

Artola, A., and W. Singer (1987). Long-term potentiation and NMDA receptors in rat visual cortex. *Nature* 330:649–652.

Bär, P.R., et al. (1984). Tetanic stimulation affects the metabolism of phosphoinositides in hippocampal slices. *Brain Research* 321:381–385.

Berger, T.W., B. Alger, and R.F. Thompson (1976). Neuronal substrate of classical conditioning in the hippocampus. *Science* 192:483–485.

Bergis, O.E., V. Bloch, and S. Laroche (1990). Enhancement of long-term potentiation in the dentate gyrus two days after associative learning in the rat. *Neuroscience Research Communications* 6:119–128.

Berridge, M.J., and R.F. Irvine (1989). Inositol phosphates and cell signalling. *Nature* 341:381–385.

Bindman, L.J., K.P.S.J. Murphy, and S. Pockett (1988). Postsynaptic control of the induction of long-term changes in efficacy of transmission at neocortical synapses in slices of rat brain. *Journal of Neurophysiology* 60:1053–1065.

Bliss, T.V.P., R.M. Douglas, M.L. Errington, and M.A. Lynch (1986). Correlation between long-term potentiation and release of endogenous amino acids from dentate gyrus of anaesthetized rats. *Journal of Physiology (London)* 377:391–408.

Bliss, T.V.P., and T. Lømo (1973). Long-lasting potentiation of synaptic transmission in the dentate area of the anaesthetized rabbit following stimulation of the perforant path. *Journal of Physiology (London)* 232:331–356.

Bliss, T.V.P., and M.A. Lynch (1988). Long-term potentiation of synaptic transmission in the hippocampus: properties and mechanisms. In P.W. Landfield and S.A. Deadwyler (eds.), *Long-Term Potentiation: From Biophysics to Behavior.* New York: Alan R. Liss, pp. 3–72.

Bloch, V., and S. Laroche (1984). Facts and hypotheses related to the search for the engram. In G. Lynch, J.L. McGaugh, and N.W. Weinberger (eds.) *Neurobiology of Learning and Memory.* New York: Guilford Press, pp. 249–260.

Bloch, V., and S. Laroche (1985). Enhancement of long-term potentiation in the rat dentate gyrus by post-trial stimulation of the reticular formation. *Journal of Physiology (London)* 360:215–231.

Buzsáki, G. (1989). Two-stage model of memory trace formation: a role for "noisy" brain states. *Neuroscience* 31:551–570.

Clements, M.P., M.L. Errington, T.V.P. Bliss, and M.A. Lynch (1990). Time-related changes in basal phosphoinositide turnover after induction of long-term potentiation in the dentate gyrus are blocked by commissural stimulation. *European Journal of Neuroscience* 2:383–387.

Collins, G.G.S., J. Anson, and G.A. Probett (1981). Patterns of endogenous amino acid release from slices of rat and guinea pig olfactory cortex. *Brain Research* 204:103–120.

Dickinson, A. (1980). *Contemporary Animal Learning Theory.* Cambridge: Cambridge University Press.

Feasey, K.J., M.A. Lynch, and T.V.P. Bliss (1986). Long-term potentiation is associated with an increase in calcium-dependent, potassium-stimulated release of (^{14}C)-glutamate from hippocampal slices: an ex vivo study in the rat. *Brain Research* 364:39–44.

Fessard, A., and T.H. Szabo (1961). La facilitation de post-activation comme facteur de plasticité dans l'établissement des liaisons temporaires. In A. Fessard, R.W. Gerard, J. Konorsky, and J.F. Delafresnaye (eds.), *Brain Mechanisms and Learning.* Oxford: Blackwell, pp. 353–371.

Iriki, A., C. Pavlides, A. Keller, and H. Asanuma (1989). Long-term potentiation in the motor cortex. *Science* 245:1385–1387.

Laroche, S., V. Bloch, V. Doyère, and C. Rédini Del Négro (1991). The significance of long-term potentiation for learning and memory. In F. Morrell, (ed.), *Kindling and Synaptic Plasticity: Legacy of G. Goddard.* Boston: Birkhäuser (in press).

Laroche, S., V. Doyère, and V. Bloch (1989). Linear relation between the magnitude of long-term potentiation in the dentate gyrus and associative learning in the rat. A demonstration using commissural inhibition and local infusion of an *N*-methyl-D-aspartate receptor antagonist. *Neuroscience* 28:375–386.

Laroche, S., M.L. Errington, M.A. Lynch, and T.V.P. Bliss (1987a). Increase in (^{3}H)glutamate release from slices of dentate gyrus and hippocampus following classical conditioning in the rat. *Behavioural Brain Research* 25:23–29.

Laroche, S., T.M. Jay, and A.M. Thierry (1990a). Long-term potentiation in the prefrontal cortex following stimulation of the hippocampal CA1/subicular region. *Neuroscience Letters* 114:184–190.

Laroche, S., N. Neuenschwander-El Massioui, J.M. Edeline, and G. Dutrieux (1987b). Hippocampal associative cellular responses: dissociation with behavioral responses revealed by a transfer-of-control technique. *Behavioral and Neural Biology* 47:356–368.

Laroche, S., C. Rédini Del Négro, M.P. Clements, and M.A. Lynch (1990b). Long-term activation of phosphoinositide turnover associated with increased release of amino acids in the dentate gyrus and hippocampus following classical conditioning in the rat. *European Journal of Neuroscience* 2:534–543.

Lynch, M.A., M.P. Clements, M.L. Errington, and T.V.P. Bliss (1988). Increased hydrolysis of phosphatidylinositol-4,5-bisphosphate in long-term potentiation. *Neuroscience Letters* 84:291–296.

Lynch, M.A., M.L. Errington, and T.V.P. Bliss (1989). Nordihydroguaiaretic acid blocks the synaptic component of long-term potentiation and the associated increase in release of glutamate and arachidonate: an in vitro study in the dentate gyrus of the rat. *Neuroscience* 30:693–701.

Matthies, H. (1989). Neurobiological aspects of learning and memory. *Annual Review of Psychology* 40:381–404.

McNaughton, B.L., et al. (1986). Long-term enhancement of hippocampal synaptic transmission and the acquisition of spatial information. *Journal of Neuroscience* 6:563–571.

Morris, R.G.M., E. Anderson, G.S. Lynch, and M. Baudry (1986). Selective impairment of learning and blockade of long-term potentiation by an *N*-methyl-D-aspartate antagonist, AP5. *Nature* 319:774–776.

Olds, J., et al. (1972). Learning centers of rat brain mapped by measuring latencies of conditioned unit responses. *Journal of Neurophysiology* 35:202–219.

Otani, S., et al. (1989). Maintenance of long-term potentiation in rat dentate gyrus requires protein synthesis but not messenger RNA synthesis immediately post-tetanization. *Neuroscience* 28:519–526.

Racine, R.J., N.W. Milgram, and S. Hafner (1983). Long-term potentiation phenomena in the rat limbic forebrain. *Brain Research* 260:217–231.

Routtenberg, A., D.M. Lovinger, and O. Steward (1985). Selective increase in phosphorylation of a 47-kDa protein (F1) directly related to long-term potentiation. *Behavioral and Neural Biology* 43:3–11.

Spear, N.E. (1978). *The Processing of Memories: Forgetting and Retention.* Hillsdale: Erlbaum.

Teyler, T.J., and P. DiScenna (1987). Long-term potentiation. *Annual Review of Neuroscience* 10:131–161.

Underwood, B.J. (1969). Attributes of memory. *Psychological Review* 76:559–573.

Wiener, S.I., C.A. Paul and H. Eichenbaum (1989). Spatial and behavioral correlates of hippocampal neuronal activity. *Journal of Neuroscience* 9:2737–2763.

20 Long-Term Potentiation and Learning and Memory

Bernard Soumireu-Mourat
and François Roman

Starting from Hebb's hypothesis in 1949, it was progressively accepted that the substrate for information storage in the central nervous system was supported by changes in synaptic efficacy, consecutive to associative learning, with the necessity of coactivity of both presynaptic and postsynaptic elements. These changes resulted in the strengthening of particular sets of connections between neurons, progressively building neural networks corresponding to specific information, whatever may be the characteristics of these networks. They were at first considered as classical on-line circuits or reverberating circuits, then progressively more as combinatorial and topographic arrays (Bloch and Laroche, 1984; Lynch, 1986). In any case, as stressed by Squire in 1986, these networks can be at the same time localized and distributed because they correspond to both specific aspects of information and relations between many neural systems involved in a whole event.

On the other hand, after its discovery by Lømo in 1966 and its first analysis by Bliss and Lømo in 1973, long-term potentiation (LTP) was largely considered as a putative mechanism of synaptic modifications involved in information encoding; indeed, LTP represents an increase in synaptic efficacy, characterized as a rapidly induced and long-lasting phenomenon, providing a possible model of the Hebbian synapse.

RELATIONSHIP BETWEEN LTP AND LEARNING: THE FACTS

A large amount of data link LTP and memory processes (Teyler and Discenna, 1987). Some data are presented in this book in such chapters as 16–19, 21 and 23. Different kinds of arguments have been provided and can be grouped along several lines.

The first group of data tends to provide direct evidence of an increase in synaptic efficacy after learning (see review in Laroche et al., 1991). Most of the data were obtained from the hippocampal formation, but more recently data have been obtained from specific cortical areas (Roman et al., 1987; see the following discussion). The data, however when considered as a whole, are still relatively controversial. In the same perspective, some recent research has tried to correlate the level of retention performance with the strength of LTP in hippocampus, suggesting a parallel decay of LTP and forgetting, and further suggesting, that LTP could constitute a predictive index of retrieval. In a similar perspective, Barnes and McNaughton (1985) showed that decay of LTP is faster in old animals than in young animals, with an interesting comparison of the rates of acquisition and forgetting of spatial information. Similarly, Ramirez and associates (1988) observed that high-performance rats showed a lower threshold of LTP than low-performance rats, suggesting that a greater learning ability was related to a higher hippocampal plasticity.

A more indirect argument is given by observations of changes in glutamate release and protein kinase C modifications after learning similar to those noted after LTP (Laroche et al., 1990). Another approach demonstrated that procedures that affect LTP also produced similar marked memory changes. Recently, it was demonstrated that activation of the *N*-methyl-D-aspartate (NMDA) receptors is required for induction of LTP. Because of this better knowledge of LTP mechanisms, the effects of NMDA receptor antagonists on learning and memory were investigated, using either competitive (APV, AP5, or AP7) or noncompetitive (MK-801) NMDA receptor blockers (see chapters 17 and 18; see also Danysz and Wroblewski, 1989). According to these authors and others, learning and memory deficits were observed after treatments with NMDA antagonists. More interestingly, Morris and coworkers (1989), considering blocking effects of AP5 on induction but not on maintenance of LTP, showed that AP5, intraventricularly delivered over long periods of time, affected new learning but had no effect on information retrieval. Looking at different results, however, the effects of such antagonists seem to be task-dependent. Moreover, although these types of data seem to indicate a parallel between effects of NMDA antagonists on LTP and on learning, they do not exclude causes of learning disturbance other than blockade of LTP. Other treatments influencing LTP have also been studied. In any case, the more indirect are the effects of the treatment on LTP, the less demonstrative are the experiments, as it is the case for steroids (Dubrovsky et al., 1987) and opioids (Derrick and Martinez, 1989).

Another line of research explored the effects of memory modulatory treatments on LTP. For instance, post-trial stimulation of the reticular formation that facilitates memory processes also enhances the amplitude of LTP induced by tetanic stimulation 2 days after conditioning (Bergis et al., 1990). But parallel effects after drugs inducing either memory facilitation (orotic acid; Krug et al., 1989) or memory disturbance (inhibitors of protein synthesis; Matthies, 1989) were also shown. More inconsistent are the data using drugs related to transmitters such as catecholamines.

Yet another approach was to study the effects of previous LTP induction on subsequent learning. Here again, data are equivocal, displaying either facilitation (Berger, 1984) or disturbance of learning performance (McNaughton and Morris, 1987), with no effect on well-learned performance (McNaughton and Morris, 1987). For these last authors, the high-frequency stimulation increased the efficacy of most of the synapses to near their maximum possible strength, leading to a saturation of the network and disruption of recently stored information or new learning.

All together, these various results seem to indicate a real link between establishment of LTP and memory processes. It might be argued, however, that a direct relationship between LTP and memory has not been clearly proved and that most of the existing data are more in favor of correlations than direct proofs of causality.

LTP AND MEMORY FORMATION: THE QUESTIONS

Examining the literature on LTP and learning and memory formation, we encounter many questions; most of them are without answers but quite exciting for future research.

A question about correlations between LTP and behavior is whether LTP exists in natural conditions and whether physiological activities are able to trigger phenomena similar to LTP. This question was raised in 1973 by Bliss and Lømo and is not completely answered. Indeed, LTP is an experimental observation triggered by electrical stimulation. Several arguments, however, seem to confirm that LTP exists in natural conditions. First, LTP is induced by short trains of repeated stimulations probably not so different from circulating impulses triggered by natural stimuli (Bloch and Laroche, 1984). Moreover, short bursts (4 spikes in about 30 milliseconds) applied to Schaffer commissural projections at 200-millisecond intervals, which represent a theta-pattern stimulation, are sufficient to induce LTP (Lynch et al., 1988). Second, electrical central stimulation was sometimes directly used as a conditioned stimulus, delivered either on perforant path (Matthies et al., 1986), cerebral peduncle (Tsukahara et al., 1981), or lateral olfactory tract (Roman et al., 1987). In all cases, the authors observed an increase in amplitude of the evoked responses, which may confirm the existence of persistent synaptic changes and thus encourages the hypothesis that LTP exists in natural conditions.

LTP was first described in hippocampus, where most available data were obtained. Progressively, it appeared that LTP might not be a unique and universal process. At least two components of LTP induced by different patterns of afferent activation have been isolated (Grover and Teyler, 1990), and phenomena close to LTP have also been distinguished, characterized by some differential aspects. For instance, mossy fiber potentiation (MFP: Harris and Cotman, 1986; Staubli et al., 1990) is not influenced by antagonists of the NMDA receptor and has not the convergence requirement typical of LTP. Even more subtle, some authors preferred not to use the word *potentiation* but rather *enhancement* because of *potentiation's* long history of specific use as meaning a nonassociative and short-lasting increase in the probability of transmitter release after tetanic stimulation (McNaughton et al., 1986; McNaughton and Morris, 1987).

By extending this point, the question is whether the different aspects of LTP are involved in several types of memory. In chapter 18, data are presented that show that spatial discrimination but not visual discrimination was affected by drugs acting on LTP induction. In a similar manner, Mondadori and coworkers (1989) reported that NMDA receptor antagonists modify task-dependent learning performance. Such differences may account for the different theories of hippocampal function (Morris et al. 1986; Rasmussen et al., 1989), and also for different implications of hippocampal LTP.

A more important point is the putative relationship between LTP found in the hippocampus and LTP observed in other structures. Recently, LTP has been observed in different cortical areas (Kuba and Kumamoto, 1990): motor cortex (Iriki et al., 1989), visual cortex (Artola and Singer, 1990), and olfactory cortex (Roman et al., 1987). The LTP found in these areas, however, differs in several aspects from hippocampal LTP (Teyler, 1989). After training rats in a series of two-odor discriminations, Roman and associates (1987) used patterned electrical stimulation of the lateral olfactory tract (LOT) as a discriminative cue. They observed that the population synaptic responses in the piriform cortex evoked by single-pulse LOT stimulation were potentiated by the training; this result was not found in rats that did not learn the discrimination task or when the stimulation was applied to naive rats. Such a result seems to indicate strongly that potentiation in the olfactory cortex is really related to information processing and storage. Given that the olfactory cortex is closely related to hippocampus, this kind of data raises the question of the possible relationship and functional importance of the existence of LTP in both hippocampus and cortex. Indeed, although it can be shown that LTP occurs in cortex after learning, the question exists whether both phenomena are independent, or what might be their relationship. In other words, it could be hypothesized that induction of LTP in hippocampus after learning might be responsible, at least partly, for appearance of potentiation in cortical regions, and so might explain the strengthening of synapses in a specified neural network. Such a hypothesis could be tested by physiological and anatomical analyses. In this kind of approach, the time of occurrence and the duration of enhancement of synaptic responses must be carefully studied; in any case, LTP may possibly reflect an intermediate mechanism that in turn may prepare more lasting changes (Bloch and Laroche, 1984). Following this line, LTP might be related to specific stages in memory formation and would constitute one of the steps to stabilize the specific network supporting information. Clearly, the importance of LTP is either as a necessary step during the formation of the network supporting the engram or as the manifestation of the activation of this same network. In this case, LTP must also be observed during retrieval, signaling activation processes in a potential network characterized by the absence of activity between storage and retrieval (Bloch and Laroche, 1984). In any case, as noted by Teyler and Discenna in 1984 and still true today, "LTP does not appear to have the longevity to account for truly long-term information storage that may span decades in some species." In fact, this question of the functional importance of LTP is not yet really solved. Again here, the question exists concerning the specificity of LTP in hippocampus, but it is probably part of the larger question of hippocampal role in memory processes. In other words, does LTP in hippocampus serve to define an information-specific network? Or is hippocampal LTP part of the activation process that allows a specific network to be "read out" somewhere else?

It will become progressively possible to know whether LTP either is involved in only some kinds of memory (Morris et al., 1989) or, on the contrary, is the counterpart of a basic process supporting memory formation.

Probably, besides neurophysiological and neurochemical studies about LTP, behavioral studies with correlative analysis of LTP will provide progressive information concerning nature, mechanisms, and the functional importance of LTP.

REFERENCES

Artola, A., and W. Singer (1990). The involvement of *N*-methyl-D-aspartate receptors in induction and maintenance of long-term potentiation in rat visual cortex. *European Journal of Neuroscience.* 2:254–269.

Barnes, C. A., and B. L. McNaughton, (1985). An age comparison of the rates of acquisition and forgetting of spatial information in relation to long-term enhancement of hippocampal synapses. *Behavioral Neuroscience,* 99:1040–1048.

Berger, T. W. (1984). Long-term potentiation of hippocampal synaptic transmission affects rate of behavioral learning. *Science* 224:627–630.

Bergis, O. E., V. Bloch, and S. Laroche (1990). Enhancement of long-term potentiation in the dentate gyrus two days after associative learning in the rat. *Neuroscience Research Communications* 6:119–128.

Bliss, T. V. P., and T. Lømo, (1973). Long-lasting potentiation of synaptic transmission in the dentate area of the anesthetized rabbit following stimulation of the perforant path. *Journal of Physiology, (London)* 232:331–356.

Bloch, V., and S. Laroche, (1984). Facts and hypotheses related to the search for the engram. In, G. Lynch, J. L. McGaugh, and N. M. Weinberger (eds.), *Neurobiology of Learning and Memory.* New York: The Guilford Press, pp. 249–260.

Danysz, W., and J. T. Wroblewski, (1989). Amnesic properties of glutamate receptor antagonists. *Neuroscience Research Communications* 5:9–18.

Derrick, B. E., and J. L. Martinez, Jr. (1989). A unique, opioid peptide–dependent form of long-term potentiation is found in the CA3 region of the rat hippocampus. In *Advances in the Biosciences,* Vol. 75. London: Pergamon Press, pp. 213–216.

Dubrovsky, B. O., M. S., Liquornik, P. Noble, and K. Gijsbers, (1987). Effects of 5-dihydrocorticosterone on evoked responses and long-term potentiation. *Brain Research Bulletin* 19:345–348.

Grover, L. M., and T. J. Teyler (1990). Two components of long-term potentiation induced by different patterns of afferent activation. *Nature* 347:477–479.

Harris, E. W., and C. W. Cotman, (1986). Long-term potentiation of guinea pig mossy fiber responses is not blocked by *N*-methyl-D-aspartate antagonists. *Neuroscience Letters* 70: 132–137.

Hebb, D. O. (1949). *The Organization of Behavior.* New York: Wiley.

Iriki, A., C. Pavlides, A. Keller, and H. Asanuma (1989). Long-term potentiation in the motor cortex. *Science* 245:1385–1387.

Krug, M., et al. (1989). Methylglucamine orotate, a memory-improving drug, prolongs hippocampal long-term potentiation. *European Journal of Pharmacology* 173:223–226.

Kuba, K., and E. Kumamoto, (1990). Long-term potentiations in vertebrate synapses: a variety of cascades with common subprocesses. *Progress in Neurobiology 34:197–269.*

Laroche, S., V. Bloch, V. Doyère, and C. Rédini Dél Négro (1991). The significance of long-term potentiation for learning and memory. In F. Morell (ed.), *Kindling and Synaptic Plasticity: The Legacy of Graham Goddard.* Boston: Birkhauser (in press).

Laroche, S., C. Rédini Del Négro, M. P. Clements, and M. A. Lynch, (1990). Long-term activation of phosphoinositide turnover associated with increased release of amino acids in the dentate gyrus and hippocampus following classical conditioning in the rat. *European Journal of Neuroscience* 2:534–543.

Lømo, T. (1966). Frequency potentiation of excitatory synaptic activity in the dentate area of the hippocampal formation. *Acta Physiologica Scandinavica* 68:128.

Lynch, G. (1986). *Synapses, Circuits, and the Beginnings of Memory.* Cambridge, Mass.: M.I.T. Press.

Lynch G., D. Muller, P. Seubert, and J. Larson (1988). Long-term potentiation: persisting problems and recent results. *Brain Research Bulletin.* 21:363–372.

Matthies, H. (1989). Neurobiological aspects of learning and memory. *Annual Review of Psychology* 40:381–404.

Matthies, H., et al. (1986). Low-frequency perforant path stimulation as a conditioned stimulus demonstrates correlations between long-term synaptic potentiation and learning. *Physiology and Behavior* 36:811–821.

McNaughton, B. L., and R. G. M. Morris. (1987). Hippocampal synaptic enhancement and information storage within a distributed memory system. *Trends in Neurosciences* 10:408–415.

McNaughton, B. L., et al. (1986). Long-term enhancement of hippocampal synaptic transmission and the acquisition of spatial information. *Journal of Neuroscience* 6:563–571.

Mondadori, C., et al. (1989). NMDA receptor antagonists can enhance or impair learning performance in animals. *Experimental Brain Research,* 75:449–456.

Morris, R. G. M., S. Davis, and S. P. Butcher (1989). The role of NMDA receptors in learning and memory. In: J. C. Watkins and G. L. Collingridge (eds.), *The NMDA Receptor.* Oxford: IRL Press, pp. 137–151.

Morris, R. G. M., J. J. Hagan, and J. N. P. Rawlins, (1986). Allocentric spatial learning by hippocampectomised rats: a further test of the "Spatial Mapping" and "Working Memory" theories of hippocampal function. *Quarterly Journal of Experimental Psychology* 38B:365–395.

Ramirez, O. A., O. A. Orsingher, and H. F. Carrer (1988). Differential threshold for long-term potentiation in the hippocampus of rats with inborn high or low learning capacity. *Neuroscience Letters.* 92:275–279.

Rasmussen, M., C. A. Barnes, and B. L. McNaughton, (1989). A systematic test of cognitive mapping, working-memory, and temporal discontiguity theories of hippocampal function. *Psychobiology* 17:335–348.

Roman, F., U. Staubli, and G. Lynch, (1987). Evidence for synaptic potentiation in a cortical network during learning. *Brain Research.* 418:221–226.

Squire, L. (1986). Mechanisms of memory. *Science* 232:1612–1619.

Staubli, U., J. Larson, and G. Lynch, (1990). Mossy fiber potentiation and long-term potentiation involve different expression mechanisms. *Synapse* 5:333–335.

Teyler, T. J. (1989). Comparative aspects of hippocampal and neocortical long-term potentiation. *Journal of Neuroscience Methods* 28:101–108.

Teyler, T. J., and P. Discenna, (1984). Long-term potentiation as a candidate mnemonic device. *Brain Research Review* 7:15–28.

Teyler, T. J., and P. Discenna (1987). Long-term potentiation. *Annual Review of Neuroscience* 10:131–161.

Tsukahara, N., Y. Oda, and T. Notsu (1981). Classical conditioning mediated by the red nucleus in the cat. *Journal of Neuroscience* 1:72–79.

V Long-Term Potentiation Rules in Neural Networks

21 Long-Term Potentiation of Entorhinal Afferents to the Hippocampus: Enhanced Propagation of Activity Through the Trisynaptic Pathway

Theodore W. Berger and Mark F. Yeckel

As other chapters in this book have reviewed, remarkable progress has been made in identifying cellular and molecular mechanisms that may underlie the induction and expression of long-term potentiation (LTP) in hippocampus. Little is known, however, about the functional consequences of LTP on the subsequent transmission of neuronal activity within the pathways containing the potentiated synapses. Effects of LTP at the network level are not necessarily related to the increase in synaptic strength that traditionally has defined LTP at the cellular level. For example, as we have discussed elsewhere (Berger and Sclabassi, 1985, 1988) and have demonstrated experimentally (Balzer et al., 1989; Berger et al., 1991), changing the input/output properties of entorhinal-dentate granule cell synapses with respect to potency (i.e., gain) also alters their input/output properties with respect to temporal order (i.e., dependence of the output on the frequency and/or pattern of the input). Furthermore, the LTP-induced changes in frequency- and pattern-dependence are not related to the number of granule cells responding to perforant path input, that is, they are independent of the increase in synaptic potency.

Another dimension of this problem derives from the fact that virtually all major intrinsic and extrinsic afferents of the hippocampus terminate within more than one of the three major subfields of the hippocampus—the dentate gyrus, the regio inferior (CA3/4 pyramidal cell field), and the regio superior (CA1/2 pyramidal cell field; Mosko et al., 1973; Steward, 1976; Hjorth-Simonsen, 1977; Swanson et al., 1978; Kiss et al., 1990). If activity of a given afferent is sufficient to induce LTP, it is likely that several populations of synapses will be potentiated, and that these populations will be distributed throughout all three hippocampal subfields. As a result, synaptic transmission will be affected at several points in the progressive propagation of activity through the intrinsic pathways of the hippocampus. The functional consequences of inducing LTP in such a distributed manner are not readily predictable given that (1) the magnitude of any changes in input/output properties (with respect to either potency or temporal order) of each subfield are not likely to be equivalent because of differences in density of innervation and/or target neuron, (2) LTP can be synapse-specific in some subfields (CA1 and dentate) but not in others (CA3; Bradler and Barrionuevo, 1989), and (3) any LTP-related changes in the input/output properties of each subfield are likely to interact because of the extensive interconnectivity between the subfields (Andersen et al., 1971b; Berger et al., 1989, 1991).

In this chapter, we review results of recent studies we have conducted on the anatomical and electrophysiological characteristics of the entorhinal afferent system in vivo, which exhibits the feature just described of terminating within all three subfields of the hippocampus. Because most past investigations have focused on monosynaptic entorhinal input to the dentate gyrus and the consequent transsynaptic influence on pyramidal cell activity, we emphasize our recent analyses of the direct, monosynaptic entorhinal projection to the pyramidal cell regions of hippocampus. We then describe the characteristics of LTP induced by tetanization of entorhinal afferents, and the effects of LTP on the propagation through the hippocampal trisynaptic pathway of activity evoked by electrical stimulation of entorhinal afferents.

INNERVATION OF THE HIPPOCAMPAL PYRAMIDAL CELL FIELDS BY ENTORHINAL AFFERENTS

The entorhinal cortex is a major source of afferents to the hippocampus and has been characterized as a focal point for the transmission of information from neocortical brain regions (Van Hoesen and Pandya, 1975; Van Hoesen et al., 1975; Insausti et al., 1987). Although the majority of previous anatomical investigations have focused on entorhinal projections to the dentate gyrus, it is well established that entorhinal afferents innervate the pyramidal cell regions as well (Ramón y Cajal, 1911; Lorente de Nó, 1934; Raisman et al., 1965; Steward, 1976; Witter et al., 1988). The distribution of entorhinal terminals in all three subfields of the hippocampus is illustrated in figure 21.1. In this experiment (Berger and Rice, 1989), wheat-germ agglutinin conjugated horseradish peroxidase (WGA-HRP) was injected into the medial entorhinal cortex of a New Zealand white rabbit, and 24 to 48 hours was allowed for anterograde transport of the tracer to terminal fields in the hippocampus. Axonal and terminal processes densely labeled with WGA-HRP can be seen in the stratum moleculare of the dentate gyrus, and they appear to extend as a continuous band into the CA3 pyramidal cell field of the regio inferior and the CA1/2 pyramidal cell field of the regio superior, in both the dorsal and the ventral hippocampus (see figure 21.1). As described previously, entorhinal afferents are highly laminated and remain within the boundaries of the stratum lacunosum-moleculare of Ammon's horn providing a restricted innervation of the outer apical dendrites of CA3 and CA1/2 pyramidal cells (see figure 21.1). The more distal segments of the apical dendrites of CA3 and CA1 pyramidal neurons and of the dendrites of dentate granule cells not labeled in this experiment are innervated by neurons of the lateral entorhinal cortex, as previously shown by Steward (1976). We have

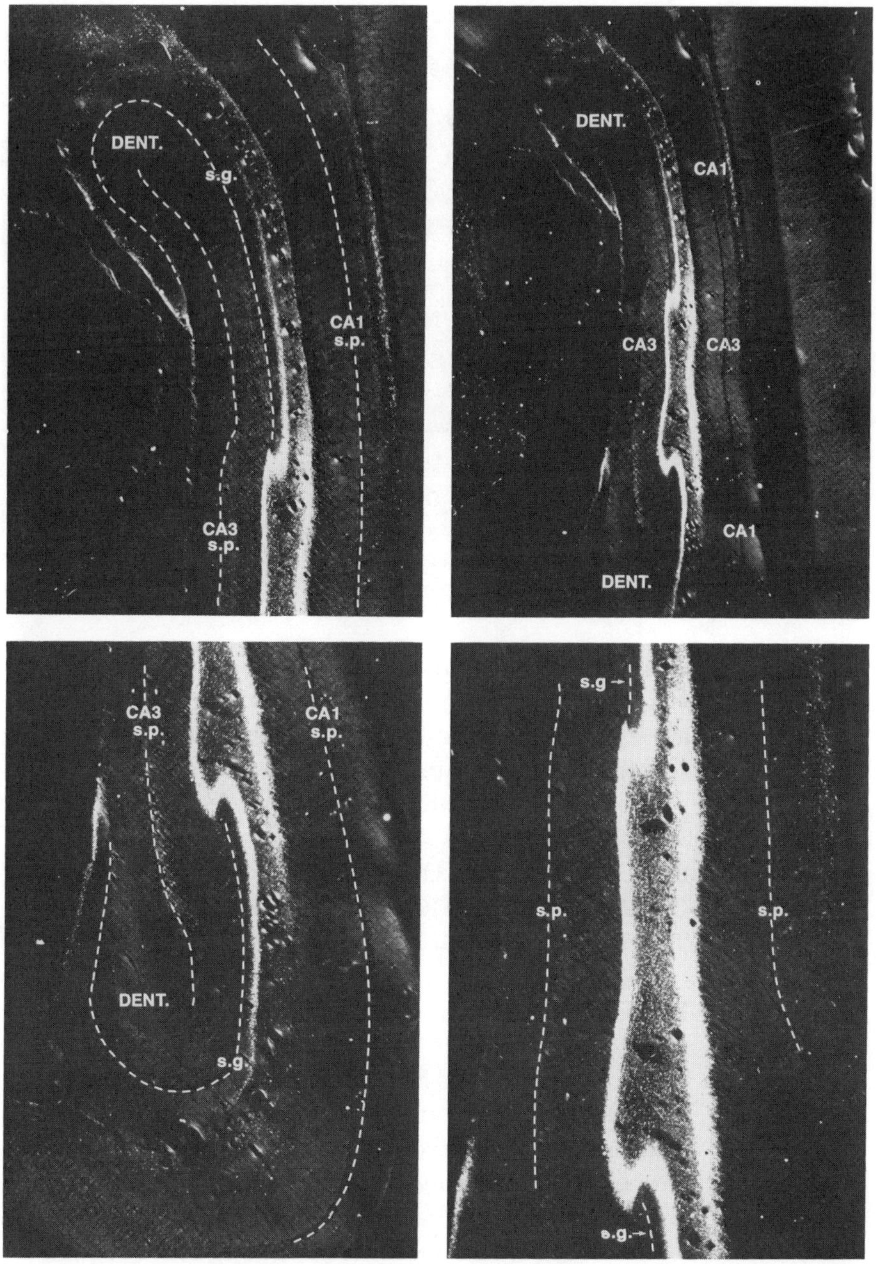

Figure 21.1 Distribution of monosynaptic afferents from the entorhinal cortex to the dentate gyrus, regio inferior, and regio superior of the hippocampus. (Left panels) Dark-field photomicrograph of anterogradely transported WGA-HRP (white, granular product) in the dorsal (upper) and ventral (lower) hippocampus after an injection of the tracer into the medial entorhinal cortex. Dashed lines indicate the center of the dentate gyrus (DENT) granule cell layer (s.g.) and pyramidal cell layers (s.p.). (Right panels) Lower-power (upper) and higher-power (lower) photomicrograph of the same section. Note the high density of labeling in the CA3 subfield and adjacent dentate gyrus and the restriction of labeled processes to the outer apical dendritic regions (stratum lacunosum-moleculare) of both CA1 and CA3.

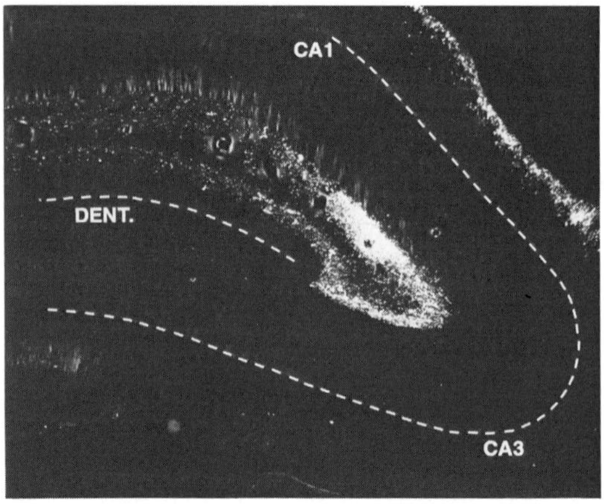

Figure 21.2 Example of nearly exclusive distribution of entorhinal cortical afferents to the CA3 pyramidal subfield. Dark-field photomicrograph showing densely labeled processes throughout the stratum lacunosum-moleculare of CA3. Only very light labeling is visible in the stratum moleculare of the dentate and the stratum lacunosum-moleculare of CA1. Dashed lines indicate the center of the granule cell and pyramidal cell layers.

found that the entorhinal neurons contained within a single injection site virtually never innervate the three principal hippocampal cell fields with an equivalent density. In fact, labeled afferents can be preferentially restricted to the stratum lacunosum-moleculare of CA3 or CA1, with little evidence for innervation of the dentate gyrus (figure 21.2).

ELECTROPHYSIOLOGICAL CHARACTERISTICS OF MONOSYNAPTIC ENTORHINAL INPUT TO HIPPOCAMPAL PYRAMIDAL NEURONS IN VIVO

Despite the apparent strength of monosynaptic input to all three subfields of the hippocampus suggested by anatomical findings, past electrophysiological studies have almost exclusively emphasized monosynaptic input to dentate granule cells. Entorhinal-induced excitation of pyramidal neurons has been described as resulting from multisynaptic propagation through the trisynaptic pathway. Direct entorhinal input to CA1 and CA3 pyramids has been characterized as insufficient for suprathreshold activation because it terminates on distal regions of the extensive apical dendritic tree. Incidental observations in vivo, however, have supported the possibility of suprathreshold excitation of hippocampal pyramidal neurons by entorhinal input (Segal, 1972; Fox and Ranck, 1981). The latter has been demonstrated in the in vitro hippocampal slice (Doller and Weight, 1982) for afferents to CA1 contained within the stratum lacunosum-moleculare, although afferents originating from brain areas other than the entorhinal occupy the same stratum (Herkenham, 1978; Berger et al., 1980). If the strength of monosynaptic entorhinal input is sufficient to generate action potential discharge of hippocampal pyramidal neurons, then the possibility of LTP induction in multiple subfields of the hippocampus becomes more likely. To resolve this issue, we conducted a series of electrophysiological studies in halothane-anesthetized New Zealand white rabbits. We electrically stimulated entorhinal axons within the angular bundle and recorded extracellularly the single unit and field potential responses evoked in the dentate, CA3, and CA1 regions of the hippocampus (Yeckel and Berger, 1990a).

As described in the classic studies of Andersen and colleagues (1960, 1966a, 1966b, 1971b), we found that impulse stimulation of entorhinal cortical axons resulted in a sequential activation of dentate granule, CA3 pyramidal, and CA1 pyramidal cells that was characteristic of the trisynaptic pathway. Sequential activation was evidenced by latencies to population and single cell responses that were progressively longer for each of the three subfields: 4 to 6 milliseconds for granule cells, 9 to 13 milliseconds for CA3 neurons, and 16 to 21 milliseconds for CA1 cells (figure 21.3). The longer latency excitations of CA3 and CA1 neurons were

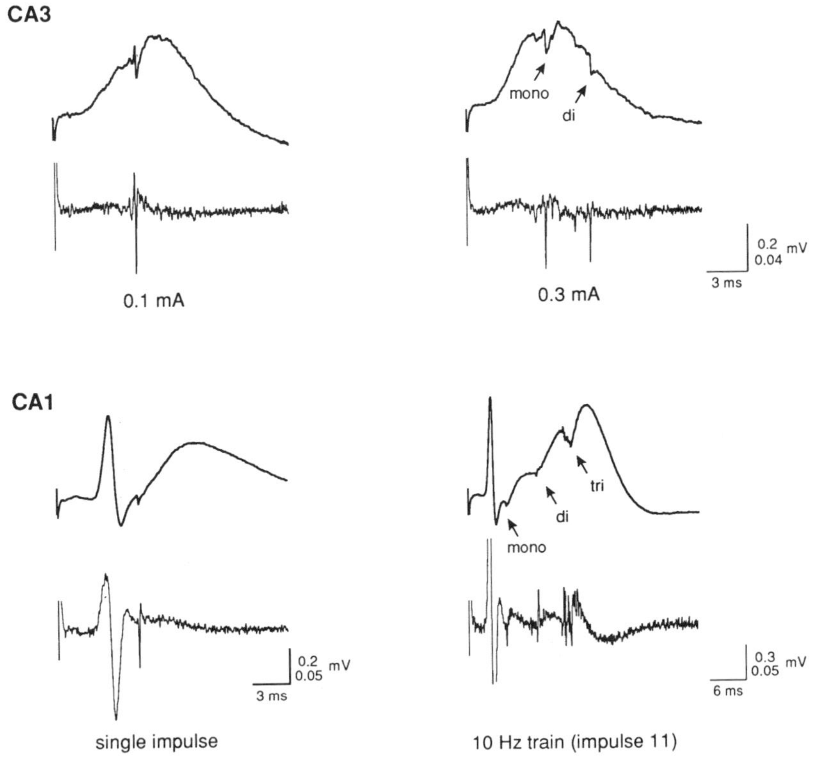

Figure 21.3 Perforant path evoked single unit and population responses in CA3 and CA1. Monosynaptic and polysynaptic responses elicited by stimulation of entorhinal axons in the angular bundle. (Top) Intensity-dependent monosynaptic and disynaptic responses; the disynaptically evoked single action potential (right) was evoked with higher stimulation intensities. (Bottom) Frequency-dependent propagation to CA1. A monosynaptically evoked action potential after single impulse stimulation of the perforant path (left); monosynaptic, disynaptic, and trisynaptic activation elicited by a 10-Hz stimulation train.

consistent with multisynaptic activation, as they could not be maintained in response to continuous stimulation with frequencies greater than 25 Hz. The latencies of pyramidal cell discharge also were consistent with the cumulative monosynaptic latencies for each of the individual pathways comprising the trisynaptic circuit: 4 to 6 milliseconds for perforant pathway input to granule cells, 4 to 7 milliseconds for activation of CA3 by mossy fiber stimulation, and 4 to 6 milliseconds for responses of CA1 cells evoked by Schaffer collateral stimulation (figure 21.4). These observations are consistent with previous characterizations of a sequential excitation of the three intrinsic hippocampal subfields due to serial organization of connectivity between dentate, CA3, and CA1 through the mossy fiber and Schaffer collateral systems (Fujita, 1962; Andersen et al., 1971b; Rawlins and Green, 1977; Herreras et al., 1987).

In addition to the long latency responses characteristic of multisynaptic activation, however, excitations of CA3 and CA1 pyramidal cells were frequently observed to occur with latencies in the range of 4 to 7 milliseconds (figure 21.3), consistent with monosynaptic input from the direct entorhinal projection. Stimulation of the perforant path also was observed

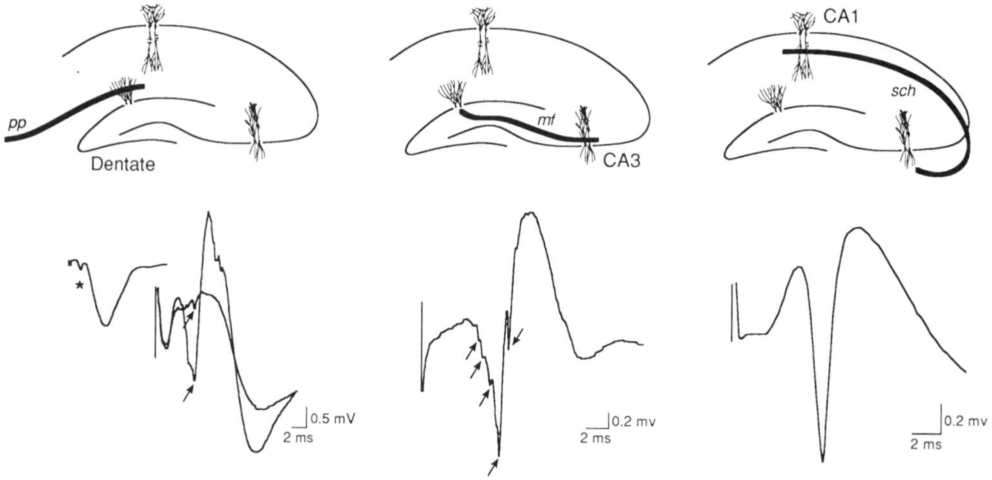

Figure 21.4 Serial propagation through the trisynaptic pathway demonstrated by monosynaptic excitation of its constituent components. (Left) Schematic diagram of entorhinal cortical input (pp-perforant path) to the hippocampal dentate gyrus. Responses of dentate granule cells evoked by single impulse stimulation of the perforant path exemplify characteristics that are classically used to identify monosynaptic excitation: left, a short latency population EPSP, recorded from stratum moleculare, preceded by the perforant path fiber volley; right, overlapped responses to subthreshold and suprathreshold stimulation intensities for population spike activation recorded in the cell body layer (arrows indicate a single action potential evoked by both intensities). (Middle) Mossy fiber (mf) input to the CA3 pyramidal cell region originating from dentate granule cells. Stimulation of granule cells resulted in monosynaptically evoked single units (arrows) and the associated population spike. (Right) Innervation of the CA1 pyramidal cell region by CA3 via the Schaffer collaterals (sch). Stimulation of CA3 axons within the stratum radiatum of CA1 resulted in a monosynaptically evoked population spike.

to elicit a response in the CA1 pyramidal cell layer that was intermediate to the short, presumed monosynaptic response and the longer trisynaptic response (see figure 21.3, lower right panel). This intermediate latency was consistent with the effects of a disynaptic pathway: monosynaptic excitation of CA3 and the subsequent excitation of CA1 via Schaffer collaterals. The possibility that the disynaptic response observed in CA3 resulted from monosynaptic excitation followed by excitation via recurrent excitatory collaterals was decreased by recording from the $CA3_c$ region, where pyramidal cells do not appear to exhibit a substantial recurrent collateralization (Lorente de Nó, 1934; Ishizuka et al., 1990).

Results of laminar analyses supported the interpretation of the short latency responses of CA3 and CA1 pyramidal cells as monosynaptic excitations evoked by entorhinal afferents. For these experiments, a recording electrode was lowered in 100-μm increments from the cell body layer of CA1 to the cell body layer of CA3 (parallel to the dendritic axes) during low-frequency, low-intensity stimulation of the angular bundle ($n = 7$). When the recording electrode was located in the cell body layer of CA1, stimulation evoked a short latency positive-going field potential—that is, a population excitatory postsynaptic potential (EPSP) consistent with a current sink generated by synaptic input terminating in the apical dendrites (Andersen et al., 1966a). If sufficient stimulation current was used, a negative-going population spike was superimposed on the population EPSP; the presence of evoked action potentials with latencies corresponding to that of the negative wave confirmed its interpretation as a population spike (Andersen et al., 1971a). When the recording electrode was moved into the apical dendritic region, the population EPSP reversed in polarity (without a change in latency) to become negative-going, consistent with an interpretation of synaptic excitation of the apical dendrites. Increasing stimulation intensity resulted in greater amplitude and onset slope of the population EPSP without decreasing onset latency, supporting an interpretation of the negativity as a dendritic response to monosynaptic, entorhinal input. The amplitude of the field EPSP became maximal in the distal apical dendritic region of CA1. The EPSP amplitude then decreased slightly as the electrode was advanced 100 to 200 μm, traversing the extreme distal ends of the CA1 dendrites, and increased to another maximum within the apical dendrites of the CA3 pyramidal field as the electrode entered the regio inferior. The polarity of the EPSP reversed again to a positive waveform as the electrode was lowered to stratum pyramidal (figure 21.5).

Small triphasic potentials (positive-negative-positive) often were detected just preceding the onset of the population EPSP (see figure 21.5, lower panel). Their latency, shape, ability to follow high frequencies of stimulation, and localization only in regions of maximum EPSP amplitude were consistent with characteristics of presynaptic fiber volleys, as reported previously for entorhinal afferents to the dentate (Lømo, 1971) and intrinsic pathways of the hippocampus (Andersen et al., 1978; Hopkins

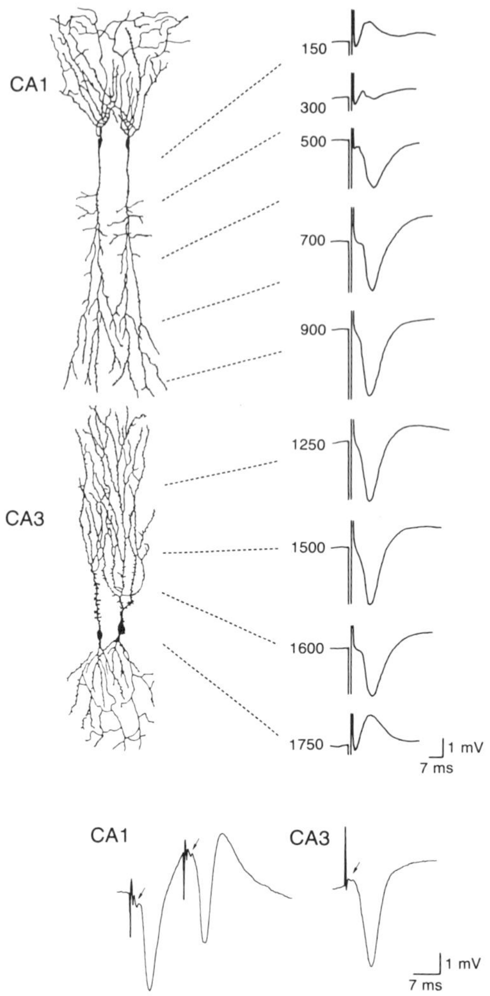

Figure 21.5 Laminar profile for perforant path evoked population EPSPs and presynaptic fiber volleys recorded in CA1 and CA3. (Upper) Low-intensity stimulation of the perforant path resulted in maximal synaptic current flow in the distal dendritic regions of CA1 and CA3. (Lower) Evoked perforant path fiber volleys (arrows) and population EPSPs recorded in stratum lacunosum-moleculare of CA1 and CA3, respectively.

and Johnston, 1988). The distance from the pyramidal cell body layer to the zone for maximum amplitude of the population EPSP and the presence of presynaptic fiber volleys was 700 to 1100 μm. When localized histologically, this corresponded to the stratum lacunosum-moleculare, the site of termination of entorhinal afferents.

The latencies of monosynaptic responses evoked in the pyramidal cell regions were compared in greater detail with those observed in the dentate gyrus. As previously noted, evoked single or multiple unitary discharges of CA1 and CA3 pyramidal neurons were routinely observed to occur with latencies consistent with monosynaptic excitation by entorhinal afferents. Evoked action potentials for CA1 pyramidal neurons were not always easily discriminated, however, because of the apparent contamination by perforant path evoked population responses generated in the dentate. In particular, when recording in the CA1 pyramidal cell layer, a short latency, positive-going waveform often obscured the perforant path evoked CA1 population spike and the unitary potentials associated with it (see figure 21.3). The variation in amplitude, latency, and shape of this positivity corresponded to that of evoked population spikes recorded in the dentate gyrus, ventral to the CA1 recording site. Subsequent experiments, in which responses of granule cells were selectively inhibited (discussed following), as well as the progressive reversal of polarity that accompanied lowering of the electrode into the dentate gyrus, identified this positivity as representing volume conducted source current generated by granule cell discharges (figure 21.6). A similar positivity was not observed in the CA3 subfield, and the possibility that the short latency population responses were volume conducted from the dentate gyrus was obviated by the fact that population spikes recorded in CA3 typically had shorter latencies than those simultaneously recorded in the dentate (two-way repeated measure ANOVA; $F = 8.64$; $df = 1,4$; $p < .05$). Despite the greater distance between the CA3 recording sites and the location of stimulation electrodes site (1.5 to 2.0 mm farther than recording sites in the dentate), population spikes recorded in CA3 were on average 417 microseconds shorter in latency (CA3: x = 4.82 milliseconds, SD = 0.49 milliseconds; dentate: x = 5.24 milliseconds, SD = 0.51 milliseconds). This relationship was not dependent on the site of recording within the dentate gyrus (figure 21.7).

Several procedures were used in an attempt to elicit monosynaptic responses of pyramidal neurons in the absence of evoked activity of direct input via the trisynaptic pathway. In one set of experiments, inhibitory input to granule cells from the contralateral dentate was used to suppress the granule cell response to excitatory entorhinal input (Buzsàki and Eidelberg, 1981; Douglas et al., 1983). Paired-impulse stimulation of entorhinal cortical axons, with a single intervening impulse delivered to the hilus of the contralateral dentate, preferentially suppressed facilitation of granule cell excitation without suppressing monosynaptic excitation of CA1 pyramidal neurons (see figure 21.6). In many cases, monosynaptic

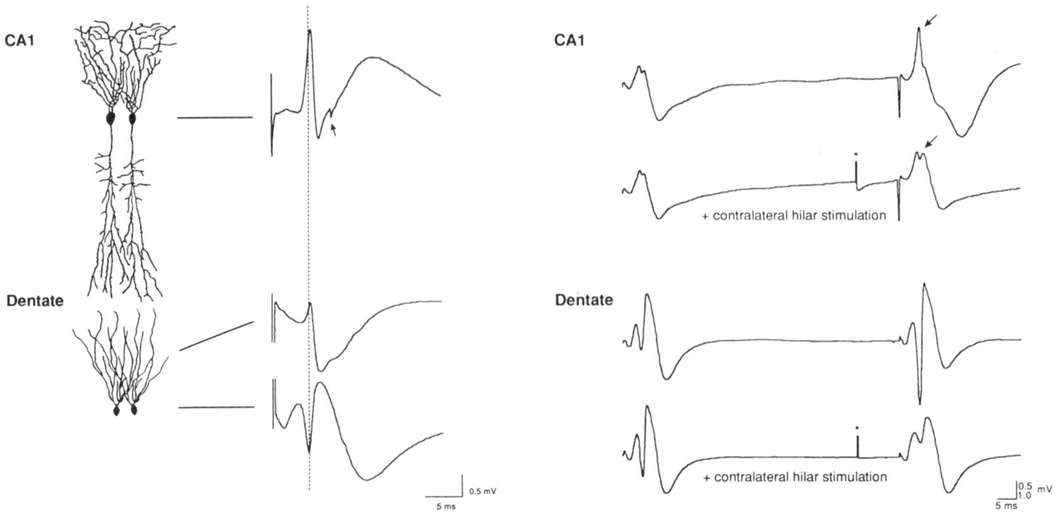

Figure 21.6 Selective inhibition of granule cell activity with contralateral hilar stimulation eliminates field propagated contamination. (Left) Diagram illustrating the sharp positive-going potential present in population potentials recorded from the CA1 pyramidal cell layer in response to stimulation of the angular bundle, and their relationship to population spikes generated by dentate granule cells. The arrow identifies a monosynaptically evoked single unit. (Right) Simultaneous recordings from CA1 and the dentate gyrus after paired-impulse stimulation (top traces). Selective inhibition of the facilitated granule cell response, and elimination of the volume-conducted signal evident in CA1, resulted when an intervening impulse of stimulation (asterisk) was given to the contralateral hilus (bottom traces). Suppression of the sharp positivity in CA1 revealed a monosynaptic population spike.

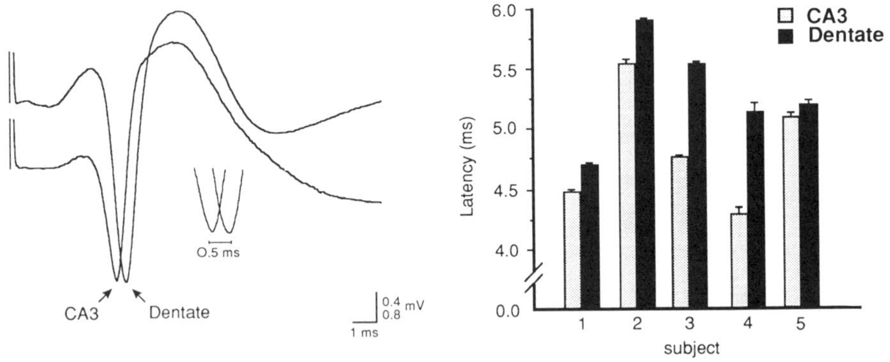

Figure 21.7 CA3 and dentate gyrus population spike latency dissociation. Averages of five evoked responses simultaneously recorded from CA3 and the dentate gyrus cell body layers. Despite being farther from the stimulation electrode, CA3 population spike latencies were shorter than those elicited in the dentate gyrus.

input to CA1 appeared to be enhanced because of the increased detectibility after elimination of the short latency, sharp positive spikes. The corresponding suppression of dentate gyrus population spikes and the elimination of the short latency positive spikes in CA1 suggest that these positive spikes represent field propagated responses from the dentate gyrus.

Pharmacological manipulations also were performed to selectively alter granule cell responsivity. Local pressure ejection of the α-aminobutyric $acid_A$ ($GABA_A$) agonist, muscimol (100 to 500 μM), into the dentate gyrus during paired impulse stimulation of the perforant path increased suppression of granule cells, particularly in response to short interstimulus intervals ($n = 5$). There was no change in the simultaneously recorded short latency pyramidal cell responses. Concomitant suppression of the late response observed in CA3 presumably resulted from decreased synaptic input from inhibited granule cell output (figure 21.8). The independence of CA3 short latency responses and monosynaptic input to granule cells, as well as the dependence of CA3 long latency responses on activation of granule cells by entorhinal afferents, was further demonstrated by application of the $GABA_A$ antagonist, bicuculline methiodide (100 to 200 μM), to

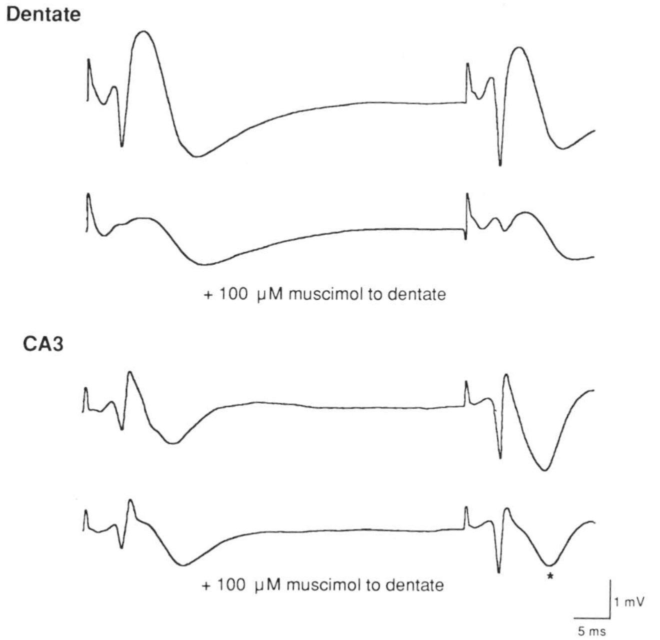

Figure 21.8 Selective inhibition of dentate granule cells with direct application of muscimol. Simultaneously recorded responses in the dentate gyrus and CA3 evoked by stimulation of entorhinal afferents. Almost complete inhibition of the dentate population spike after muscimol application (top traces). There was no apparent effect on monosynaptic excitation of CA3 pyramidal cells; there was a decrease in the late negative wave (asterisk), reflecting a decrease in disynaptic activation via mossy fibers originating in the dentate gyrus (bottom traces).

granule cells ($n = 2$). Disinhibition of granule cells resulted in increased responsivity to entorhinal input and associated increases in activation of CA3 long latency responses; short latency, monosynaptic responses in CA3 were not affected.

The entorhinal cortex and pyramidal cell regions of the hippocampus are reciprocally connected (Lorente de Nó, 1934; Hjorth-Simonsen, 1971; Swanson and Cowan, 1977), and responses characteristic of antidromic invasion were observed in some preparations (Leung, 1979). In agreement with anatomical and physiological evidence demonstrating stronger projections to the entorhinal cortex from CA1 than from CA3 (Hjorth-Simonsen, 1971; Andersen et al., 1973; Swanson, 1981), antidromic activation occurred exclusively in regio superior. Nevertheless, the possibility that CA3 neurons were activated antidromically at sites temporal to the recording electrode cannot be excluded (West et al., 1975). Antidromic responses were clearly distinguishable from monosynaptic, orthodromic responses, as they: (1) were elicited with latencies (2 to 3 milliseconds) that were shorter than those for monosynaptic activation, (2) were not preceded by a positive-going wave indicative of synaptic activation, (3) were less variable than orthodromic responses, and (4) followed impulses during high-frequency stimulation (200 Hz) of the perforant path with a one-to-one correspondence; monosynaptic orthodromic responses did not.

Antidromic activation of the pyramidal cell regions raises the possibility that the presumed monosynaptic responses evoked by excitation of entorhinal afferents represented orthodromic input from excitatory collaterals of pyramidal cells (Lebovitz et al., 1971; Miles and Wong, 1986; Christian and Dudek, 1988a, 1988b; Sayer et al., 1990). It also is possible that monosynaptic excitation of CA1 resulted from antidromic activation of CA3 neurons and subsequent propagation via Schaffer collaterals. Therefore, in several preparations in which both antidromic and orthodromic activation of CA1 pyramidal neurons were recorded simultaneously, hippocampal efferents to retrohippocampal regions were transsected at a site posterior to the recording electrode and anterior to the stimulating electrode ($n = 5$). The tip of a finely tapered surgical blade was inserted into the hippocampus just ventral to the CA1 pyramidal cell layer and moved mediolaterally to transect all fibers carried in the alveus, stratum oriens, and stratum pyramidal. The antidromic spike elicited in the CA1 pyramidal layer was recorded at several different locations in the dorsal hippocampus, and was used as an index of the extent to which hippocampal efferents to retrohippocampal regions were successfully transsected. Results showed that this procedure completely eliminated antidromic input to this subfield (and presumably the entire dorsal hippocampus), sparing orthodromic activation through fibers terminating more ventrally.

Of particular interest was a comparison of the relative strengths of monosynaptic and trisynaptic input originating from one set of entorhinal cortical axons (one stimulation site) to CA1 pyramidal neurons. Results showed that suprathreshold, long latency responses of CA1 pyramidal cells attributable to trisynaptic pathway excitation were seen only rarely when using low-frequency stimulation (0.2 Hz; singles or pairs). In contrast, suprathreshold monosynaptic responses were always observed. Monosynaptic discharges were sometimes followed by two waves of subthreshold excitation (population EPSPs only) at latencies corresponding to disynaptic input via monosynaptic entorhinal excitation of CA3 (9 to 12 milliseconds) and trisynaptic input, reflecting sequential excitation starting with entorhinal activation of the dentate gyrus (16 to 21 milliseconds). Propagation of perforant path input through the trisynaptic pathway to CA1 reached suprathreshold levels only in response to perforant path stimulation with higher frequencies of 5 to 15 Hz (figure 21.9; also see Andersen, 1975). Analogous observations were made with respect to monosynaptic and disynaptic input to CA3 pyramidal cells. Recording sites were varied along the longitudinal axis of the hippocampus for a distance of 4 mm (i.e., perpendicular to the orientation of the trisynaptic pathway) as well as perpendicular to the longitudinal axis from CA3 to the CA1/subicular border (i.e., parallel to the orientation of the trisynaptic pathway). The predominance of low-frequency monosynaptic excitation

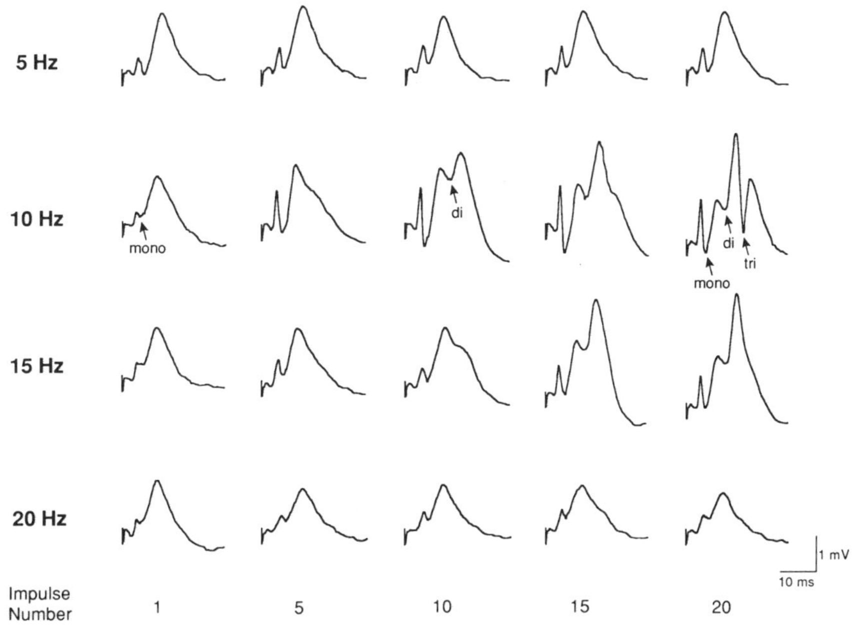

Figure 21.9 Frequency-dependent excitation of CA1 pyramidal cells by perforant path stimulation. Trains of stimulation impulses were given at various frequencies (5–20 Hz; 20 impulses). Suprathreshold disynaptic and trisynaptic activation of CA1 pyramidal cells occurred when 10–15 Hz trains of stimulation impulses were given to entorhinal afferents (arrows point to population spikes).

and a 5 to 15-Hz frequency facilitation of trisynaptic excitation were characteristic of pyramidal neurons sampled at all locations. Thus, this result is not specific to a particular pair of stimulation-recording locations.

The results of these experiments demonstrate that an afferent volley from the entorhinal cortex induces nearly simultaneous monosynaptic excitation of all three subfields of the hippocampus. Furthermore, for any given subpopulation of pyramidal neurons, monosynaptic input from entorhinal afferents predominates over disynaptic and trisynaptic input. Based on these findings, we have proposed a new conceptualization for the functional organization of the hippocampus: excitatory input from the entorhinal cortex initiates a two-phase, feedforward excitation of CA1 pyramidal cells, with the dentate providing feedforward excitation of CA3, and both the dentate and CA3 providing feedforward excitation of CA1 (figure 21.10; Yeckel and Berger, 1989).

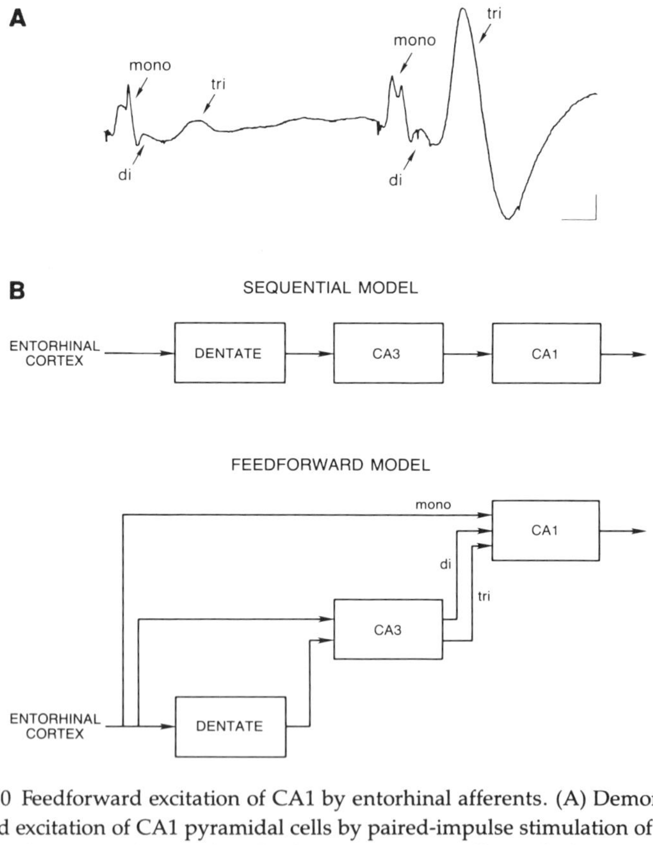

Figure 21.10 Feedforward excitation of CA1 by entorhinal afferents. (A) Demonstration of feedforward excitation of CA1 pyramidal cells by paired-impulse stimulation of input from the entorhinal cortex. Arrows identify the monosynaptically evoked population spikes (mono), followed by a disynaptically evoked single action potential (di; second impulse), and the trisynaptic (tri) population EPSP (calibration; 10 ms and 1 mV). (B, top) Schematic representation of the traditional model of sequential propagation of activity through the trisynaptic pathway. (Bottom) Schematic representation of the proposed model of two-phase feedforward excitation of CA1 pyramidal cells.

LTP OF MONOSYNAPTIC ENTORHINAL INPUT TO HIPPOCAMPAL PYRAMIDAL NEURONS

Many investigations have demonstrated LTP of monosynaptic entorhinal afferents to the dentate gyrus (Bliss and Lømo, 1973; Douglas and Goddard, 1975; McNaughton et al., 1978). Given the high probability that at least some entorhinal cortical neurons project to both the dentate gyrus and CA3, and given the apparent strength of the direct entorhinal projection to CA3 pyramidal cells, we examined the possibility that LTP could be expressed by the monosynaptic entorhinal innervation of CA3 (Yeckel and Berger, 1989). Results showed that tetanizing stimuli of 400 Hz (10 trains of 10 impulses; 1 train/10 seconds) substantially increased the apparent efficacy of this projection, and that characteristics of the potentiation were very similar to that observed in the dentate gyrus in a number of respects: probability of induction, time-course, and magnitude of increase. In several experiments ($n = 12$) simultaneous recordings were made from the cell body layers of both the dentate gyrus and CA3. Evoked population spikes were evaluated in response to pairs of stimulation impulses (20- to 200-millisecond interstimulation intervals) delivered at a low frequency (0.2 Hz). Input/output functions for an average of five evoked responses to the first impulse of each pair were evaluated before and 30 to 60 minutes after high-frequency tetanus. LTP was operationally defined as a sustained increase in amplitude that exceeded standard deviations when compared with control responses evoked by stimulation intensities that produced 20 to 50% of the maximal amplitude. In the same 10 animals, LTP was induced in both cell fields (figure 21.11). The time-course for potentiated responses was similar for the two cell fields; LTP appeared to be induced after four or five tetanization trains, with maximal potentiation appearing approximately 10 to 20 minutes later and remaining relatively stable for at least another 30 minutes.

Monosynaptic LTP of CA3 pyramidal neurons by entorhinal afferents also was similar to LTP of the dentate gyrus with respect to its dependence on activation of NMDA receptors (Yeckel and Berger, 1990c). Pressure ejection (15-millisecond impulses; 5 to 15 psi) of d-APV (50 to 100 μM) reversibly blocked LTP of the entorhinal to CA3 projection ($n = 10$). In addition, it was possible to selectively block LTP in either CA3 or the dentate gyrus with focal application of d-APV (figure 21.12). The NMDA dependence for entorhinal input to CA3 is consistent with autoradiographs showing NMDA receptor binding in stratum lacunosum moleculare of this subfield (Monaghan and Cotman, 1985).

In contrast to the similarities just described for the entorhinal LTP of the dentate and CA3, several differences were evident between LTP observed for entorhinal input and the LTP observed for mossy fiber input. As has been previously demonstrated (Harris and Cotman, 1986), mossy fiber LTP of CA3 was not blocked by APV (figure 21.13). In a number of

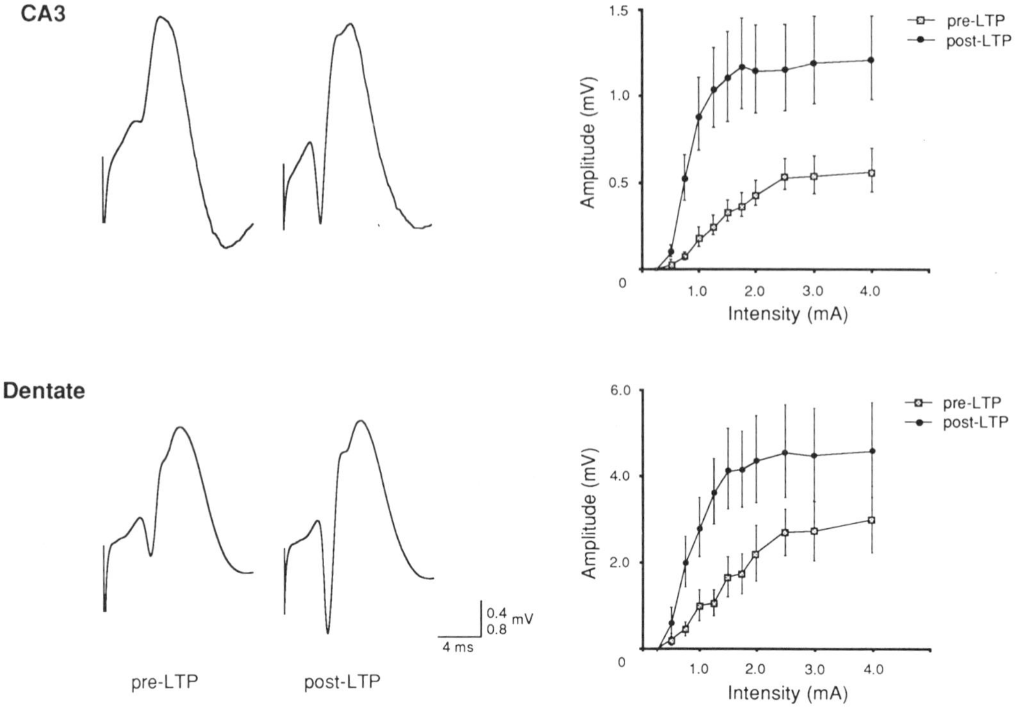

Figure 21.11 Long-term potentiation of CA3 pyramidal cells and granule cells of the dentate gyrus by entorhinal afferents. (Left) Averages of five responses simultaneously recorded from CA3 and the dentate gyrus before and 30 min after the induction of perforant path LTP. (Right) Summary input/output graphs for ten animals in which LTP was induced.

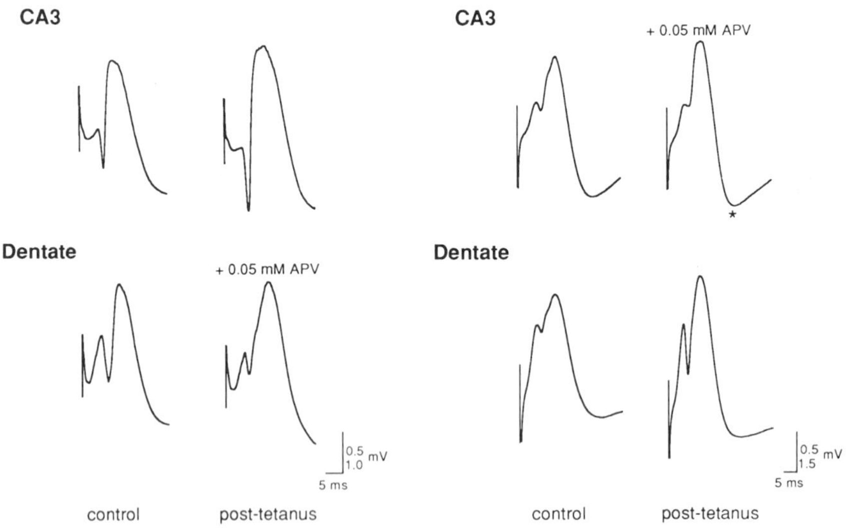

Figure 21.12 Selective blockade of induction of perforant path LTP. Focal injection of the NMDA antagonist d-APV reversibly blocked perforant path LTP. (Right) APV-sensitive blockade of LTP in the dentate gyrus (and selective induction of LTP in CA3). (Left) APV-sensitive blockade of LTP in CA3. The asterisk reflects an increase in disynaptic input from the selectively potentiated granule cells. All waveforms are averages of five responses.

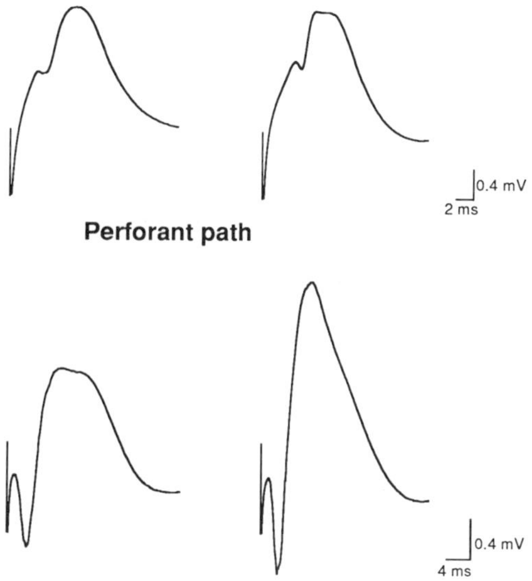

Figure 21.13 NMDA-independent LTP of CA3 by mossy fiber input. Pressure-ejection of d-APV into the CA3 subfield did not block mossy fiber LTP of CA3; however, perforant path LTP of the same subpopulation of CA3 neurons was blocked. Waveforms are averages of five responses.

experiments ($n = 5$), stimulation electrodes were placed simultaneously in the angular bundle to activate entorhinal afferents, the ipsilateral stratum lucidum to activate mossy fibers, and the contralateral CA3 pyramidal cell field to activate commissural input. LTP could be successfully induced in any of the three afferent systems, and APV blocked LTP of perforant path and commissural inputs but not LTP of mossy fibers. In addition, LTP observed after tetanus of the mossy fibers was not input-specific (Yamamoto and Chujo, 1978; Bradler and Barrionuevo, 1989): induction of mossy fiber LTP also enhanced CA3 pyramidal cell responses to nontetanized, commissural afferents (i.e., heterosynaptic LTP) though did not alter the potency of entorhinal afferents. In addition, heterosynaptic LTP did not result when entorhinal afferents were tetanized (Yeckel and Berger, 1990b; including the possibility that it might be polysynaptically mediated, as has been reported; Buzsàki, 1988).

Another difference between entorhinal and mossy fiber input was the observation that different stimulation parameters produced maximal LTP for the two pathways. Tetanization, using lower frequencies (less than 100 Hz; 3 trains, 1-second duration every 10 seconds), was found to induce more robust mossy fiber LTP than higher frequency trains (400 Hz; 10 trains of 10 impulses/10 seconds), irrespective of the order with which they were given. In contrast, LTP of CA3 by entorhinal afferents was maximal with higher tetanization frequencies (400 Hz). The difference between the magnitudes of increase for 100 or 400 Hz tetanization was not as dramatic as the difference observed for mossy fiber LTP. Finally, LTP of entorhinal input was evident soon after the tetanization trains began (independent of frequency), whereas potentiation of mossy fiber input was much slower to develop (see Yamamoto and Chujo, 1978), in some cases taking 5 to 10 minutes after completion of the tetanization trains before potentiation was observed.

ENHANCED PROPAGATION OF ACTIVITY THROUGH THE TRISYNAPTIC PATHWAY AFTER LTP OF ENTORHINAL AFFERENTS

Repetitive stimulation of hippocampal pathways has long been known to alter neuronal transmission through its intrinsic pathways (Andersen, 1960; Gloor et al., 1964; Andersen and Lømo, 1966; Herreras et al., 1987). As we have previously described, long latency single unit and population discharges, characteristic of serial propagation through the trisynaptic pathway, were evoked reliably with 10-Hz stimulation trains (see figure 21.9). Occasionally, disynaptic and trisynaptic population EPSPs were elicited with lower frequencies of stimulation (< 5 Hz), or with pairs of impulses (60-millisecond interstimulus interval). Lower frequencies of stimulation trains (< 5 Hz; < 30 impulses) rarely evoked suprathreshold long latency responses, regardless of intensity.

Changes in the propagation of activity through the hippocampus were evaluated after the induction of entorhinal LTP. Trains of stimulation (10 Hz; 15 to 30 impulses), with intensities that evoked greater than 50% maximal response, were delivered to the perforant path. The number of impulses necessary to evoke suprathreshold disynaptic and trisynaptic responses, as well as the maximal amplitude polysynaptic response, was determined. Monosynaptic LTP of the hippocampal subfields by entorhinal afferents was then induced (400 Hz protocol). After the induction of LTP (30 to 60 minutes), 10 Hz stimulation trains were again delivered to perforant path fibers. Results showed that increasing the synaptic strength for monosynaptic input from entorhinal afferents significantly decreased the number of impulses necessary to evoke suprathreshold activation of disynaptic and trisynaptic responses in the pyramidal cells (CA3: $n = 5$; CA1: $n = 5$). Additionally, the amplitude of the maximally evoked polysynaptic response was profoundly increased post-LTP (figure 21.14). The change in propagation of activity through the trisynaptic pathway was not specific to responses evoked by 10 Hz trains; it also occurred in those cases when a pair of impulses resulted in polysynaptic excitation (figure 21.15).

Additional experiments were performed to determine whether this phenomenon could be accounted for simply by an increase in the potency of entorhinal input to dentate granule cells. In one series of experiments, LTP was induced either in monosynaptic entorhinal afferents to CA3 (and

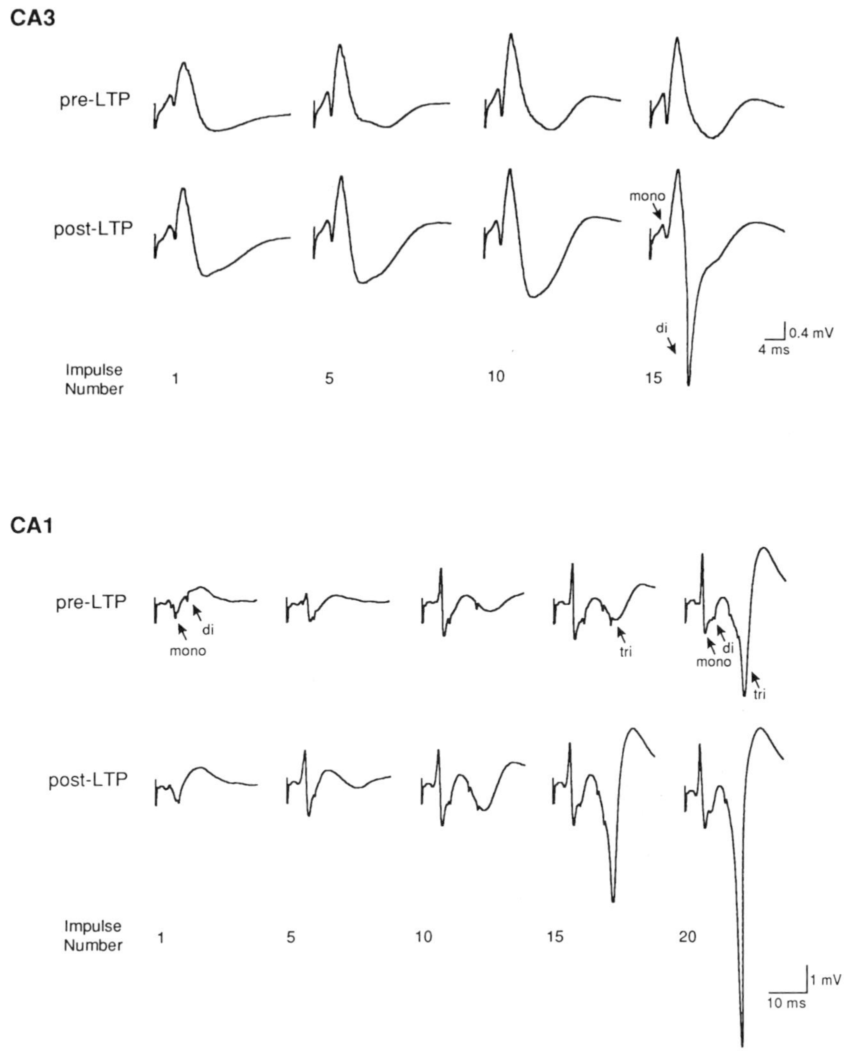

Figure 21.14 Propagation of pyramidal cells following LTP of entorhinal afferents. Disynaptic and/or trisynaptic responses were evoked in CA3 and CA1 when 10-Hz stimulation trains were applied to entorhinal afferents. (Upper) There was a substantial increase in disynaptic activation of CA3 after the induction of perforant path LTP. Fifteen impulses were given; every fifth response is displayed. (Lower) Disynaptic and trisynaptic input to CA1 was similarly increased after LTP of the hippocampal subfields by entorhinal afferents. Twenty impulses were given; every fifth response is shown. Arrows indicate evoked responses.

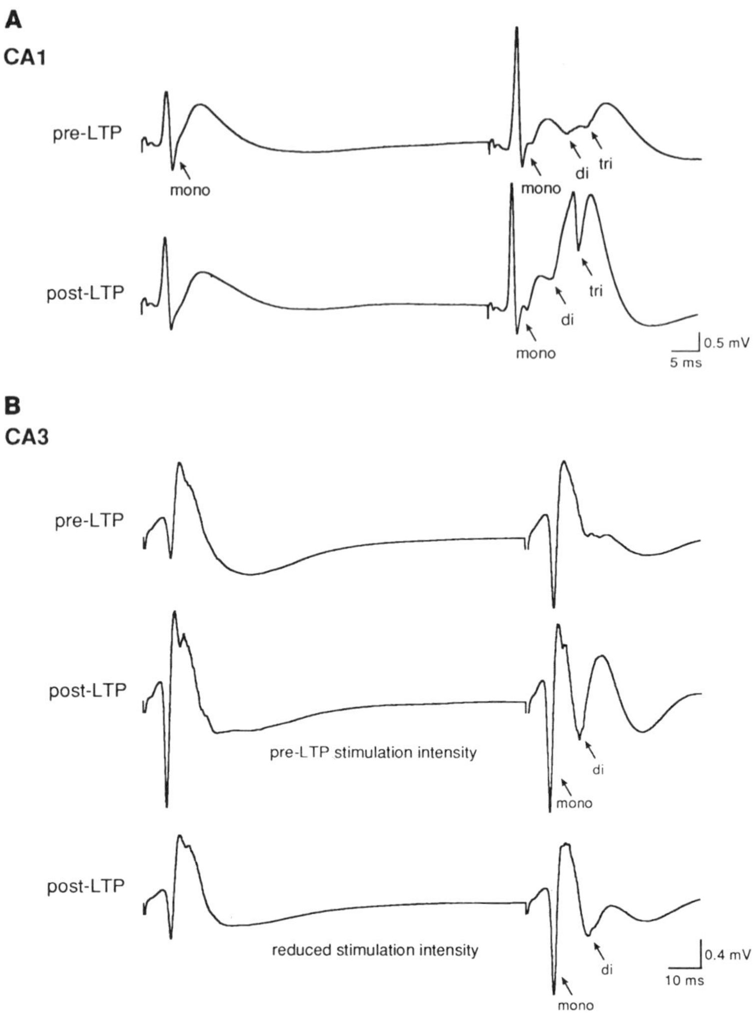

Figure 21.15 Perforant path LTP increases propagation to CA1 and CA3 elicited by pairs of impulses. (A) Responses evoked in CA1 by a pair of impulses before and after entorhinal LTP. (B) Disynaptic propagation to CA3, evoked by a pair of impulses to entorhinal axons, remained enhanced when the stimulation intensity was reduced to evoke pre-LTP amplitude monosynaptic responses in the dentate gyrus. All traces are averages of five responses.

thus also monosynaptic input to the dentate) or in mossy fiber afferents to CA3, and the magnitude of perforant path evoked disynaptic input to CA3 was assessed. It was found that mossy fiber LTP increased disynaptic input to CA3 only slightly. This finding was in contrast to the robust effect of perforant path LTP (figure 21.16).

In a final set of experiments, the intensity of stimulation was reduced after the induction of LTP so as to evoke dentate population spikes with amplitudes equivalent to those obtained prior to tetanization. This presumably approximately equated the number of granule cells activated before and after the induction of LTP. Results indicated that transsynaptic propagation was still enhanced (figures 21.15 and 21.16). In addition, when pre-LTP intensities were used post-LTP, there was little change in facilitation in response to both pairs and trains of impulses. This result suggests that LTP-induced enhancement of transsynaptic propagation

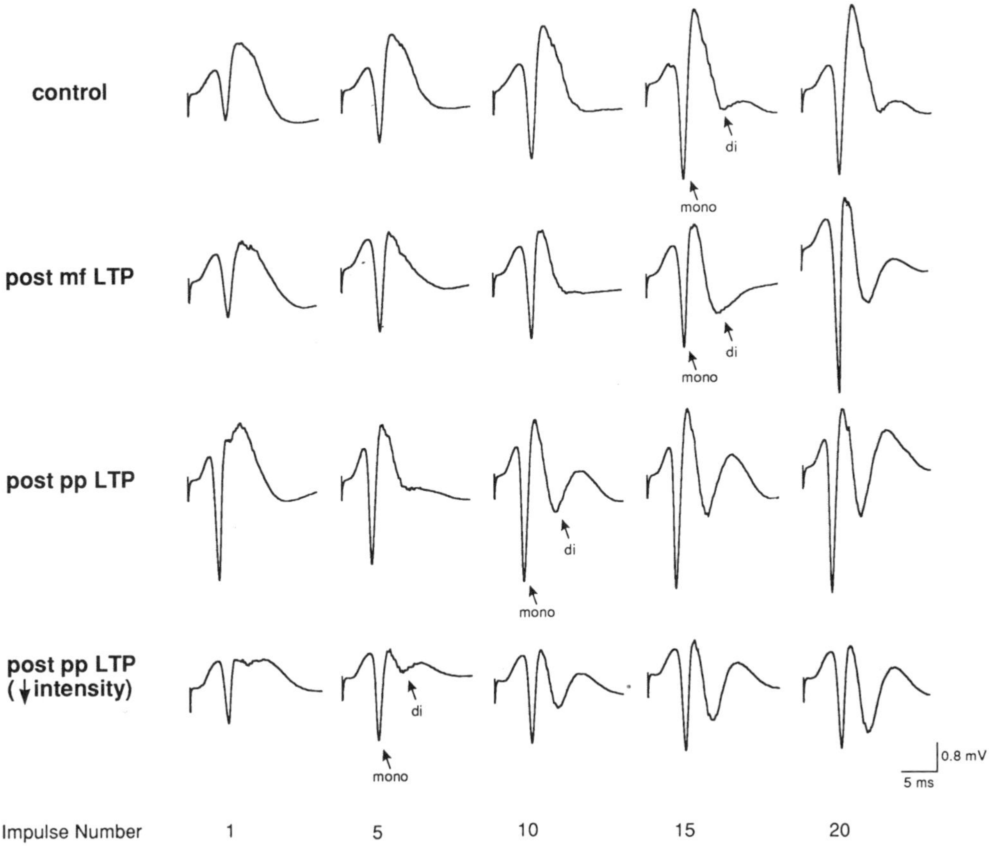

Figure 21.16 Transsynaptic propagation to CA3 after LTP of a single cell field, and after LTP of distributed subfields. Disynaptic input to CA3 pyramidal cells, evoked with 10-Hz stimulation trains to entorhinal afferents, was evaluated after mossy fiber LTP and after perforant path LTP. The magnitude of disynaptic excitation was considerably greater when synaptic input to multiple subfields was potentiated (i.e., perforant path LTP). This also occurred when the stimulation intensity was reduced to evoke pre-LTP amplitude monosynaptic responses.

does not result from changes in local recurrent excitatory and inhibitory circuitry, and instead, more likely reflects an increase in synaptic strength distributed across multiple cell regions.

DISCUSSION

In this chapter, we attempt to address experimentally the possibility that potentiating several subsets of synapses distributed throughout a network of multiple, interconnected populations of neurons will alter the functional interactions among those populations, and thus, the propagation of activity through the network. The experiments reviewed here only begin to investigate this possibility with respect to the hippocampus, but they do demonstrate that LTP of entorhinal afferents, which terminate in each of the three hippocampal subfields, alters the relative magnitude of feedforward excitation of CA1 pyramidal neurons by dentate granule and CA3 pyramidal cells. In considering these initial findings, several issues can be identified that are important not only for ultimately interpreting these specific data, but also for clarifying at a more general level the problem of the effect of LTP on the functional dynamics of neural networks.

Nonparallel Topographic Organizations for Entorhinal Projections to Dentate and CA3

For example, the proposed feedforward model (see figure 21.10) makes an implicit assumption of convergence between monosynaptic and multisynaptic entorhinal projections to any one subpopulation of hippocampal pyramidal neurons. With respect to disynaptic input to CA3, this assumption requires at least that the topographies of monosynaptic entorhinal input to dentate and CA3 parallels that of mossy fiber input to CA3. Anatomical evidence from the injection of tracers into either the entorhinal or the dentate (Swanson et al., 1978; Wyss, 1981; Witter and Groenewegen, 1984; Amaral and Witter, 1989) suggest some significant disparities between the topographic organizations of these two systems. The obvious difficulty with attempting to address this question by studying each projection system individually is the inherent variability in data collected from different preparations and the comparability of terminal fields (e.g., entorhinal projections to the dentate) and injection sites (e.g., in the dentate to map mossy fiber projections to CA3) to reconstruct multisynaptic circuitry. In an attempt to circumvent these limitations, we (Berger and Rice, 1989) recently have enhanced the sensitivity of procedures for transsynaptic transport of WGA-HRP (Itaya et al., 1983) so that after injection of the tracer into the entorhinal cortex, several things occurred: (1) the distribution of monosynaptic projections could be identified by terminal labeling in the dendritic regions of the dentate and pyramidal cell regions, (2) the distribution of granule cells presumably receiving the densest innervation could be identified by the presence of

WGA-HRP transsynaptically transported to the granule cell layer, and (3) the distribution of CA3 pyramidal cells receiving input from the WGA-HRP filled granule cells could be identified by the presence of labeled mossy fibers.

Because sensitivity decreases progressively with distance from the injection site, the population of CA3 cells receiving monosynaptic and disynaptic entorhinal input almost certainly is underestimated. Nonetheless, comparisons of the septotemporal extent of label in the stratum lacunosum moleculare and stratum lucidum of CA3 indicate, for the ventral hippocampus, that considerable overlap exists between the monosynaptic and disynaptic projections (i.e., label can be detected in both strata of the same section) but that the maximum density of label for each pathway is found at different septotemporal planes. These preliminary findings indicate that the assumption of parallel topographies for the direct and indirect pathways to CA3 pyramidal cells is not warranted, and also suggest that the number of CA3 neurons receiving convergent monosynaptic and disynaptic input could vary substantially depending on the degree of synchronous discharge among dentate granule cells. The massive recruitment of granule cells in response to 10-Hz stimulation, and the enhanced rhythmicity of granule cell firing during performance of goal-directed and learned behaviors (Rose et al., 1983; Berger and Weisz, 1987) are relevant to this possibility.

Convergence of Monosynaptic and Multisynaptic Inputs to CA1

The issues with respect to convergence onto CA1 pyramidal neurons are more complex for several reasons. First, any differences in topographies of the monosynaptic, disynaptic, and trisynaptic pathways will increase the possibility of lack of convergence or of patterns of convergence that are difficult to predict. Analyses have shown that the topography of entorhinal projections to CA1 is ordered with respect to the CA1-subiculum axis (parallel to the plane of the cell body layer), in contrast to the topography of projections to dentate and CA3, which is ordered parallel to the dendritic axis (perpendicular to the planes of the cell body layers; Steward, 1976). In addition, evidence suggests that the cells of origin for entorhinal projections to the dentate and CA3 arise from layer II, whereas those projecting to CA1 arise from layer III (Steward and Scoville, 1976). Assuming that the degree of correlated activity within a layer is greater than that between layers, the probability of convergence at the level of CA1 may depend to a greater extent on temporal coherence of the monosynaptic and multisynaptic inputs compared to CA3.

Expression of Different Forms of LTP within Different Subsets of Hippocampal Synapses

Although long-lasting enhancement of synaptic efficacy is a defining characteristic of LTP (Bliss and Lømo, 1973), at least two forms of the phenomenon have been identified and appear to be specific to particular subsets of hippocampal synapses. LTP of both afferents to the proximal apical dendrites of CA1 pyramidal cells and perforant path afferents to dentate granule cells requires activation of NMDA receptors, conjunctive depolarization of presynaptic and postsynaptic elements, and is specific to the synapses tetanized (Andersen et al., 1980; Wigström and Gustaffson, 1981; Collingridge et al., 1983). In contrast, LTP of mossy fiber input to CA3 pyramidal neurons is not dependent on NMDA receptor function, can be induced in the absence of postsynaptic depolarization (Zalutsky and Nicoll, 1990), and is expressed in nontetanized afferents (Yamamoto and Chujo, 1978; Bradler and Barrionuevo, 1989, 1990). Global functional properties of the hippocampus should be affected differently depending on which form of LTP is induced. Because it appears that the optimal induction parameters differ for homosynaptic and heterosynaptic LTP, the possibility exists that different patterns of afferent activity could lead to the selective induction of homosynaptic or heterosynaptic LTP (in different pathways), and thus have fundamentally different consequences for network function. It is clear from results of ongoing experiments (Yeckel and Berger, 1990b) that homosynaptic and heterosynaptic LTP are not mutually exclusive, given that both can be expressed by CA3 cells simultaneously. The importance of the specificity of the induction requirements for LTP can be seen in the data reviewed here: despite the fact that 10-Hz stimulation of entorhinal axons resulted in the massive recruitment of dentate granule cells and subsequent depolarization of mossy fiber terminals and CA3 pyramidal cells, this mode of stimulation never resulted in the induction of LTP in the mossy fiber–CA3 pathway. This remained true even after LTP of entorhinal input, which resulted in even more widespread recruitment of granule cell and mossy fiber discharge, and enhancing excitation CA3 neurons via the direct pathway as well.

SUMMARY

Entorhinal cortical afferents to the hippocampus should prove a useful model system for studying experimentally the effects of LTP on neural network function. Entorhinal cortical input is capable of monosynaptic, suprathreshold excitation of dentate granule, CA3 and CA1 pyramidal cells. Tetanization of the angular bundle leads to the induction of NMDA-receptor dependent LTP of entorhinal input to at least the dentate and CA3 components of the trisynaptic pathway (CA1 not yet examined). Thus, this system provides the basis for investigating the consequences of inducing LTP at multiple sites distributed throughout a neural network. As suggested by the experiments reviewed here, the enhancement of excitatory input to each of the three hippocampal subfields may become amplified during the cascading propagation of activity through the intrinsic circuitry connecting those subfields. As also has been demonstrated here, it is possible to selectively induce LTP of entorhinal input to one subfield only, allowing study of the consequences of potentiating a more anatomically localized subset of synapses. The latter case is particularly interesting given that the transformational properties (i.e., dependence of output on temporal characteristics of the input) of each of the three hippocampal subfields are determined in part by feedback from the other subfields (Berger et al., 1989). Any changes in the transformational properties of one subfield resulting from the induction of LTP (e.g., due to changes in the relative strengths of excitatory and inhibitory inputs) are likely to alter the transformational properties of other subfields as well, and thus, the functional properties of the entire hippocampal system. Such dynamics are not likely to be revealed by studies of LTP in vitro, where interconnectivity is eliminated among the cell fields as well as between principal neurons and interneurons (Amaral and Witter, 1988; Berger et al., 1989).

ACKNOWLEDGMENTS

This research was supported by National Science Foundation (BNS 86-17107), Office of Naval Research (N00014-90-J-4000), Air Force Office of Scientific Research (88-NL-289), and National Institutes of Mental Health (MH00343). M. Yeckel was supported by a training grant from the National Institutes of Mental Health (MH18273).

REFERENCES

Amaral, D. G., and M. P. Witter (1989). The three-dimensional organization of the hippocampal formation: a review of anatomical data. *Neuroscience* 31:571–591.

Andersen, P. (1960). Interhippocampal impulses II. Apical dendritic activation of CA1 neurons. *Acta Physiologica Scandinavica* 48:178–208.

Andersen, P. (1975). Organization of hippocampal neurons and their interconnections. In R. L. Isaacson and K. H. Pribram (eds.), *The Hippocampus*, Vol. I. New York: Plenum Press, pp. 55–176.

Andersen, P., B. H. Bland, and J. D. Dudar (1973). Organization of hippocampal output. *Experimental Brain Research* 17:152–168.

Andersen, P., T. V. P. Bliss, and K. K. Skrede (1971a). Unit analysis of hippocampal population spikes. *Experimental Brain Research* 13:208–221.

Andersen, P., T. V. P. Bliss, and K. K. Skrede (1971b). Lamellar organization of hippocampal excitatory pathways. *Experimental Brain Research* 13:222–238.

Andersen, P., B. Holmqvist, and P. E. Voorhoeve (1966a). Entorhinal activation of dentate granule cells. *Acta Physiologica Scandinavica* 66:448–460.

Andersen, P., B. Holmqvist, and P. E. Voorhoeve (1966b). Excitatory synapses on hippocampal apical dendrites activated by entorhinal stimulation. *Acta Physiologica Scandinavica* 66:461–472.

Andersen, P., and T. Lømo (1966). Mode of activation of hippocampal pyramidal cells by excitatory synapses on dendrites. *Experimental Brain Research* 2:247–260.

Andersen, P., et al. (1978). Functional characteristics of unmyelinated fibres in the hippocampal cortex. *Brain Research* 144:11–18.

Andersen, P., et al. (1980). Possible mechanisms for long-lasting potentiation of synaptic transmission in hippocampal slices from guinea-pigs. *Journal of Physiology* 302:463–482.

Balzer, J. R., R. J. Sclabassi, and T. W. Berger (1989). Nonlinear response properties of dentate granule cells are not dependent on mean frequency after long-term potentiation of entorhinal cortical input. *Society for Neuroscience Abstracts* 15:403.

Berger, T. W., T. P. Harty, G. Barrionuevo, and R. J. Sclabassi (1989). Modeling of neuronal through experimental decomposition. In V. Z. Marmarelis (ed.), *Advanced Methods of Physiological System Modeling*, Vol. II. New York: Plenum Press, pp. 113–128.

Berger, T. W., and P. Rice (1989). Comparison of direct and indirect input to the hippocampal regio inferior from the entorhinal cortex using transsynaptic transport of WGA-HRP. *Society for Neuroscience Abstracts* 15:402.

Berger, T. W., and R. J. Sclabassi (1985). Nonlinear systems analysis and its application to study of the functional properties of neural systems. In J. H. McGaugh and G. Lynch (eds.), *Memory Systems of the Brain*. New York: Guilford Press, pp. 120–133.

Berger, T. W., and R. J. Sclabassi (1988). Long-term potentiation and its relation to hippocampal pyramidal cell activity and behavioral learning during classical conditioning. In P. W. Landfield and S. A Deadwyler (eds.), *Long-Term Potentiation: From Biophsics to Behavior*. New York: Alan R. Liss, pp. 467–497.

Berger, T. W., and D. J. Weisz (1987). Single unit analysis of hippocampal pyramidal and granule cells and their role in classical conditioning of the rabbit nictitating membrane response. In I. Gormezano, W. F. Prokasy, and R. F. Thompson (eds.), *Classical Conditioning*, 3rd ed. Hillsdale, N.J.: Lawrence Erlbaum Associates, pp. 217–253.

Berger, T. W., et al. (1980). Reciprocal anatomical connections between hippocampus and subiculum in the rabbit: evidence for subicular innervation of regio superior. *Brain Research* 183:265–276.

Berger, T. W., et al. (1991). Nonlinear systems analysis of network properties of the hippocampal formation. In J. W. Moore and M. Gabriel (eds.), *Neurocomputation and Learning: Foundations of Adaptive Networks*. Cambridge, Mass: MIT Press (in press).

Bliss, T. V. P., and T. Lømo (1973). Long-lasting potentiation of synaptic transmission in the dentate area of the anaesthetized rabbit following stimulation of the perforant path. *Journal of Physiology* 232:331–356.

Bradler, J., and G. Barrionuevo (1989). Long-term potentiation in hippocampal CA3 neurons: tetanized input regulates heterosynaptic efficacy. *Synapse* 4:132–142.

Bradler, J. E., and G. Barrionuevo (1990). Heterosynaptic correlates of long-term potentiation induction in hippocampal CA3 neurons. *Neuroscience* 35:265–271.

Buzsàki, G. (1988). Polysynaptic long-term potentiation: a physiological role of the perforant path-CA3/CA1 pyramidal cell synapse. *Brain Research* 455:192–195.

Buzsàki, G., and E. Eidelberg (1981). Commissural projection to the dentate gyrus of the rat: evidence for feed-forward inhibition. *Brain Research* 230:346–350.

Christian, E. P., and F. E. Dudek (1988a). Characteristics of local excitatory circuits studied with glutamate microapplication in the CA3 area of rat hippocampal slices. *Journal of Neurophysiology* 59:90–109.

Christian, E. P., and F. E. Dudek (1988b). Electrophysiological evidence from glutamate microapplications for local excitatory circuits in the CA1 area of rat hippocampal slices. *Journal of Neurophysiology* 59:110–123.

Collingridge, G. L., S. J. Kehl, and H. McLennan (1983). Excitatory amino acids in synaptic transmission in the Schaffer collateral–commissural pathway of the rat hippocampus. *Journal of Physiology* 334:33–46.

Doller, H. J., and F. F. Weight (1982). Perforant pathway activation of hippocampal CA1 striatum pyramidale neurons: electrophysiological evidence for a direct pathway. *Brain Research* 237:1–13.

Douglas, R. M., and G. V. Goddard (1975). Long-term potentiation of the perforant path–granule cell synapse in the rat hippocampus. *Brain Research* 86:205–215.

Douglas, R. M., B. L. McNaughton, and G. V. Goddard (1983). Commissural inhibition and facilitation of granule cell discharge in fascia dentata. *Journal of Comparative Neurology* 219:285–294.

Fox, S. E., and J. B. Ranck (1981). Electrophysiological characteristics of hippocampal complex-spike cells and theta cells. *Experimental Brain Research* 41:399–410.

Fujita, Y. (1962). Synaptic activation of dentate granule cells and its effect upon pyramidal cells in rabbit. In P. Passouant (ed.), *Physiolgie De L'Hippocampe.* Paris: CNRS, pp. 47–69.

Gloor, P., C. L. Vera, and L. Sperti (1964). Electrophysiological studies of hippocampal neurons. III. Responses of hippocampal neurons to repetitive perforant path volleys. *Electroencephalography and Clinical Neurophysiology* 17:353–370.

Harris, E. W., and C. W. Cotman (1986). Long-term potentiation of guinea pig mossy fiber responses is not blocked by *N*-methyl-D-aspartate antagonists. *Neuroscience Letters* 70:132–137.

Herkenham, M. (1978). The connections of the nucleus reuniens thalami: evidence for a direct thalamo-hippocampal pathway in the rat. *Journal of Comparative Neurology* 177:589–610.

Herreras, O., J. M. Solis, R. Martin Del Rio, and J. Lerma (1987). Characteristics of CA1 activation through the hippocampal trisynaptic pathway in the unanaesthetized rat. *Brain Research* 413:75–86.

Hjorth-Simonsen, A. (1971). Hippocampal efferents to the ipsilateral entorhinal area: an experimental study in the rat. *Journal of Comparative Neurology* 142:417–438.

Hjorth-Simonsen, A. (1977). Distribution of commissural afferents to the hippocampus of the rabbit. *Journal of Comparative Neurology* 176:495–514.

Hopkins, W. F., and D. Johnston (1988). Noradrenergic enhancement of long-term potentiation at mossy fiber synapses in the hippocampus. *Journal of Neurophysiology* 59:667–687.

Insausti, R., D. G. Amaral, and W. M. Cowan (1987). The entorhinal cortex of the monkey. II. Cortical afferents. *Journal of Comparative Neurology* 264:356–395.

Ishizuka, N., J. Weber, and D. G. Amaral (1990). Organization of intrahippocampal projections originating from CA3 pyramidal cells in the rat. *Journal of Comparative Neurology* 295:580–623.

Itaya, S. K., G. W. Van Hoesen, and C. L. Barnes (1983). Anterograde transsynaptic transport of WGA-HRP in the limbic system of rat and monkey. *Brain Research* 398:397–402.

Kiss, J., A. J. Patel, and T. F. Freund (1990). Distribution of septohippocampal neurons containing parvalbumin or choline acetyltransferase in the rat brain. *Journal of Comparative Neurology* 298:362–372.

Lebovitz, R. M., M. Dichter, and W. A. Spencer (1971). Recurrent excitation in the CA3 region of cat hippocampus. *International Journal of Neuroscience* 2:99–108.

Leung, L.-W. S. (1979). Potentials evoked by alvear tract in hippocampal CA1 region of rats. II. Spatial field analysis. *Journal of Neurophysiology* 42:1571–1589.

Lømo, T. (1971). Patterns of activation in a monosynaptic cortical pathway: the perforant path input to the dentate area of the hippocampal formation. *Experimental Brain Research* 12:18–45.

Lorente de Nó, R. (1934). Studies of the structure of the cerebral cortex. II. Continuation of the study of the ammonic system. *Journal of Psychology and Neurology* 46:113–177.

McNaughton, B. L., R. M. Douglas, and G. V. Goddard (1978). Synaptic enhancement in fascia dentata: cooperativity among coactive afferents. *Brain Research* 157:277–293.

Miles, R., and R. K. S. Wong (1986). Excitatory synaptic interactions between CA3 neurones in the guinea-pig hippocampus. *Journal of Physiology* 373:397–418.

Monaghan, D. T., and C. W. Cotman (1985). Distribution of *N*-methyl-D-aspartate-sensitive L-[$_3$H] glutamate binding sites in rat brain. *Journal of Neuroscience* 5:2909–2919.

Mosko, S., G. Lynch, and C. W. Cotman (1973). The distribution of septal projections to the hippocampus of the rat. *Journal of Comparative Neurology* 152:163–174.

Raisman, G., W. M. Cowan, and T. P. S. (1965). The extrinsic afferent, commissural and association fibres of the hippocampus. *Brain Research* 88:963–995.

Ramón y Cajal, S. (1911). *Histologie du Systeme Nerveux: De l'Homme et Des Vertebres, II.* Paris: A. Maloine.

Rawlins, J. N. P., and K. F. Green (1977). Lamellar organisation in the rat hippocampus. *Experimental Brain Research* 28:335–344.

Rose, G., D. Diamond, and G. S. Lynch (1983). Dentate granule cells in the rat hippocampal formation have the behavioral characteristics of theta neurons. *Brain Research* 266:29–37.

Sayer, R. J., M. J. Friedlander, and S. J. Redman (1990). The time course and amplitude of EPSPs evoked at synapses between pairs of CA3/CA1 neurons in the hippocampal slice. *Journal of Neuroscience* 10:826–836.

Segal, M. (1972). Hippocampal unit responses to perforant path stimulation. *Experimental Neurology* 35:541–546.

Steward, O. (1976). Topographic organization of the projections from the entorhinal area to the hippocampal formation of the rat. *Journal of Comparative Neurology* 167:285–314.

Steward, O., and S. Scoville (1976). Cells of origin of entorhinal cortical afferents to the hippocampus and fascia dentata of the rat. *Journal of Comparative Neurology* 169:347–370.

Swanson, L. W. (1981). A direct projection from Ammon's horn to prefrontal cortex in the rat. *Brain Research* 217:150–154.

Swanson, L. W., J. M. Wyss, and W. M. Cowan (1978). An autoradiographic study of the organization of intrahippocampal association pathways in the rat. *Journal of Comparative Neurology* 181:681–716.

Van Hoesen, G. W., and D. N. Pandya (1975). Some connections of the entorhinal (area 28) and perirhinal (area 35) cortices of the rhesus monkey. I. Temporal lobe afferents. *Brain Research* 95:1–24.

Van Hoesen, G. W., D. N. Pandya, and N. Butters (1975). Some connections of the entorhinal (area 28) and perirhinal (area 35) cortices of the rhesus monkey. II. Frontal lobe afferents. *Brain Research* 95:25–38.

West, J. R., S. Deadwyler, C. W. Cotman, and G. Lynch (1975). Time-dependent changes in commissural field potentials in the dentate gyrus following lesions of the entorhinal cortex in adult rats. *Brain Research* 97:215–233.

Wigström, H., and B. Gustafsson (1981). Increased excitability of hippocampal unmyelinated fibres following conditioning stimulation. *Brain Research* 229:507–513.

Witter, M. P., and H. J. Groenewegen (1984). Laminar origin and septotemporal distribution of entorhinal and perirhinal projections to the hippocampus in the cat. *Journal of Comparative Neurology* 224:371–385.

Witter, M. P., A. W. Griffioen, B. Jorritsma-Byham, and J. L. M. Krijnen (1988). Entorhinal projections to the hippocampal CA1 region in the rat: an underestimated pathway. *Neuroscience Letters* 85:193–198.

Wyss, J. M. (1981). An autoradiographic study of the efferent connections of the entorhinal cortex in the rat. *Journal of Comparative Neurology* 199:495–512.

Yamamoto, C., and T. Chujo (1978). Long-term potentiation in thin hippocampal sections studied by intracellular and extracellular recordings. *Experimental Neurology* 58:242–250.

Yeckel, M. F., and T. W. Berger (1989). Long-term potentiation of monosynaptic entorhinal cortical input to CA3 and CA1 pyramidal neurons of the hippocampus. *Society for Neuroscience Abstracts* 15:402.

Yeckel, M. F., and T. W. Berger (1990a). Feedforward excitation of the hippocampus by afferents from the entorhinal cortex: redefinition of the role of the trisynaptic pathway. *Proceedings of the National Academy of Science USA* 87:5832–5836.

Yeckel, M.F., and T.W. Berger (1990b). An *in vivo* comparison of the induction of long-term potentiation for perforant path, mossy fiber, and commissural input to CA_3 pyramidal cells. *Abstracts of the Fourth Conference on the Neurobiology of Learning and Memory* 4:57.

Yeckel, M.F., and T.W. Berger (1990c). NMDA-dependent LTP of monosynaptic entorhinal input to CA3 and the dentate gyrus alters propagation of activity through the trisynaptic pathway. *Society for Neuroscience Abstracts* 16:491.

Zalutsky, R. A., and R. A. Nicoll (1990). Comparison of two forms of long-term potentiation in single hippocampal neurons. *Science* 248:1619–1624.

22 Hebbian Modifications in Hippocampal Neurons

Thomas H. Brown, Anthony M. Zador, Zachary F. Mainen, and Brenda J. Claiborne

Long-term potentiation (LTP) is a rapid and persistent form of synaptic enhancement. First discovered in the hippocampus by Bliss and Lømo (1973) almost two decades ago, LTP is being intensively investigated by a large number of laboratories. We now know that LTP is not unique to the hippocampus and that there are several varieties of LTP.

One form of LTP resembles a hypothetical synaptic modification that was proposed 40 years ago by the Canadian psychologist Donald Hebb (Hebb, 1949). What has become known as the "Hebb synapse" has long been postulated to serve as a substrate for aspects of the organization of perception and behavior as well as cognitive learning. A large body of theoretical work has demonstrated that interesting forms of associative learning and self-organization can emerge from networks of simple processing elements that are interconnected by formal representations of Hebbian synapses (see Anderson, 1985; Kohonen, 1989; Linsker, 1990).

This chapter is concerned with Hebbian modifications in hippocampal neurons. We begin by defining a Hebbian synapse and then show that at least one form of hippocampal LTP can be considered a biological instance of a Hebbian modification. Next we develop a biophysical model of this Hebbian form of LTP and discuss some conclusions based on simulations of this model. Finally, we illustrate an approach for developing a neurobiologically based theory of associative learning and self-organization.

CONCEPT OF A HEBBIAN SYNAPSE

Hebb's Ideas and Its Antecedents

Underlying the 40-year-old idea of the Hebb synapse was the belief that certain forms or aspects of learning and memory result from use-dependent synaptic modifications. Donald Hebb's (1949) pivotal contribution was the postulation of a particular kind of synaptic modification as the substrate for learning and memory. His idea has come to be known as "Hebb's postulate" for learning (Stent, 1973). In his influential work, *The Organization of Behavior*, Hebb (1949) expressed this postulate as follows:

"When an axon of cell A is enough to excite cell B, or repeatedly or consistently takes part in firing it, some growth process or metabolic change takes place in one or both cells such that A's efficiency, as one of the cells firing B, is increased."

By "efficiency" Hebb meant what we now call "efficacy" or "synaptic strength." In brief, a Hebbian synapse strengthens when the presynaptic and postsynaptic elements tend to be coactive.

Hebb's postulate can be seen as the synthesis of two earlier ideas about memory. The first has roots in Aristotle's *laws of association,* which sought to explain the conditions under which associations between thoughts were formed. The American psychologist William James (1890) proposed that the most basic law of association was the *law of neural habit,* which maintained that if two "elementary brain processes" are active at the same time, then each will tend to "propagate its excitement into the other." James did not suggest a cellular correlate or substrate for these elementary brain processes. The second idea concerns the physical nature of the changes underlying memory. The Italian neuroanatomist Eugenio Tanzi (1893) proposed that the synapse might be the locus of the modification, an idea that was later advanced by Cajal (1911). Hebb's postulate can be seen as the synthesis of the law of neural habit and the synaptic hypothesis for memory.

Contemporary Concept of a Hebbian Modification

Hebb's postulate has been influential in a range of fields, including psychology, neuroscience, and neural network theory (or connectionism, as it is sometimes called). In the 40 years since Hebb published his monograph, the concept of a Hebbian modification has undergone considerable evolution.

The contemporary concept of a Hebbian modification can be characterized by three key features (Brown et al., 1990). First, the process is *local,* meaning that all the information that is necessary for the modification is available to the synapse as a consequence of ordinary synaptic transmission. Specifically, there is no special external "teacher signal" that instructs change on a synapse-by-synapse basis. This is in contrast to many of the so-called supervised learning schemes, such as the back propagation algorithm.

Second, the process is *interactive.* The change depends on activity on both sides of the synaptic cleft. It involves a true interaction, in the statistical sense, between presynaptic and postsynaptic activity. Processes that depend on either presynaptic or postsynaptic activity alone, or on a linear superposition of the consequences of presynaptic and postsynaptic activity, are termed "noninteractive." The nature of the interaction can involve a *conjunctive-type* rule, where the simple co-occurrence of presynaptic and postsynaptic activity causes strengthening, or a *correlational-type* rule, where the synaptic enhancement depends on the covariance, or some other statistical measure of the association, between presynaptic and postsynaptic activity.

Third, the mechanism is *time-dependent*. For the modification to occur, the presynaptic and postsynaptic events must occur in the correct temporal relationship to each other. The timing of presynaptic and postsynaptic events play an essential role in determining the change. This contrasts with many of the supervised learning schemes, such as the back-propagation algorithm.

Generalized Hebbian Modification and Related Terminology

To summarize thus far, a *strictly Hebbian modification* uses a time-dependent, local, and interactive mechanism to increase synaptic efficacy as a function of the correlation or conjunction between presynaptic and postsynaptic activities. Note that Hebb did not discuss the conditions under which synaptic efficacy should *decrease*. It is clear that, in the absence of a mechanism for synaptic weakening, the synaptic strength could tend to increase without bound, or else saturate at some asymptotic value. A *generalized Hebbian modification* includes both Hebb's original enhancement process plus one or more processes that cause synaptic weakening (Brown et al., 1990). Some known biological processes that lead to synaptic strengthening and weakening are listed in table 22.1. Also indicated are presynaptic and postsynaptic activity conditions that may cause the synaptic change.

Before proceeding further, we should define some of the terms introduced in table 22.1. As already indicated, *long-term synaptic potentiation* (LTP) refers to the ease with which synaptic stimulation causes a rapid and persistent increase in synaptic strength. Similarly, *long-term synaptic depression* (LTD) refers to synaptic stimulation's causing a rapid and persistent decrease in synaptic strength. The terms LTP and LTD do not imply any particular mechanism. Rather, they are generic categories of synaptic activity–modification relationships. There may be several varieties of LTP and LTD, and both phenomena may be present at the same synapse.

If a synaptic change occurs in a stimulated pathway, the result is referred to as a *homosynaptic* modification. Both homosynaptic LTP and LTD have been reported. If stimulation of one pathway causes a change in a pathway that was not stimulated, the result is termed a *heterosynaptic* modification. Both heterosynaptic LTP and LTD have been reported. It is sometimes useful to distinguish a third kind of activity-modification

Table 22.1 Terms in the Modification Equation and Possible Biological Correlates

Biological Correlate	Presynaptic Activity	Postsynaptic Activity	Synaptic Change
Long-term potentiation	+	+	+
Homosynaptic depression	+	−	−
Heterosynaptic depression	−	+	−
Passive decay	−	−	−

relationship. An *associative* modification is a synaptic change that occurs in one stimulated pathway as a function of the interaction between that pathway and another pathway (see Barrionuevo and Brown, 1983; Kelso and Brown, 1986). Both associative LTP and LTD have been reported (reviewed in Brown et al., 1990).

Mathematical Formulations of a Hebbian Modification

Hebb did not give his postulate in mathematical terms. Although many "neural network" models incorporate a Hebbian modification, researchers do not generally agree on the precise mathematical form of the algorithm. What the algorithms have in common is that they share the three features mentioned earlier. Most can be expressed in the following form:

$$\frac{dw_{ij}}{dt} = F[a_i(t), a_j(t), w_{ij}(t)] \qquad (22.1)$$

where t is time; $w_{ij}(t)$ is the connection strength (w stands for "weight") at time t from the jth (presynaptic) element to the ith (postsynaptic) element; $a_j(t)$ and $a_i(t)$ are some measures or functions of, respectively, incoming (presynaptic) and outgoing (postsynaptic) activity; and F[•] is some functional of these activities.

We defer until later discussion of the biophysical interpretation of concepts such as "connection strength" and "activity measure." It is the form of $F[\bullet]$, which represents the interactive nature of the modification rule, that varies in different models. Several forms of $F[\bullet]$ have been reviewed elsewhere (Brown et al., 1990).

Here we focus on a special case that has served as a starting point for many modeling studies because of its mathematical tractability and because it may lend itself to a neurophysiological interpretation. Specifically, let F[•] be of the form:

$$F[a_i(t), a_j(t)] = F[\alpha(a_i(t) - A_i)(a_j(t) - A_j)] \qquad (22.2)$$

where A_i, A_j, and α are constants and $a_i(t)$ and $a_j(t)$ are defined as for equation (22.1). If $F[\bullet]$ is a linear functional, then equation (22.2) can be rewritten as follows:

$$F[\alpha(a_i(t) - A_i)(a_j(t) - A_j)] =$$
$$\alpha F[a_i(t)a_j(t)] - \beta F[a_i(t)] - \gamma F[a_j(t)] - \delta \qquad (22.3)$$

where β, γ, and δ depend upon A_i, A_j, and α.

Brown and associates (Kairiss et al., 1988) previously noted that it is possible to relate the terms in equation (22.3) to the four processes shown in table 22.1. In this case, the first term on the right hand side could correspond to an interactive form of LTP; the second term to homosynaptic depression; the third term to heterosynaptic depression; and the fourth to passive decay. Note that if $F[\bullet]$ is the expectation value $E\{\}$, and A_j and A_i are, respectively, the average presynaptic and postsynaptic activities, then equations (22.2) and (22.3) represent the *covariance* of presynaptic and postsynaptic activities (Sejnowski, 1977). It may be convenient to generalize equation (22.3) as follows:

$$F[a_i(t), a_j(t)] = \alpha[a_i(t)a_j(t)] - \beta[a_i(t)] - \gamma[a_j(t)] - \delta \qquad (22.4)$$

where $\alpha[\bullet]$. $\beta[\bullet]$, and $\gamma[\bullet]$ now represent distinct functionals rather than constants, and the other terms have their previous meanings.

PHYSIOLOGY OF HEBBIAN SYNAPSES

We now know that there are several forms of LTP (Briggs et al., 1985a, 1985b; Baxter et al., 1985; Brown et al., 1989). The form that has been most extensively studied is the variety that occurs in the *Schaffer collaterall/commissural* (Sch/com) synaptic input to the pyramidal neurons of hippocampal region CA1 (figure 22.1). This laboratory and others have shown that the induction of LTP in the Sch/com synapses satisfies our definition of a Hebbian modification (figure 22.2; Kelso et al., 1986; Malinow and Miller, 1986; Wigström et al., 1986). At the moment there is some question about whether a non-Hebbian form of LTP also occurs in the hippocampus (Jaffe and Johnston, 1990; Zalutsky and Nicoll, 1990). He we summarize some of the key aspects of the physiology of LTP in the Sch/com synapses of the hippocampus. More extensive reviews are published elsewhere (Brown et al., 1989, 1990).

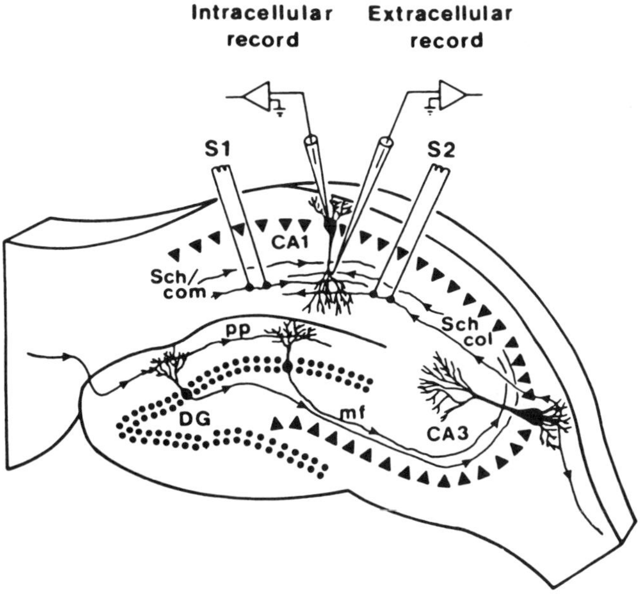

Figure 22.1 Hippocampal brain slice. Schematic illustration of the experimental arrangement used to examine LTP in the CA1 region of a hippocampal brain slice. Intracellular and extracellular recordings can be used to test the response to two or more sets of synaptic inputs. With suitable positioning of the stimulating electrodes (located at S1 and S2 in this example), different Schaffer/commissural (Sch/com) synaptic inputs can be independently and separately activated. (From Brown and Zador, 1990.)

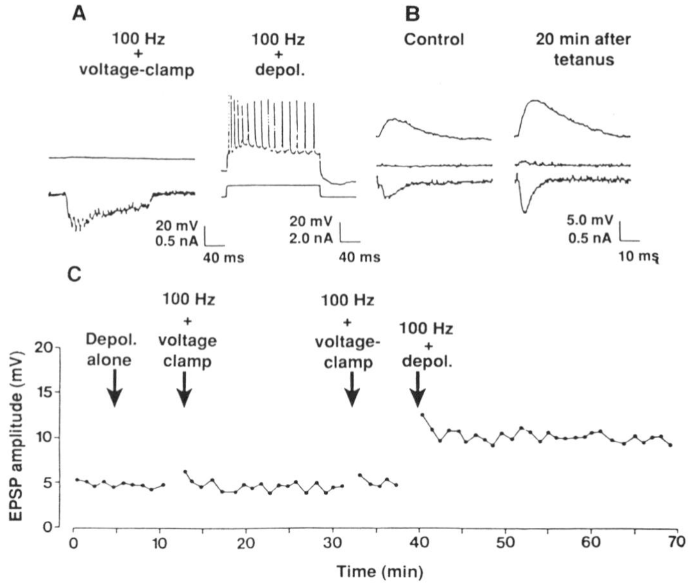

Figure 22.2 Demonstration of Hebbian mechanism. The experiment demonstrates that the induction of LTP in the Sch/com synapses is controlled by a Hebbian mechanism. The experimental arrangement was similar to that illustrated in figure 22.1. Current- and voltage-clamp recordings were done in a pyramidal cell of region CA1. The synaptic responses were produced by stimulating a Sch/com input. (A; left) Voltage-clamp record of inward synaptic currents (lower trace) and membrane potential (upper trace) during a high-frequency train of synaptic stimulations. (Right) Current-clamp recording of postsynaptic action potentials (upper trace) produced by an outward current step (lower trace), which was sometimes paired with the synaptic stimulation train. (B) Current-clamp (top trace) and voltage-clamp (bottom trace) records before and 20 min after pairing synaptic stimulation with the outward current step. The middle trace is the membrane potential during the voltage clamp. (C) The excitatory postsynaptic potential (EPSP) amplitudes are plotted as a function of the time. Arrows denote the occurrence of three manipulations: an outward current step alone (Depol. alone) or synaptic stimulation trains delivered while applying either voltage clamp (100 Hz + voltage-clamp) or an outward current step (100 Hz + depol.). Each point is the average of five consecutive EPSP amplitudes. (From Kelso et al., 1986.)

Postsynaptic [Ca^{2+}]

An early step in the induction of LTP at Sch/com synapses is thought to involve an increase in the postsynaptic [Ca^{2+}] (Dunwiddie and Lynch, 1979). This increase in [Ca^{2+}] is believed to trigger a sequence of biochemical events that ultimately leads to the synaptic modification (reviewed in Brown et al., 1988a). The initial evidence pointing to the importance of a rise in the [Ca^{2+}] was a report suggesting that it was difficult or impossible to induce LTP in cells that had been injected with the calcium chelator ethyleneglycol *bis* (β-aminoethylether)-N,N^1-tetra-acetic acid (EGTA) (Lynch et al., 1983). A more recent and complementary line of evidence came from studies of cells that were injected with the photolabile Ca^{2+} chelator nitr-5. Photolysis of nitr-5 reduces its affinity for Ca^{2+}.

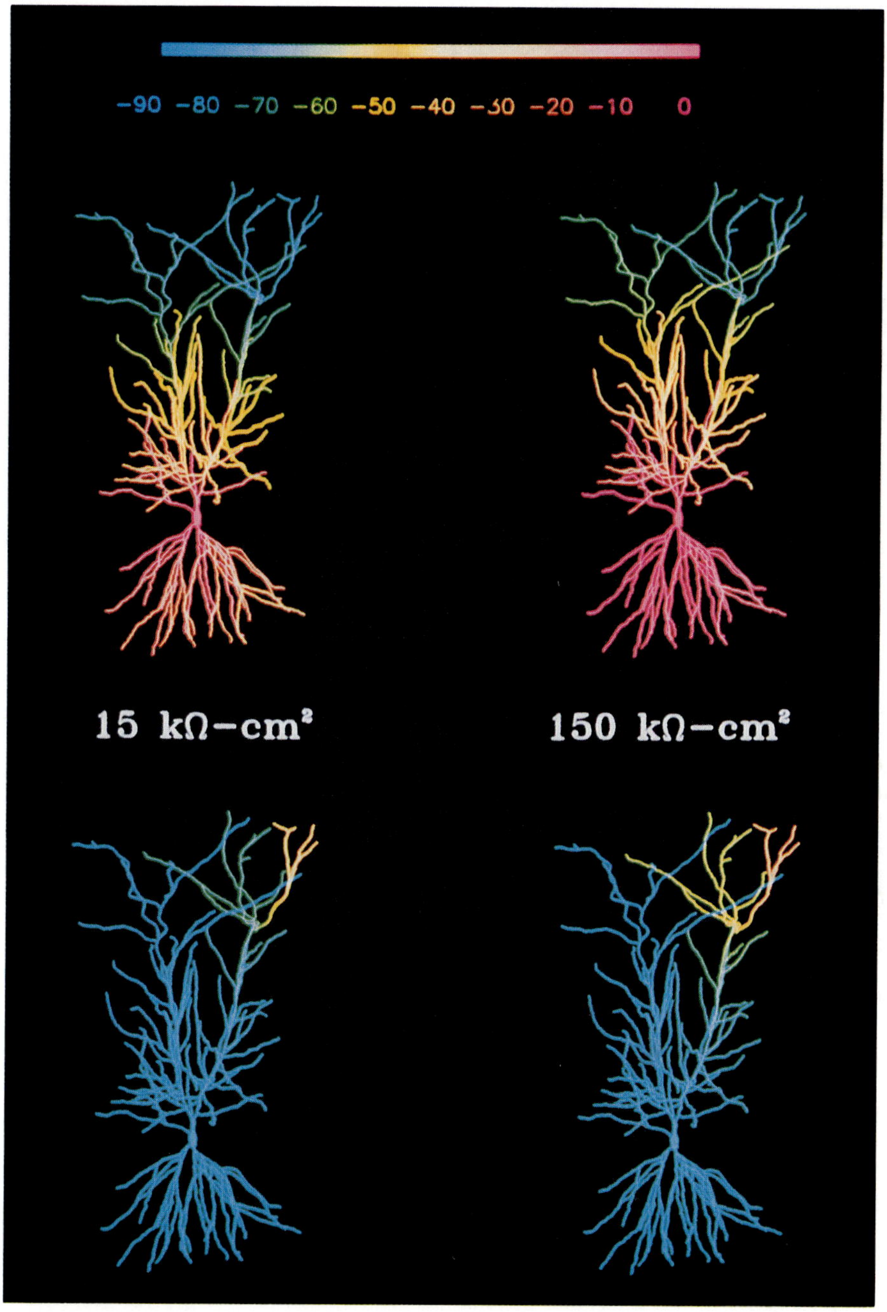

Plate 1 Voltage gradients in pyramidal neurons. Illustration that pyramidal neurons are not isopotential in the transient case even when R_m is made very large. (Top) Color illustrates voltage gradients 16 milliseconds after somatic voltage-clamp to 0 mV (see color scale at top). The simulation used a 3000-compartment anatomically reconstructed region CA1 neuron (Claiborne et al., 1991). Simulations using both a low (R_m = 15 kΩ-cm²; left) and a high (R_m = 150 kΩ-cm²; right) value for membrane resistivity showed substantial voltage gradients. (Bottom) Voltage gradients following synchronous activation of 25 synapses ($\gamma_{\text{AMPA-PEAK}}$ = 0.5 nanoseconds at 300 Hz for 10 milliseconds/three stimuli). The synapses were distributed with uniform probability across two branches in the upper right corner of the dendritic tree. The neuron is shown at the moment of peak voltage response, 26 milliseconds after the onset of the first synaptic stimulus. As indicated, there were substantial voltage gradients. This was true using both a low (R_m = 15 kΩ-cm²; left) and a high (R_m = 150 kΩ-cm²; right) value for membrane resistivity.

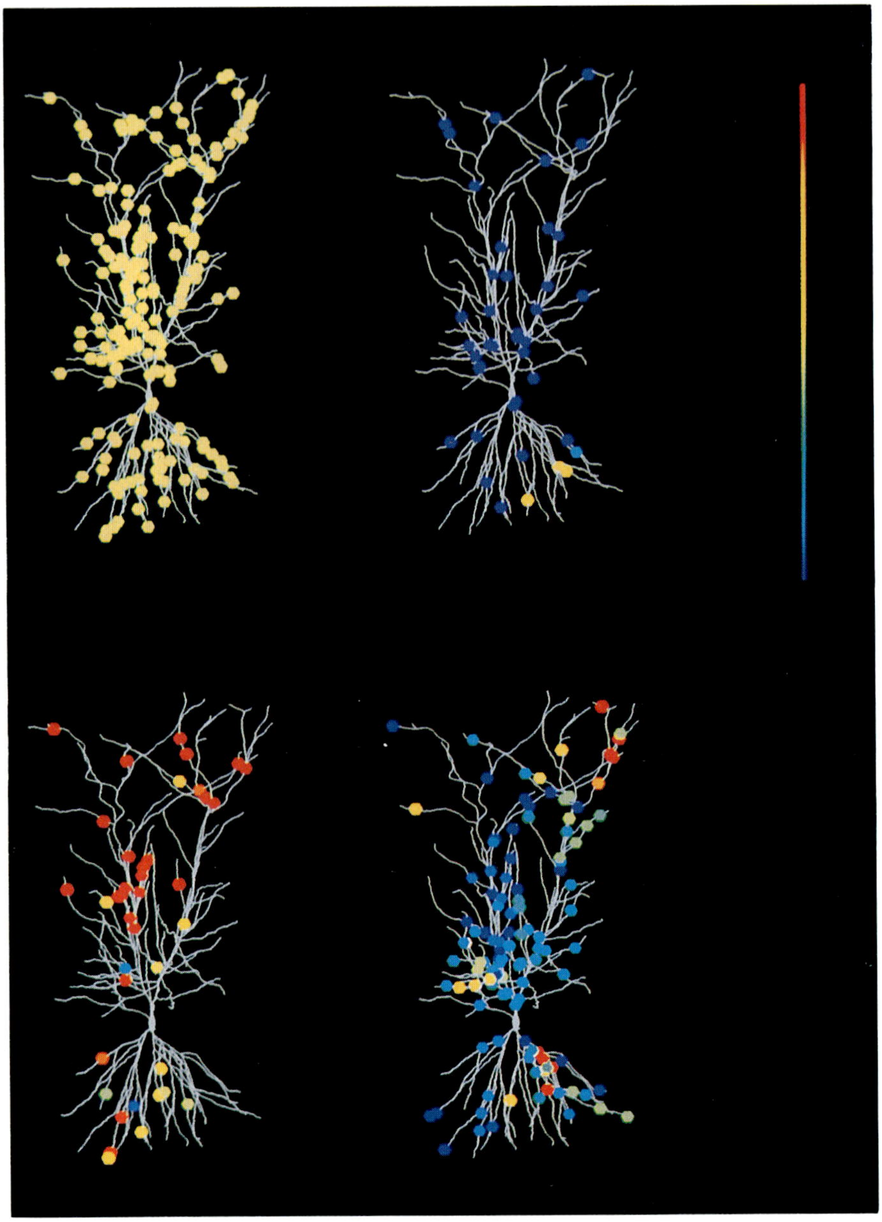

Plate 2 Pattern selection and cluster formation. The environment of the neuron consisted of five patterns of 40 synapses (upper left) selected at random from a total set set of 3500 synapses. The synapses belonging to one pattern were uniformly depressed (upper right) while most of those in a different pattern were enhanced (lower left). We also commonly observed the formation of local clusters of potentiated synapses (lower right). In this particular simulation, each pattern consisted of 120 synapses. (From Mainen et al., 1990.)

If the nitr-5 is preloaded with Ca^{2+}, then photolysis can be used to cause a jump in the postsynaptic [Ca^{2+}]. Using this approach, Malenka and coworkers (1988) reported that illumination of cells injected with nitr-5 caused an increase in excitatory postsynaptic potential (EPSP) amplitude. This chemically induced change is interesting even if the mechanism ultimately proves not to be identical to the mechanism responsible for LTP.

Role of NMDA Receptors

Other evidence that implicates an increase in the postsynaptic [Ca^{2+}] comes from studies of the role of the *N*-methyl-D-aspartate (NMDA) subclass of glutamate receptor. It is known that this channel has a substantial permeability to Ca^{2+} (Mayer and Westbrook, 1987) and that activation of NMDA receptors causes an increase in intracellular [Ca^{2+}], as determined by optical measurements using Ca^{2+}-sensitive dyes (MacDermott et al., 1986; Mayer et al., 1987). Furthermore, Collingridge and coworkers (1983) discovered that LTP cannot be induced in the Sch/com synapses when the NMDA receptor is blocked by the selective antagonist 2-amino-5-phosphonovalerate (AP5). As illustrated in figure 22.3, AP5 prevents LTP induction but does not prevent the expression of LTP that has already been induced, nor does it block ordinary synaptic transmission. It is worth pointing out that the density of NMDA receptors in region CA1 of the hippocampus is among the highest in the brain (Monaghan and Cotman, 1985).

How does Ca^{2+} influx through the NMDA receptor-gated channel relate to the Hebbian nature of LTP induction? It turns out that this channel has just the kind of gating properties needed to account for a Hebb-type conjunctive mechanism. The NMDA conductance is a function of both glutamate binding to the receptor site and the voltage across the channel (Nowak et al., 1984; Mayer et al., 1984; Jahr and Stevens, 1987; Cull-Candy and Usowicz, 1987). The voltage dependence results from the fact that the NMDA channels are normally partially blocked by Mg^{2+} and the fact that this channel block is gradually relieved as the membrane is depolarized. Thus, the conjunction of presynaptic activity (to cause glutamate release) and a sufficient amount of postsynaptic depolarization (to relieve the channel block) allows Ca^{2+} influx into the postsynaptic cell.

Role of AMPA Receptors

To integrate this information about the NMDA conductance with the results shown in figure 22.3, we need to consider a second subclass of glutamate receptor–gated channel. The α-amino-3-hydroxy-5-methyl-4-isoxazoleproprionate (AMPA) receptor–gated channel is more conventional in two respects. First, the conductance increase produced by glutamate binding to the AMPA receptor is not voltage-dependent. Second, the channel is not permeable to Ca^{2+}. The pharmacology of the

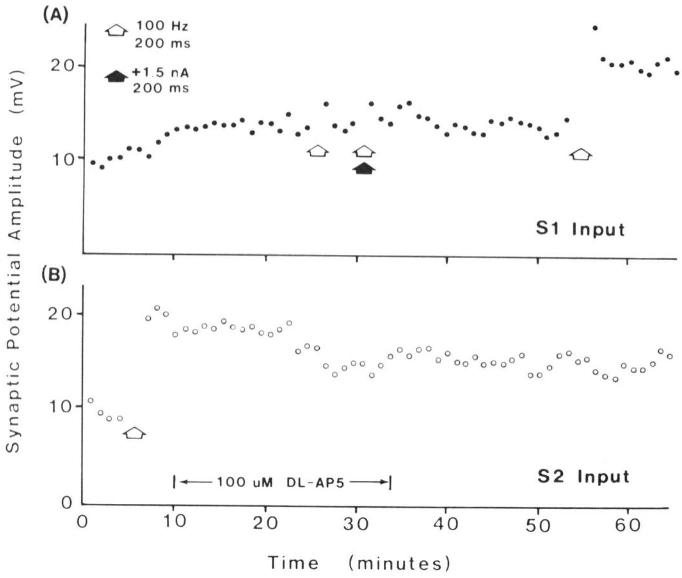

Figure 22.3 Effect of AP5. The experiment shows that AP5 prevents the induction of LTP in the Sch/com synapses but it does not prevent the expression of LTP that has already been induced nor does it block synaptic transmission in an unpotentiated pathway. There are two sets of Sch/com inputs, as illustrated in figure 22.1, whose response amplitudes are plotted in the upper and lower graphs. (A) Bath application of 100 μM of DL-AP5 did not attenuate the EPSPs produced by stimulating the S1 pathway. However, the drug did prevent the induction of LTP in this pathway. The tetanic stimulation consisted of three 100-Hz trains each lasting for 100 msec each. The trains were either unpaired (open arrow) or paired (open and solid arrow) with simultaneous outward current steps (1.5nA, 200 msec). Once the drug was washed out, LTP could be induced in this pathway. Because this was a strong synaptic input, it was not necessary to pair the train with an outward current step. (B) The addition of DL-AP5 did not block the expression of LTP in the S2 pathway that was induced prior to the addition of the drug. (From Brown et al., 1989.)

AMPA receptor is also different from that of the NMDA receptor. The AMPA receptor is not blocked by AP5, but it is blocked by 6-cyano-2, 3-dihydroxy-7-nitroquinoxaline (CNQX) (Honore et al, 1988). Turning to the results in figure 22.3, we see that AP5 prevents LTP induction, but that the expression of previously induced LTP can occur in the presence of this drug. A simple interpretation would be that the induction of LTP requires NMDA receptor activation, but that the expression of LTP only requires AMPA receptors.

Results by two laboratories (Muller et al., 1988; Kauer et al., 1988) have raised the possibility that *only* AMPA receptors can express LTP. Of course, at negative membrane potentials, the NMDA current would normally be very small, owing to the Mg^{2+} block of the channel. It might therefore seem inconsequential whether the NMDA conductance can or cannot display LTP. There are, however, at least two reasons why it may be important to know whether the NMDA conductance is capable of displaying LTP. The first reason is that one cannot assume that the NMDA conductance plays no role in normal synaptic transmission. There is evidence, in the visual cortex of the cat, that the NMDA conductance may in fact play an essential role in normal synaptic transmission (DeFreitas and Stryker, 1990). Even in the hippocampus, there is no compelling basis for the widespread belief that the NMDA conductance does not participate in normal synaptic transmission. Our simulations suggest that if several synapses that are electrotonically near each other are repetitively stimulated at about the same time, the voltage at the subsynaptic membrane can easily reach the level that allows a significant NMDA current. The design of the experiment illustrated in figure 22.3 was not appropriate for detecting this effect.

The second reason concerns the locus of the modification responsible for the expression of LTP. It has been suggested that if the expression of LTP is entirely restricted to the AMPA conductance, then it becomes difficult to understand how LTP could result from an increase in neurotransmitter release. More transmitter release, it is argued, should increase both the AMPA and the NMDA conductance. We will not review the theoretical arguments and counter arguments here, because the outcome does not bear critically on the rest if this paper. Furthermore, it is possible to skip over this debate and question the original inference that the NMDA currents cannot potentiate. Three laboratory directors (T. Brown, G. Collingridge, and R. Malinow) have indicated that they have seen LTP of NMDA currents in the hippocampus.

Locus of the Change

We already know that, in some synapses, the expression of LTP involves a presynaptic modification that increases transmitter release. In the rat sympathetic ganglion, this was shown using a reliable and specific assay for acetylcholine (Briggs et al., 1985a, 1985b). In the crayfish neuromuscular junction, this was shown using a quantal analysis (Baxter et al., 1985). Neither of these results is controversial. Several laboratories, including ours (Xiang et al., 1990), are currently attempting to perform a full quantal analysis of LTP in the hippocampus. Unpublished data from two laboratories (Bekkers and Stevens, 1990; Malinow and Tsien, 1990) seem consistent with a presynaptic mechanism for LTP expression in the Sch/com synapses.

In our view, the issue is whether LTP expression *always* involves a presynaptic modification. At the moment, we cannot rule out the possibility that postsynaptic modifications may contribute to the expression of LTP in some synapses. Perhaps the most hotly contested case is the Sch/com synapse. In these synapses, as we have already indicated, some key aspects of the induction of the modification appear to be initiated on the postsynaptic side of the synaptic cleft. Some have regarded this as evidence that the changes responsible for the expression of LTP must also reside on the postsynaptic side of the cleft. In contrast, Brown and colleagues (1988a, 1988b, 1989) argued that it is not unreasonable to entertain the possibility of a *retrograde signal* from the postsynaptic side of the cleft to the synaptic terminal, and unpublished work from the laboratory of Timothy Bliss is certainly consistent with this idea. It is clear that exciting work remains to be done in this area of retrograde signals, a topic to which we will return later in this paper.

FOUNDATIONS OF A BIOPHYSICAL MODEL OF LTP INDUCTION

For the last several years, we have been developing a biophysical model of the Hebbian mechanism (Brown et al., 1988, 1989) as part of a more general theoretical effort. The biophysical model consists of separate electrical and Ca^{2+} components (compare Gamble and Koch, 1987), as illustrated in figure 22.4. It allows analysis of Ca^{2+} influx, transport, and buffering following activation of synapses located on the head of a dendritic spine (Zador et al., 1990). Here we discuss some of the biophysical justifications underlying the formulation of the model. Holmes and Levy (1990) have recently reported simulations that make somewhat different assumptions.

NMDA Current

Total synaptic current was the sum of separate NMDA and AMPA components. The NMDA conductance was a function of both time and membrane potential. The voltage-dependence was derived from a model in which the binding rate constant of Mg^{2+} to the site of channel block varied

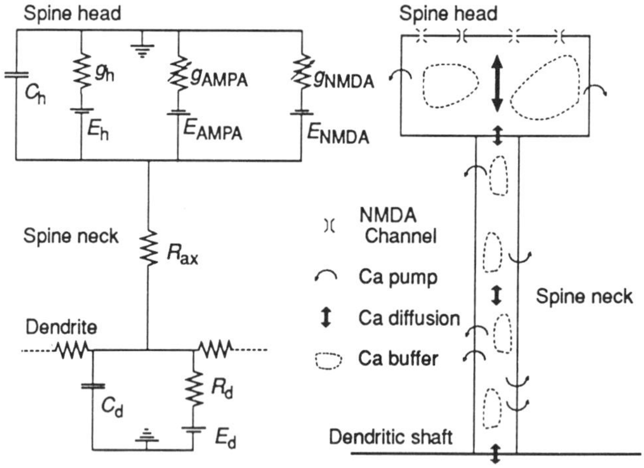

Figure 22.4 Biophysical model of spine. The model has an electrical component (*left*) and a chemical component (*right*). The electrical component incorporates both an NMDA conductance (equation [22.5]) and a non-NMDA (or AMPA) conductance (equation [22.10]). In some simulations, a perfect voltage clamp was applied to the spine head. In other simulations, the spine was attached to a 3000-compartment anatomically reconstructed neuron (Claiborne et al., 1991). The chemical component of the model simulated Ca^{2+} influx, transport, and buffering. Ca^{2+} entered the spine through channels located only on the distal spine head and then diffused along the length of the spine to the dendritic shaft. Diffusion was limited by binding to saturable membrane pumps and cytosolic buffers. (From Zador et al., 1990.)

as a function of voltage (Ascher and Nowak, 1988; Jahr and Stevens, 1990a, 1990b). Specifically,

$$I(t) = (V_m - E_{\mathrm{syn}})\left\{ g_n \frac{\exp(-t/\tau_1) - \exp(-t/\tau 2)}{1 + \eta\,[\mathrm{Mg}^{2+}]\exp(-\gamma V_m)} \right\}, \tag{22.5}$$

with $\tau_1 = 80$ msec, $\tau_2 = 0.67$ msec, $\eta = 0.33$/mM, $\gamma = 0.06$/mV, $E_{\mathrm{syn}} = 0$ mV, and $g_n = 0.2$ nS. These parameters were based on voltage-clamp studies of synaptic currents in the hippocampal slice (Nobre et al., 1990) and on single-channel recordings from cultured hippocampal neurons (Jahr and Stevens, 1990a, 1990b). Short trains of synaptic stimulations were modeled as the sum of these conductance waveforms.

Equation (22.5) is an expression of Ohm's law for a battery (represented by the term in parentheses) in series with a time- and voltage-dependent conductance (represented by the term in curly brackets). The proportionality constant g_n is used to adjust the overall conductance. The numerator of the term in curly brackets expresses the intrinsic time-dependence of the conductance. The constants τ_1 and τ_2 jointly determine the time-to-peak and decay time of the synaptic current. These constants were fit to the empirically measured time-course of the synaptic current. The double exponential form can arise as the solution of a pair of coupled differential equations representing two opposing processes. One possible pair of opposing processes is the binding and unbinding of neurotransmitter from the receptor after release of neurotransmitter. Slow unbinding of glutamate from the NMDA receptor has recently been reported to account for the long decay time of the NMDA current (Lester et al., 1990).

The denominator of the term in curly brackets expresses the voltage-dependent Mg^{2+} block of the channel. This expression represents the probability that a channel is open (ignoring the time-dependence owing to neurotransmitter binding) and is therefore proportional to the average number of open channels. It can be derived from a three-state model (Jahr and Stevens, 1990a, 1990b; compare Ascher and Nowak, 1988) in which the channel can make transitions from the open state (O) to either of two nonconducting states—a closed state (C) and a blocked state (B):

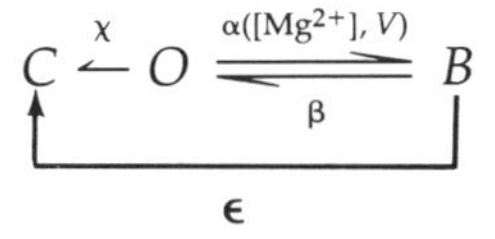

Here the rate constants ϵ, β and χ have units msec^{-1}, and α, in units of $\mathrm{mM}^{-1}\mathrm{msec}^{-1}$, depends on $[\mathrm{Mg}^{2+}]$ and V.

Although this kinetic scheme does not imply a specific physical model, the following interpretation provides an intuitive basis. In the closed state, the channel is nonconducting because there is no neurotransmitter bound to the receptor. In the blocked state, the channel is nonconducting because a magnesium ion is bound to the channel. The transition rate from the open to the blocked state—the rate of binding of a magnesium ion to some site on the receptor channel protein located within the applied membrane field—depends linearly on $[Mg^{2+}]$ and exponentially on the membrane voltage:

$$\alpha([Mg^{2+}], V) = [Mg^{2+}] \exp(\gamma V - \rho) \tag{22.6}$$

where γ is the same as in equation (22.5), ρ is dimensionless, and $[Mg^{2+}]$ is the extracellular concentration in millimolar (mM) of magnesium ions. The transition from the blocked to the closed state depends on the single rate constant ϵ, although the actual process probably occurs in at least two steps.

This scheme represents one of the simplest possible models for channel block. It is similar to that proposed for block at other channels, including block of acetylcholine (ACh) receptor channels by the lidocaine derivatives QX-222 and QX-314 (Neher and Steinbach, 1978). The model of block by local anesthetics differs from the above three-state model only in that the ACh receptor channel does not appear to undergo a direct transition from the blocked to the closed state ($\epsilon = 0$). The equation derived from the three-state model of NMDA receptor channel block provides a good fit to the measured *I-V* relationship for the NMDA current at physiological concentrations (> 0.5 mM) of Mg^{2+} in both culture (Jahr and Stevens, 1990b) and acute slice (Nobre et al., 1990) preparations, although a four-state model is required to account for very low Mg^{2+} concentrations (Jahr and Stevens, 1990b).

The voltage-dependence in this three-state model can be expressed in terms of the four rate constants:

$$g_{\text{NMDA}}(V) \propto \frac{1}{1 + \alpha\epsilon/\chi(\beta + \epsilon)} \approx \frac{1}{1 + \alpha\epsilon/\chi\beta} \tag{22.7}$$

where the approximation is valid if $\beta \gg \epsilon$. Using this approximation and equation (22.6), the constant η in equation 22.5 can be expressed in terms of the rate constants:

$$\eta = \frac{\epsilon \exp(-\rho)}{\chi\beta} \tag{22.8}$$

Calcium Component of NMDA Current

Ion permeation through the NMDA receptor channel has not been carefully examined. The calcium component of the NMDA current was assumed to be a fixed fraction of the inward current (equation [22.5]) at membrane potentials more negative than the synaptic reversal potential and zero at membrane potentials more positive:

$$I_{\text{Ca}} = \begin{cases} \phi I_{\text{NMDA}} & V_m < E_{\text{syn}} \\ 0 & V_m \geq E_{\text{syn}} \end{cases} \tag{22.9}$$

with $\phi = 0.02$. This simple equation captures some key features of certain plausible models of ion permeation. More complex quantitative formulations have been proposed for the ACh channel (Lewis and Stevens, 1979; Quartararo et al., 1987; Decker and Dani, 1990). Although there are not yet comparably detailed quantitative models of NMDA receptor channel permeability, we do not anticipate that a more complete formulation would substantially affect the simulation results reported in this chapter.

AMPA Current

The AMPA current was represented by a so-called "alpha function" (Jack et al., 1975):

$$I(t) = (V_m - E_{syn})\, \kappa\, g_p t \exp(-t/t_p) \tag{22.10}$$

where $\kappa = e/t_p$, $t_p = 1.5$ milliseconds, $E_{syn} = 0$ mV, and the peak conductance $g_p = 0.5$ nanosiemens (Brown and Johnston, 1983; Brown et al., 1988b). The time-dependence, $t \exp(-t/t_p)$, represents the solution to a pair of coupled differential equations in which the rate constants of the two opposing processes are equal. The calcium component of the current through AMPA channels is negligible (Mayer and Westbrook, 1987) and was ignored.

Ca^{2+} Diffusion

In our model, Ca^{2+} entered through NMDA receptor–gated channels located on the distal part of a spine head. It then diffused along the length of the spine to the dendritic shaft. Ca^{2+} was also buffered and pumped in each compartment. The $[Ca^{2+}]$ at the shaft was generally fixed at the assumed resting value ($[Ca^{2+}]_{rest} = 0.05$ μM), although in some simulations it was fixed at a higher value (1.0 μM; see the following). For purposes of Ca^{2+} transport and buffering (see figure 22.4), the spine geometry was modeled as a short cylindrical head at the end of a long cylindrical neck. The following radii (r) and lengths (l) were used: $r_{neck} = 0.05$ μm; $l_{neck} = 1.0$ μm; $r_{head} = 0.25$ μm; $l_{head} = 0.30$ μm.

Because the spine was modeled as a cylinder of variable diameter, symmetry permitted simplification of the general diffusion equation,

$$\frac{\partial[Ca^{2+}]}{\partial t} = D\nabla^2 [Ca^{2+}] \tag{22.11}$$

to its one-dimensional form,

$$\frac{\partial[Ca^{2+}]}{\partial t} = D\,\frac{\partial^2 [Ca^{2+}]}{\partial x^2} \tag{22.12}$$

where $D = 0.6$ μ^2/ms. Here radial diffusion has been ignored. These continuum equations (equations [22.11] and [22.12]) can be derived as the limiting case of an isotrophic random walk (Brownian motion) for a large number of noninteracting particles. At the resting concentration in the spine head when the average number of free ions is about two, this continuum approximation might introduce a source of error. However, the conclusions discussed involve concentrations at least an order of magnitude higher, when the continuum approximation should be valid.

Ca^{2+} Pumps

There is little quantitative evidence regarding the density and properties of Ca^{2+} pumps in neurons of the mammalian brain. Reported densities range from 1×10^{-14} μmol/μm^2 in sarcoplasmic reticulum—1/5 the maximum theoretical membrane density of a protein that size (Hille, 1984)—to 4×10^{-16} μmol/μm^2 in squid axon. We modeled two separate pumps for Ca^{2+} extrusion from the spine lumen. Both obeyed saturable first-order Michaelis-Menton kinetics:

$$\frac{\partial [Ca^{2+}]_{pump}}{\partial t} = -K_{max}\, P_s \frac{A}{V} \frac{[Ca^{2+}]}{[Ca^{2+}] + K_d} + J_{leak} \frac{A}{V} \tag{22.13}$$

where $K_{max} = 0.2$/ms is the Ca^{2+} turnover rate, P_s the surface density, A/V the ratio of surface area to volume, J_{leak} the leak flux of Ca^{2+}, and K_d the dissociation constant. Two different pump systems were considered: a higher-affinity ($K_d = 0.5$ μM) lower-capacity pump and a lower-affinity ($K_d = 20$ μM) higher-capacity pump. The leak flux (J_{leak}) was determined by setting the net flux due to the pump to 0 at $[Ca^{2+}]_{rest}$.

Nonuniform Pump Density In some simulations (Zador et al., 1990), the higher-affinity pump was included at a uniform density ($P_s = 5 \times 10^{-16}$ μmol/μm^2) throughout the spine membrane, but the density of a lower-affinity ($K_d = 20$ μmol) pump was nonuniform. The density was lower ($P_s = 1 \times 10^{-15}$ μmol/μm^2) in the distal 1/3 of the spine neck and in the spine head than in the rest of the spine neck ($P_s = 5 \times 10^{-15}$ μmol/μm^2). The higher density at the base of the spine neck was intended to reflect the contribution of the spine apparatus (Harris and Stevens, 1989; Harris et al., 1989), which may be rich in pump molecules.

Uniform Pump Density In other simulations, the density of the lower-affinity pump was distributed uniformly ($P_s = 1.5 \times 10^{-15}$ μmol/μm^2). The results were quantitatively different, but qualitatively similar. The conclusions drawn from our model do not depend on whether the pumps are uniformly distributed.

Ca^{2+} Buffers

Calmodulin is present at high concentrations at the postsynaptic density, and it has been suggested that a Ca^{2+}-calmodulin–dependent protein kinase, CamKII, may play an important role in LTP induction (reviewed in Kennedy, 1989). We included in our model a fixed concentration (100.0 μM) of an immobile saturable buffer with a kinetic scheme based on one proposed for calmodulin. Ca^{2+} binding to four equivalent sites was assumed to be sequential and noncooperative. The binding and unbinding rate constants were in the range of those reported for calmodulin (see Zador et al., 1990). The following kinetic scheme used:

$$Ca_0 B \underset{k_R}{\overset{k_F}{\rightleftharpoons}} Ca_1 \cdot B \underset{k_R}{\overset{k_F}{\rightleftharpoons}} Ca_2 \cdot B \underset{k_R}{\overset{k_F}{\rightleftharpoons}} Ca_3 \cdot B \underset{k_R}{\overset{k_F}{\rightleftharpoons}} Ca_4 \cdot B$$

with $k_F = 0.05/\mu\text{M/msec}$ and $k_R = 0.5/\text{msec}$ and $\sum_{x=0}^{4} \text{Ca}_x \cdot B = B_{\text{TOTAL}} = 100.0\ \mu\text{M}$.

To simplify discussion, we assumed that the amount of synaptic enhancement depended upon the peak [CaM-Ca_4]. However, many other measures of CaM-Ca_4 activity (such as its time integral), or even measures of other Ca^{2+}-dependent enzymatic processes, gave qualitatively similar results. The critical assumption is that the relation between the [Ca^{2+}] and the amount or probability of LTP is monotonic.

Simulations

The equations describing electrical and chemical dynamics were advanced independently, and at the end of each time step electrical current was converted to ionic flux through Faraday's constant. These equations were discretized and then solved using alternating implicit-explicit steps (Hines, 1984; Mascagni, 1989). A custom simulator, written in C, was used to simulate Ca^{2+} dynamics. When the full dendritic complexity was included in the simulations, we used NEURON, a compartmental simulator based on CABLE (Hines, 1989).

SIMULATIONS OF A BIOPHYSICAL MODEL OF LTP INDUCTION

Phenomenology of LTP Induction

Our biophysical model accounted for three key aspects of the phenomenology of LTP induction in the Sch/com input to region CA1 pyramidal neurons—the conjunctive requirement, the input specificity, and the requirement for temporal contiguity.

Conjunctive Requirements Stimulation of a weak synaptic input, consisting of only a few synapses, will not generally cause LTP in that input. To induce LTP, the cell must be strongly depolarized during or shortly after the stimulation. This strong depolarization can be supplied either by another synaptic input to the cell (Barrionuevo and Brown, 1983; Kelso and Brown, 1986) or by passing an outward current through a recording electrode (see figure 22.2; Kelso et al., 1986).

What is absolutely clear is that LTP induction in the Sch/com synapses requires the conjunction of presynaptic stimulation with sufficient postsynaptic depolarization (see figure 22.2). This is the *sine qua non* of a Hebbian synapse. Figure 22.5 illustrates the voltage dependence of the NMDA current along with the free [Ca^{2+}] and the [CaM-Ca_4]. In each simulation, the peak [CaM-Ca_4] was recorded following a train of three presynaptic stimuli during voltage clamp of the subsynaptic membrane. The peaks were plotted as a function of holding potential in figure 22.5. Peak values increased only slightly at holding potentials less than about −60 mV, but increased rapidly as the holding potential was varied from

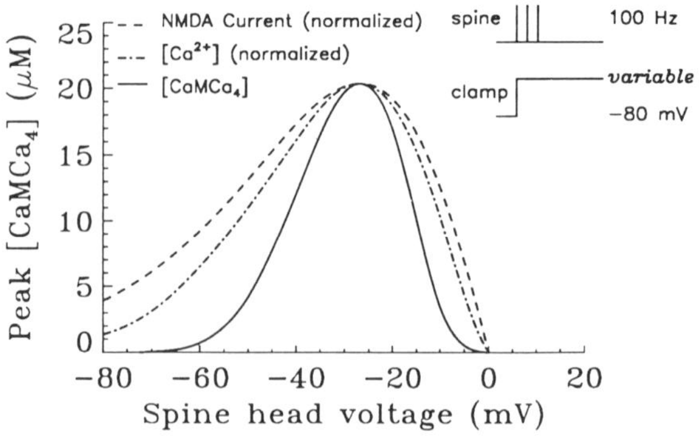

Figure 22.5 Voltage dependence of postsynaptic responses. The effects of voltage at the spine head are shown for three measures of the postsynaptic response—the peak NMDA current (normalized), the peak [Ca^{2+}] (normalized), and the peak [CaM-Ca_4]. The input consisted of a train of three presynaptic stimuli applied at 100 Hz. The voltage at the spine head was clamped to potentials ranging from −80 mV to 0 mV. To facilitate comparisons, the curves for [Ca^{2+}] and NMDA current have been scaled so that their maximum values superimpose on the maximum value for [CaM-Ca_4]. The ordinate is thus only appropriate for the [CaM-Ca_4]. Note that [Ca^{2+}] and [CaM-Ca_4] are *steeper* functions of voltage than I_{NMDA}. (From Zador et al., 1990.)

−60 to −30 mV. These results provide a quantitative basis for the conjunctive requirement.

It has been suggested (Bliss and Lynch, 1988; Wickens, 1988) that if NMDA receptors were colocalized with AMPA receptors on the spine head, as in the present model, then activation of even a single synapse would provide sufficient depolarization at the spine head to cause LTP induction. If this were the case, then the synapses would not appear to be Hebbian. There would be no conjunctive requirement. Therefore, according to this argument, the NMDA receptors must not be colocalized with the AMPA receptors on the spine head. The quantitative issue concerns the depolarization at the spine head owing to a single input. Is the depolarization so large that LTP would be expected to occur in response to the weakest possible input?

In other words, does our model predict *obligate LTP*? The amount of depolarization will depend on both the size of the peak synaptic conductance change g_p and the input impedance at the spine head (Brown et al., 1988b). We previously evaluated this issue using a simplified (compare Traub, 1983) model of a hippocampal neuron (Zador et al., 1990). For the parameters that we used, activation of a single afferent did not lead to a substantial increase in [CaM-Ca_4]. We have subsequently examined this matter using a very detailed representation of the electrotonic structure of the neuron (Mainen et al., 1990; Claiborne et al., 1991). In these simulations the model of the postsynaptic cell was obtained by combining estimates of membrane and axoplasmic resistivity with a very accurate 3-D anatomical reconstruction (Claiborne et al., 1991).

Figure 22.6 shows the depolarization at the unclamped spine head after

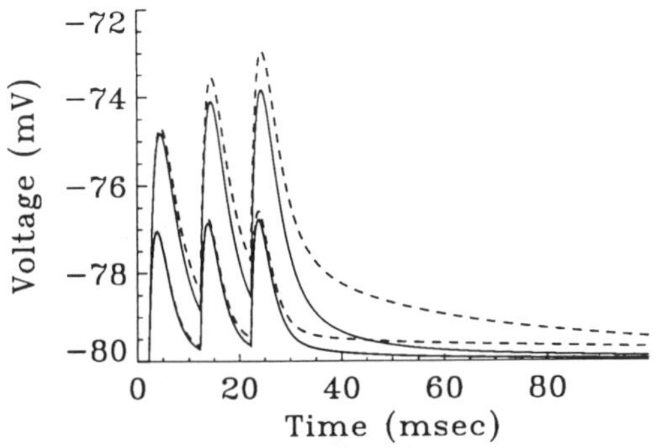

Figure 22.6 Peak voltage at spine head. Illustration that a single synapse does not drive the voltage at the spine head into the voltage range required to generate a large NMDA current. The synapse, which was located on the head of a spine head, was activated at 100 Hz for 30 msec. The spine was attached to a 3000-compartment electrotonic model of the neuron. The compartmental model was based on a detailed anatomical reconstruction of a hippocampal pyramidal neuron from the CA1 region (Claiborne et al., 1991). Two different values were used for specific membrane resistivity (R_m = 15 kΩ-cm^2, solid lines; R_m = 150 kΩ-cm^2, dashed lines). The spine was located in either of two different locations on the dendritic tree (distal synapses, top two traces; proximal synapses, lower two traces). Comparison with figure 22.5 indicates that the depolarization resulting from this synaptic stimulation would not lead to a substantial increase in the [Ca^{2+}]. (From Zador and Brown, unpublished data.)

the same stimulus that was used in figure 22.5. Over a wide range of membrane parameters and synaptic locations, the peak voltage at the spine head never exceeded -70 mV. Figure 22.5 illustrates that this depolarization is not sufficient to cause a large increase in [CaM-Ca_4]. Recent reports (Malinow and Tsien, 1990; Bekkers and Stevens, 1990) that g_p may be substantially smaller than the value used in these simulations strengthens the argument. We conclude that obligate LTP is not a necessary consequence of colocalizing NMDA and AMPA receptors on the spine head.

Input Specificity LTP induction at Sch/com synapses appears to be limited to just those synapses that satisfy the conjunctive requirement for potentiation. This finding has been demonstrated in experiments in which two input pathways are stimulated independently (see figure 22.1). The synaptic terminations from these two pathways may be very close on the dendritic tree. If tetanic stimulation of only one of these pathways is paired with strong postsynaptic depolarization, then only that pathway becomes potentiated. The unpaired pathway remains unpotentiated (Barrionuevo and Brown, 1983; Kelso et al., 1986; Kelso and Brown, 1986). These experiments suggest that, to the limits of experimental resolution, LTP induction is specific to a particular synaptic input. Heterosynaptic LTP of neighboring synapses has not been reported in the CA1 region.

Figure 22.7 shows the simulated spatiotemporal dynamics of [Ca^{2+}] and

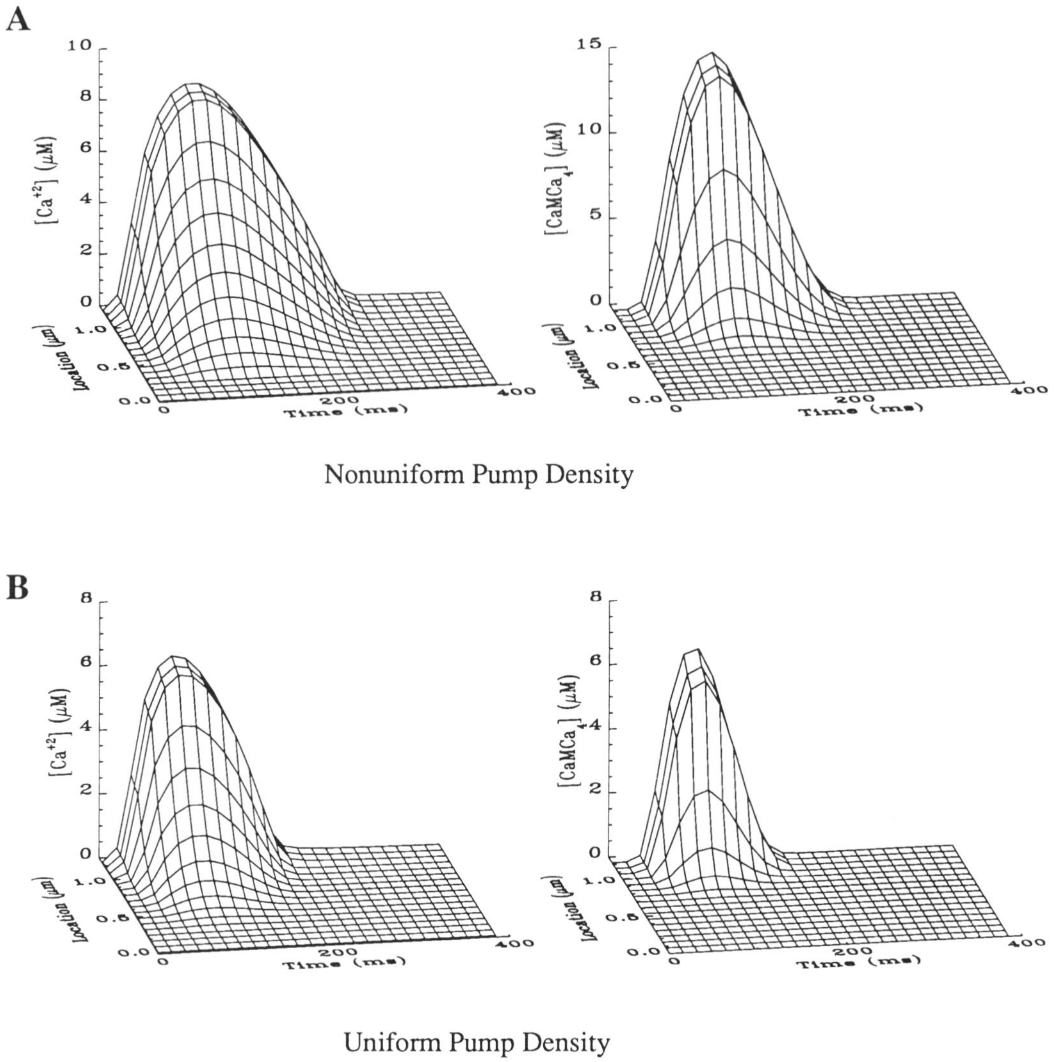

Figure 22.7 Spatiotemporal dynamics of postsynaptic responses. The spatial distribution and time-course are shown for the peak [Ca^{2+}] (*left*) and for the peak [CaM-Ca_4] (*right*). The Z axis is distance from the dendritic shaft (distance along the spine). The input consists of three presynaptic stimuli delivered at 100 Hz while the postsynaptic voltage at the spine head was clamped to −40 mV. The peak changes in [Ca^{2+}] and [CaM-Ca_4] are restricted mainly to the spine head, where they are amplified. Note that the [CaM-Ca_4] transient is a steeper function of distance and time than the [Ca^{2+}] transient. (A) The surfaces show the results for a nonuniform low-affinity pump density ($P_s = 1 \times 10^{-15}$ μmol/μm^2 and $P_s = 5 \times 10^{-15}$ μmol/μm^2). (B) Similar results are shown for a uniform low-affinity pump density ($P_s = 3 \times 10^{-15}$ μmol/μm^2). (From Zador et al., 1990; Zador and Brown, unpublished data.)

[$CaM-Ca_4$] after synaptic activation. Concentration changes were effectively limited to a single spine, which implies that the changes were specific to a single synapse because there do not appear to be multiple terminations on spines in the CA1 region (Brown and Zador, 1990). The spine may thus provide a mechanism for achieving the postsynaptic input specificity observed at Sch/com synapses. Because each spine maintains its own microenvironment distinct form that of neighboring spines, synaptic enhancement can be highly selective. The same results were obtained for both a nonuniform (figure 22.7a) and a uniform pump density (figure 22.7b). In both cases, a large change at the spine head resulted in only a very small change at the dendritic shaft.

This account of input specificity assumes that the molecular events that control the induction of LTP and its expression can be adequately understood from the perspective of the dendritic spine. In its current form, our computational model does not address the possibility that the expression of LTP is ultimately controlled or triggered by a retrograde signal, as suggested by Brown and associates (1988b, 1989). If a retrograde signal turns out to be important, then the explanation of input specificity would have to take into account spatiotemporal aspects of the production and action of the signal and the conditions under which it produces a modification. Although there is certainly no proof that retrograde LTP signals exist, it is not unreasonable to imagine that there is a two-way communication process across the synaptic cleft. If this supposition is correct, then the explanation of LTP may have to take into account the dynamics of this communication.

Temporal Contiguity To be effective in inducing LTP, presynaptic stimulation and postsynaptic depolarization must occur at about the same time (Kelso et al., 1986; Brown et al., 1989). Our model, however, predicts that they do not have to be perfectly synchronous. The slow unbinding of glutamate from the NMDA receptor suggests the possibility that LTP induction should occur even if postsynaptic depolarization follows neurotransmitter release by tens of milliseconds. Figure 22.8 illustrates that this "trace period" may in fact last longer than 40 milliseconds. This prediction may explain a number of experimental observations regarding the induction of LTP by sequential synaptic inputs (Brown et al., 1989; Steward et al., 1988; Larsen and Lynch, 1989).

Role of Spines in LTP Induction

Our computer simulations suggest three important ways in which the microphysiology of the spine may play an important role in LTP induction: by creating a separate microenvironment for second messenger signals, by amplifying these signals, and by steepening the voltage dependence of the overall mechanism for LTP induction.

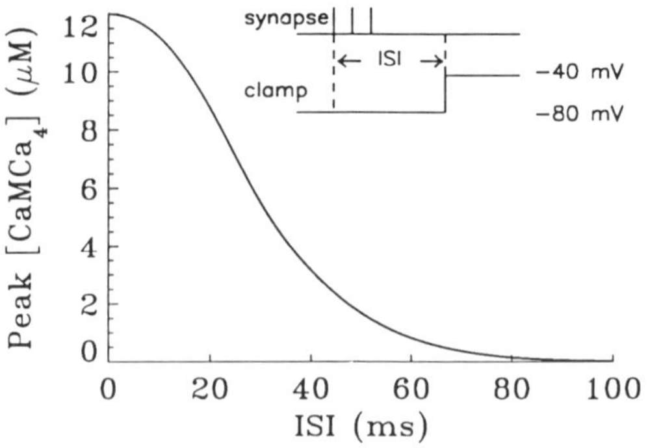

Figure 22.8 Interstimulus interval effects. Peak [CaM-Ca_4] in the subsynaptic compartment is shown as a function of the delay in the onset of postsynaptic depolarization. The interstimulus interval (ISI) is the interval between the onset of the synaptic stimulation and the onset of postsynaptic activity. A train of three presynaptic stimuli was applied at 100 Hz. The postsynaptic depolarization consisted of voltage clamp to −40 mV. A substantial increase in the peak [CaM-Ca_4] can occur even with an ISI greater than 20 msec. Precise synchrony of presynaptic and postsynaptic activity is thus not required, but there is a narrow time window. (From Zador et al., 1990.)

Creation of a Separate Microenvironment The simulations illustrated in figure 22.7 show that spines can compartmentalize the postsynaptic Ca^{2+} signals. Specifically, they appear to restrict the transient increase in the [Ca^{2+}] to the region of the subsynaptic membrane. This finding was extremely robust with respect to variations in parameters. The spines also served to isolate the subsynaptic membrane concentration changes at the dendritic shaft. For example, when dendritic [Ca^{2+}] was stepped to a constant value of 1 μM, the change at the subsynaptic membrane was negligible (Zador et al., 1990). This isolation effect was observed with either a nonuniform or a uniform pump distribution, which may help explain why Ca^{2+} influx through dendritic Ca^{2+} channels opened during prolonged postsynaptic depolarization is not sufficient to induce LTP (Kelso et al., 1986; compare Regehr et al., 1989). Compartmentalization and isolation can be regarded as two aspects of the same phenomenon—the creation of a synapse-specific microenvironment that can control synaptic plasticity. The existence of this microenvironment may contribute to the input specificity observed in the Sch/com synapses.

In our simulations, the isolation of the subsynaptic membrane from [Ca^{2+}] changes initiated in the dendritic shaft depended on the presence of pumps in the spine neck and head. The effect could not be achieved through buffers, which affected only the rate at which the steady-state subsynaptic [Ca^{2+}] was reached, but not its final value. It is important to appreciate that the model does not predict isolation under all possible experimental circumstances. Under conditions of very large or prolonged increases in dendritic [Ca^{2+}], factors such as energetic rundown of pumps could attenuate the degree of isolation of the subsynaptic membrane (compare Segal et al., 1990).

Amplification of Second Messenger Signals The simulations show that spines *amplify* the small Ca^{2+} fluxes through the NMDA receptor channel into large changes in [Ca^{2+}]. Amplification may help achieve a [Ca^{2+}] high enough for the induction of LTP. This amplification depended primarily on the restriction of Ca^{2+} to the small volume of the subsynaptic compartment. The amount of amplification, as monitored by the peak [Ca^{2+}] attained at the spine head during a train of synaptic stimuli, could be varied over a wide range by altering the concentrations of Ca^{2+} pumps and buffers over a reasonable physiological range. The spine microphysiology may thus regulate the accumulation of the second messengers that lead to the induction of LTP. This regulation could provide a mechanism for adaptive control of the overall plasticity.

Steepening the Voltage-dependence of the Mechanism Spines may *steepen* the voltage-dependence of the processes underlying LTP induction. The voltage dependence that we have assumed for the NMDA receptor-gated channel is not very steep (see figure 22.5). The current at -80 mV was only 4.4 times less than at -40 mV. Both [Ca^{2+}] and the concentration of activated calmodulin varied as steeper functions of voltage than the NMDA current. Further experimental analysis is needed to determine whether the voltage dependence of LTP induction is greater than can be explained directly by the properties of the NMDA receptor–gated channel.

New View of Spine Function

The present suggestion that spines play a critical role in the regulation of Ca^{2+} dynamics contrasts with the more traditional approach to spine function that has emphasized electrotonic effects. One previous proposal (Diamond et al., 1970) is that the large spine axial resistance isolates synapses from electrical activity at the dendritic shaft and at neighboring spines. This idea of electrical isolation is not consistent with theoretical results that predict essentially complete voltage transfer from the dendritic shaft to the spine head (Brown et al., 1988b; Carnevale and Johnston, 1982). Another previous hypothesis is that modulation of the spine axial resistance, possibly through changes in spine neck geometry, mediates changes in synaptic efficacy (compare Chang, 1952; Rall, 1970) underlying the expression of hippocampal LTP (Bliss and Lømo, 1973; Koch and Poggio, 1983). The extent to which axial resistance can in fact control synaptic efficacy depends on the ratio of this resistance to the inverse of the peak synaptic conductance (Brown et al., 1988b, 1989; Koch and Poggio, 1983; Wilson, 1984). Simulations have suggested that this critical ratio may not be sufficiently large to allow significant control of synaptic efficacy in hippocampal neurons (Brown et al., 1988b; Harris and Stevens, 1989). It may therefore be appropriate to shift attention to the role of spines in regulating second messengers.

HEBBIAN COMPUTATIONS IN NODES AND NEURONS

Theoretical studies have shown that interesting forms of associative learning and self-organization can emerge in networks in which the connections among nodes can change according to a Hebbian algorithm (Anderson, 1985; Hopfield, 1984; Kohonen, 1989; Linsker, 1990; reviewed in Brown et al., 1990). We have been interested in the relationship between the kinds of modifications that occur in these artificial neural networks and those that might be expected to occur in neurobiological systems. The main reason for creating the biophysical model of the Hebbian synapse was to incorporate it into a detailed representation of a hippocampal neuron. Before we do so, it is perhaps worthwhile to compare neurons and nodes.

Processing Elements or "Nodes"

In artificial neural networks, the processing elements (PEs) are generally simple summation nodes whose output is typically the weighted sum of the inputs passed through a transfer function:

$$a_i^{t+1} = \theta\left(\sum_{j=1}^{N} w_{ij}^t \, a_j^t\right) \tag{22.14}$$

where the output a_i of the ith element at time $t + 1$ is equal to the sum of N inputs a_j at time t weighted by associated "synaptic weights" w. This sum is then passed through the (often sigmoidal) transfer function $\theta(\bullet)$. The popularity of equation (22.14) and its variants stems in large part from their mathematical tractability. The successes of network models in solving many real-world tasks (see Sejnowski and Rosenberg, 1986) attests to the computational power of these simple systems.

Nodes Versus Neurons

The summation node or PE (equation [22.14]) does not capture the *temporal, spatial,* and *stochastic* complexity inherent in the dynamics of neurons. The much richer temporal behavior of neurons results both from their passive membrane properties and from the abundance of voltage- and ligand-gated channels. The spatial extent of the dendritic tree adds a second complexity because it permits local interactions among subsets of inputs. Inclusion of this complexity in a PE requires higher-order interactions among inputs. *Sigma-pi* units (Durbin and Rumelhart, 1989) actually do include second- and higher-order multiplicative terms of the form $[w_{ijk} \, a_j \, a_k]$. The quantal nature of synaptic transmission gives rise to stochastic complexity that is also not captured in the typical node (equation [22.14]).

NEUROBIOLOGY OF HEBBIAN COMPUTATIONS

The differences between nodes and neurons may have interesting computational implications. With respect to Hebbian computations, we would like to know what kinds of new possibilities or rules emerge when we consider the actual neurobiology. Our initial approach has been at the single neuron level. The plan is to gain some insights at this level before scaling up to the circuit level.

The Single-Neuron Model

CA1 pyramidal neurons were simulated on a Sun 4/330 workstation using a customized version of NEURON, a compartmental simulator developed by Michael Hines (Hines, 1989). In the beginning, we did not worry about the complexity of the simulations because run times on NEURON scale linearly with the number of compartments. But soon we were simulating neurons with 64,000 compartments, and it became clear that we needed to simplify our spine model for LTP induction. The problem is that there are more than 10^4 spines on these pyramidal neurons and our spine model, which takes into account Ca^{2+} dynamics, is computationally expensive. We have therefore begun to explore various ways to simplify the synaptic modification algorithm. Here we describe one example of such a simplification.

The Parameter Space

As we began to appreciate the magnitude of this theoretical effort, it seemed appropriate to step back and appraise the size and complexity of parameter space that requires exploration. Based on preliminary simulations, we decided that the initial problem at the single-neuron level was to understand the interactions among three categories of variables—the neuronal morphology and membrane physiology, the spatial and temporal relations among the inputs to the neuron, and the nature of the synaptic learning mechanism. Most of our effort to date has involved wrestling with these three categories.

Neuronal Morphology and Physiology Anatomical measurements were obtained from three-dimensional reconstructions of hippocampal neurons (Mainen et al., 1990; Claiborne et al., 1991). Both dentate granule cells and CA1 pyramidal cells were used. Here we will focus on the CA1 pyramidal neurons. Each pyramidal neuron was described by a tree structure consisting of a set of short cylinders. The end of each cylinder was specified by a three-dimensional location (XYZ coordinate) and a diameter. The original morphometric data consisted of 3000 to 4000 coordinate-diameter pairs. Usually these 3000 to 4000 cylinders were collapsed into 300 to 400 compartments. A correction factor was applied to the membrane area based on an estimate for spine density of 2/μm (Claiborne et al., 1991). For the simulations illustrated here, the usual parameter values were R_m = 70 kΩ-cm^2 (15 − 150 kΩ-cm^2 range), C_m = 1 μF/cm^2, R_i = 200 Ω-cm (compare Brown et al., 1981; 1988b). It seemed to us to make sense to try to comprehend the linear case before introducing voltage-dependent conductances. Each simulated neuron received 3000 to 20,000 synaptic contacts, which were distributed randomly across the dendritic tree. The peak synaptic conductances were subject to a Hebbian form of enhancement and one or more forms of depression. The equations governing the modification process are discussed in the following section.

Statistical Structure of the Environment The model neurons were placed in a structured environment that consisted of various spatiotemporal patterns of synaptic activation. In one of the simplest cases, discussed next, 5 to 10 groups of synapses were randomly selected from a total set of 3500. Among simulations, the groups ranged in size from 30 to 200 synapses, but within a simulation the size was usually constant. In each simulated epoch of 100 milliseconds, one group of synapses was stimulated synchronously with parameters known to induce LTP in hippocampal neurons (three tetanic stimulations at 300 Hz). Synaptic stimulation was represented by the sum of separate AMPA and NMDA currents (equations [22.10] and [22.5]). This correlated synaptic activity within a group could be thought of as representing a "feature" in the input space of the neuron. The features were presented sequentially, and their synapses were modified after each epoch. Presentation of the complete set of patterns constituted a trial. Before the first trial, all of the synaptic conductances were identical.

Synaptic Modification Rule A generalization of equation (22.4) was used to model synaptic plasticity:

$$\frac{dw_{ij}}{dt} = \{\alpha[a_i(t), a_j(t)] - \beta[a_i(t)] - \gamma[a_j(t)] - \delta\} \tag{22.15}$$

The value of the peak AMPA conductance $g_{\text{AMPA - PEAK}}$ was related to the synaptic weight w_{ij} by equation (22.16):

$$g_{AMPA\,-\,PEAK} = \frac{g_{max}}{1 + e^{-\sigma(W_{ij}\,-\,0.5g_{max})}} \tag{22.16}$$

where σ determines the steepness of the sigmoid and g_{max} is a constant. The value $g_{\text{AMPA - PEAK}}$ was updated for every synapse at the end of a simulation epoch. The maximum possible value of the NMDA conductance was set initially to a fixed fraction (0.2) of the peak AMPA conductance. In some situations the NMDA conductance remained fixed at this initial value, while in others it was a constant fraction of peak AMPA conductance.

As noted earlier, the terms on the right-hand side of equation (22.15) can possibly be related to the biological mechanisms of table 22.1. The first term, $\alpha[a_i(t), a_j(t)]$, represents an interactive process for synaptic enhancement. We used a simplified form of the single-spine model of Ca^{2+} dynamics just described to compute the concentration of Ca^{2+}-activated calmodulin. Synaptic potentiation was assumed to be proportional to the time integral of this concentration over a simulation epoch:

$$\alpha[a_i(t), a_j(t)] = \alpha \int_{\text{epoch}} [\text{CaM-Ca}_4^{2+}]\, dt \qquad (22.17)$$

Equation (22.15) also contains two terms for use-dependent synaptic depression. The function $\beta[a_j(t)]$ represents the contribution of homosynaptic depression based on some measure of presynaptic activity. Following the hypothesis that homosynaptic depression involves activation of the "Q2 receptor" (Bear and Cooper, 1990), we interpreted this term as a linear function of the time integral of the AMPA conductance:

$$\beta[a_j(t)] = \beta \int_{\text{epoch}} g_{\text{AMPA}}(t)\, dt \qquad (22.18)$$

where $g_{\text{AMPA}}(t)$ is the conductance of the AMPA component of the response at time t, which is given by equation (22.10). The quantity g_{AMPA} can be considered a measure of presynaptic activity because it is insensitive to postsynaptic voltage. Because the quantity $\beta[a_j(t)]$ is subtracted, and its magnitude increased with $g_{\text{AMPA}}(t)$, it provides negative feedback on weights that are approaching large values.

The function $\gamma[a_j(t)]$ represents the contribution of heterosynaptic depression. Postsynaptic activity was represented by local depolarization. This term was calculated as a linear function of the time integral of the difference between the resting membrane potential V_{rest} and the local potential at the subsynaptic membrane V_{syn}:

$$\gamma[a_j(t)] = \gamma \int_{\text{epoch}} [V_{\text{syn}}(t) - V_{\text{rest}}(t)]\, dt \qquad (22.19)$$

The key difference between this term and the postsynaptic activity in an ordinary bilinear equation arises from the voltage gradients in dendrites. A node is a point, meaning that the "activity" or "activation" of the node is the same at all simultaneous inputs. By contrast, as we show next, in a hippocampal neuron there can be steep voltage gradients along the dendritic tree. For some kinds of computations, these voltage gradients may not be important. In considering Hebbian synapses, however, the postsynaptic membrane potential is obviously critical. Because of the electrotonic structure of the neuron, for a given input pattern, the voltages at the subsynaptic membrane are not the same for the various synapses. The actual subsynaptic voltages are dependent on the precise electrotonic relationships among the active synapses.

The constant δ represents a passive decay process operating at a constant rate throughout simulation time. This term is the simplest form of depression. Unlike the heterosynaptic and homosynaptic depression terms just described above there is no difference between the biological and the strictly nodal interpretation of passive decay.

Simulation Results

The parameter space that we are exploring is obviously large and complex. What is already clear is that there are strong interactions among the three categories of variables—those associated with the neuron, the environment, and the learning rule. For instance, the average level of depolarization in response to a single input pattern could be adjusted using any combination of changes to the membrane resistance, pattern size, or peak synaptic conductance (as well as many other parameters).

Voltage Gradients in Hippocampal Dendrites Because LTP induction is controlled in part by postsynaptic voltage, it matters whether the cells are isopotential. If the cells are isopotential, the dendrites play no computational role with respect to the signaling of voltage and we can represent the electrical properties of the neuron using a single compartment. On the other hand, if there are steep voltage gradients, the electrotonic structure of the postsynaptic cell can play an important role in determining Hebbian modifications.

The magnitude of voltage gradients in the dendritic tree depends on assumptions about membrane properties, such as the membrane resistivity R_m. In the steady state, we can anticipate that the gradients will decrease as R_m increases (Jack et al., 1975). At the moment, there is some controversy over the value of R_m. Estimates based on whole-cell recordings are substantially higher than those based on recordings using "sharp electrodes." In one set of simulations (color plate 1) we let R_m vary from 15 to 150 kΩ-cm^2.

These simulations revealed that even if R_m is as high as 150 kΩ-cm^2, hippocampal pyramidal neurons are not isopotential. This is shown in color plate 1 for two kinds of perturbations—a voltage step applied to the cell soma (top) and the activation of a group of synapses (bottom). Thus, the location of a synaptic input on the dendritic tree is an important determinant of plasticity.

Pattern Selection and Cluster Formation. Our initial explorations of synaptic plasticity have focused on the self-organization of Hebbian synapses in response to a structured environment (Mainen et al., 1990). The most general result was that the average synaptic strength increased for some patterns and decreased for others (see color plate 2). Some patterns "win" and others "lose," in spite of each having the same number of synapses with the same initial conductances. We do not yet understand all of the factors and rules that determine winning and losing. One can surmise that the patterns that eventually win are those in which the synapses have a "favorable" electrotonic location, meaning that the synapses within the pattern tend to be electrotonically near each other. Because of the heterosynaptic depression term, the electrotonic location relative to other winning patterns is also presumably relevant. Following this line of thought, an "unfavorable" location would be one in which the synapses are not electrotonically near each other and/or they are electrotonically near a winning pattern. We have just begun to develop methods for evaluating these intuitions.

The overall result is that each neuron becomes selective to a particular subset of its original feature space. This spontaneous or unsupervised "tuning" of the neuron to particular features is sensitive to the initial number and spatial distribution of synapses as well as to temporal correlations with other patterns. If instead of presenting the patterns sequentially, two patterns co-occur, the probability is greatly increased that synapses in these coincident patterns will be strengthened, a fact that seems relevant to associative forms of learning. The rate, extent, and type of pattern selection is also highly dependent on the details of the modification rule. Depending on the rule, the degree of selection can be modest or extreme. In an extreme case, a small number of patterns can take control of the activity of the neuron. The degree to which the neuron focuses on very restricted features in the original input space seems to be a function of both the nature of modification rule and the spatiotemporal structure of the input patterns.

Thus far, we have been considering self-organization in terms of gross pattern selection—winning and losing. Examined in this way, pattern selection can be evaluated by taking the sum of the synaptic conductances for the pattern or simply by looking at the synaptic potential produced by the pattern in the cell body. These overall measures do not, however, reveal the details of what happens during the process of self-organization. If one looks more closely at the data with proper graphics it is possible to get a feeling for the dynamics of the process. Intuitively, one might expect that a Hebbian synaptic mechanism "could cause the formation of spatial domains (mosaics) of enhancement among electrotonically proximal and functionally related synapses" (Brown et al., 1988). Indeed, within a feature one sees clusters of strengthened synapses that are near each other (see color plate 2). These feature clusters can occur within either a winning or a losing pattern. We sometimes see a feature cluster form and then disappear. By watching the formation and disappearance of feature clusters we are hoping to gain some insight into the rules.

Implications for Computation

The formation of feature clusters provides a specific example of how a neurobiologically realistic model can exhibit behavior that is more interesting and complex than that exhibited by a simple summation node. In considering differences between PEs and neurons, earlier we identified three broad categories that might be computationally important. One category of difference that we suggested could be important concerns space. A PE is a point, meaning that there is no spatial aspect to the internal computations performed by a PE. A PE does not have dendrites, which raises this question: what is the computational function of dendrites?

Interactions Among Inputs Of course, it is easy to think of many possible functions for dendrites that have no computational importance. Part of the motivation underlying our simulations is to develop ideas about the specific kinds of computations that dendrites enable. The results illustrated in color plate 2 demonstrate one consequence of dendrites that could be important for Hebbian learning. In particular, the electrotonic structure of the neuron allows a kind of interaction among synaptic inputs that cannot occur in the kind of PE represented by equation (22.14). Input-dependent spatial inhomogeneity enables complex interactions among Hebbian synapses. This finding is true even for the purely passive case that we have illustrated here, but it will obviously become even more important when we introduce the varieties of active membrane that are known to be present on these neurons.

Hot Spots and Cold Spots There is evidence that voltage-gated Ca^{2+} channels and other voltage-dependent channels are distributed nonuniformly in hippocampal neurons (Jones et al., 1989; Regehr et al., 1989). Especially interesting are the possible computational consequences of "hots spots" and "cold spots" on the dendrites. By hot spots we mean either of two kinds of membrane patches—one that contains a conductance that increases after depolarization and that has a reversal potential that is much more positive than the resting potential, or one that contains a conductance that decreases after depolarization and that has a reversal potential near or more negative than the resting potential. By cold spots we mean just the opposite.

We can anticipate two consequences of these local nonlinearities. First, they will obviously influence the formation of feature clusters. Second, they will allow regions of a dendrite to make *decisions* about subsets of the inputs that were previously selected by clustering. We are currently exploring our intuition that the addition of active membrane to the dendrites will allow single pyramidal neurons to learn nonlinear pattern separations. One possible implication is that single neurons may be able to extract higher-order features from the input space.

SUMMARY AND CONCLUSIONS

We began this paper by introducing the bilinear equation (equations [22.3] and [22.4]) for a generalized Hebbian modification. This equation was then loosely interpreted in terms of some neurobiological processes (table 22.1). What we have seen is that the bilinear equation takes on a greater complexity in the context of the electrotonic structure of pyramidal neurons. The kind of self-organization that we illustrated in pyramidal neurons (see color plate 2) cannot occur in a simple summation node.

In this respect, a single hippocampal neuron may behave more like a network of summation nodes—a *micronet*. Once we have some understanding of self-organization and associative changes in linear models of pyramidal neurons, it will become important to introduce nonlinearities into the dendritic membrane. This overall effort has both theoretical and practical implications. It is a necessary first step toward the creation of a computational theory of learning that is well-grounded in cellular neurobiology. It is also important for efforts to implement neurobiologically inspired computations in analog VLSI (see Mead, 1989).

ACKNOWLEDGMENTS

We thank Daniel Johnston for useful comments on this manuscript. This research was supported by grants from the Office of Naval Research, the Defense Advanced Research Projects Agency, and the Air Force Office of Scientific Research.

REFERENCES

Anderson, J.A. (1985). In W. B. Levy, J. A. Anderson, and S. Lehmkuhle (eds.), *Synaptic Modification, Neuron Selectivity, and Nervous System Organization*. Hillsdale, N.J.: Lawrence Erlbaum Associates.

Ascher, P., and Nowak L. (1988). *Journal of Physiology (London)* 399:247–266.

Barrionuevo, G., and T. H. Brown (1983). *Proceedings of the National Academy of Sciences USA* 80:7347–7351.

Baxter, D. A., G. D. Bittner, and T. H. Brown (1985). *Proceedings of the National Academy of Sciences USA* 82:5978–5982.

Bear, M., and L. N. Cooper (1990). In M, Gluck and D. E. Rumelhart (eds.), *Neuroscience and Connectionist Theory*. Hillsdale, N.J.: Lawrence Erlbaum Associates.

Bekkers, J. M., and C. F. Stevens (1989). *Nature (London)* 341:230–233.

Bekkers, J. M., and C. F. Stevens (1990). *Nature (London)* 346:724–729.

Bliss, T. V. P., and T. Lømo (1973). *Journal of Physiology (London)* 232:331–356.

Bliss, T. V. P., and M. A. Lynch (1988). In P. W. Landfield, and S. A. Deadwyler (eds.), *Long-Term Potentiation: From Biophysics to Behavior*. New York: Alan R. Liss, pp. 3–72.

Briggs, C. A., T. H. Brown, and D. A. McAfee (1985a). *Journal of Physiology (London)* 359:503–521.

Briggs, C. A., D. A. McAfee, and R. E. McCaman (1985b). *Journal of Physiology (London)* 363:181–190.

Brown, T. H, P. F. Chapman, E. W. Kairiss, and C. L. Keenan (1988a). *Science*. 242:724–728.

Brown, T. H., et al. (1988b). In P. W. Landfield, and S. A. Deadwyler (eds.), *Long-Term Potentiation: From Biophysics to Behavior.* New York: Alan R. Liss, pp. 197–260.

Brown, T. H., et al. (1989). In J. H. Byrne and W. O. Berry (eds.), *Neural Models of Plasticity* San Diego: Academic Press, pp. 266–306.

Brown, T. H., R. A. Fricke, D. H. Perkel (1981). *Journal of Neurophysiology* 46:812–827.

Brown, T. H., and D. Johnston (1983). *Journal of Neurophysiology* 50:487–507.

Brown, T. H., E. W. Kairiss, and C. L. Keenan (1990). *Annual Review of Neuroscience* 13:475–512.

Brown, T. H., and A. M. Zador (1990). In G. M. Shepherd (ed.), *The Synaptic Organization of the Brain.* New York: Oxford University Press, pp. 346–388.

Cajal, S. Ramon y (1911). *Histologie du System Nerveux,* Vol. 2. Paris: Maloine.

Carnevale, N. T., and D. Johnston (1982). *Journal of Neurophysiology* 47:606–621.

Chang, H–T. (1952). *Cold Spring Harbor Symposium on Quantitative Biology* 17:189–202.

Claiborne, B. J., A. M. Zador, Z. F. Mainen, and T. H. Brown (1991). Computational Models of Hippocampal Neurons. In T. McKenna, J. Davis, and S. F. Zornetzer (eds.), *Single Neuron Computation.* San Diego: Academic Press.

Collingridge, G. L., S. J. Kehl, and H. McLennan (1983). *Journal of Physiology (London)* 334:19–31.

Cull-Candy, S. G., and M. M. Usowicz (1987). *Nature (London)* 325:525–528.

DeFreitas, J. B., and M. P. Stryker (1990). *Society for Neuroscience Abstracts* 16:798.

Diamond J., E. G. Gray, and G. M. Yasargil (1970). In P. Andersen and J. K. S. Jensen (eds.), *Excitatory Synaptic Mechanisms.* Oslo: Universitetsforlaget, pp. 213–222.

Decker, R. E., and J. A. Dani (1990). *Journal of Neuroscience* 10:3413–3420.

Doerner, D., T. A. Pitler, and B. E. Alger (1988). *Journal of Neuroscience* 11:4069–4078.

Dunwiddie, T., and G. Lynch (1978). *Journal of Physiology* 276:353–367.

Dunwiddie, T., and G. Lynch (1979). *Brain Research* 169:103–110.

Durbin, R., and D. E. Rumelhart (1989). *Neural Computation* 1: 133–142.

Forsythe, I. D., and G. L. Westbrook (1988). *Journal of Physiology (London)* 396:515–533.

Gamble, E., and C. Koch (1987). *Science* 236:1311–1315.

Harris, K. M., F. E. Jensen, and B. H. Tsao (1989). In V. Chan-Palay and C. Kohler (eds.), *The Hippocampus—New Vistas.* New York: Alan R. Liss, p. 32–52.

Harris, K. M., and J. K. Stevens (1989). *Journal of Neuroscience* 9:2982–2997.

Hebb, D. O. (1949). *The Organization of Behavior.* New York: Wiley.

Hille, B. (1984). *Ionic Channels of Excitable Membranes.* Sunderland, Mass: Sinauer.

Hines, M. (1984). *International Journal of Bio-Medical Computation* 15:69–76.

Hines, M. (1989). *International Journal of Bio-Medical Computation* 24:55–68.

Holmes, W. R., and W. B. Levy (1990). *Journal of Neurophysiology* 63:1148–1168.

Honore, T., et al. (1988). *Science* 241:701–703.

Hopfield, J. J. (1984). *Proceedings of the National Academy of Science USA* 81:3088–3092.

Jack, J., A. Noble, and R. W. Tsien (1975). *Electrical Current Flow in Excitable Membranes.* London: Oxford University Press.

Jaffe, D., and D. Johnston (1990). *Journal of Neurophysiology* 64:948–960.

Jahr, C. E., and C. F. Stevens (1987). *Nature* 325:522–525.

Jahr, C. E., and C. F. Stevens (1990a). *Journal of Neuroscience* 10:1830–1837.

Jahr, C. E., and C. F. Stevens (1990b). *Journal of Neuroscience* 10:3178–3182.

James, W. (1890). *Psychology: Briefer Course.* Cambridge: Harvard University Press.

Jones, O. T., D. L. Kunze, and K. J. Angelides (1989). *Science* 244:1189–1193.

Kairiss et al. (1988). *Society for Neuroscience Abstracts* 14:832.

Kauer, J.A., R. C. Malenka, and R. A. Nicoll (1988). *Neuron* 1:911–917.

Keenan, C. L., A. C. Nobre, B. C. Claiborne, and T. H Brown (1990). *Society for Neuroscience Abstracts* 16:660.

Kelso, S. R., and T. H. Brown (1986). *Science* 232:85–87.

Kelso, S. R., A. H. Ganong, and T. H. Brown (1986). *Proceedings of the National Academy of Science USA* 83:5326–5330.

Kennedy, M. B. (1989). *Cell* 59:777–787.

Koch, C., and T. Poggio (1983). *Proceedings of the Royal Society (London)* 218:455–477.

Kohonen, T. (1989). *Self-organization and Associative Memory.* Berlin: Springer-Verlag.

Larsen, J., and G. Lynch (1989). *Brain Research* 489:49–58.

Lester, R. A. J., J. D. Clements, G. L. Westbrook, and C. E. Jahr (1990). *Nature (London)* 346:565–567.

Lewis, C. A., and C. F. Stevens (1979). In C. F. Stevens and R. W. Tsien (eds.), *Membrane Transport Processes.* New York: Raven Press, pp. 133–151.

Linsker, R. (1990). *Annual Review of Neuroscience* 13:257–282.

Lynch, G., et al. (1983). *Nature* 305:719–721.

MacDermott, A. B., et al. (1986). *Nature* 321:519–522.

Mainen, Z. M., A. M. Zador, B. Claiborne, and T. H. Brown (1990). *Society for Neuroscience Abstracts* 16:492.

Malenka, R. C., J. A. Kauer, R. S. Zucker, and R. A. Nicoll (1988). *Science* 242:81–84.

Malinow, R., and J. P. Miller (1986). *Nature* 320:529–530.

Malinow, R., and R. W. Tsien (1990). *Nature* 346:177–180.

Mascagni, M. V. (1989). In C. Koch and I. Segev (eds.): *Methods in Neuronal Modeling: From Synapses to Networks.* Cambridge Mass: MIT Press, pp. 439–484.

Mayer, M. L., et al. (1987). *Journal of Neuroscience* 7:3230–3244.

Mayer, M. L., G. L. Westbrook, and P. B. Guthrie (1984). *Nature* 309:261–263.

Mayer, M. L., and G. L. Westbrook (1987). *Journal of Physiology (London)* 394:501–527.

Mead, C. (1989). *Analog VLSI and Neural Systems.* Reading, MA: Addison-Wesley.

Monaghan, D. T., and C. W. Cotman (1985). *Journal of Neuroscience* 5:2909–2919.

Muller, D., M. Jolly, and G. Lynch (1988). *Science* 242:1694–1697.

Neher, E., and J. H. Steinbach (1978). *Journal of Physiology (London)* 277:153–176.

Nobre, A. C., Z. Xiang, A. M. Zador, and T. H. Brown (1990). *Society for Neuroscience Abstracts* 16:492.

Nowak, L., et al. (1984). *Nature* 307:462–465.

Qian, N., and T. J. Sejnowski (1989). *Biological Cybernetics* 62:1–15.

Quartararo, N., P. H. Barry, and P. W. Gage (1987). *Journal of Membrane Biology* 97:137–159.

Rall, W. (1970). In P. Andersen and J. K. S. Jensen (eds.), Oslo: Universitetsforlaget, pp. 175–187.

Regehr, W. G., J. A. Connor, and D. W. Tank (1989). *Nature* 341:533–536.

Richardson, T. L., R. W. Turner, and J. J. Miller (1987). *Journal of Neurophysiology* 58:981–996.

Segal, M., P. Guthrie, and S. B. Kater (1990). *Society for Neuroscience Abstracts* 16:468.

Sejnowski, T. J. (1977). *Journal of Theoretical Biology* 69:385–389.

Sejnowski, T. J., and C. R. Rosenberg (1986). *JHU/EECS–86/01* 32.

Squire, L. R. (1987). *Memory and the Brain.* New York: Oxford University Press.

Stanton, P. K., and T. J. Sejnowski (1989). *Nature* 339:215–218.

Stent, G. S. (1973). *Proceedings of the National Academy of Science USA* 70:997–1001.

Steward, O., G. White, D. Korol, and W. B. Levy (1988). In P. W. Landfield and S. A. Deadwyler (eds.), *Long-Term Potentiation: From Biophysics to Behavior*. New York: Alan R. Liss, pp. 139–166.

Tanzi, E. (1893). *Rivista Sperimentale Freniatria e di Medicina Legale* 19:419–472.

Traub, R. D. (1982). *Neuroscience* 7:1233–1242.

Wickens, J. (1988). *Progress in Neurobiology* 31:507–528.

Wigström, H., B. Gustafsson, Y.-Y. Huang, and W. C. Abraham (1986). *Acta Physiologica Scandinavia* 126:317–319.

Wilson, C. J. (1984). *Journal of Neuroscience* 4:281–297.

Xiang, Z., et al. (1990). *Society for Neuroscience Abstracts* 16:492.

Yamada, K. A., J. M. Dubinsky, and S. M. Rothman (1989). *Journal of Neuroscience* 9:3230–3236.

Zador, A., C. Koch, T. H. Brown (1990). *Proceedings of the National Academy of Science USA* 87:6718–6722.

Zalutsky, R. A., and R. A. Nicoll (1990). *Science* 248:1619–1624.

23 Possible Computations of Primary Sensory Cortex: Hypotheses Based on Computer Models of Olfaction and Audition

Richard Granger, Alberto Cobas, and Gary Lynch

The physiological phenomenon of synaptic long-term potentiation (LTP) has characteristics that make it a candidate mechanism for long-term memory: it is rapidly induced, specific, and extremely long-lasting; it has been found to occur in brain structures presumed to be involved in long-term memory in human beings and other animals, including paleocortex (Roman et al., 1987; Jung et al., 1991), archicortex (Bliss and Lømo, 1973; Staubli and Lynch, 1987), and neocortex (Lee 1982; Artola and Singer, 1987; Iriki et al., 1989); and behavioral learning can be blocked by pharmacological manipulations that block LTP (Staubli et al., 1987; Staubli et al., 1989).

Given that behavioral learning and memory involves more than single cells or synapses, aggregate function of networks of neurons must be investigated, via theoretical and empirical approaches, to understand the processes by which LTP in identified brain circuitry might give rise to memory. We have undertaken a line of research intended to study such aggregate function in hopes of drawing out ways in which the operation of LTP in telencephalic networks might underlie aspects of learning and memory. Our research effort begins with physiological function in anatomical structures, and attempts to find coherent processing characteristics that emerge. It is worth noting a subtle advantage of this relatively "bottom-up" approach: it has the capability of suggesting emergent memory processes that may not have been focused on in behavioral or psychological studies. This ability to discover novel aggregate phenomena serves to contrast the present approach with some other modeling efforts, in which circuit-level explanations are sought for prespecified function that those circuits are presumed to subserve. The bottom-up modeling approach has recently led to an example of this form of discovery: simulation of the olfactory bulb–olfactory cortex system led to identification of a previously unsuspected memory phenomenon, which is therefore now hypothesized to be a feature of this system. In short, cyclic processing between simulations of the olfactory cortex and its primary input structure, olfactory bulb, resulted in a number of emergent network properties that translate into behavioral abilities, including the ability to classify cues by similarity (Lynch and Granger, 1989), to extract constituent components from compounds or mixtures (Granger et al., 1989), and to sequentially or iteratively recognize finer-grained detail comprising a cue, via hierarchical clustering over successive sampling cycles (Ambros-Ingerson, et al., 1990). Specific predictions from these hypotheses have recently been tested with positive results in behavioral (Granger et al., 1991) and physiological studies (McCollum et al., 1991), and further tests are in progress.

One interesting issue raised by these findings is the question of generality of the findings; in particular, the extent to which they might apply to systems other than olfaction. Olfactory paleocortex (piriform cortex) is a presumed phylogenetic precursor to neocortex, raising questions of possibly analogous anatomical, physiological, and functional shared properties between these cortical organizations. To study these possibilities, we have constructed models of principal portions of the auditory system, including the ventral and magnocellular divisions of the thalamic medial geniculate nucleus (MGv and MGm), the six-layered primary auditory neocortex (AI), and connectivity between and intrinsic to these structures. These computer models have been used to simulate physiological findings in the auditory system, to investigate possible roles of LTP in these findings, and to raise questions of potential auditory function based on these hypotheses.

BACKGROUND: PALEOCORTEX

Anatomy of the Olfactory Bulb–Olfactory Cortex System

Figure 23.1A schematically illustrates the primary circuitry of the olfactory bulb–olfactory cortex system; we briefly outline it here. The primary olfactory receptors in the nose innervate the apical dendrites of the primary excitatory cells (mitral/tufted, or M/T, cells) in the olfactory bulb. These dendrites are arranged in groups (glomeruli), with the dendrites of roughly 120 M/T cells in each glomerulus. The M/T cells range in firing threshold such that the most superficial M/T cells are most easily fired and the deeper ones less readily activated (Schneider and Scott, 1983). Thus, more intense receptor activation of a glomerulus tends to recruit more of the M/T cells in a patch, whereas less intense stimuli will recruit fewer. This threshold gradient enables each glomerulus to encode the intensity of its input by the number of cells firing, effectively transforming frequency coded receptor firing into spatially coded bulb M/T cell response (Antón et al., 1991). The M/T cells also have very long oblique dendrites, which make dendrodendritic synapses with inhibitory granule cells in the bulb. This arrangement has been hypothesized to serve a "normalizing" function in the bulb, that is, keep the overall activity in the bulb (in terms of number of M/T cells firing) at an approximately constant rate during inspiration (Kauer, 1987; Ambros-Ingerson et al., 1990). Approximate spatial topology from receptors to bulb is preserved, such that a recognizable spatial pattern of activation on the surface of the bulb is observed

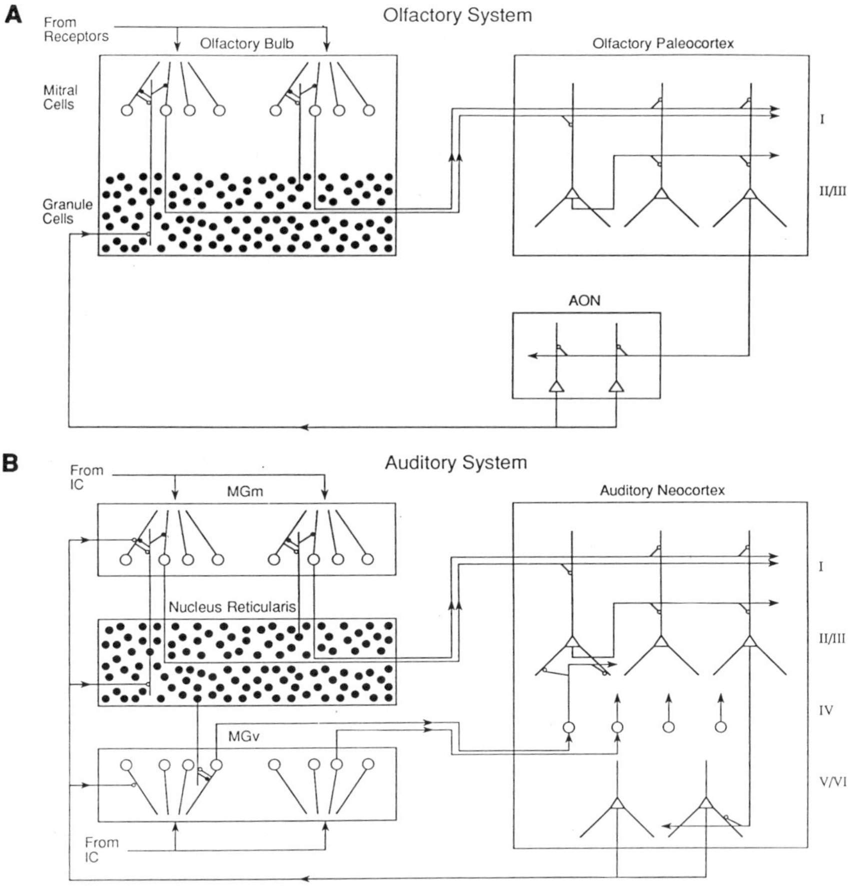

Figure 23.1 Identification of paleocortical anatomy embedded in neocortical anatomy. (A) Olfactory bulb and paleocortex. Primary excitatory (mitral) cells in the olfactory bulb are grouped in a glomerular organization; each glomerulus receives input from the olfactory receptors; some gross topography is preserved from receptors to bulb. Mitral cells are inhibited by granule cells and excite them via dendrodendritic synapses. Mitral cell axons innervate layer I olfactory cortex, synapsing sparsely and nontopographically with the apical dendrites of layer II/III cells. The axons of layer II/III cells contact basal dendrites of local layer II/III cells, then collateralize in layer I and make contact with the apical dendrites of these cells. Layer II/III cells also project to the anterior olfactory nucleus (AON), which despite its name has a laminar structure. It projects back to the inhibitory (granule) cell layer in the bulb.

(B) Medial geniculate and auditory neocortex. Primary excitatory cells in the magnocellular division of the medial geniculate (MGm) are grouped in a glomerular organization; each glomerulus receives input from the inferior colliculus (IC); some gross topography is preserved from IC to MGm. MGm cells are inhibited by GABAergic cells from nucleus reticularis thalami, and in turn excite them, via dendrodendritic synapses. MGm cell axons innervate layer I auditory cortex, synapsing sparsely and nontopographically with the apical dendrites of layer II/III cells. The axons of layer II/III cells contact basal dendrites of local layer II/III cells, then collateralize in layer I and make contact with the apical dendrites of these cells. Layer II/III cells also project to layer V/VI cells, which project back to the inhibitory nucleus reticularis, as well as projecting back to MGm directly.

In addition, primary excitatory cells in the ventral division of the medial geniculate (MGv) are grouped in a glomerular organization; topography from IC to MGv is highly preserved. MGv cells are inhibited by GABAergic projections from nucleus reticularis. MGv projects topographically to layer IV auditory cortex, which in turn projects vertically to layer III. The feedback projections from neocortical deep layer cells also innervate MGv.

across animals for given odors; the characteristic pattern for a given odor is enlarged or shrunk for higher or lower concentrations of the odor (Kauer, 1987).

Olfactory cortex (paleocortex) consists of three cell layers with a superficial molecular or connectivity layer; the deepest "layer" (layer IV) is somewhat nuclear in structure and is alternately referred to as the endopiriform nucleus. The most superficial cell layer, layer II, consists of primary excitatory cells in a densely packed cell layer, with many fewer relatively short-axon inhibitory interneurons; the broader layer III consists of more classical pyramidal neurons in a more loosely packed arrangement. The long output axons of the bulb M/T cells form an axon bundle called the lateral olfactory tract (LOT), which innervates layer I of paleocortex, contacting the apical dendrites of cortical layer II and III cells. These contacts are extremely sparse (probability of contact between a given LOT axon and cortical dendrite is less than 0.1) and nontopographic. Layer II/III cells are arranged into "patches" by the radial axonal arborization of the inhibitory interneurons in cortex. Simulation work has shown that these patches can operate effectively as "competitive" or "winner-take-all" patches (i.e., only the most strongly activated excitatory cell within a patch will be permitted to fire, whereas all others will be inhibited; Coultrip et al., 1991). Cortical cells emit axons that collateralize in layer I and flow both posteriorly (toward entorhinal cortex) and anteriorly back to bulb. These latter axons project back to the inhibitory granule cell layer in olfactory bulb, both directly and via anterior olfactory nucleus (AON), providing inhibitory feedback from cortex to bulb.

Architecture and Operation of the Olfactory System Simulation

Elements of the Simulation and Their Operating Rules Simulation studies have incorporated scaled-down versions of the circuitry illustrated in figure 23.1A and just discussed. In short, two networks, bulb and cortex, consisting of distinct architectures and physiologies, are extensively connected via both feedforward and feedback projections.

The bulb simulation contains 400 projection (M/T) units (simulated neurons), divided into 40 separate groups, each of which receives an input from one group of peripheral receptor axons (Mori, 1987). The intensity of an input is reflected in the number of cells within the appropriate group (or groups in the case of multicomponent cues) that it activates. The (excitatory) mitral projection cells in the bulb have been shown to have extremely long oblique dendrites that form dendrodendritic contacts with a dense granule cell inhibitory network (Mori, 1987). We adopt an assumption made by others (e.g., Kauer, 1987) that this excitatory-inhibitory arrangement serves to normalize the output of the bulb (i.e., the total number of M/T cells that are activated is reasonably constant across cues with different intensities and compositions). The inhibitory neurons (granule and probably periglomerular) are represented in the model by a single layer of cells and are innervated by randomly organized excitatory feedback from the cortex. The strength of the simulated feedback contacts is set during a "development" period in which hundreds of cues are presented and the strength of feedback synapses allowed to vary according to a correlational ("Hebb") rule.

The mitral cells of the bulb project sparsely and nontopographically to the outermost layer of olfactory cortex via the lateral olfactory tract (LOT), both biologically and in the simulation. The cortex is simulated as a layer of 1000 excitatory layer-II cells that are assumed in the model to be arranged into patches of 20 cells each by the radial axonal arborizations of local (feedback) inhibitory interneurons. The modeled neurons sum the voltages from their active synaptic inputs and require different amounts of depolarization for discharges, bursts of discharges, and for induction of synaptic change via LTP. A more detailed simulation of individual patches has shown that active cells triggering inhibitory interneurons can suppress firing by other cells in a patch; because of this, typically only one or two cells in a patch will discharge in response to bulbar inputs, making each patch into a "competitive" (or modified "winner-take-all") arrangement of the type discussed by many authors (e.g., von der Malsburg, 1973; Grossberg, 1976; Rumelhart and Zipser, 1985). Such an arrangement is assumed in the present simulation. Each cortical cell receives input from the LOT and from a feedforward associational system generated by the cortical neurons themselves, in both the cortex and the simulation. The operating rules for the model are based on physiological data reported in the literature.

The entire system works in synchrony with a 4- to 7-Hz (theta) sampling pattern that is characteristic of small mammals (Macrides, 1975). Bulb mitral cells (those neurons innervated by the peripheral receptors and that project to the cortex) receive inputs presented repetitively for brief periods. Inputs to the cortical network arise from the resultant synchronous bursting in a subset of mitral cells, yielding cyclic activity in relatively discrete "operation cycles" time-locked to the sampling rhythm.

Effects of LTP-based Learning on the Olfactory Simulation Sparse random connectivity in the simulation selectively activates those cortical cells whose dendrites are most connected to the input lines that are active. Learning increments active synapses on sufficiently depolarized cells via a rule based on LTP (Lynch and Granger, 1989), which has been shown to produce a measurable increment in synaptic strength during even a single 50-millisecond burst of activity (Larson and Lynch, 1989); that is, during each operation cycle in the model. Learning requires only a few training trials per cue, as in rapid olfactory learning in mammals (Slotnick and Katz, 1974; Staubli et al., 1987). Input lines shared across many similar input cues, and thus participating in many learning episodes, will strengthen their target synapses more than lines that participate in relatively fewer episodes. The result is that cortical dendrites (which can be viewed as vectors being moved by synaptic learning) become increasingly well-tuned to those inputs containing the shared subset (i.e., those inputs that are sufficiently similar to constitute members of a cluster). We have shown that this circuit will generate cell-firing responses that group learned cues by similarity. That is, for a given threshold of input similarity among a set of cues, outputs are identical for all of the cues, whereas below that similarity threshold, outputs are much less similar than corresponding inputs (Lynch and Granger, 1989). This form of *unsupervised* learning is to be distinguished from *supervised* learning, in which categorization information is provided to the learner.

As mentioned, feedback from the cortex to the bulb inhibitory layer in the model (see figure 23.1) is trained via a correlational rule during an earlier "developmental" period, via a Hebb rule coarsely correlating activity in the cortex with activity in the bulb. The feedback then selectively inhibits the mitral cells in those bulb patches (see figure 23.1) that are most responsible for the cortical output response, via relatively long-lasting inhibition, which has been shown to exist in the olfactory bulb (Nicoll, 1969). Resulting renormalization of bulb activity maintains the total number of firing mitral cells at a roughly constant level. This renormalization thus recruits additional mitral cells in remaining (uninhibited) bulb patches to fire to compensate for those selectively inhibited by the feedback. Thus, the pattern of mitral cell firing on the next operation cycle (roughly 200 milliseconds later) is distinct spatially from the previous pattern. This in turn activates a distinct set of cortical cells. This sampling cycle (bulb activation → cortical activation → inhibitory feedback → renormalization) can be repeated until the bulb is sufficiently inhibited to be largely quiescent. The sequence of cortical responses after the initial (first-sample) response becomes progressively different for different cues, increasingly approximating a given cue, thus producing unique encodings for individuals.

Simulation of Paleocortex Performs Hierarchical Clustering It has been shown that simplification of this operation of the paleocortical simulation gives rise to a novel and efficient algorithm for hierarchical clustering. In particular, Ambros-Ingerson, Granger, and Lynch (1990) showed that a simplified algorithm could operate to first identify clusters in arbitrary data, and then inhibitory feedback would "mask" the initial bulb inputs, uncovering smaller components of the bulb response, which in turn would be clustered by the cortex on the next cycle of operation. The algorithm has recently been shown to perform effective clustering on speech databases (Leen et al., 1990), a soybean database (Leuchtenberg et al., unpublished data), and a sonar database (Keren et al., unpublished data). The number of units in the network needed to store n inputs is a linear function of the number of inputs. Thus, the algorithm is linear in the number (n) and dimensionality (N) of inputs: the space complexity of the algorithm is $O(nN)$. The time complexity of the algorithm is dependent on summation of inputs in patches, computations of winners in patches, and synaptic weight changes. Thus, on a serial processor, the training time of the network per presentation is $O(nN,)$ and on a suitable parallel processor, the time complexity is $O[\log n(\log n + \log N)]$, because of the inherent parallelism of the algorithm (Ambros-Ingerson, et al., 1990). Moreover, the algorithm lends itself to efficient hardware implementation (Hammerstrom, 1988).

These findings also raise the hypothesis that approximate hierarchical clustering of this form will emerge as a fundamental property of memories based (at least in part) on correlational or Hebbian synaptic modifications in networks of the type found in the bulbar-cortical system. Human subjects in perceptual studies robustly recognize objects first at categorical levels and subsequently at successively subordinate levels (Rosch et al., 1976), suggesting the presence of structured memories that are organized and searched hierarchically during recognition.

Paleocortex as Precursor to Neocortex

Identification of Paleocortical Circuitry Embedded in Neocortex The auditory thalamocortical system has an organization roughly schematized in figure 23.1B. Inferior colliculus innervates both magnocellular and ventral subdivisions of the medial geniculate nucleus (MGm and MGv). MGv contains narrowly tuned cells, which retain the topography of the colliculus, and is the major lemniscal, tonotopic input to auditory cortex, topographically innervating cortical layer IV.

In contrast, the projection from IC to MGm is nontopographic, and MGm contains cells with very broad frequency tuning. MGm projects sparsely and nontopographically primarily to layer I of auditory cortex, contacting dendrites of layer II/III cells; it does not project to layer IV.

The functional circuitry within auditory cortex has been well delineated by physiological studies in which intracellular recordings have been obtained from neurons whose type and laminar position were verified by intracellular staining (Mitani and Shimokouchi, 1985; Mitani et al., 1985). Excitatory input from the MGv is projected to layer IV. This in turn projects excitation to layers II/III. Finally, cells in these superficial layers project excitatory effects to the large pyramidal output neurons in layers V/VI. The deep layers in turn project back to the two thalamic nuclei, both directly and via the nucleus reticularis thalami, consisting of predominantly inhibitory cells.

It can be seen that a subset of this anatomical architecture finds close analogy with the olfactory system as previously described. In particular, the MGm is organized into glomerular structures bearing some resemblance to those in the bulb, and they project sparsely and nontopographically to layer I of the cortex, innervating the apical dendrites of layer II and III cells. The layer II and III cells in turn project back to their input structure (MGm), via layer V in this case, rather than via the anterior olfactory nucleus. And, as in the olfactory system, this feedback projection targets inhibitory cells (nucleus reticularis in thalamus, analogously with granule cells in the bulb), rather than just directly targeting the excitatory cells in the input structure (thalamus or bulb). In this architectural context, then, the auditory cortex anatomical scheme adds the topographic thalamic nucleus (MGv), projecting to the topographic cortical cell layer (IV), which in turn projects upwards to layers II and III and the deep layer output cells (V and VI), which receive their projections from the superficial cell layers. It is worth noting that the plasticity present in the superficial layers of the olfactory cortex appears to be intact in the superficial auditory neocortex, and that the added topographic system (MGv → layer IV → deep layer III) does not exhibit plasticity in the adult (see, e.g., Fox et al., 1989; Artola and Singer, 1987; Bode-Greuel and Singer, 1989).

Identification of Physiological Characteristics of Paleocortex in the Auditory System Operation of the olfactory bulb–olfactory cortex system to give rise to the computational characteristics just described involves repetitive sampling of an olfactory stimulus, driving the system at a fixed rhythm, in synchrony. The rhythmic synchronous activation of olfactory cortex in turn drives feedback inhibition to the bulb, selectively inhibiting (masking) the bulb response such that the second sample or cycle of bulb activity is distinct from the first cycle, and the resulting cortical response is also distinct. It is this successive feedforward excitation–feedback inhibition cycle that gives rise to the successive hierarchical components that are "read out" by the olfactory system.

Auditory stimuli are rapid and transient compared to olfactory stimuli, and any possibility of behavioral repetitive sampling of auditory stimuli seems remote. Nonetheless, the massive anatomical feedback pathway from auditory cortex to thalamus suggests that cyclic activity is inherent to the operation of this system. Moreover, studies have shown that reversible inactivation of auditory cortex suppresses late reverberatory thalamic responses; that is, those that are probably due to corticothalamic feedback (Ryugo and Weinberger, 1978). These feedback pathways are myelinated, raising the possibility that extremely rapid cyclic activity between thalamus and cortex could be present during normal processing of auditory cues (on the order of 10 milliseconds per thalamocortical processing cycle). Thus, it is possible that cyclic feedforward excitation–feedback inhibition activity of a sort related to that hypothesized for the olfactory system could be present in the auditory system, in this form that is now decoupled from any notion of behavioral repetitive sampling. Instead, internal clocking (possibly at rates significantly higher than the theta rhythm) could provide synchronous cyclic activity in the thalamocortical system. It is worth noting in this regard that synchronous oscillations in the 40-Hz range have been identified in primary visual cortex (Gray et al., 1989; Gray and colleagues, however, observed no corresponding oscillatory activity in the primary thalamic afferent to visual cortex, the lateral geniculate nucleus. Clearly further exploration of this point is in order, in part to investigate possible effects of the paralysis used in these experiments, and to explore other stimuli that might be more likely to require multiple cycles of processing.)

As we just stressed, plasticity is present in the superficial layers of the auditory cortex, as it is in the same layers of paleocortex; this plasticity is accompanied by the presence of *N*-methyl-D-aspartate (NMDA) receptors in the superficial layers, whereas the added topographic system (MGv to layer IV) is not plastic in the adult, and does not exhibit NMDA receptors in the adult animal (Monaghan and Cotman, 1985).

POSSIBLE COMPUTATIONAL IMPORTANCE OF EMPIRICAL FINDINGS IN THE AUDITORY SYSTEM: THREE PATHWAYS

In light of the relationships just identified between paleocortex and neocortex, the following three sections focus on three of the major anatomical pathways in the auditory thalamocortical system, with a discussion of their potential computational importance. The three anatomical pathways of the auditory system that have been isolated and discussed are (1) the converging afferents to layer II/III cells, from MGm and from layer IV; (2) the projection from superficial (II/III) to deep (V/VI) layers; and (3) the back-projection from cortex to the thalamic medial geniculate nucleus, via the thalamic reticular nucleus.

Convergent Topographic and Nontopographic Input to Layer II/III Auditory Cortex

Layer II/III cells are innervated via their apical dendrites by MGm axons, and via their basal dendrites by layer IV cells. The MGm input is sparse and nontopographic, whereas the input from layer IV is denser and topographic. For a given frequency *F*, there will be a relatively circumscribed region of layer II/III that will receive input from layer IV, corresponding to that tonotopic region of layer IV that is preferentially activated by frequency *F*. In contrast, most of layer II/III will be activated by MGm input corresponding to *F* because that input is relatively diffuse and lacking in topographic organization. It is anticipated, then, that the layer II/III cells that will be most activated will be those that vertically receive layer IV input because they will be receiving convergent input from both layer IV and MGm, whereas other regions of layers II/III will only be receiving MGm input.

The sparse random connectivity of the MGm inputs to layers II/III cells will differentially activate the set of II/III cells in the activated region, thereby giving rise to a range of activation levels (depolarizations) in the set of cells. The presumed presence of extensive lateral inhibition in layer II/III cells, largely via basket and chandelier cells in this layer, can give rise to "competition" among the excitatory cells: once a cell has risen to its spiking threshold, it activates feedback inhibition, which in turn will tend to damp the activity in other excitatory cells within the axonal arborization of the activated inhibitory cells. The result can be a form of "winner-take-all" competition, in which only the most-depolarized cell within a region is able to spike or burst in response to a given input, whereas others are inhibited (Coultrip et al., 1991).

A number of researchers have shown that synaptic plasticity in a winner-take-all arrangement gives rise to the computational effect of *clustering* of inputs, as described by many researchers (von der Malsburg, 1973; Grossberg, 1976; Rumelhart and Zipser, 1985). The clustering effect in the context of the olfactory cortex is described in Granger et al., 1989; and Ambros-Ingerson, Granger and Lynch (1990).

The phenomenon of clustering can be readily described in terms of auditory cues. Assume a set of stimuli centered around a given frequency F. Synapses will be strengthened on the dendrites of a cell that wins the competition on F within the tonotopic region corresponding to F. The probability is thus increased that this cell will then win subsequent competitions on the same or very similar inputs (e.g., within a range $[F + \epsilon]$ to $[F - \epsilon]$ for some small frequency ϵ), since these inputs will be similar to each other by virtue of activating input axons in common with each other. If the active synapses are enhanced each time the cell "wins" and responds to a new similar input, it's response properties should be broadened: its probability of response to stimuli within the frequency range should increase. This broadening or increased bandwidth means that there is now a set of similar cues all of which will elicit response from this cell. Thus, this cell responds to any of these cues; this corresponds to those cues having been grouped into a cluster.

Changes in tone frequency correspond to variation along a single dimension, raising the question of other qualitative (e.g., complex tones) and quantitative (e.g., volume) dimensions of variation. In particular, simple tone triads (chords) are readily learned and recognized (e.g., A major [A-C#-E], A minor [A-C-E]). The tonotopic localization of individual tones in layer IV would seem to prevent convergence of the constituent notes in a chord onto any target cell. It is worth noting in this regard that the combinatorial connectivity from MGm to layer I can serve the purpose of creating unitary representations of composite chords in primary auditory cortex. Indeed, these convergent-divergent afferents allow a set of disparate tone inputs to converge on shared targets, and the plasticity in these synapses allows for learning of the coactivity of the set of tones, raising the possibility that such composites could be encoded in primary cortex.

Projection from Superficial to Deep-layer Cells
Layer II/III cells project to the (predominantly basal) dendrites of layer V and VI cells; a vertical organization (and thus tonotopy) is preserved. For a given deep cell, its best frequency (BF) will fall within the frequency range corresponding to the vertical columnar organization defined by the tonotopic layer IV. The farther an input frequency gets from the BF for this cell, the less excitation will be present in this column from layer IV, which in turn will contribute less to layer II/III. (This may provide a partial explanation for the "V" shaped intensity/frequency response curves often found in recording studies.) As previously described, it is assumed that layer II/III contains lateral-inhibition competitive circuitry. Thus, two different tones within a frequency range may activate different populations of superficial cells within the vertical column corresponding to this frequency range. After training on a conditioning stimulus (CS) near the BF for an identified deep cell, the cell will often exhibit "retuning"; that is, it will now respond more strongly to the CS than to the BF. Intermediate retuning effects, in which the cell's response to the CS is increased but not so as to exceed its response to the initial BF, are even more common (see Weinberger et al., 1990). Assuming the competitive arrangement in the superficial layers, we may hypothesize that a particular population of superficial cells preferentially responds to the BF initially, and another population that responds most to some similar but distinct CS tone. The CS shares axons with the BF because it is a nearby tone. Training on the CS can be assumed to strengthen synapses activated by the CS, which can cause the cells that formerly responded to the CS to now "win" the competition for the BF as well, and lateral inhibition can then inhibit response of the previous BF cells. Then deep cells will be activated by different input populations before and after training, which can provide an intuitive account of the retuning effects. It is worth noting that this account does not require synaptic weakening; synaptic strengthing in a system with lateral inhibition is sufficient.

Feedback from Cortical Deep Cells to Thalamus
The deep layer cortical cells project back to both the topographic and nontopographic thalamic projection nuclei, MGv and MGm, as well as projecting to nucleus reticularis, which in turn sends a GABAergic projection to both of these nuclei. The very size of these feedback projections raises the question of functionality: the feedback projections are at least as large as the feedforward thalamocortical pathways. Excitatory and inhibitory corticothalamic feedback will presumably produce quite a different pattern of thalamic response to a given input, which in turn will be fed forward to cortex again. The resulting cortical response will then presumably also differ from the initial cortical response to the stimulus. Because both the feedforward and feedback pathways are myelinated, this sequence from thalamus to cortex back to thalamus and to cortex

again can occur very rapidly (within tens of milliseconds), and can thus instigate a brief *sequence* of cortical response to a single stimulus, rather than a single response. The resulting longer-latency cortical responses may have interesting functional characteristics, in light of valuable computational properties identified in the analogous olfactory cortico-bulbar system. We outline some of these computational properties here, in the context of some of their possible behavioral and physiological correlates.

Long-latency Response Characteristics in Discrimination Tasks The simple observation that more difficult discrimination tasks evoke longer-latency behavioral responses raises the question of whether these responses might be delayed by further cortical processing, accompanied by longer-latency cortical responses. Because longer-latency cortical responses can allow the time required for corticothalamic feedback activity, the possibility is raised that this activity may play a role in difficult sensory discrimination tasks. Studies in the analogous olfactory bulb–olfactory cortex system are illustrative in this regard. Two primary computational results have emerged from studies of this system: *extraction of "hidden" signals,* and *hierarchical organization of learned data.*

Extraction of Constituents of Complex Cues Animals and human beings are capable of extracting constituents of complex cues, such as shapes in a composite picture or tones from a chord. Simulation studies in the olfactory system have raised the suggestion that this ability might arise from processing involving feedback from cortex to its input structure (bulb in the olfactory system; thalamus for other sensory systems). For instance, after training on the combination of two frequencies *FG,* will the constituent tones *F* and *G* alone be recognized? Interestingly, in the olfactory system, lacking any topographic organization, this proves not to be the case in general, though recognition of *previously learned* constituents occurs (Staubli et al., 1989). It may be the case in topographic modalities that constituents can be recognized without pretraining.

When complex tone *FG* is presented, two regions or columns of cortex are activated, corresponding to the tonotopic regions for frequencies *F* and *G*. Within those regions, however, the nontopographic MGm input to the superficial layers will preferentially activate cells that receive the most innervation from the combination *FG.* As illustrated in figure 23.2, these cells may or may not be the union or intersection of the cells that would be selected by either *F* or *G* alone. Figure 23.3 illustrates the effect of presenting composite stimuli: intuitively, the idea is that there will be cells receiving insufficient activation from either *F* or *G* alone to respond, but the convergent combination of both *F* and *G* together could cause strong activation of such a cell—stronger than that of cells that would respond to either *F* or *G* alone. If the same cells are selected for the composite as for the constituents, then no obvious physiological correlate of the discrimination task is suggested. If, however, different cells are selected for the

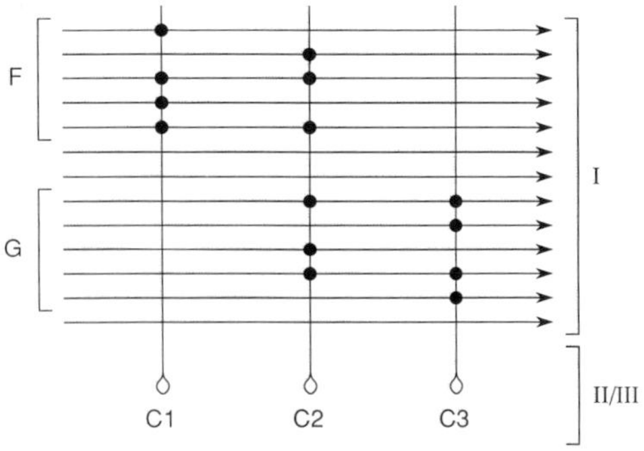

Figure 23.2 Differential cellular activation by a composite cue versus by its constituents. Layer I (connectivity layer) and II/III (cell body layers) of auditory cortex. Axons from MGm are labeled according to their activity in response to tone frequencies *F* and *G*. (The axon assignments are shown grouped together, though in nontopographic MGm this need not be the case. This grouping is made for pedagogical enhancement; if the axons were shown distributed across the field of layer I, the argument would not be different.) Because of the sparse, random connectivity in layer I, different cells are differentially activated by inputs. In particular, cell C1 will be most strongly activated by frequency *F*, since it has most synapses in common with those input axons activated by that frequency. Likewise, cell C3 will be most strongly activated by frequency *G*. However, the composite stimulus *FG* will activate cell C2 more strongly than either C1 or C3, owing to the connectivity. Given strong lateral inhibition, the cells responding to the conditions *F*, *G*, and *FG* could all be distinct from each other.

composite than for the constituents, then the deep cell response also will be different for the composite versus the constituents. In this case, training on the composite will not train *F* or *G* cells, and presentation of the constituents will not necessarily activate strengthened synapses. This would mean that neither the same tuning responses nor behavioral recognition should occur to the constituents.

The effect of pretraining can be studied via composite discrimination experiments. If animals are not able to recognize constituents, then after being trained on *FG*+ versus *FH*−, they will nonetheless not be able to respond to *G*+ alone because different cells will have been involved.

If, instead, pretraining is performed on *F*, and then discrimination training is performed on *FG*+ versus *FH*−, then it is predicted that the animal should recognize *G*+. The hypothesis involves corticothalamic feedback. Pretraining on *F* involves the selective strengthening of synapses on those cells that respond to *F*. Subsequent training on *FG* versus *FH* will activate those input lines that now have strengthened contacts with *F*-selective cells, so those cells should preferentially respond to both *FG* and *FH*. Paradoxically, this pretraining on *F* should therefore make the discrimination *FG* versus *FH* more difficult to learn because the two cues should now evoke more similar cortical responses than would have been evoked in the absence of pretraining on *F*.

It is hypothesized that this discrimination can be accomplished via corticothalamic feedback: after the predominantly *F* response from cortex to either composite *FG* or *FH*, feedback (which is topographic) can inhibit

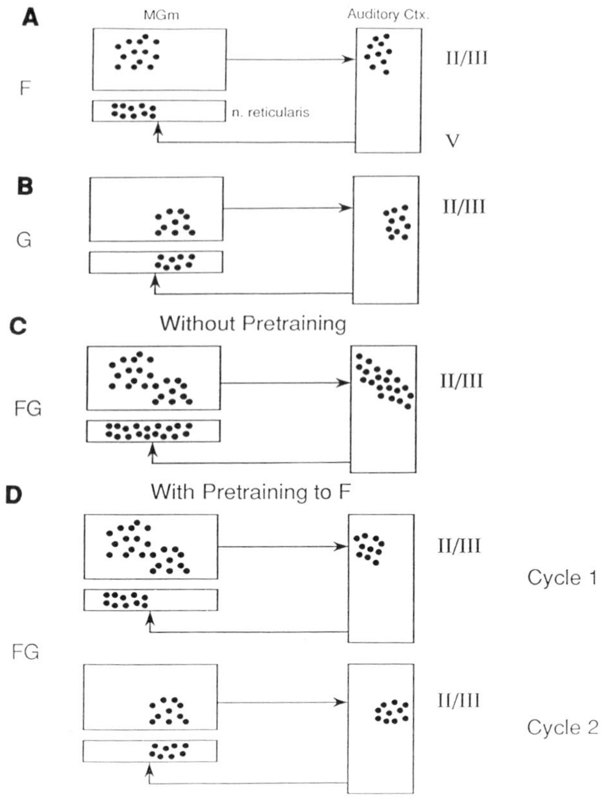

Figure 23.3 Effect of pretraining on thalamocortical cyclic processing and recognition of constituents of composite cues. Schematic illustration of the spatial pattern of cell firing in MGm and in auditory cortex layer II/III cells in response to frequencies *F* and *G*, is shown in parts A and B. It is seen that the responses are spatially distinct. The cortical response results in a relatively topographic corticothalamic feedback response to nucleus reticularis which preferentially targets the region corresponding to the cortical activation. Since nucleus reticularis cells are GABAergic, they will then preferentially inhibit those thalamic cells that gave rise to the cortical response; thus on the next feedforward cycle of activity from thalamus to cortex, there should be very little response.

Part C of the figure schematically illustrates the effect of presentation of the composite cue *FG*. Most of both regions (corresponding to *F* and *G*) in MGm are activated, giving rise to feedforward activation of most of both *F* and *G* regions in cortex; the resulting corticothalamic feedback reflects the cortical activity and activates most of the region corresponding to both *F* and *G*.

Part D illustrates the effect of presentation of composite cue *FG* after training on tone F alone. The training on F will have strengthened pathways from those F cells in MGm to cells in layer II/III auditory cortex. Thus presentation of *FG* should correspond to presentation of a previously-learned signal (*F*) together with background noise (*G*). It is assumed that the cortical response will reflect the strengthened pathway, and thus the cortical response is expected to resemble that which would have appeared in response to the presentation of *F* alone (in the absence of the "noise" *G*).

By the above set of hypotheses, this "*F*"-like cortical response should then give rise to a corticothalamic feedback also corresponding to *F*. This in turn should selectively inhibit the *F* portion of the thalamic response, but have little effect on the *G* portion. Thus the next thalamocortical feedforward response should largely reflect *G*, the remainder of the feedback inhibition operation. This should show up as a longer-latency cortical tuning response.

the thalamic response corresponding to that cortical *F* response. The remainder will be a thalamic signal that is quite different for *FG* versus *FH*, corresponding to either *G* or *H*. If this is the case, the learning should thus be accompanied by long-latency cortical responses that correspond to the remaining constituent *G* or *H*. Analysis of long-latency responses in composite cue discrimination experiments thus might uncover properties of corticothalamic feedback in processing of these complex cues.

Successive Hierarchical Discrimination The previous discussion relates primarily to the dissection of composite cues into their constituent components, an effect that is hypothesized to arise, as described, from the cyclic feedback processing of the auditory thalamocortical system. That same cyclic processing can give rise to an additional effect, and one of equal computational interest, when viewed from the point of view of making very difficult (i.e., fine-grained) discriminations. Such discriminations are those that arise when an animal is asked to discriminate between two tones that are extremely close to each other (e.g., frequency F versus frequency $F + \epsilon$ where ϵ is a very small increment in frequency); or asked to discriminate between two complex tones (chords) that contain many elements in common (e.g., tone *FGHIJ* versus *FGHIK*). In these fine-grained discrimination tasks, one possibility is that the inherent discrimination power of the (feedforward) thalamocortical system is sufficient to distinguish between the two: such proposals arise, for instance, in studies of "coarse-coding" (e.g., Rumelhart and McClelland, 1986). An alternative proposal (Ambros-Ingerson et al., 1990) forwards the hypothesis that the same set of (sparsely coded) cells are reused across cycles of activity involving inhibitory feedback (of the corticothalamic type just described) yielding increasingly finer-grained distinction among groups of cues over cycles. Intuitively, the processing is as follows. Difficult discriminations are those involving similar cues (e.g., *FGHIJ* versus *FGHIK*); such sets of cues are similar by virtue of sharing a large component of their input lines (*FGHI* in this case). Training enhances synaptic strength of those input lines that tend to recur; these are precisely those that are shared and thus occur in the inputs more often than the nonshared portions. Feedforward recognition in the cortex will identify first the strengthened portions of the input (as in the previous case of component recognition, in which the pretrained *F* portion of the composite *FG* yielded a cortical response first). The inhibitory feedback will then selectively mask the thalamic portion of the cue that gave rise to this cortical response. The thalamic remainder is then precisely the portion of the input that is different between the similar cues (*J* versus *K*). Thus, subsequent feedforward response will distinguish between the two cues. In other words, the cyclic thalamocortical processing hypothesized here would sequentially (over successive cycles) yield cortical responses first to large components and then to successively smaller components of an input, offering increasingly finer-grained discriminations among similar stimuli. This effect should show up in the form of longer-latency response in cortex (and thalamus) in difficult discrimination tasks; simpler discriminations may not require cyclic processing.

Discussion

The neocortex, by far the largest structure in the human brain, is surprisingly regular in anatomical structure; with few exceptions, there are approximately 80,000 neurons per square millimeter (Rockel et al., 1980), arranged in laminae with relatively consistent input-output assignation (Rockland and Pandya, 1979; Maunsell and Van Essen, 1983; Shanks et al., 1985). The very size and regularity of the neocortex has led to suggestions that functionally similar or even identical subunits may comprise the neocortex, with the predominant differences being only what the afferents are to a specific region (see, e.g., Hubel and Wiesel, 1977; Mountcastle, 1978, for a discussion). The arrangement of topographic and nontopographic thalamic nuclei specific to each of the three major sensory modalities (vision, audition and somatosensory) and their feedforward (thalamocortical) and feedback (corticothalamic) projections is also surprisingly regular (see Herkenham, 1986, for a review). Indeed, Sur and colleagues (e.g., Roe et al., 1990) have found that changing the inputs of the MG-A1 system to retinal instead of cochlear pathways induce, in auditory cortex, visual representations analogous to those normally found in the primary visual cortex. Physiologically, dominant synchronous rhythmic activity has been found throughout the neocortex (Freeman and Van Dijk, 1978; Gray et al., 1989). Despite these tantalizing suggestions, characterization of a computational construct that could have such regularity of design and yet such computational power has proven elusive. We have attempted to integrate a range of anatomical and physiological findings in the olfactory and auditory systems, in hopes of identifying unifying principles that might suggest how advanced perceptual processing might emerge from regular cortical architectures of the kind described. We have forwarded the hypothesis that normal function of bulbar-paleocortical and thalamic-neocortical systems may give rise to sequential factorization of cues into increasingly finer-grained components. This hypothesis leads to a number of predictions, many of which are testable. Tests of some such predictions have been carried out in the olfactory system with positive results. Testing of the hypothesis in the auditory system clearly relies on further elaboration of the hypothesis in this neocortical system, and raises the possibility that some shared properties and principles of operations of paleocortical and neocortical systems may be identified by further simulation and analysis.

REFERENCES

Ambros-Ingerson, J., R. Granger, and G. Lynch. (1990). Simulation of paleocortex performs hierarchical clustering. *Science* 247:1344–1348.

Antón, P. S., G. Lynch, and R. Granger (1991). Computation of frequency-to-spatial transform by olfactory bulb glomeruli (*submitted*).

Artola, A., and W. Singer (1987). Long-term potentiation and *N*-methyl-D-aspartate receptors in rat visual cortex. *Nature* 330:649–652.

Bliss, T. V. P., and T. Lømo (1973). Long-lasting potentiation of synaptic transmission in the dentate area of the anesthetized rabbit following stimulation of the perforant path. *Journal of Physiology (London)* 232:334–356.

Bode-Greuel, K., and W. Singer (1989). The development of *N*-methyl-D-aspartate receptors in cat visual cortex. *Developments in Brain Research* 46:197–204.

Coultrip, R., R. Granger, and G. Lynch (1991). A cortical model of winner-take-all competition via lateral inhibition. *Neural Networks* (in press).

Fox, K., H. Sato, and N. Daw (1989). The localization and function of NMDA receptors in cat and kitten visual cortex. *Journal of Neuroscience* 9:2443–2454.

Freeman, W. J., and B. Van Dijk (1978). Spatial patterns of visual cortical fast EEG during conditioned reflex in a rhesus monkey. *Brain Research* 422:267–276.

Granger, R., J. Ambros-Ingerson, and G. Lynch. (1989). Derivation of encoding characteristics of layer II cerebral cortex. *Journal of Cognitive Neuroscience* 1(1):61–87.

Granger, R., et al. (1991). Behavioral tests of a prediction from a cortical network simulation. *Psychological Science* (in press).

Gray, C. M., P. Konig, A. K., Engel, and W. Singer (1989). Oscillatory responses in cat visual cortex exhibit inter-columnar synchronization which reflects global stimulus properties. *Nature* 338:334–337.

Grossberg, S. (1976). Adaptive pattern classification and universal recoding: I. Parallel development and coding of neural feature detectors. *Biological Cybernetics* 23:121–134.

Hammerstrom, D. (1988). The connectivity analysis of simple association or how many connections do you need? In D. Z. Anderson (ed.), *Neural Information Processing Systems.* New York: American Institute of Physics, pp. 338–347.

Herkenham, M. (1986). New perspectives on the organization and evolution of nonspecific thalamocortical projections. In A. Peters and E. G. Jones (ed.), *Cerebral Cortex,* vol. 5. New York: Plenum Press, pp. 403–445.

Hubel, D. H, and T. N. Wiesel. (1977). Functional architecture of macaque monkey cortex. *Proceedings of the Royal Society (London)* 198:1–59.

Iriki, A., C. Pavlides, A. Keller, and H. Asanuma, (1989). Long-term potentiation in the motor cortex. *Science,* 245:1385–1387.

Jung, M., J. Larson, and G. Lynch (1991). Long-term potentiation of monosynaptic EPSPs in rat piriform cortex in vitro. *Synapse* (in press).

Kauer, J. S. (1987). Coding in the olfactory system. In T. E. Finger (ed.), *Neurobiology of Taste and Smell.* John Wiley, pp. 205–231.

Larson, J., and G. Lynch (1989). Theta pattern stimulation and the induction of LTP: the sequence in which synapses are stimulated determines the degree to which they potentiate. *Brain Research* 489:49–58.

Lee, K. (1982). Sustained enhancement of evoked potentials following brief, high-frequency stimulation of the cerebral cortex in vitro. *Brain Research* 239:617–623.

Leen, T. K., R. Cole, D. Hammerstrom, and J. Inouye (1990). Speech recognition with a cortex model: Preliminary results and outlook. Technical report, Oregon Graduate Institute, Beaverton, Ore. 97006–1999.

Lynch, G., and R. Granger (1989). Simulation and analysis of a cortical network. *Psychology of Learning and Motivation* 23:205–241.

Macrides, F. (1975). Temporal relationships between hippocampal slow waves and exploratory sniffing in hamsters. *Behavioral Biology* 14:295–308.

Maunsell, J. H. R., and D. C. Van Essen (1983). The connections of the middle temporal visual area (mt) and their relationship to a cortical hierarchy in the macaque monkey. *Journal of Neuroscience* 3:2563–2586.

McCollum, J., et al. (1991). Short latency single unit processing in olfactory cortex. *Journal of Cognitive Neuroscience* (in press).

Mitani, A., et al. (1985). Morphology and laminar organization of electrophysiologically identified neurons in the primary auditory cortex in the cat. *Journal of Comparative Neurology* 235:430–447.

Mitani, A., and M. Shimokouchi (1985). Neuronal connections in the primary auditory cortex: An electrophysiological study in the cat. *Journal of Comparative Neurology* 235:417–429.

Monaghan, D. T., and C. W. Cotman (1985). Distribution of *N*-methyl-D-aspartate–sensitive 1–[^{3}h] glutamate–binding sites in rat brain. *Journal of Neuroscience* 5:2909–2919.

Mori, K. (1987). Membrane and synaptic properties of identified neurons in the olfactory bulb. *Progress in Neurobiology* 29:275–320.

Mountcastle, V. B. (1978). An organizing principle for cerebral function: the unit module and the distributed system. In G. M. Edelman and V. B. Mountcastle (eds.), *The Mindful Brain*. Cambridge, Mass: MIT Press, pp. 199–212.

Nicoll, R. (1969). Inhibitory mechanisms in the rabbit olfactory bulb: dendrodendritic mechanisms. *Brain Research* 14:157–172.

Rockel, A. J., R. W. Hiorns, and T. P. S. Powell (1980). The basic uniformity in structure of the neocortex. *Brain* 103:221–244.

Rockland, K. S., and D. N. Pandya (1979). Laminar origins and terminations of cortical connections of the occipital lobe in the rhesus monkey. *Brain Research* 179:3–20.

Roe, A. W., S. L. Pallas, J. -O., Hahm, and M. Sur, (1990). A map of visual space induced in primary auditory cortex. *Science* 250:818–820.

Roman, F., U. Staubli, and G. Lynch (1987). Evidence for synaptic potentiation in a cortical network during learning. *Brain Research* 418:221–226.

Rosch, E., et al. (1976). Basic objects in natural categories. *Cognitive Psychology* 8:382–439.

Rumelhart, D. E., and J. McClelland (1986). *Parallel Distributed Processing*. Cambridge, Mass: MIT Press.

Rumelhart, D. E., and D. Zipser (1985). Feature discovery by competitive learning. *Cognitive Science* 9:75–112.

Ryugo, D. K., and N. M. Weinberger (1978). Differential plasticity of morphologically distinct neuron populations in the medial geniculate body of the cat during classical conditioning. *Behavioral Biology* 22:275–301.

Schneider, S. P., and J. W. Scott (1983). Orthodromic response properties of rat olfactory bulb mitral and tufted cells correlate with their projection patterns. *Journal of Comparative Physiology* 50:319–333.

Shanks, M. F., R. C. A. Pearson, and T. P. S. Powell (1985). The ipsilateral cortico-cortical connexions between the cytoarchitectonic subdivisions of the primary somatic sensory cortex in the monkey. *Brain Research Review* 9:67–88.

Slotnick, B. M., and H. M. Katz (1974). Olfactory learning-set formation in rats. *Science* 185:796–798.

Staubli, U., D. Fraser, R. Faraday, and G. Lynch (1987). Olfaction and the "data" memory system in rats. *Behavioral Neuroscience* 101(6):757–765.

Staubli, U., and G. Lynch (1987). Stable hippocampal long-term potentiation elicited by "theta" pattern stimulation. *Brain Research* 435:227–234.

Staubli, U., O. Thibault, M. DiLorenzo, and G. Lynch (1989). Antagonism of NMDA receptors impairs acquisition but not retention of olfactory memory. *Behavioral Neuroscience* 103(1):54–60.

von der Malsburg, C. (1973). Self-organization of orientation sensitive cells in the striate cortex. *Kybernetik* 14:85–100.

Weinberger, N. M., et al. (1990). Retuning auditory cortex by learning: A preliminary model of receptive field plasticity. *Concepts in Neuroscience* 1:91–132.

24 A Theorist's Search for Simplicity in Memory

John G. Taylor

This chapter attempts to address some of the theoretical questions raised in this book and their possible solutions. Included in the title of this chapter is the word *simplicity,* one of this chapter's themes. The complexities and uncertainties of memory that arise when the results of one group are compared against those of another, or when a group's results are exposed to careful questioning are overwhelming. But the subject itself is complex. To make progress in understanding such a subject it is essential to bring order and simplicity to it, even if from only one perspective.

This chapter covers three areas: First, we present some of the major theoretical questions in the field today. Then frameworks within which these problems might be tackled are outlined and, finally, possible answers to some of the questions raised earlier are conjectured.

THE QUESTIONS

Memory involves many structures in the brain. First we examine the global or large-scale questions, and then, moving down the scale, we ultimately address questions at the molecular level.

At the global level, the main question is, What is the form of the knowledge being stored? Is that form, for example, of a spatial character only, or is there also a temporal element? The current literature heavily emphasizes the spatial aspect of the input (e.g., in terms of spatial maps developed in the hippocampus). Can there be manipulation, in time, of the inputs to determine the temporal features of relevance?

There are also other aspects of memory storage. Is target material of greatest importance, or is context playing a role (as it is known to do in certain situations)? What importance should be assigned to context? What are the mechanisms by which context is incorporated into stored memories?

Other questions arise in the area of the mixing of modalities. Although various candidate brain regions have been suggested for this activity, what does mixing mean? Does it include context in different modalities?

Related to the latter is the problem of the actual coding of the input information. Recent results from the cat visual cortex (Gray and Singer,

1989) indicate that there may be use of the temporal properties of the firing pattern, and in particular the phase of oscillatory activity. Is this used in storage (as has been suggested to be one of the roles of the theta rhythm in the hippocampus; McNaughton and Morris, 1987)?

A further and closely related question concerns memory storage. Is it stored in terms of an increase; (or decrease; Stanton and Sejnowski, 1989; Artola et al., 1990) of connection weights? Are other parameters describing neuronal activity also involved? Where is memory stored? It is becoming accepted that the hippocampus is crucial for certain types of memory, but not for others. Thus, specific or episodic memory (Tulving, 1983) seems to require an intact hippocampus in human beings, but that organ is not needed for the storage of procedural skills. It is also accepted, however, that the nearby cortex—and not the hippocampus—is the final receptacle of episodic memory storage. How is such storage achieved? And how is such long-term memory retrieved?

There are many questions about the details of wiring diagrams that must be answered before it is possible to build realistic models of memory storage and retrieval. In chapter 21, Berger and Yeckel indicate that there are new connections in the hippocampus (monosynaptic and disynaptic circuits) that are being discovered. How can these circuits be incorporated into models of hippocampal activity during memory storage or retrieval?

At a more atomic level we come to the single neuron. The beautiful simulations of Brown and coworkers in chapter 22 indicate some of the potential complexity of a single pyramidal neuron. The compartmental structure of the neuron indicates that it may indeed function as a separate computing unit in its own right, instead of only being a simple decision node in a large parallel computer. But what are the principles of such computation? Can they be reduced to the rules already extracted from the simple model of the neuron as a binary decision unit and presently being actively explored by the neural net community? If not, what are the important extra features that the latter community is missing?

The more complicated neurons discussed in chapter 22 only have extra compartments. What if an active membrane is added to that model? Is computing power further increased? And what about interneurons: can these also be modeled at such a complex level?

Last, but certainly not least, are the synapses. They can be described presynaptically in terms of vesicle distribution functions and release probability functions. On the postsynaptic side there are receptor efficiences and conductances of spine structures. The modification of these by activity is one of the core investigations of LTP research. What is actually occurring at these presynaptic and postsynaptic sites?

These questions may only be answerable, not just by synapse analyses, but by analysis at the level of channel openings and closings, controlled by potential-dependent dynamics. Such channel dynamics may have important effects at a global level on the effectiveness of memory storage. Such an effect has been found, using a simple model, in an analysis of the storage of temporal sequences (Reiss and Taylor, 1991). How much detail must be added?

These questions lead us to what some regard as one of the central questions facing brain research today: At what level should we attempt to explain the brain? Working at the most detailed level will guarantee that nothing is left out of the models. But then the extreme danger of never seeing the forest for the trees exists, which has already been encountered in attempts to model all the activities of neurons with active membrane and compartments and many ionic currents.

The general structure of the models are clear. They correspond to a set of coupled nonlinear stochastic time-delayed differential equations for the membrane potentials x_i (i denoting the label of the neuron or the compartment on that neuron) and "weight" variables w_i, of form

$$\begin{aligned} dx_i/dt &= G_i[(w_j), (I_j), (x_j)] \\ dw_i/dt &= F_i[(w_j), (I_j), (x_j)] \end{aligned} \qquad (24.1)$$

where F_i and G_i are some nonlinear functions that may be possible to specify, but that are surely so complicated as to preclude any analytic solution to the set of equations (24.1). The weights w_i denote many variables: channel concentration variables for many ions, such as Ca^{2+}, postsynaptic efficacies of *N*-methyl-D-aspartate (NMDA) and other receptors, probability distributions for various transmitter vesicles, spine dimensions, and axonal nerve impulse time delays.

The nonlinearities of the sets of functions F_i and G_i are determined by a set of Hodgkin-Huxley equations, each with at least four variables. These equations are applicable not only to the axon hillock compartment but also to the regions of active membrane, which may be distributed over various dendrites and the soma.

As previously noted, the only way to solve such a complicated system of equations is to simulate them on a large computer. But the results may be highly dependent on some of the details of the model and not give any indication as to what the information powers of the system actually are.

The problem here is that one would like to be able to work at different levels, which are somewhat separated from each other. Thus, one would hope that the main effects of molecular processes at synapses could be approximated by changes in fewer variables. A simpler model would then arise, which could be used to describe the single neuron, to a good approximation, when it is active in a large net.

Such a separation of levels has been achieved in materials science, where one does not need to include the details of quark physics, such as quantum chromodynamics, to consider the electronic properties of, for example, metals. It may be that such a separation of levels in the brain does not exist. It is possibly a useful strategy, however, to attempt to search for such a separation. We follow that approach here. In particular, we proceed by starting with the simplest neuron model, adding complexity. We are thus assuming that there are at least two levels, that of the neuron and that of its subneuronal processes (such as synaptic channels, nonlinear membrane, compartmental structure).

Thus, our program is to go from simple to complex. In the process we wish to see how the complexity that has been added affects the processing powers of the system built from the increasingly complex neurons.

THE FRAMEWORKS

As we add complexity to the simple binary decision neuron of McCulloch and Pitts (1943) and of Caianiello (1961), we have to enlarge the mathematical structure used to incorporate the added properties. The additional features we wish to add are (1) vesicular transmission, (2) leaky integrator membrane, (3) geometry, and (4) nonlinearity.

We need to place each of these properties into a different mathematical framework to be able to construct a set of equations describing the corresponding neuron. The details of the mathematical structures involved are beyond the scope of this chapter, but a brief survey with additional references is provided here. The moral as to what each of the additional features is allowing the net made up of such neurons to accomplish as an information processor will also be discussed.

Noisy Neurons

The essential variables at a synapse are of two forms: presynaptic, which describe the amount of chemical transmitter, and postsynaptic, which quantify the transmitter uptake.

Because we want to work at as simple a level as possible we call the presynaptic variable q, denoting the amount of transmitter released into the cleft at any time. The postsynaptic variable is quantified by the efficiency of uptake and is denoted by the single parameter ϵ. The postsynaptically effective amount of transmitter can therefore be given by the parameter

$$w = q\epsilon \tag{24.2}$$

which is the usual connection weight used in artificial neural net analysis.

Because q is a random variable it has an associated distribution function $p(q)$, which contains a spontaneous release contribution and a contribution arising from release produced by the arrival of a nerve impulse at a synaptic bouton (Taylor, 1972). We neglect the former component and only discuss the latter. This contribution may be of one-vesicle or binomial form, or even of compound binomial form if there are several axon collaterals on the same neuron.

The mathematical framework used to describe such activity is that of random iterative networks (Bressloff and Taylor, 1990b). The nature of this framework is given in terms of a simple extension of the original Caianiello (1961) equations. If the activity of a neuron is described by the variable $u(t)$ (1 if the neuron is active and O if it is not), then these equations describe the temporal development of the activity variables, in discrete time, as

$$(t + 1) = Y[\Sigma w_{ij} u_j (t) - s_i] \tag{24.3}$$

where $Y(x)$ is the step function, with value 1 if x is positive and 0 if not. The parameter s_i is the usual threshold of the ith cell. Then equation (24.3) states that the ith cell fires if the total activity arriving on it at a previous time step is greater than the threshold value.

In the light of equation (24.2) it is necessary to choose a new value for the connection weights at each time step, these being drawn as random variables with distribution functions determined by the functions $p_{ij}(q_{ij})$, one for each synapse. Thus, at each time step the iteration of equation (24.3) is random (to within the distributions p_{ij}); hence the epithet "random iteration networks."

It is also possible to make not only the variables q_{ij} but also the thresholds s_i to be stochastic. In that way it is possible to include the spin-glass approach to neural nets, which has been popular recently among the physics community following the seminal paper of Hopfield (1982). This model is obtained in particular by choosing the distribution function for the variables s_i to be

$$p(s) = d/ds(1 + e^{-s/T})^{-1} \tag{24.4}$$

where T is an effective temperature. It is through such a variable that physicists' intuition can be released to transfer to neural nets some of the concepts of statistical physics. The resulting system looks like a lattice of spins (the nodes of the lattice being the neurons, the spin being up for an active neuron, down for an inactive one). The bonds between the nodes are constantly fluctuating because of the distribution functions $p(q)$; they can therefore be regarded as annealed and not quenched (as is usual in the spin-glass approach).

This approach has been developed to analyse pattern storage under a variety of learning rules (Bressloff and Taylor, 1990b), again extending much of the spin-glass approach to neural nets to the case of synaptic noise. An interesting aspect of this approach is that it has proven possible to develop a hardware realization of such synaptic noise by means of the pRAM (Gorse and Taylor, 1989), which is a RAM, at each address of which there is stored not either a 0 or 1 but a real number between 0 and 1. A 1 is generated when that address is accessed, with probability given by the number stored there.

Gorse and Taylor (1989) proved the pRAM theorem, which states that "every random iterative net is implementable by some pRAM net." Moreover, such nets are in general implementing higher-order neurons. These have terms in their activity such as $\Sigma_{j,k} w_{ijk} u_j u_k$ extending the activity variable in the step function on the right of equation (24.3). This nonlinearity, in addition to the stochasticity, seems to give increased storage capacity powers to the net.

It should also be mentioned that the pRAM has been built in hardware (Clarkson et al., 1989), so that it is possible to directly run a hardware model of the stochastic and nonlinear features of neurons (the nonlinear features are discussed more fully later).

Noisy neurons of this form can be trained in a variety of ways. At this point it is perhaps appropriate to comment generally on learning in artificial neural network (ANN) research.

In general, there are three distinct types of training schemes used in ANN work:

1. Supervised learning, in which the net is required to output a set of desired targets for a given set of inputs. Such training in general leads to both long-term potentiation (LTP) and long-term depression (LTD). That is true, for example, if the training uses a gradient descent method in which the weight w is changed by the amount δw, to reduce an error E (depending on w), by

$$\delta w = (\text{const}).dE/dw \tag{24.5}$$

The sign of the right hand side of equation (24.5) is not guaranteed to be positive, which leads to the possibility of LTD. If LTD is absent in hippocampus, then it just reduces the relevance of gradient descent learning to real brain simulations (and does not negate the approach of gradient descent per se).

2. Reinforcement or reward training, in which a reward is given to a neuron if it produces a value that leads to success in the output of the net, which leads to both LTP and LTD in the standard algorithms. It is to be remarked that designing a purely hardware version of pRAM reinforcement learning is easy (Gorse and Taylor, 1990).

3. Unsupervised learning rules of a Hebbian type, which in general lead to both LTP and LTD unless especially designed to avoid LTD. This may, in particular, be achieved in the case of sparse nets.

It should be added that there are few attempts to deal with the separate presynaptic and postsynaptic aspects of learning. There is the discussion of Bressloff and Taylor (1990b) already alluded to, as well as the purely deterministic approach of Gardner-Medwyn (1989), in which there are different time courses for the two factors. That there are two factors is natural in the noisy neural model of Taylor (1972), as is clear from equation (24.2).

Having given a brief account of the approaches to learning at the simplest level of ANNs, the conclusion reached by Gorse and Taylor (1989, 1990) and Clarkson and coworkers (1989), (and from the analyses of spin-glass theorists) is that intrinsic noise at synapses and thresholds helps a net to (1) avoid "false" solutions to desired input-output transformations, and (2) to learn to generalize as part of the learning process. This feature is sometimes called "learning in noise." Such an approach allows the net to experience a range of inputs that do not coincide with the original training set because of the internal noise modifying it.

Leaky Integrators

Numerous methods have been tried in the ANN approach to store temporal sequences. Various past-state buffers have been tried (direct storage, the use of temporal windows, time delays, etc.), as well as the use of feedback to capture the effect of earlier activity on the net.

The simplest form of connection weight matrix w_{ij} to store a sequence of patterns $[\xi\ (t)]$ (with t as the time) is by means of the value

$$w_{ij} = \Sigma\ \xi\ (t + 1)\xi\ (t) \tag{24.6}$$

This form of weight matrix produces the transition

$$\xi_i\ (t) \rightarrow \xi_i\ (t + 1) \tag{24.7}$$

if the net is set up in the initial state ξ (see equation [24.1]).

The difficulty with the rule shown in equation (24.6) is that the sequence has to be learned beforehand for the net to be constructed. A method has been set up (Reiss and Taylor, 1990) to train a net composed of leaky integrator neurons to build the connection matrix (see equation [24.6]; together with terms for earlier histories than purely one time step earlier, given by equation [24.6]). This approach uses the time-dependent equation for the activity $A_i(t)$ for the ith leaky integrator neuron as

$$A_i\ (t + 1) = (1 - d)A_i\ (t) + I_i\ (t) \tag{24.8}$$

where I_i is the input at time t, and d is the decay constant of the neuron.

The structure of the system to achieve this is shown in figure 24.1 and is discussed in more detail elsewhere (Reiss and Taylor, 1991). The net L is a net of leaky integrator neurons which acts to store a past history. This history is then fed onto the net M by means of plastic synapses. At the same time the input is fed directly onto the net M to act as a "teacher" of the output of the net M. There is also assumed to be feedback from M to L.

The teaching of the adaptive weights on the net M is performed so that the output from M is as close as possible to the direct "teaching" input coming onto it. Thus, if the inputs are denoted by $I(1)$, $I(2)$, . . . , and the output of the net M at time t by $M(t)$, then the training rule achieves the condition

$$M(t) = I(t + 1) \tag{24.9}$$

If at some time only the input $I(1)$ is fed to the net L, say, and then nothing, then pattern completion will occur. This is because the output from M at $t = 1$ is $I(2)$, which is then fed back to L by the assumed feedback lines, to lead to the output $I(3)$, and so on. In other words, the whole sequence is generated starting with only the first pattern.

Finally, the training rule is a simple delta-type rule:

$$\delta w_{ij} = [I_i\ (t + 1) - \mathrm{out}_i\ (t)]\mathrm{out}_j\ (t) \tag{24.10}$$

where i denotes label of the neuron of the net M and j denotes the neuron in the net L. Increases in the weight matrix cause the output of the ith cell to be closer to the next input. Note that the rule in equation (24.10) could avoid LTD if it were clipped.

It was shown (Reiss and Taylor, 1991) that this system learns fast, has no assumption on sequence length, and allows for disambiguation such as occurs in the sequence ABCBD. . . Moreover, it is biologically realistic in terms of the neurons it incorporates. It is even possible to relate the architecture, as shown in figure 24.1, to that of the hippocampus, especially as described by Berger and colleagues (see chapter 21). The net L is to be interpreted as the dentate gyrus, and the net M is CA3.

There are two features to be discussed further in this interpretation. The first is the detailed biological implementation of the learning rule in equation (24.10), which may be seen to be achieved (Reiss and Taylor, 1990) by means of the inhibitory feedback of CA3 cells (through inhibitory interneurons) onto themselves. The first factor in the learning rule in equation (24.10) then arises from the difference between the direct perforant path input distally onto the CA3 cell (denoted in equation [24.10] by $I[t + 1]$) and the output of the cell, which arises from the inhibitory interneuron. The second factor in equation (24.10) is that of the activity arriving at the mossy synapse. It is the latter synapse that was regarded as modifiable by Reiss and Taylor (1990). Addition of modifiability of the synapses onto the dentate gyrus (net L of figure 24.1) and those of the perforant path (pp) onto the CA3 cells are to be regarded as enhancing the powers of the system.

The other aspect requiring some discussion is the new architecture described by Berger in chapter 21. In particular there is an apparent repeat of the circuitry of figure 24.1 in that shown in figure 21.10B. The simplest interpretation of the new structure is that there is a repeat of the original "teaching" structure of figure 24.1 by the system of figure 21.10B. Indeed the addition of the subiculum may add a further teaching stage to the whole system. Modifiability of the synapses on the dentate gyrus and CA1 are expected to make the system even more effective (and with higher capacity).

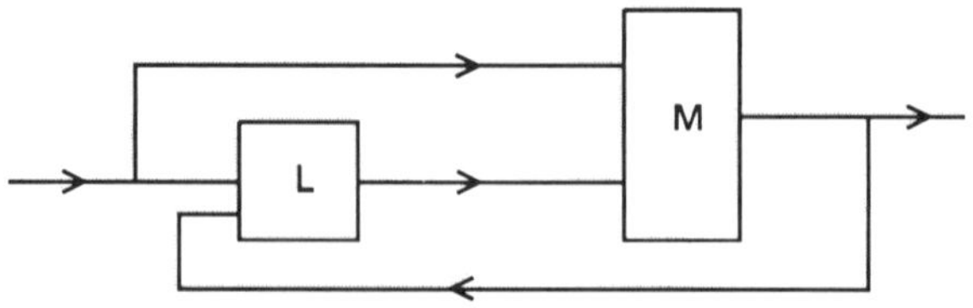

Figure 24.1 The architecture of the system of Reiss and Taylor (1991) used for temporal sequence storage. The net L is composed of leaky integrator neurons, and acts as a buffer for the inputs coming from the left. The synapses of the neurons of L onto the net M are adaptive, by the rule in equation (24.10). The input is also fed onto the net M to act as a "teacher." The mode of action is more fully discussed in the text.

The moral of this analysis is that the hippocampus can be regarded as a system ideally built to store temporal sequences. This storage depends on the use of leaky integrator neurons because they are required to buffer the past history on their surface in the learning process. It is interesting to note that it is not easy to discern a similar type of teaching structure in the cortex; that may indicate the need for a specialized structure to help later, more permanent storage of temporal sequences in nearby cortex.

It may also be appropriate to point to another algorithm for learning temporal sequences (Taylor, 1991), which uses a much richer structure of the neurons. It assumes that there are independent weights for the different time-delays, so that the activity develops not as in equation (24.8). Rather, the Caianiello equations of (24.3) become

$$u_i\ (t\ +\ 1)\ =\ \Upsilon\ (\Sigma_{j,\ r\ =\ 0}{}^{R} w_{ijr}\ u_j\ (t\ -\ r)\ -\ s_i) \tag{24.11}$$

where the weights w_{ijr} are all independent. It is then possible to introduce training rules for these weights (Taylor, 1990a), such as

$$\delta w_{ijr}\ =\ (\text{const})u_i(t)\ u_j(t\ -\ r)e^{-r/a} \tag{24.12}$$

with some decay constant.

It is also possible to determine the capacity of the net (equation [24.11]), using standard arguments (Reis and Taylor, 1991; Taylor, 1990). Thus, for uncorrelated patterns the capacity is $2RN$ for all-to-all connections; there is a corresponding increase in the case of sparse connectivity.

This question of capacity of the net for the storage of temporal sequences is important. In general, for all-to-all connectivity that quantity is of the order of N, the number of neurons in the net. That was shown by simulation (Reiss and Taylor, 1991). As just noted the capacity can be increased by sparse connectivity, for example, to be of value of about $N^2/(1nN)^2$ (Gardner, 1988). It is important to note that there is not an increase of total information stored by such a change in connectivity, but actually a decrease.

If we use the capacity value of about N, a value of N of about 5×10^6, and a new pattern every 300 milliseconds (corresponding to the time interval at which there is a change of visual focus) then the saturation point is reached after about 4 weeks. The time to reach capacity is reduced proportionally with any reduction of N. Thus, it is of interest to determine if keeping an animal awake for a long enough period would lead to symptoms of saturation. These symptoms would be expected to be a drastic reduction in learning powers or in long-term memory storage potential.

Finally, it is relevant to note that there is a system, the accessory olfactory bulb, that does not appear to need the hippocampus to lay down new memories. This process has recently been analyzed (Keverne and Taylor, 1991). The modification of the transfer function when learning occurs has been considered there, and experiments to detect the resulting changes have been suggested (which are presently being performed).

Compartmental Neurons

One of the most effective ways of handling the complex geometry of a neuron's surface is to split it up into compartments (Perkel et al., 1981). The detailed simulations of such neurons, with up to 30,000 compartments, is described by Brown (see chapter 22). In this brief account we consider what we would expect to be the information-handling strategies that will be produced by such complexity.

A simple way to understand what may be occurring is to look at the expression that replaces the right side of equation (24.11). The desired expression may be obtained by now regarding the indices i,j as the compartment labels. The weights lose their separate r-dependence, except for acquiring a factor $\exp[(r - 1)M]_{ij}$, where M is the matrix connecting the compartments to each other (Bressloff and Taylor, 1990a). The detailed form of M is not given here, but note that it has diagonal elements given by the decay constant of the relevant compartment. The off-diagonal terms only connect adjacent compartments and have about the same size as the diagonal ones. These facts lead to the value for the factor mentioned above of order

$$e^{-r/a}(r - 1)^R/R! \tag{24.13}$$

where R is the number of compartments from the synapse of interest (the jth) to the axon hillock, and a is a common time-constant. The term in equation (24.13) has a maximum value for the time delay r equal to Ra. This means that there is a delay of the time of impact of a synaptic input onto the axon hillock of value proportional to the distance of the former from the latter. That is not unexpected; the accuracy of the result can be improved if the geometry of the cell is included more carefully.

This result has relevance to the learning of temporal sequences. It allows the cell to learn those sequences that have separate patterns arriving at synapses appropriately distanced from the axon hillock. Thus, a signal arriving at a distal synapse, with a later signal arriving at a proximal one, could allow the coincidence to be learned by the latter synapse. It is clear that such features can be investigated in detail in an analytic fashion, and so one can probe the manner in which different learning rules lead to the learning of particular temporal aspects of inputs.

It may be of interest to add here that although the weights arising in the compartmental model do not have independent values for different earlier times along the lines of those in the step function in equation (24.11), it is possible to consider the effective weights, as measured at the axon hillock, as having the form of that equation. The possibility of these being trained independently arises from possible modifications of the membrane constants as well as the synaptic weights per se. The number of adaptive parameters entering in this manner will depend on the details of the learning rules at synaptic level; here is a clear bridge from the subneuronal level to the neuronal level that has as yet been only little explored.

Nonlinear Neurons

That nonlinearity is the essence of a neuron's response is already clear by the presence of the step function in Caianiello's equations (24.3). Does further nonlinearity help?

It is well known that nonlinear neurons have an exponentially increasing capacity in the number n of their inputs because they have 2^n independent weights. In general, the nonlinearities introduced by the output process do not, however, lead to an increase in the number of trainable parameters. Neither does the inclusion of active membrane appear to achieve that increase. Thus, we do not pursue that type of nonlinearity further here (although note that it might be important in the detailed study of cortical oscillations; Mannion and Taylor, 1991).

CONJECTURED SOLUTIONS

Let us now try to deduce a few answers to the questions raised at the beginning of this chapter.

We consider the knowledge being stored as being both spatial and temporal and have indicated in the previous section in what manner we regard tests of the temporal properties of the stored material as important as that of the spatial aspects.

It is possible that target and contextual material are being processed in the hippocampus, and suggest that the dentate gyrus, as the input net, is the most appropriate place to look at the effect of varied context on unit activity.

We cannot comment at this point on the nature of the coding of the input. It is relevant to note that the coding may well have been chosen to be most effective to allow the learning rule to work (and vice versa). That interplay is a feature that is worth exploring.

The detailed manner of the storage process has been covered by a number of chapters in this book. The associative nature of the process is clearly one which those working in artificial neural nets should take increased notice.

Storage in the hippocampus, with later storage in nearby cortex, seems accepted. This leads to the need to determine the lifetime for hippocampal storage. Figures quoted in this book cover quite a range of values; a reliable upper limit would be of great interest to relate to the questions of capacity mentioned in the previous section. Such capacity values are independent of the learning algorithm, so this avenue of exploration does not need to wait on clarification of the situation about LTP and LTD to make progress.

Let me add that it is important to understand the process of permanent storage in the cortex from hippocampal input. It seems to need a resonant type of feedback-feedforward activity so that the temporal sequences stored in hippocampus are appropriately transferred to cortex. That process of transfer is a challenge to theorist and experimentalist alike. The correlated activity reported in chapter 16 may be an indication of this process at work.

In conclusion, I hope I have shown how various simple rules (about temporal sequence storage, the use of noise, effects of cell geometry, capacity, and so on) may be extracted from the various features of cell activity. The application of these to help further understand memory processes may lead to new insights. It seems a valuable avenue to explore further.

REFERENCES

Artola, A., S. Bröcher, and W. Singer (1990). *Nature* 347:69.

Bressloff, P.C. and J.G. Taylor (1990a). "Discrete Time Models of Networks with Synaptic Noise." General Electric Company preprint.

Bressloff, P.C., and J.G. Taylor (1990b). *Physical Review* 41:1126.

Caianiello, E. (1961). *Journal of Theoretical Biology* 1:209.

Clarkson, T., D. Gorse, and J.G. Taylor (1989). In *Proceedings of the First IEE Conference on Artificial Neural Networks,* IEE Publications. London, p. 310.

Gardner, E. (1988). *Journal of Physics Mathematical and General* 21:257.

Gardner-Medwyn A.R. (1989). *Proceedings of the Royal Society (London).* B:238:137.

Gorse, D., and J.G. Taylor (1989). *Physica* D34:90.

Gorse, D., and J.G. Taylor (1990). "Universal Stochastic Learning Automata." University College preprint.

Gray, C.M., and W. Singer, (1989). *Proceedings of the National Academy of Science USA* 86:1698–1702.

Hopfield J.J. (1982). *Proceedings of the National Academy of Science USA* 79:2554–2558.

Keverne, E.B. and J.G. Taylor (1991). Accessory olfactory learning. *Biological Cybernetics* 64:301.

Lopes da Silva, F.H., M.P. Witter, P.H. Boeijinga, and A.H.M. Lohman (1990). *Physiology Review* 70:453.

Mannion, C.L.T. and J.G. Taylor (1991). Coupled excitable cells. In Mannion and Taylor (eds.), *NCM '90: Neural Computation.* London: Springer Verlag (in press).

McCulloch, W.S., and W. Pitts (1943). *Bulletin of Mathematics and Biophysics* 5, 115–133.

McNaughton, B.L. and R.G. Morris (1987). *Trends in Neuroscience* 10:408–415.

Perkel, D., B. Mulloney, and R.W. Budelli (1981). *Neuroscience* 6:823.

Reiss, M., and J.G. Taylor (1990). "Does the Hippocampus Store Temporal Sequences?" Kings College London preprint.

Reiss, M., and J.G. Taylor (1991). "Storing Temporal Sequences." Kings College London preprint. *Neural Networks (in press).*

Stanton, P.K., and T. Sejnowski (1989). *Nature* 339:215.

Taylor, J.G. (1972). *Journal of Theoretical Biology* 36:513.

Taylor, J.G. (1990). In *Proceedings of the International Conference on Artificial Neural Networks* Paris: Kluwer Academic, p. 952.

Taylor, J.G. (1991). "Neural Network Capacity for Temporal Sequence Storage." *International Journal of Neural Systems (in press).*

Tulving, E. (1983). *Elements of Episodic Memory.* Oxford: Clarendon Press.

25 Computational Approaches to Network Processing and Plasticity

Yves Frégnac

LEVELS OF COMPLEXITY

One of the central questions facing the modeler is that of the level of description at which he or she should attempt to explain long-term changes in brain processing. A tentative approach in describing rules of synaptic plasticity is to go from simple to complex and evaluate progressively how each level of complexity that has been added affects the processing and adaptive powers of the overall network. This chapter reviews recent computational approaches applied to the understanding of synaptic plasticity and network processing in the hippocampus and the olfactory system.

MODELING OF THE NEURONAL ELEMENTS

A first step is to define a useful and modulary representation of neuronal integration. Neurons can be seen first as simple binary decision units (McCulloch and Pitts, 1943), to which several features might be added. Some general parameters are used to characterize synaptic noise (spontaneous or afferent to each neuron), or random variations in firing thresholds by defining a "temperature" (see also Burnod and Korn, 1989), which allows the application of statistical physics tools to the study of random iterative networks (Little, 1974; Gorse and Taylor, 1988; see also chapter 24). Introduction of noise in the elements of a learning set serves two main functions: (1) to avoid false solutions (trap of the global energy function of the network in a local minimum), and (2) to learn to generalize convergence when randomly modifying an initial training set.

Time-processes can also be incorporated, by explicitly modeling traces of past activity in membrane properties ("leaking integrator"), or by introducing feedback connections that allow a delayed re-entry of the effect of earlier input on the net. Real neurons act as leaky integrators in that they store the postsynaptic effects produced in previous fractions of seconds by past activity in the afferents. Different models have explored ways in which persistence of the activity of a sequence of patterns allows for the direct storage of the sequence (Reiss and Taylor, 1990). A basic assumption developed by Taylor is that the leaky integrators hold the incoming activity long enough for the net to learn the transitions between the patterns of sequence. Interestingly, theoretical considerations discussed in detail in Reiss and Taylor suggest an almost neuroanatomical partition of the global network into two separate assemblies (see the section Specificity of the Network Architecture later in this chapter).

More detailed representations of neuronal elements can be applied, especially in the case of stereotyped patterns in the geometry of real neurons and their connections. Brown and colleagues (Brown et al., 1990; Zador et al., 1990), using both in situ biophysical estimates of membrane conductances and correlated morphology of the individual neurons, have been able to quantitatively simulate the spatiotemporal functioning of subdivisions of the hippocampus. Electrotonic modeling allows the description of specific paths of lesser attenuation, according to the geometry of the cell and its regional membrane properties. An interesting application would be to assess to what extent the temporal frequency of propagated input and its site of entry can affect the geometry of the isopotential domains of each responsive unit, and consequently the graph of connections instantaneously activated by a burst of activity arising in one point of the net.

This type of study shows the need for a better description of compartmentalization in the neuronal structures. How many individual compartments are needed to fully describe one cell? Can we simplify dendritic branching? Less accessible to experimenters is a representative model of the synaptic locus of interaction, and more especially that of dendritic spines. Detailed biophysical models (Zador et al., 1990) suggest that spines might help the compartmentalization of transient changes in calcium level to just the synapses that satisfy the conjunctive requirement for synaptic modification (review in Brown et al., 1990). In spite of earlier models based on electrotonic properties of the spine apparatus, more attention should be given to the role of the microphysiological properties of spines in regulating calcium-dependent second messengers.

Similar biophysical approaches can be found in computational approaches modeling nonlinearities and amplification processes triggered by the activation of *N*-methyl-D-aspartate (NMDA) receptor–mediated synaptic conductances (Holmes and Levy, 1990). Systematic timing studies in asynchronous stimulation of a pair of inputs, one weakly excitatory and the other strongly excitatory, paired with calcium videomicroscopy, might be of importance in defining sequential processes leading to peak concentrations of postsynaptic calcium in the spine head, which appear as a major measure of the probability of induction of LTP.

ALGORITHMS OF SYNAPTIC PLASTICITY

Standard correlation matrix techniques and learning algorithms of associative memories have been applied to model synaptic competition in the spatial domain in different cortical structures (in hippocampus: review in

Brown et al., 1990; in visual cortex: Bienenstock et al., 1982; review in Frégnac and Shulz, 1991) and account for the temporal and input specificity of potentiation of synaptic links during LTP. Less attention, however, has been devoted to modeling the learning of temporal sequences. Among various classes of time-delayed models based on the Hopfield-Kohonen approach (Hopfield, 1982; Kohonen, 1988), auto-associative sequential memories can be constructed using a simple architecture of two interconnected nets (see the section Specificity of the Network Architecture) and a correction error rule where the message originating from feedback projections from the output adaptive net is subtracted from the incoming input.

WHAT GOES UP MUST COME DOWN

Most algorithms of synaptic plasticity use, in addition to Hebbian rules of reinforcement of active connections, additional rules of normalization that require depression of certain synapses. It is somehow surprising that long-term depression (LTD) of synaptic efficacy, either homosynaptic or heterosynaptic, has not been studied with the same attention as long-term potentiation (LTP) in various parts of the brain, with the notable exception of cerebellum (Ito et al., 1982; Crépel and Krupa, 1989; Crépel and Jaillard, 1991). Are the conditions under which the strength of a synapse between two neurons is reduced with use the obverse face of the "long-term potentiation coin" (Stevens, 1990)? Neural network modeling of associative nets predicts such down-regulation, and behaviorally, habituation and extinction are possible correlates of depression in responsiveness of synapses (Morris and Willshaw, 1989).

Initial reasoning, originating mainly from modelers (Sejnowski, 1977), predicts during LTP a concomitant depression in the transmission efficacy of synapses, the activity of which was uncorrelated in time with that of the tetanized pathway. Heterosynaptic depression was first observed in the dentate hippocampus (Lynch et al., 1977; Levy and Stewart, 1983; Stanton and Sejnowski, 1989), and a related form of "depotentiation" linked to a persistent low level of afferent activity was more recently described in CA1 (Staubli and Lynch, 1988). A functional role for this type of plasticity was found in kitten visual cortex, which could explain the cortical effects of monocular occlusion on binocular interaction: "crossed" or "heterosynaptic" LTD was found to be induced after persistent stimulation of the optic nerve (in vivo: Tsumoto and Suda, 1979, or in vitro: Kimura et al., 1989). Recent observations by Tamura and coworkers (1990) suggest the importance of tonic afferent activity from both eyes in the probability of induction of LTD: a possible scheme is that low-frequency inputs of the nonconditioned pathway, out of phase with the tetanic stimulation of the conditioned pathway, are necessary to induce LTD (see also Stanton and Sejnowski, 1989).

Multiplication of high-frequency stimulation protocols have led to the occasional report, more complex to interpret, of LTD of transmission efficacy of tetanized pathways, which may be induced using the same parameters of afferent stimulation as those claimed to be effective in triggering LTP. In vitro studies using low-frequency pairings with postsynaptic depolarization in the sensorimotor cortex (Bindman et al., 1988) or bursts of high-frequency stimulation applied in the white matter in visual cortex (Berry et al., 1989), or intracortically in the frontal cortex (Hirsch and Crépel, 1990) induce both LTP and LTD. More recently reunifying schemes have been proposed that rely on voltage dependency of different plasticity thresholds. Dual stimulation studies in hippocampus suggest that potentiation of the weak pathway is seen when strong input follows the weak input. Depression has been shown to occur when the paired stimulations are applied in the reverse order, and could be linked with the consecutive hyperpolarizing phase after the tetanus corresponding to the strong stimulus (Stanton and Sejnowski, 1989). Recent intracellular in vitro studies both in hippocampus (Chattarji et al., 1989; Sejnowski et al., 1989; Stanton and Sejnowski, 1989) and in visual cortex (Frégnac et al., 1990) suggest that hyperpolarization paired with afferent stimulation may lead to synaptic depression of the active pathway in a major number of cases, whereas pairing with postsynaptic depolarization leads to potentiation of the same pathway (but see Stevens, 1990, and Hvalby, unpublished observations). A similar scenario of voltage dependency has been proposed by Artola and coworkers (1990), who also described in a recent report independent voltage thresholds in LTD and LTP. The plasticity thresholds found in their experimental situation, however, were reached in succession when depolarizing the postsynaptic neuron more and more strongly.

Taken globally, and in spite of some important interstudy differences, studies by Sejnowski and collaborators (Stanton and Sejnowski, 1989; Chattarji et al., 1989; Sejnowski et al., 1990), Artola and colleagues (1990), as well as our own work (Frégnac et al., 1990) showed that identical parameters of tetanic stimulation can induce either LTP or depression of excitatory postsynaptic potentials (EPSPs) at the same synaptic locus, depending on the level of depolarization of the target neuron (figure 25.1). Partial evidence both from hippocampus and visual cortex suggests that this type of homosynaptic depression could involve phosphoinositide metabolism triggered by activation of quisqualate metabotropic receptors (review in Sladeczek et al., 1988). These findings are further supported by independent biochemical studies (Palmer et al., 1988) suggesting that second messenger systems linked to NMDA and non-NMDA ("ibotenate") receptors could be antagonistic. NMDA would inhibit phosphoinositide turnover (stimulated by excitatory aminoacids) in a calcium-dependent fashion, and its activation would protect synapses from depression. In that respect low-frequency stimulation of previously tetanized pathways could lead to "depotentiation" if one assumes that NMDA receptor activation is no longer reached during a reduced level of afferent activity. On the

MODELS VISUAL CORTEX / HIPPOCAMPUS

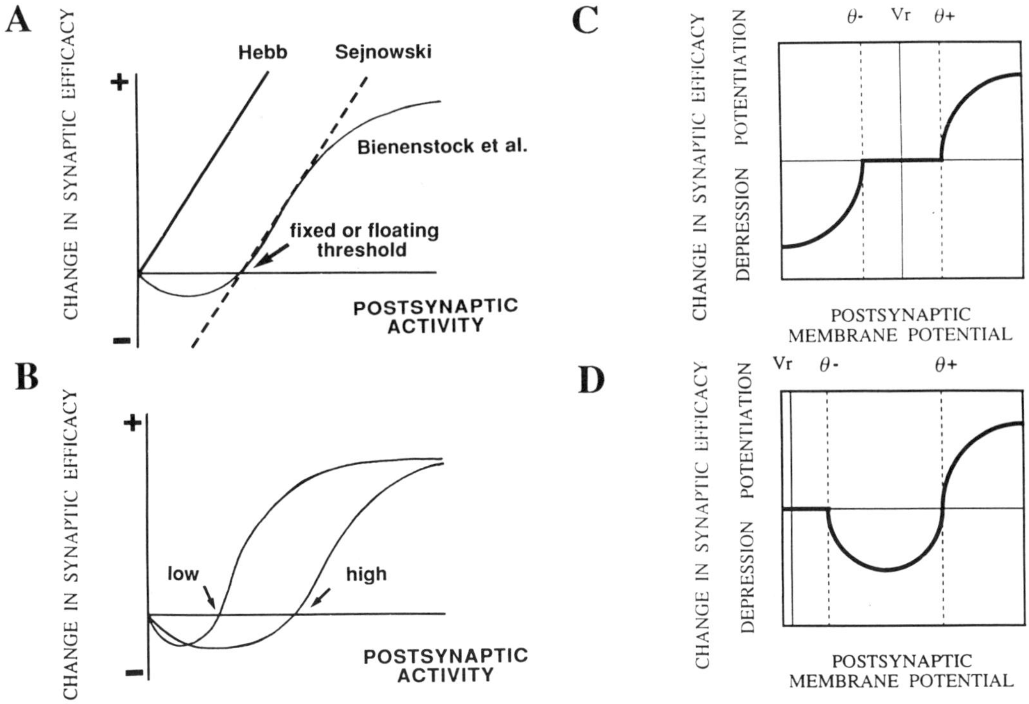

Figure 25.1 Postsynaptic dependency of plasticity thresholds for LTP and LTD. Theoretical models of self-organization suppose that synaptic change is controlled by both presynaptic and postsynaptic factors. (Left panel) Comparison between Hebbian scheme of plasticity (Hebb, 1949) and the covariance rule (Sejnowski, 1977), which has been applied successfully to hippocampus and visual cortex. (A) Changes in synaptic efficacy predicted by Hebb's postulate and by the covariance algorithm are plotted for a given input level, as a function of postsynaptic activity. Hebb's postulate predicts only positive changes in synaptic efficacy, which increase linearly with postsynaptic activity. In contrast, the covariance hypothesis predicts either increase or decrease in synaptic efficacy, depending on where the instantaneous postsynaptic activity reaches a fixed threshold value (Sejnowski, 1977). (B) Bienenstock et al. (1982) proposed a slightly different plasticity algorithm, where the threshold deciding for the sign of the synaptic modification is floating and depends on past activity of the cell, which avoids too rapid divergence of the synaptic gain towards extreme values following maintained periods of very low or high postsynaptic activity. Diagram in B is the same as in A, showing the behavior of the modification function used by Bienenstock et al. (1982) for two levels of mean postsynaptic activity (low and high). These authors assume that the modification sign threshold increases (high) or decreases (low) faster than the mean postsynaptic activity. (Right panel) Schematic representation of change in synaptic efficacy as a function of the postsynaptic membrane potential imposed during pairing or tetanus, predicted (C) from our electrophysiological findings (Frégnac et al., 1990) and those of Sejnowski et al. (Stanton and Sejnowski, 1989), and (D) from experiments by Artola et al. (1990). Synaptic potentiation corresponds to positive ordinates, synaptic depression to negative ones.

C demonstrates a "read-only" synaptic state around the resting membrane potential (Vr), where the test-PSP is supposed to be unaffected by the associative conditioning procedure, and of *two* plasticity thresholds above which ($\theta +$) potentiation occurs and below which ($\theta -$) depression occurs. A similar dependence hypothesized by Artola et al. (D), assumes a shift in the abcissa, where depression and potentiation are observed for postsynaptic membrane potential levels more depolarized than the resting level.

other hand, blockade of NMDA process is not sufficient to reveal depression per se: presynaptic activity uncoupled from postsynaptic NMDA receptor activation is not sufficient to reduce synaptic strength (Goldman et al., 1990). According to different teams, changes in membrane potential (moderate postsynaptic depolarization or hyperpolarization) are necessary at the time of synaptic activation to trigger LTD, which requires further experimental clarification.

Postsynaptic calcium concentration associated with repetitive synaptic input might be a more relevant index than the actual postsynaptic potential (which is nevertheless recorded at the soma and not at the synaptic locus) and may play a key role in switching the direction of long-term changes in synaptic efficacy toward either LTP or LTD (Kimura et al., 1990; review in Tsumoto, 1990). These latter data, which show, at least in visual cortex, that chelation of free calcium in the postsynaptic cell leads to LTD when associated with tetanic inputs, are in fact supported by independent models based initially on theoretical considerations. Lisman and collaborators (Lisman and Goldring, 1988; Lisman, 1989) supposed that the quantitative level of input-dependent increase of calcium in the postsynaptic cell regulates autophosphorylation of CaMll and transforms LTP into LTD if the influx of calcium is not strong enough. These theoretical and experimental studies agree with the hypothesis that heterosynaptic depression and homosynaptic depression could underly a common activity dependent postsynaptic phenomenon, which may be overcome or converted into LTP, when synaptic activity is associated with a larger increase in calcium concentration (review in Bindman et al., 1991).

SPECIFICITY OF THE NETWORK ARCHITECTURE

As noted by Taylor in chapter 24, details of wiring diagram must be answered before it is possible to build realistic models of memory storage and retrieval. Several central structures have been modeled, taking into account the neuroanatomical specificity of their structure (Haberly and Bower, 1989; Berger et al., 1988a, 1988b; Ambros-Ingerson et al., 1990), and simulation studies stress the importance of both feedforward layering and feedback connections in establishing associative memories in both the spatial and temporal domains. In the model presented by Taylor, a two-subnet architecture is hypothesized: the first net is composed only of leaky integrators and acts as a teacher. It feeds an associative net in a feedforward manner where modifications of synaptic weights should produce an output to be the closest to the next message on the input lines. The dual separation between the leaky integrator set and the associative memories makes use of specific feedback from the modifiable set output on the leaky integrator input. Such recurrent architecture can be made more complex by repeating this pattern at different stages of intergration in the processing stream; the biological plausibility of this scheme has been extensively discussed in chapters 21 and 24.

A second consequence of feedback connections could be to impose rhythmicity in neuronal dynamics. Successive cycles of activity could be seen as computing cycles, and a remarkable modeling approach by Ambros-Ingerson and colleagues (1990) suggests that this sequential process could allow some sort of principal component analysis and extraction or "clustering" of hierarchical structures. A major step operated by the feedback loop is to subtract the winners from the next input line, allowing the strengthening of synapses to occur for links less prominent in the hierarchy. Thus, its main action is to counteract the strengthening of the initial hot spots induced by LTP (otherwise winners take all), to be able to explore the input space completely during the following sampling cycles. Consequently, exploration through a series of excitation and inhibition cycles leads to the identification of the multilevel statistical structure of the novel input. In this respect it may be interesting to compare the use of oscillations in systems showing stereotyped architecture as well as stereotyped sampling modes (sniffing) such as the olfactory system and the hippocampal formation, and in complex neocortical nets randomly fed by visual input (review in Frégnac, 1991). Synchronization seems to occur at very distinct rhythms (4 to 7 Hz for the theta rhythm in the hippocampal formation, 50 Hz in visual cortex; Gray and Singer, 1989) and could correspond to different types of organization and function in inhibitory feedback loops.

A third issue to be tackled by a joint effort of experimenters and theoreticians is to separate the result of direct synaptic activation and the subsequent modulatory influence of the network excited by the initial input. Nonlinear system analysis techniques (first-order and second-order kernel analysis) have been applied to the hippocampal perforant path–dentate projection, and give new insights on the action of serial organization (Sclabassi et al., 1988; Berger et al., 1988a, 1988b). Feedback loops may be conjectured to introduce nonlinearities in accordance with the length of their projection.

A fourth unsolved problem is the modulation of adaptive control linked to the level of recruitment of inhibitory constraints. LTP and LTD outcome has been shown at least in visual cortex to depend on the level of intracortical inhibition and/or the strength of the tetanizing stimulus (Artola et al., 1990), which supports a modulatory action of "unseen" units during the tetanus. Simulation studies have developed a new concept of apparent or "effective" connectivity, which may be useful in separating network plasticity from synaptic plasticity (Aertsen et al., 1988). Although most models of formal neurons ignore plasticity in inhibitory synapses, it should not be taken as a fixed constraint because high-frequency trains of nervous activity have been reported to affect inhibitory processes or induce synchronization processes in the hippocampal assembly (Miles and Wong, 1987; Traub et al., 1989). Interestingly, in repetitive sampling models of the olfactory system, the strength of inhibitory synapses is allowed to vary according to a Hebbian rule, operating during a "developmental" phase.

CONCLUSION

The study of complex problems, such as memory formation, benefits from the use of simple putative elementary principles of plasticity, operating at a local level (the synapse) and uniformally across the cell assembly. Hippocampus and the olfactory system offer a variety of experimental networks where similar generic algorithms of potentiation can be implemented using different cascades of second messenger processes put into play through the activation of synaptic and/or voltage conductances. On the other hand, the intimate knowledge of the organization of a neuronal structure, its decomposition into identified feedforward and feedback streams, associated with the biophysical recomposition of the elementary computing units, might help us understand why different forms of LTP and LTD could exist in separate or identical loci. "Teleonomic" approaches, which attribute a specific function to the predominance of a given type of synaptic plasticity, give hope of finding novel classes of algorithms that could reveal which "project" ("teleonomy") the structure was built for. In this latter case, computational capacities of the system are no longer embodied by the plastic properties of individual synapses and spines, but rather by the network architecture which may serve a specific cognitive function. How various properties of memory might emerge from "design features of circuits" (Ambros-Ingerson et al., 1990) is a question best suited to neuroanatomical models and simulation studies of the workings of our hippocampal and sensory cortices.

ACKNOWLEDGMENTS

In vitro work reviewed in figure 25.1 was supported by North Atlantic Treaty Organization and International Human Frontier Science Program Organization grants to Y. Frégnac, and National Institutes of Health support to M. J. Friedlander.

REFERENCES

Aertsen, A. M. H. J., G. L. Gerstein, M. Habib, and G. Palm (1988). Dynamics of neuronal firing correlation: modulation of "effective" connectivity. *Journal of Neurophysiology* 61:900–917.

Ambros-Ingerson, J., R. Granger, and G. Lynch (1990). Simulation of paleocortex performs hierarchical clustering. *Science* 247:1344–1348.

Artola, A., S. Bröcher, and W. Singer (1990). Different voltage-dependent thresholds for inducing long-term depression and long-term potentiation in slices of the rat visual cortex. *Nature* 347:69–72.

Berger, T. W., J. L. Eriksson, D. A. Ciarolla, and R. J. Sclabassi (1988b). Nonlinear systems analysis of the hippocampal perforant path–dentate projection. I. Comparison of random train and paired impulse stimulation. *Journal of Neurophysiology* 60(3):1095–1109.

Berger, T. W., J. L. Eriksson, D. A. Ciarolla, and R. J. Sclabassi (1988b). Nonlinear systems analysis of the hippocampal perforant path–dentate projection. I. Comparison of random train and paired impulse stimulation. *Journal of Neurophysiology* 60(3):1095–1109.

Berry, R. L., T. J. Teyler, and H. Taizhen (1989). Induction of LTP in the rat primary visual cortex: tetanus parameters. *Brain Research* 481:221–227.

Bienenstock, E., L. N. Cooper, and P. Munro (1982). Theory for the development of neuron selectivity: orientation specificity and binocular interaction in visual cortex. *Journal of Neuroscience* 2:23–48.

Bindman, L., G. Christofi, K. Murphy, and A. Nowicki (1991). Long-term potentiation (LTP) and depression (LTD) in the neocortex and hippocampus: an overview. In T. W. Stone (ed.), *Aspects of Synaptic Transmission.* London: Taylor Francis (in press).

Bindman, L. J., K. P. S. J. Murphy, and S. Pockett (1988). Postsynaptic control of the induction of long-term changes in efficacy of transmission at neocortical synapses in slices of rat brain. *Journal of Neurophysiology* 60(3):1053–1065.

Brown, T. H., A. H. Ganong, E. W. Kairiss, and C. L. Keenan (1990). Hebbian synapses: biophysical mechanisms and algorithms. *Annual Review of Neuroscience* 13:475–511.

Burnod, Y., and H. Korn (1989). Consequences of stochastic release of neurotransmitters for network computation in the central nervous system. *Proceedings of the National Academy of Science USA* 86:352–356.

Chattarji, S., P. K. Stanton, and T. J. Sejnowski (1989). Commissural synapses, but not mossy fiber synapses, in hippocampal field CA3 exhibit associative long-term potentiation and depression. *Brain Research* 495:145–150.

Crépel, F., and D. Jaillard (1991). Pairing of pre- and postsynaptic activities in cerebellar Purkinje cells induces long-term changes in synaptic efficacy: an in vitro study. *Journal of Physiology (London)* 432:123–141.

Crépel, F., and M. Krupa (1988). Activation of protein kinase C induces a long-term depression of glutamate sensitivity of cerebellar Purkinje cells: an in vitro study. *Brain Research* 458:397–401.

Frégnac, Y., and D. Shulz (1991). Models of synaptic plasticity and cellular learning in mammalian visual cortex. In V. Casagrande and P. Shinkman (eds.), *Advances in Neural and Behavioral Development.* Neural Ablex Publishers, pp. 97–109.

Frégnac, Y., D. Smith, and M. J. Friedlander (1990). Postsynaptic membrane potential regulates synaptic potentiation and depression in visual cortical neurons. *Society for Neuroscience Abstracts* 16:798.

Frégnac, Y., D. Smith, and M. J. Friedlander (1990). Postsynaptic membrane potential regulates synaptic potentiation and depression in visual cortical neurons. *Society for Neuroscience Abstracts* 16:798.

Goldman, R. S., L. E. Chavez-Noriéga, and C. F. Stevens (1990). Failure to reverse long-term potentiation by coupling sustained presynaptic activity and *N*-methyl-D-aspartate receptor blockade. *Proceedings of the National Academy of Science USA* 87:7165–7169.

Gorse, D., and J. G. Taylor (1988). On the equivalence and properties of noisy neural and probabilistic ram nets. *Physics Letters* 131(6):326–332.

Gray, C. M., and W. Singer (1989). Stimulus-specific neuronal oscillations in orientation columns of cat visual cortex. *Proceedings of the National Academy of Science USA* 86:1698–1702.

Haberly, L. B., and J. M. Bower (1989). Olfactory cortex: model circuit for study of associative memory. *Trends in Neurosciences* 12(7):258–264.

Hebb, D. O. (1949). *The Organization of Behavior.* New York: Wiley.

Hirsch J. C., and F. Crépel (1990). Use-dependent changes in synaptic efficacy in rat prefrontal neurons in vitro. *Journal of Physiology (London)* 427:31–49.

Holmes, W. R., and W. B. Levy (1990). Insights into associative long-term potentiation from computational models of NMDA receptor–mediated calcium influx and intracellular calcium concentration changes. *Journal of Neurophysiology* 63:1148–1168.

Hopfield, J. J. (1982). Neural networks and physical systems with emergent collective computational abilities. *Proceedings of the National Academy of Science USA* 79:2554–2558.

Ito, M. (1989). Long-term depression. *Annual Review of Neuroscience* 12:85–102.

Ito, M., M. Sakurai, and P. Tongroach (1982). Cerebellar climbing fibre induced depression of both mossy fibre responsiveness and glutamate sensitivity of cerebellar Purkinje cells. *Journal of Physiology (London)* 324:113–134.

Kimura, F., A. Nishigori, T. Shirokawa, and T. Tsumoto (1989). Long-term potentiation and *N*-methyl-D-aspartate receptors in the visual cortex of young rats. *Journal of Physiology (London)* 414:125–144.

Kimura, F., T. Tsumoto, A. Nishigori, and Y. Yoshimura (1990). Long-term depression but not potentiation is induced in Ca^{2+}-chelated visual cortex neurons. *Neuro-Report* 1:65–68.

Kohonen, T. (1988). *Self-organization and Associative Memory,* 2nd ed. Berlin: Springer-Verlag.

Levy, W. B., and O. Stewart (1983). Temporal contiguity requirements for long-term associative potentiation/depression in the hippocampus. *Neuroscience* 8:791–797.

Lisman, J. (1989). A mechanism for the Hebb and the anti-Hebb processes underlying learning and memory. *Proceedings of the National Academy of Science USA* 86:9574–9578.

Lisman, J. E., and M. A. Goldring (1988). Feasibility of long-term storage of graded information by the Ca^{++}/calmodulin-dependent protein kinase molecules of the post-synaptic density. *Proceedings of the National Academy of Science USA* 85:5320–5324.

Little, W. A. (1974). The existence of persistent states in the brain. *Mathematics and Bioscience* 19:101–120.

Lynch, G., T. V. Dunwiddie, and V. K. Gribkoff (1977). Heterosynaptic depression: a postsynaptic correlate of long-term potentiation. *Nature* 266:737–739.

McCulloch, W. S., and W. Pitts (1943). A logical calculus of the ideas immanent in nervous activity. *Bulletin of Mathematics and Biophysics* 5:115–133.

Miles, R., and R. K. S. Wong (1987). Latent synaptic pathways revealed after tetanic stimulation in the hippocampus. *Nature* 329:724–726.

Morris, R. G. M., and D. J. Willshaw (1989). Must what goes up come down? *Nature* 339:175–176.

Palmer, A., D. T. Monaghan, and C. W. Cotman (1988). Bidirectional regulation of phosphoinositide metabolism by glutamate receptors: stimulation by two classes of quisqualate receptors and inhibition by NMDA receptors. *Molecular Brain Research* 4:161.

Pockett, S., N. H. Brookes, and L. J. Bindman (1990). Long-term depression at synapses of rat hippocampus can be induced by bursts of postsynaptic activity. *Experimental Brain Research* 80:196–200.

Reiss, M., and J. G. Taylor (1991). "Storing temporal sequences." Kings College London preprint.

Sclabassi, R. J., et al. (1988). Nonlinear systems analysis of the hippocampal perforant path-dentate projection. I. Theoretical and interpretational considerations. *Journal of Neurophysiology* 60(3):1066–1076.

Sejnowski, T. J. (1977). Storing covariance with non-linearly interacting neurons. *Journal of Mathematics and Biology* 4:303–321.

Sejnowski, T. J., S. Chattarji, and P. K. Stanton (1989). Induction of synaptic plasticity by Hebbian covariance in the hippocampus. In *The Computing Neuron*. R. Durbin, C. Miall and G. Mitchison (eds.), Reading, MA: Addison-Wesley, pp. 105–124.

Sladeczek, F., M. Recasens, and J. Bockaert (1988). A new mechanism for glutamate receptor action: the phosphoinositide (PI) hydrolysis. *Trends in Neuroscience* 11(12):545–549.

Stanton, P. K., and T. J. Sejnowski (1989). Associative long-term depression in the hippocampus induced by Hebbian covariance. *Nature* 339:215–218.

Staubli, U., and G. Lynch (1988). Stable depression of potentiated synaptic responses in the hippocampus induced by low frequency stimulation. *Society for Neuroscience Abstracts* 14:566.

Stevens, C. F. (1990). A depression long awaited (News and Views). *Nature* 347:16.

Tamura, H., Y. Hata, and T. Tsumoto (1990). Long-term potentiation and depression in kitten visual cortex studied in vivo. *Society for Neuroscience Abstracts* 16:985.

Traub, R. D., R. Miles, and R. K. S. Wong (1989). Model of the origin of rhythmic population oscillations in the hippocampal slice. *Science* 243:1319–1325.

Tsumoto, T. (1990). Long-term potentiation and depression in the cerebral neocortex (Minireview). *Japan Journal of Physiology* 40:573–593.

Tsumoto, T., and K. Suda (1979). Cross-depression: an electropysiological manifestation of binocular competition in the developing visual cortex. *Brain Research* 168:190–194.

Zador, A., C. Koch, and T. H. Brown (1990). Biophysical model of a Hebbian synapse. *Proceedings of the National Academy of Science USA* 87:6718–6722.

Index